Acute Lung Injury: Pathophysiology, Prevention and Treatment

Acute Lung Injury: Pathophysiology, Prevention and Treatment

Editor: Violet Murphy

AMERICAN
MEDICAL PUBLISHERS
www.americanmedicalpublishers.com

AMERICAN
MEDICAL PUBLISHERS
www.americanmedicalpublishers.com

Cataloging-in-Publication Data

Acute lung injury : pathophysiology, prevention and treatment / edited by Violet Murphy.
p. cm.
Includes bibliographical references and index.
ISBN 979-8-88740-568-1
1. Lungs--Wounds and injuries. 2. Respiratory distress syndrome, Adult. 3. Lungs--Wounds and injuries--Pathophysiology. 4. Respiratory distress syndrome, Adult--Prevention. 5. Lungs--Wounds and injuries--Treatment. 6. Respiratory distress syndrome, Adult--Treatment. I. Murphy, Violet.
RC776.R38 A28 2023
616.24--dc23

American Medical Publishers,
41 Flatbush Avenue,
1st Floor, New York,
NY 11217, USA

ISBN 979-8-88740-568-1 (Hardback)

Contents

Preface IX

Chapter 1 **Circulating Skeletal Troponin During Weaning from Mechanical Ventilation and their Association to Diaphragmatic Function** 1
Savino Spadaro, Francesca Dalla Corte, Gaetano Scaramuzzo, Salvatore Grasso, Gilda Cinnella, Valentina Rosta, Valentina Chiavieri, Valentina Alvisi, Rosa Di Mussi, Carlo Alberto Volta, Tiziana Bellini and Alessandro Trentini

Chapter 2 **Pulmonary Interstitial Matrix and Lung Fluid Balance from Normal to the Acutely Injured Lung** 10
Egidio Beretta, Francesco Romanò, Giulio Sancini, James B. Grotberg, Gary F. Nieman and Giuseppe Miserocchi

Chapter 3 **Right Ventricular Function in Acute Respiratory Distress Syndrome: Impact on Outcome, Respiratory Strategy and Use of Veno-Venous Extracorporeal Membrane Oxygenation** 28
Matthieu Petit, Edouard Jullien and Antoine Vieillard-Baron

Chapter 4 **Effects of Different Levels of Variability and Pressure Support Ventilation on Lung Function in Patients with Mild-Moderate Acute Respiratory Distress Syndrome** 36
Lorenzo Ball, Yuda Sutherasan, Martina Fiorito, Antonella Dall'Orto, Lorenzo Maiello, Maria Vargas, Chiara Robba, Iole Brunetti, Davide D'Antini, Pasquale Raimondo, Robert Huhle, Marcus J. Schultz, Patricia R. M. Rocco, Marcelo Gama de Abreu and Paolo Pelosi

Chapter 5 **Monitoring Expired CO_2 Kinetics to Individualize Lung-Protective Ventilation in Patients with the Acute Respiratory Distress Syndrome** 46
Fernando Suárez-Sipmann, Jesús Villar, Carlos Ferrando, Juan A. Sánchez-Giralt and Gerardo Tusman

Chapter 6 **The Renin-Angiotensin System as a Component of Biotrauma in Acute Respiratory Distress Syndrome** 57
Katharina Krenn, Verena Tretter, Felix Kraft and Roman Ullrich

Chapter 7 **Airway Pressure Release Ventilation with Time-Controlled Adaptive Ventilation (TCAV™) in COVID-19: A Community Hospital's Experience** 70
Philippe Rola and Benjamin Daxon

Chapter 8 **Astrocytes Downregulate Inflammation in Lipopolysaccharide-Induced Acute Respiratory Distress Syndrome: Applicability to COVID-19** 79
Michal Izrael, Kfir Molakandov, Ariel Revel, Shalom Guy Slutsky, Tehila Sonnenfeld, Julia Miriam Weiss and Michel Revel

Chapter 9 **Mechanical Ventilation in Pediatric and Neonatal Patients** 92
Michaela Kollisch-Singule, Harry Ramcharran, Joshua Satalin, Sarah Blair, Louis A. Gatto, Penny L. Andrews, Nader M. Habashi, Gary F. Nieman and Adel Bougatef

Chapter 10 **Unsuccessful and Successful Clinical Trials in Acute Respiratory Distress Syndrome: Addressing Physiology-Based Gaps** 105
Jesús Villar, Carlos Ferrando, Gerardo Tusman, Lorenzo Berra, Pedro Rodríguez-Suárez and Fernando Suárez-Sipmann

Chapter 11 **Assessment of Alveolar Macrophage Dysfunction using an *in vitro* Model of Acute Respiratory Distress Syndrome** 115
Rahul Y. Mahida, Aaron Scott, Dhruv Parekh, Sebastian T. Lugg, Kylie B. R. Belchamber, Rowan S. Hardy, Michael A. Matthay, Babu Naidu and David R. Thickett

Chapter 12 **Gene Therapy for Acute Respiratory Distress Syndrome** 127
Jing Liu and David A. Dean

Chapter 13 **Static and Dynamic Measurements of Compliance and Driving Pressure** 161
Pierre Tawfik, Muhammad K. Hayat Syed, Firas S. Elmufdi, Michael D. Evans, David J. Dries and John J. Marini

Chapter 14 **MicroRNA-7 Deficiency Ameliorates the Pathologies of Acute Lung Injury through Elevating KLF4** 168
Juanjuan Zhao, Chao Chen, Mengmeng Guo, Yijin Tao, PanPan Cui, Ya Zhou, Nalin Qin, Jing Zheng, Jidong Zhang and Lin Xu

Chapter 15 **Aerobic Exercise Attenuates Acute Lung Injury through NET Inhibition** 181
Yue Shi, Tingting Liu, David C. Nieman, Yanqiu Cui, Fei Li, Luyu Yang, Hui Shi and Peijie Chen

Chapter 16 **Preventing Ventilator-Associated Lung Injury: A Perioperative Perspective** 192
Satoshi Kimura, Nicoleta Stoicea, Byron Rafael Rosero Britton, Muhammad Shabsigh, Aly Branstiter and David L. Stahl

Chapter 17 **Gut-Lung Crosstalk in Sepsis-Induced Acute Lung Injury** 198
Xin Zhou and Youxia Liao

Chapter 18 **Protective Effects of Anti-IL17 on Acute Lung Injury Induced by LPS in Mice** 209
Renato Fraga Righetti, Tabata Maruyama dos Santos, Leandro do Nascimento Camargo, Luciana Ritha Cássia Rolim Barbosa Aristóteles, Silvia Fukuzaki, Flávia Castro Ribas de Souza, Fernanda Paula Roncon Santana, Marcus Vinicius Rodrigues de Agrela, Maysa Mariana Cruz, Maria Isabel Cardoso Alonso-Vale, Isabella Santos Genaro, Beatriz Mangueira Saraiva Romanholo, Edna Aparecida Leick, Milton de Arruda Martins, Carla Máximo Prado and Iolanda de Fátima Lopes Calvo Tibério

Chapter 19 **Inflammatory Caspases Drive Pyroptosis in Acute Lung Injury....224**
Bohao Liu, Ruyuan He, Lin Zhang, Bo Hao, Wenyang Jiang, Wei Wang and Qing Geng

Permissions

List of Contributors

Index

Preface

Acute lung injury (ALI) is a form of acute respiratory failure that causes disruption of epithelial and endothelial barriers in the lungs. The severe form of acute lung injury manifests as adult respiratory distress syndrome (ARDS). Some common symptoms of acute lung injury are severe dyspnoea, tachypnoea, and resistant hypoxaemia, bowel perforation, and sepsis syndrome. Appropriate diagnostic tests such as blood or urine cultures, and bronchoalveolar lavage are performed for examining a patient for underlying conditions, particularly pneumonia, sepsis, pancreatitis or transfusion related lung injury. Treatment strategy for acute lung injury consists of treatment of the underlying disease, mechanical ventilation for elimination of carbon dioxide and securing oxygenation, and adjunctive procedures for treating specific pulmonary pathologies. This book outlines the pathophysiology, prevention and treatment of acute lung injury in detail. A number of latest researches have been included to keep the readers up-to-date with the global concepts in this area of medicine. Students, researchers, experts and all associated with the study of this medical condition will benefit alike from this book.

The researches compiled throughout the book are authentic and of high quality, combining several disciplines and from very diverse regions from around the world. Drawing on the contributions of many researchers from diverse countries, the book's objective is to provide the readers with the latest achievements in the area of research. This book will surely be a source of knowledge to all interested and researching the field.

In the end, I would like to express my deep sense of gratitude to all the authors for meeting the set deadlines in completing and submitting their research chapters. I would also like to thank the publisher for the support offered to us throughout the course of the book. Finally, I extend my sincere thanks to my family for being a constant source of inspiration and encouragement.

Editor

1

Circulating Skeletal Troponin During Weaning from Mechanical Ventilation and their Association to Diaphragmatic Function

Savino Spadaro [1†], Francesca Dalla Corte [1,2†], Gaetano Scaramuzzo [1], Salvatore Grasso [3], Gilda Cinnella [4], Valentina Rosta [5], Valentina Chiavieri [1], Valentina Alvisi [1], Rosa Di Mussi [3], Carlo Alberto Volta [1], Tiziana Bellini [5] and Alessandro Trentini [5]*

[1] Department of Translational Medicine, Anesthesia and Intensive Care, University of Ferrara, Ferrara, Italy, [2] Department of Anesthesia and Intensive Care Medicine, Humanitas Clinical and Research Center-Istituto di Ricovero e Cura a Carattere Scientifico (IRCCS), Milan, Italy, [3] Department of Emergency and Organ Transplantation, University of Bari, Bari, Italy, [4] Department of Medical and Surgical Sciences, University of Foggia, Foggia, Italy, [5] Section of Medical Biochemistry, Molecular Biology and Genetics, Department of Biomedical and Specialist Surgical Sciences, University of Ferrara, Ferrara, Italy

***Correspondence:**
Savino Spadaro
spdsvn@unife.it

† These authors have contributed equally to this work and share first authorship

Background: Patients with acute respiratory failure (ARF) may need mechanical ventilation (MV), which can lead to diaphragmatic dysfunction and muscle wasting, thus making difficult the weaning from the ventilator. Currently, there are no biomarkers specific for respiratory muscle and their function can only be assessed trough ultrasound or other invasive methods. Previously, the fast and slow isoform of the skeletal troponin I (fsTnI and ssTnI, respectively) have shown to be specific markers of muscle damage in healthy volunteers. We aimed therefore at describing the trend of skeletal troponin in mixed population of ICU patients undergoing weaning from mechanical ventilation and compared the value of fsTnI and ssTnI with diaphragmatic ultrasound derived parameters.

Methods: In this prospective observational study we enrolled consecutive patients recovering from acute hypoxemic respiratory failure (AHRF) within 24 h from the start of weaning. Every day an arterial blood sample was collected to measure fsTnI, ssTnI, and global markers of muscle damage, such as ALT, AST, and CPK. Moreover, thickening fraction (TF) and diaphragmatic displacement (DE) were assessed by diaphragmatic ultrasound. The trend of fsTnI and ssTnI was evaluated during the first 3 days of weaning.

Results: We enrolled 62 consecutive patients in the study, with a mean age of 67 ± 13 years and 43 of them (69%) were male. We did not find significant variations in the ssTnI trend ($p = 0.623$), but fsTnI significantly decreased over time by 30% from Day 1 to Day 2 and by 20% from Day 2 to Day 3 ($p < 0.05$). There was a significant interaction effect between baseline ssTnI and DE [$F_{(2)} = 4.396$, $p = 0.015$], with high basal levels of ssTnI being associated to a higher decrease in DE. On the contrary, the high basal levels of fsTnI at day 1 were characterized by significant higher DE at each time point.

Conclusions: Skeletal muscle proteins have a distinctive pattern of variation during weaning from mechanical ventilation. At day 1, a high basal value of ssTnI were associated to a higher decrease over time of diaphragmatic function while high values of fsTnI were associated to a higher displacement at each time point.

Keywords: acute hypoxemic respiratory failure, assisted mechanical ventilation, biomarker, diaphragm, diaphragmatic ultrasound, skeletal troponin, weaning

INTRODUCTION

Ventilatory support is an essential life-saving therapy for intensive care patients with acute respiratory failure (1). However, most patients under mechanical ventilation (MV) experience deleterious impact of mechanical ventilation on the diaphragm (2). The balance between lung and diaphragm protection remains challenging. As known, MV can trigger a sustained change in muscle fibers biochemistry (3), ultimately leading to diaphragmatic atrophy (4). Experimental evidence suggest that signs of increased oxidative stress and diaphragm fiber proteolysis may arise as early as 12 h from MV initiation (5). Ventilator induced diaphragmatic dysfunction (VIDD) (6) has a rapid onset, is related to the duration of ventilation support (7) and affects the clinical outcome (8–11). The diaphragm seems to be more susceptible to fast disuse atrophy, as compared to peripheral skeletal muscles (e.g., pectoralis muscle and latissimus dorsi) (12). In order to minimize VIDD, it has been suggested to implement assisted modes as soon as clinically feasible and safe (13), to minimize patient-ventilator asynchronies (14) and to avoid excessive expiratory braking (15, 16), despite definitive evidence are not available.

In critically ill patients, no bedside tools are available to monitor the muscular function except for ultrasound, which is non-invasive but highly operator-dependent (17). Phrenic nerve stimulation, which would be the "gold standard," is invasive, complex and thus limited in the routine clinical application.

Specific circulating biomarkers for skeletal muscles have been recently identified. In contrast with non-specific muscular markers, like creatine kinase (CPK), specific markers could potentially open the possibility to provide real time information on the integrity of different types of muscular fibers (18). Slow- and fast-twitch skeletal troponin I (ssTnI and fsTnI) have been shown to be promising markers of damage to slow oxidative (Type I) and fast glycolytic (Type II) muscular fibers (19, 20), respectively.

In a previous report in healthy subjects undergoing an inspiratory threshold loading trial (21), fsTnI was regarded as an early marker, more sensitive than CK, of subclinical diaphragmatic damage. Furthermore, recent data suggest the use of these markers for evaluating subclinical muscular damage (22), since their circulating level are influenced by both muscular mass and amount of muscle disruption.

It is not clear what happens to the circulating levels of skeletal troponin in patients with acute respiratory failure (ARF) undergoing mechanical ventilation, especially during the early phase of weaning. Therefore, the primary aim of the present study was to describe the trend of circulating skeletal troponins during the early part of weaning in a population of mechanically ventilated critically ill patients. Moreover, we hypothesized that values of skeletal troponin beyond normality could be associated to diaphragmatic dysfunction. To test this hypothesis, we compared ultrasound derived diaphragmatic parameters with the baseline levels and the trend of plasma skeletal troponins to determine if they could serve as early markers of diaphragmatic atrophy/ventilator over assistance.

METHODS

Study Population

This is a longitudinal, single-center, observational cohort study, conducted over a 24-months period (March 2017 to March 2019) in the ICU of the S. Anna University Hospital, Ferrara, Italy. The study was approved by the ethics committee of our institution (Azienda Ospedaliero-Universitaria Ferrara Ethic Committee, number of ethical approval 131084). Informed consent was obtained from each patient or next of kin. All consecutive patients recovering from acute hypoxemic respiratory failure (AHRF) with an expected length of mechanical ventilation of 72 h or more were screened for study inclusion. The inclusion criteria were: age 18 years or older, ventilation in assisted mode, Richmond Agitation Sedation Scale (RASS) between −1 and +1. Exclusion criteria were: history of neuromuscular disease, continuous infusion of muscle-paralyzing agents in the last 48 h, diaphragm atrophy or paralysis, abnormal values of myocardial and muscular damage markers at ICU admission, presence of moderate/severe acute kidney injury (23) at ICU admission, presence of thoracotomy, pneumothorax or pneumomediastinum, pregnancy.

Study Protocol

All patients were enrolled at the beginning of weaning from MV and therefore when able to trigger the ventilator. Specifically, the patients were studied from the 1st (defined Day 1) to the 3rd day (defined Day 3) since the switch from the beginning of assisted mode ventilation (PSV). The following data were collected: mode of mechanical ventilation, ventilator parameters [i.e., pressure support, positive end-expiratory pressure (PEEP), inspired oxygen fraction (FiO_2)], breathing pattern [i.e., tidal volume (V_T), respiratory rate (RR)] and the occlusion pressure at 100 ms (P0.1), defined as the negative pressure measured 100 ms after the initiation of an inspiratory effort. All included patients underwent a daily ultrasonographic evaluation of the diaphragmatic function. Arterial blood samples were collected right after ultrasound measurements to evaluate arterial blood gasses and circulating markers. Creatinine was collected each day during the study period to evaluate the onset of moderate/severe acute kidney injury (23).

Mechanical Ventilation Setting

Patients with ARF were included in the study within 24 h after the initiation of assisted mechanical ventilation (i.e., pressure support ventilation, PSV) according to the attending physicians' judgment. The readiness to sustain PSV was based on the following criteria: (a) improvement of the condition leading to acute respiratory failure, (b) positive end-expiratory pressure (PEEP) lower than 10 cm H_2O and inspiratory oxygen fraction (FiO_2) lower than 0.5, (c) Richmond Agitation Sedation Scale (RASS) between −1 and +1, with no sedation or with low dose of continuous infusion of sedation (i.e., propofol 0.5–1.5 mg/kg/h and/or remifentanil 0.03–0.05 mg/kg/min or dexmedetomidine (0.3–1.0 µg/kg/h), (d) ability to trigger the ventilator, (e) hemodynamic stability (with norepinephrine $\leq$ 0.1 µg/kg/min or equivalent), (f) normothermia.

Pressure support ventilation was set to meet the following targets: V_T of 6–8 mL/kg/PBW, with RR 20–30 bpm. Pressure support (PS) was decreased if V_T > 8 mL/kg/PBW and/or RR < 20 while it was increases if V_T < 6 mL/kg PBW and/or RR > 30 and/or in the presence of respiratory distress (e.g., marked use of the accessory muscles). PEEP and then FiO_2 were increased if SpO_2 was < 90%, while FiO_2 and then PEEP were decreased if SpO_2 was > 96%. The PEEP and FiO_2 levels in use before the study were left unchanged. Patients returning into controlled mechanical ventilation due to deteriorating respiratory mechanics or general clinical conditions were excluded from the clinical study.

Ultrasonography

Ultrasonographic assessments were performed by a single well-trained physician (F.D.C.) by using the same ultrasonography machine (M-Turbo, SonoSite, Inc., USA). All measurements were performed in patients lying in the semi-recumbent position and on the right side. Diaphragmatic excursion (DE) was evaluated using a 3.5 to 5-MHz convex ultrasound probe using a subcostal approach (24–26).

Diaphragmatic thickness and thickening fraction were assessed using a 12-MHz linear ultrasound probe by using an intercostal approach, as previously described (27, 28). Diaphragm thickening fraction (TFdi) was measured in M-mode as TFdi = $[(T_{EI}\text{-}T_{EE})/T_{EE}] \times 100$, where T_{EE} and T_{EI} correspond to the thickness of the diaphragm at the end of expiration and inspiration, respectively. Normal diaphragmatic function was defined as the presence of a DE $\geq$ 10 mm (28) or a TFdi $\geq$ 30% (29).

Serum Sampling and Quantification of Skeletal Troponins

Serum samples were obtained from the arterial blood in anticoagulant-free tubes by centrifugation at 1,500 rpm for 10 min after clotting and stored in aliquots at −80°C until assay. To avoid possible loss of bioactivity, samples were analyzed within 3 months from the collection and thawed only once. Slow skeletal Troponin I (ssTnI, Mybiosource, Cat. No. MBS2510383) and fast skeletal Troponin I (fsTnI, Mybiosource, Cat. No. MBS927961) were assayed by commercially available ELISA kits according to manufacturer's instructions. Specific technical details can be found elsewhere (22).

Myoglobin, Creatine Kinase (CPK) and creatinine were determined by routine analysis from the hospital's clinical laboratory. The concentration of aldolase, aspartate aminotransferase (AST), and alanine aminotransferase (ALT) were assayed on undiluted serum samples by coupled spectrophotometric enzymatic assays on a Tecan Infinite M200 (Tecan Group Ltd., Männedorf, Switzerland) as detailed elsewhere (22).

Demographic and Clinical Data Collection

Demographics, anthropometrics, comorbidities, information, and causes of hospitalization were recorded into study-specific case report forms and database. Simplified Acute Physiology Score II (SAPSII) values, etiology, diagnosis, and severity of AHRF, days on mechanical ventilation before study enrollment were collected for each patient. Sequential organ failure assessment (SOFA) was calculated daily throughout the study observation period. Finally, days of mechanical ventilation, ICU length of stay, hospital length of stay, ICU mortality, and 28-days mortality were recorded as outcome data.

Statistical Analysis

Given the observational nature of this pilot study we enrolled a convenience sample size of consecutive patients matching inclusion criteria over a 2-year period based on previous studies (30). Continue variables are expressed as mean ± standard deviation or medians [interquartile range] depending on their distribution, whereas categorical variables are presented as frequencies and percentages. The Shapiro-Wilk test was used to assess the assumption of normality. Categorical data were compared using the χ^2 test or Fisher exact test as appropriate. Unpaired Student's *t*-tests or Mann-Whitney *U*-tests for data with normal or non-normal distribution, respectively, were used to compare continuous variables.

Mixed ANOVA was used to test differences in breathing parameters, diaphragmatic ultrasound measurements and sTnI serum levels among different time points [24 h (Day 1), 48 h (Day 2) and 72 h (Day 3) from assisted mechanical ventilation initiation], after log transformation of variables. In this case, statin use and other variables like sex, age (centered to the mean of 67 years), and BMI (centered to the mean of 28.4 Kg/m^2) were included in the model as covariates to correct for possible confounding factors. The subjects were divided into two groups based on the presence of higher of lower values than the median of biomarkers at baseline (ssTnI = 66 pg/mL, fsTnI = 31 pg/mL, CK = 68 U/L, myoglobin = 151 ng/mL). Then, we performed a mixed ANOVA by using these groups as between-subject variable to observe the possible interaction between low/high levels of biomarkers at baseline on respiratory effort parameters.

Correlation between diaphragmatic ultrasound measurements and circulating muscle functionality biomarkers

TABLE 1 | Patients' clinical characteristics at ICU admission.

Variables	Patients ($N = 62$)
Age, years	67 ± 13
Male sex, *n* (%)	43 (69)
BMI, kg/m²	28.4 ± 5.5
SAPS II score at admission	42 [35–49]
Smoker, *n* (%)	
Actual	18 (29)
Former	6 (10)
Comorbidities, *n* (%)	
Heart diseases	16 (26)
Hypertension	37 (60)
Chronic cardiac ischemia	7 (11)
COPD	9 (15)
Diabetes	13 (21)
CKD	5 (8)
Reason for MV initiation, *n* (%)	
AHRF	29 (47)
Sepsis	6 (10)
Septic shock	18 (29)
Hemorrhagic shock	4 (6)
Coma	4 (6)
Cardiogenic shock	1 (2)
Outcomes	
Days spent on MV	10 [6–16]
ICU LOS	13 [8–19]
Hospital LOS	31 [15–53]
28-days mortality	10 (16)

BMI, body mass index, SAPS, simplified acute physiology score, COPD, chronic pulmonary obstructive disease, CKD, chronic kidney disease, AHRF, acute hypoxemic respiratory failure, ICU, intensive care unit, LOS, length of stay.

TABLE 2 | Skeletal troponin and "traditional" muscle damage parameters during the study period.

Variables	Day 1	Day 2	Day 3	*p*-value
ssTnI, pg/mL	66 [15–164]	55 [18–140]	51 [18–154]	0.623
fsTnI, pg/mL	31 [5–90]	18 [5–76]	13 [2–67]	<0.05
CK, U/L	68 [26–243]	55 [21–176]	44 [15–104]	<0.0001
Myoglobin, ng/mL	151 [57–276]	85 [40–153]	79 [41–126]	<0.0001
AST, U/L	5.4 [1.6–10.9]	3.4 [1.3–9.7]	3.9 [1.3–10.6]	0.226
ALT, U/L	4.8 [2.1–20.8]	5.3 [2.2–13.8]	6.1 [2.2–13.2]	0.617
Aldolase, U/L	4.5 [3.2–5.7]	3.9 [3.3–5.6]	4.2 [3.4–5.7]	0.789

ssTnI, slow skeletal troponin I, fsTnI, fast skeletal troponin I, AST, aspartate aminotransferase, ALT, alanine aminotransferase, CK, creatine kinase.

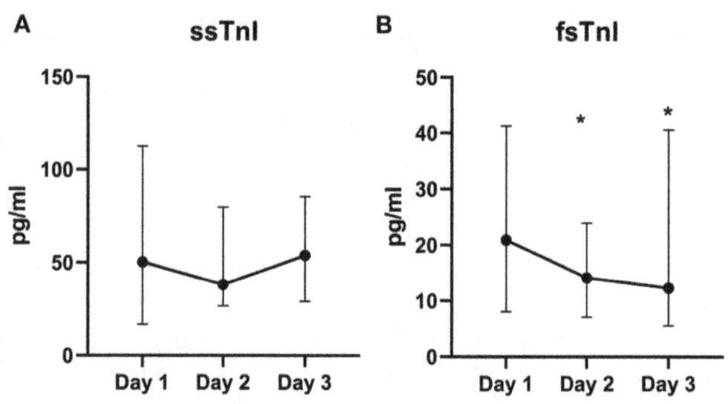

FIGURE 1 | Skeletal TnI serum levels over the study period. Value of ssTnI **(A)** were not different over time, whereas fsTnI **(B)** significantly decreased within the time frame of the study ($p < 0.05$ for within-subjects linear trend). The dots represent the median whereas the upper and lower bars the upper and lower 95% confidence interval, respectively. *$p < 0.05$ vs. T0.

were assessed by multivariate linear mixed-effects models, as stated elsewhere (31). sTnI values were tested as predictors of "normal diaphragmatic function" determined by diaphragmatic ultrasound through receiver operator characteristic (ROC) curves. For each ROC curve, sensitivity, specificity, accuracy, and optimal cut-off point using Youden's index were calculated. Statistical analyses were performed using SPSS 20.0 statistical software (SPSS Inc., Chicago, IL). In all statistical analyses, a 2-tailed test was performed and the $p \leq 0.05$ was considered statistically significant.

RESULTS

Patient Population

A total of 62 consecutive patients were included in the study after 1 [1-3] days from ICU admission. The main clinical characteristics of patients at admission are shown in **Table 1**. Their mean age was 67 ± 13 years old and 43 (69%) were male. Their median SAPSII score was 42 [35-49], resulting in a 29% predicted mortality. The most frequent causes for ICU admission were acute hypoxemic respiratory failure (AHRF) (43%), sepsis (37%), ARDS (24%) and hemorrhagic shock (9%). The median time spent on invasive mechanical ventilation was 10 [6−16] days, and their median ICU length of stay was 13 [8−19] days. No patient developed moderate/severe acute kidney injury during the study period.

Skeletal Troponin and "Classic" Muscle Damage Parameters

We did not find significant variations in the ssTnI trend ($p = 0.623$). On the contrary, fsTnI significantly decreased over time by 30% from Day 1 to Day 2 and by 20% from Day 2 to Day 3, $p < 0.05$, within-subjects linear contrast: $p < 0.05$ (**Table 2** and **Figure 1**). Of note, by correcting the values for the use of statin as a confounding factor, fsTnI still significantly decreased over time ($p < 0.05$). However, when considering the other confounding factors (sex, centered age, and centered BMI), the fsTnI trend was not significant.

A decreasing trend over time was also detected for myoglobin ($p < 0.0001$), with a 45% decrease from Day 1 to Day 2 and almost a 30% decrease from Day 2 to Day 3. Similar data were also observed for CPK, which showed a significant decrease over time (**Table 2**, $p < 0.0001$) with almost 20% lower values each following day. None of the other traditional markers (aldolase, AST, and ALT) showed significant variations within the study.

Of note, by correcting the values of both myoglobin and CPK for statin use the variables remained significant ($p = 0.011$ and $p < 0.001$, respectively), whereas they lose their significance in the fully corrected model.

Ventilation Parameters and Clinical Variables Over Time

Respiratory parameters and gas exchange remained stable throughout the study. The number of patients requiring the use of vasoactive drugs decreased over time (Day 1: 48%, Day 2: 37%, Day 3: 29%, **Table 3**).

TABLE 3 | Clinical and mechanical ventilation parameters during the study period.

	Day 1	Day 2	Day 3	*p*-value
Pressure support, cmH_2O	9 ± 4	9 ± 3	8 ± 4	0.036
PEEP applied, cmH_2O	8 ± 3	8 ± 3	8 ± 3	0.211
Respiratory rate, bpm	15 ± 5	16 ± 6	17 ± 5	0.548
V_E, L/min	7.5 ± 2.0	7.5 ± 2.0	8.1 ± 2.1	0.418
Cdyn, ml/cmH_2O	59 [40–70]	53 [39–64]	56 [40–74]	0.433
PaO_2/FiO_2	228 [156–293]	208 [153 –305]	230 [153 –280]	0.799
MAP, mmHg	83 [75–95]	85 [73–96]	83 [76–93]	0.740
SOFA score	6 [3–8]	5 [3–7]	4 [3–7]	0.852
Vasoactive drug use, *n* (%)	30 (48)	23 (37)	18 (29)	-
Steroid use, *n* (%)	26 (42)	29 (47)	26 (42)	-

PEEP, positive end-expiratory pressure, V_E, minute ventilation, Cdyn, dynamic compliance, PaO_2/FiO_2, oxygen partial arterial tension/inspired oxygen fraction, MAP, mean arterial pressure, SOFA, sequential organ failure assessment.

Skeletal Troponin and Diaphragmatic Ultrasound

We found a significant interaction effect between baseline ssTnI levels and DE [$F_{(2)} = 4.396$, $p = 0.015$], indicating that the observed decrease in DE over time was dependent on the baseline levels of ssTnI. In particular, subjects with high basal levels of ssTnI had a greater decrease in DE when compared to those with low ssTnI basal levels, identified by the steeper slope in **Figure 2A**. We did not find any significant interaction between baseline fsTnI levels and the DE trend [$F_{(2)} = 0.662$, $p = 0.518$, **Figure 2B**]. However, contrary to what observed for ssTnI, patients characterized by high basal levels of fsTnI had a higher DE at each time point than those with low fsTnI basal levels (log transformed variables: Day 1 mean difference: −0.356, $p = 0.006$, Day 2: −0.332, $p = 0.014$, Day 3: −0.102, $p = 0.102$). CK and myoglobin, did not any correlation with DE despite their decrease over time (data not shown). The TFdi trend was not influenced by the baseline levels of any of the measured muscular biomarkers.

Finally, we evaluated whether the frequency of patients developing diaphragmatic dysfunction (defined as DE < 1 cm at Day 3) was different between those demonstrating higher or lower levels of muscular biomarkers at Day 1 (i.e., higher or lower of the median serum concentration). The frequency of patients developing diaphragmatic dysfunction at Day 3 was independent from both ssTnI (40.6% of subjects each group, Fisher's exact test, $p = 1$), fsTnI (low fsTnI vs. high fsTnI: 47.1 vs. 35.3%, $p = 0.460$) (**Supplementary Figure 1**), CPK or myoglobin. When diaphragmatic dysfunction was evaluated by TFdi (i.e., <30%), the results were similar. We did not find any significant correlation between inspiratory effort parameters and muscular biomarkers within-subjects (e.g., at each time point,

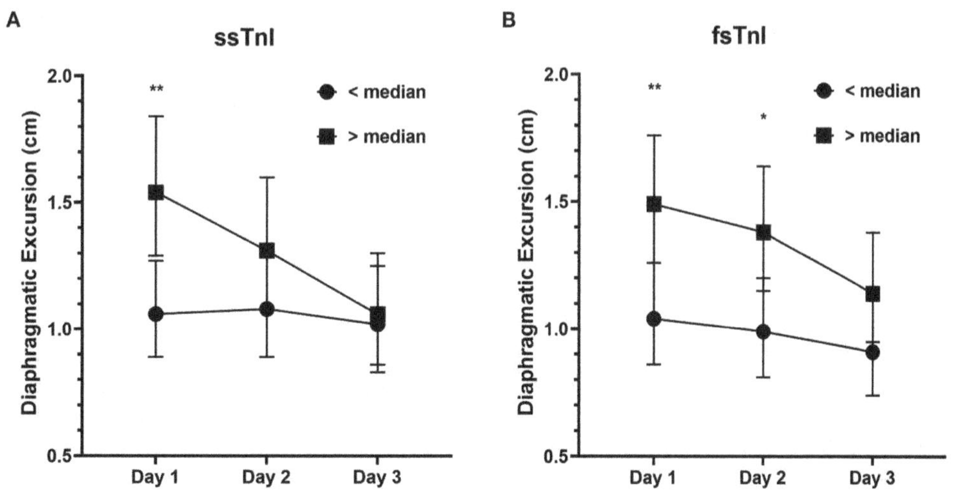

FIGURE 2 | Diaphragmatic excursion (cm) in patients with high or low median levels of skeletal troponins. **(A)** The decrease in diaphragmatic excursion was more prominent in patients with higher basal levels of ssTnI (i.e., >median) denoting the influence of ssTnI basal levels on DE. On the contrary, fsTnI basal levels **(B)** did not influence the decrease in DE. The dots represent the geometric means whereas the upper and lower bars the upper and lower 95% confidence interval, respectively. **$p < 0.01$, *$p < 0.05$.

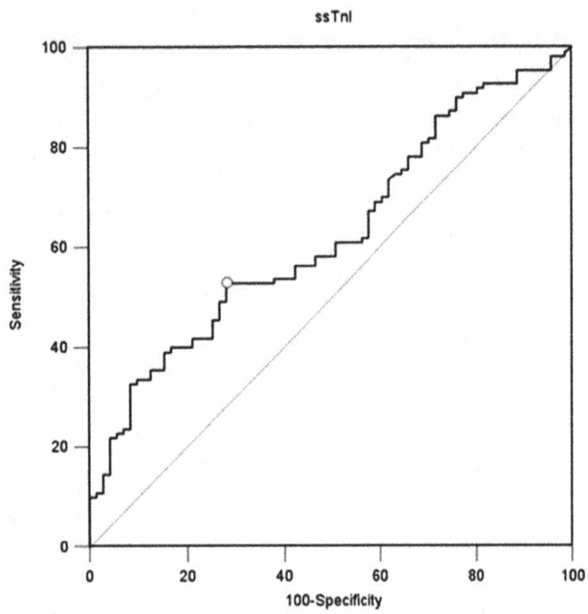

FIGURE 3 | ROC curve analysis for ssTnI as a predictor of normal diaphragmatic function as assessed by diaphragmatic ultrasound (diaphragmatic displacement ≥ 10 mm).

Supplementary Table 1). The only exception was for myoglobin, which showed a positive within-subjects relationship with both DE and TFdi ($r = 0.464$, $p = 0.001$ and $r = 0.462$, $p = 0.001$, respectively). Interestingly, ssTnI and fsTnI showed a significant between-subjects positive correlation with DE and TEE (for ssTnI $r = 0.332$, $p = 0.038$ for DE and $r = 0.346$, $p = 0.027$ for TEE and for fsTnI $r = 0.445$, $p = 0.005$ for DE and $r = 0.400$, $p = 0.009$ for TEE). As such, this indicates that subjects with higher serum levels of skeletal troponins had higher DE and TEE values. Instead, CK correlated only with TEE ($r = 0.381$, $p = 0.016$) and P0.1 ($r = 0.657$, $p = 0.002$).

Skeletal Troponins as Diaphragmatic Function Predictors

A value of ssTnI > 60.06 pg/mL was found to detect a DE ≥ 10 mm (AUC-ROC = 0.628, 95% CI = 0.551 to 0.696, $p = 0.003$) with sensibility 53 [43–62] % and specificity 72 [60–82] % (**Figure 3**). A value of fsTnI > 46.81 pg/mL was found to detect a DE ≥ 10 mm (AUC-ROC = 0.619, 95% CI = 0.545 to 0.689, $p = 0.004$) with sensibility 38 [29–48] % and specificity 83 [72–90] % (**Figure 4A**). A value of fsTnI > 18.29 pg/mL was found to detect a TFdi ≥ 30% (AUC-ROC = 0.617, 95% CI = 0.541 to 0.688, $p = 0.006$) with sensibility 59 [49–68] % and specificity 67 [55–76] % (**Figure 4B**).

DISCUSSION

In this study we described the trend of circulating skeletal troponin in a population of mechanical ventilated ICU patients during the early phase of weaning from mechanical ventilation. We found that (1) the fast but not the slow isoform of skeletal troponin decreased over time within the first 3 days of weaning, (2) patients with higher levels of ssTnI on day 1 had a higher decrease of diaphragmatic excursion while (3) patients with higher basal fsTnI had higher DE (4) both fsTnI and ssTnI showed a significant positive between-patients correlation with both DE and TFdi while no correlation was found between myoglobin and CPK levels and ultrasound-derived parameters.

Critical illness-associated diaphragm weakness can affect up to 64% of patients within 24 h after intubation (32) and up to 80% of patients requiring prolonged mechanical ventilation (33). However, to the best of our knowledge, no serum biomarker has been suggested to specifically diagnose and monitor the development of respiratory muscles damage. A major limitation of traditional serum biomarkers (i.e., CK, lactate dehydrogenase, myoglobin, AST) is that they have a large normal reference range for healthy subjects (19) and thus, low levels of injury in the individual patient may go undetected. In addition, although these markers are useful for the study of muscle-related diseases, they suffer from a low specificity in detecting solely the damage to skeletal muscles, since an increase of these proteins may also be related to myocardial injury (34).

We hereby describe for the first time the trend of circulating skeletal troponin during the early phase of weaning. We found that the fast skeletal troponin decreased over time during the 3 days of observation but not the slow isoform. The discrepancy between the circulating values of these two isoforms is not new and has been recently found in patients with neuromuscular disease (35). Elevations in both ssTnI and fsTnI have been recorded in severe trauma and ischemia (36), therefore suggesting that the increase of ssTnI into circulation may require muscle injury beyond the damage caused by defective contraction or, in our case, by mechanical ventilation. We might then speculate that an increase in fsTnI could be a marker of muscle overload, rather than a sign of loss of muscular mass caused by ischemia or direct muscular trauma. At the same time, the very decrease of ssTnI below the "normal threshold" could indicate a diaphragm dysfunctionality or muscular mass loss, given the found relationship between DE and ssTnI.

In fact, both fsTnI and ssTnI, but not the other classical markers of muscular damage, were positively correlated with ultrasonographic measurements of diaphragmatic displacement. In particular, subjects with higher levels of these two markers had both higher diaphragmatic excursion and diaphragmatic thickness at end-expiration.

Recently, Dres et al. (37) showed that the use of parasternal intercostal muscle ultrasound was responsive to respiratory load and a greater parasternal intercostal muscle thickening under pressure support ventilation was associated with diaphragm dysfunction. Accordingly, it could be interesting to investigate the relative contribution of parasternal intercostal muscle in relationship of skeletal troponin kinetics.

Our study population seemed to maintain clinical stability over time, with stable levels of mechanical ventilation assistance (i.e., pressure support and PEEP) and no substantial changes in respiratory mechanics and gas exchange. The values of P0.1 (ranging between 1.4 and 1.2) were relatively low and

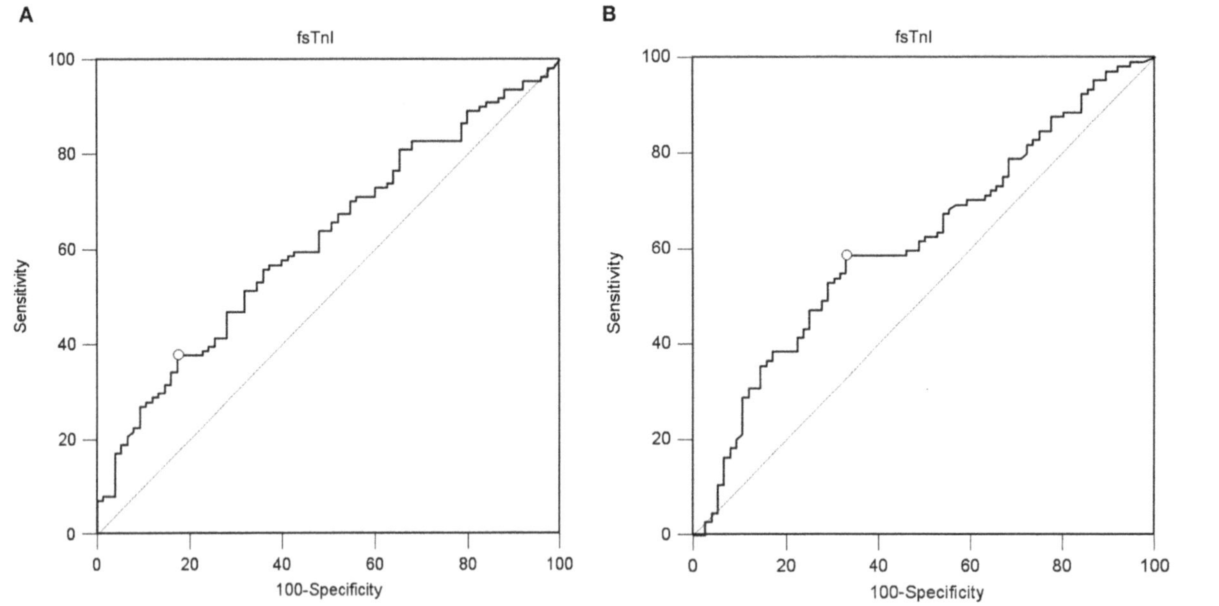

FIGURE 4 | ROC curve analysis for fsTnI as a predictor of normal diaphragmatic function as assessed by diaphragmatic ultrasound (**A**, diaphragmatic excursion ≥ 10 mm, **B**, diaphragmatic thickening fraction ≥ 30%).

both median values of diaphragmatic excursion and thickening fraction were below the thresholds for diaphragmatic weakness (9, 28, 38) indicating that a "diaphragm protective" mechanical ventilation was maintained (39). Nevertheless, we found an increasing trend of patients presenting a diaphragmatic dysfunction, as assessed by ultrasound, over time. These findings prompt the need of a continuous and accurate monitoring of respiratory muscle function during the ICU stay (40).

Diaphragmatic ultrasound is a non-invasive tool to assess the function of the diaphragm, but the technique is time consuming and highly operator dependent. Therefore, dosing fsTnI and ssTnI could potentially increase the number of patients screened for diaphragmatic dysfunction, improve the use of human resources, and allow this assessment also when and where an expert sonographer is not available.

Our study has relevant limitations. First, it is a single-center designed study with a small sample size. Nevertheless, this is a pilot study aiming at describing for the first time the trend of a novel serum marker in a general ICU population of patients recovering from AHRF and our study population might be used as a reference for normal values for a general ICU population during the early phases of their ICU stay. Second, we compared serum skeletal troponin levels only to diaphragmatic dysfunction, without taking into account global muscular mass or performing direct measurements of limb function. However, since the diaphragm is more sensitive to iatrogenic injury caused by MV (12), we decided to focus on this peculiar muscle after a relatively short period of controlled mechanical ventilation (i.e., 1 [1–3] days). Further studies are needed to assess whether the two isoforms of skeletal troponin are associated to systemic muscle wasting, sarcopenia and extradiaphragmatic wasting during ICU stay (41). Third, patients' population (i.e., patients recovering from AHRF from several causes) is representative of a general ICU population, but little is known on patients' diaphragmatic function before ICU admission. Fourth, we have followed patients for a relatively short time compared to their median ICU length of stay (i.e., 13 [8–19] days), the latter issue is related to the need to perform a time consuming, expensive and not readily available analysis for skeletal troponin serum levels. Finally, we have not studied patients both during controlled mechanical ventilation and during unassisted spontaneous breathing. Further studies are needed to assess skeletal troponin trend during the whole respiratory failure treatment, from complete assistance to complete weaning from mechanical ventilation.

CONCLUSIONS

Circulating fast and slow skeletal troponin have specific and different trends in the early phase of weaning from mechanical ventilation and they correlate with ultrasound derived diaphragmatic assessment parameters. The fsTnI decreased during the early phase of weaning while high initial values of ssTnI are associated to a higher decrease of diaphragmatic displacement over time. Further studies are needed to confirm the relationship between these novel biomarkers, protective mechanical ventilation and weaning outcome.

AUTHOR CONTRIBUTIONS

SS, AT, FD, SG, TB, and CV were involved in the conception and the design of the study, analyzed the data, and wrote the paper. VC, VR, and VA collected the data. FD performed the statistical work. RD, GC, AT, and FD contributed to the analysis of the data, SS, FD, AT, SG, GC, TB, and CV contributed to the critical revision of the manuscript for important intellectual content. All authors read and approved the final manuscript.

ACKNOWLEDGMENTS

We are immensely grateful to Prof. Franco Laghi for their comments and suggestions that greatly improved the manuscript.

REFERENCES

Brochard L, Slutsky A, Pesenti A. Mechanical ventilation to minimize progression of lung injury in acute respiratory failure. *Am J Respir Crit Care Med.* (2017) 195:438–42. doi: 10.1164/rccm.201605-1081CP

Di Mussi R, Spadaro S, Mirabella L, Volta CA, Serio G, Staffieri F, et al. Impact of prolonged assisted ventilation on diaphragmatic efficiency: NAVA versus PSV. *Crit Care.* (2016) 20:1. doi: 10.1186/s13054-015-1178-0

Jaber S, Petrof BJ, Jung B, Chanques G, Berthet J-P, Rabuel C, et al. Rapidly progressive diaphragmatic weakness and injury during mechanical ventilation in humans. *Am J Respir Crit Care Med.* (2011) 183:364–71. doi: 10.1164/rccm.201004-0670OC

Levine S, Nguyen T, Taylor N, Friscia ME, Budak MT, Rothenberg P, et al. Rapid disuse atrophy of diaphragm fibers in mechanically ventilated humans. *N Engl J Med.* (2008) 358:1327–35. doi: 10.1056/NEJMoa070447

Hudson MB, Smuder AJ, Nelson WB, Bruells CS, Levine S, Powers SK. Both high level pressure support ventilation and controlled mechanical ventilation induce diaphragm dysfunction and atrophy. *Crit Care Med.* (2012) 40:1254– 60. doi: 10.1097/CCM.0b013e31823c8cc9

Vassilakopoulos T, Petrof BJ. Ventilator-induced diaphragmatic dysfunction. *Am J Respir Crit Care Med.* (2004) 169:336–41. doi: 10.1164/rccm.200304-489CP

Hermans G, Agten A, Testelmans D, Decramer M, Gayan-Ramirez G. Increased duration of mechanical ventilation is associated with decreased diaphragmatic force: a prospective observational study. *Crit Care.* (2010) 14:R127. doi: 10.1186/cc9094

Goligher EC, Dres M, Patel BK, Sahetya SK, Beitler JR, Telias I, et al. Lung- and diaphragm-protective ventilation. *Am J Respir Crit Care Med.* (2020) 202:950–61. doi: 10.1164/rccm.202003-0655CP

Goligher EC, Dres M, Fan E, Rubenfeld GD, Scales DC, Herridge MS, et al. Mechanical ventilation-induced diaphragm atrophy strongly impacts clinical outcomes. *Am J Respir Crit Care Med.* (2018) 197:204–13. doi: 10.1164/rccm.201703-0536OC

Spadaro S, Grasso S, Mauri T, Dalla Corte F, Alvisi V, Ragazzi R, et al. Can diaphragmatic ultrasonography performed during the T-tube trial predict weaning failure? The role of diaphragmatic rapid shallow breathing index. *Crit Care.* (2016) 20:305. doi: 10.1186/s13054-016-1479-y

Di Mussi R, Spadaro S, Volta CA, Bartolomeo N, Trerotoli P, Staffieri F, et al. Continuous assessment of neuro-ventilatory drive during 12 h of pressure support ventilation in critically ill patients. *Crit Care.* (2020) 24:652. doi: 10.1186/s13054-020-03357-9

van Hees HWH, Schellekens WJM, Andrade Acuña GL, Linkels M, Hafmans T, et al. Titin and diaphragm dysfunction in mechanically ventilated rats. *Intensive Care Med.* (2012) 38:702–9. doi: 10.1007/s00134-012-2504-5

Jubran A, Grant BJB, Laghi F, Parthasarathy S, Tobin MJ. Weaning prediction: esophageal pressure monitoring complements readiness testing. *Am J Respir Crit Care Med.* (2005) 171:1252–9. doi: 10.1164/rccm.200503-356OC

Mojoli F, Iotti GA, Arnal J-M, Braschi A. Is the ventilator switching from inspiration to expiration at the right time? Look at waveforms! *Intensive Care Med.* (2016) 42:914–5. doi: 10.1007/s00134-015-4174-6

Pellegrini M, Hedenstierna G, Roneus A, Segelsjö M, Larsson A, Perchiazzi G. The diaphragm acts as a brake during expiration to prevent lung collapse. *Am J Respir Crit Care Med.* (2017) 195:1608–16. doi: 10.1164/rccm.201605-0992OC

Volta CA, Dalla Corte F, Ragazzi R, Marangoni E, Fogagnolo A, Scaramuzzo G, et al. Expiratory flow limitation in intensive care: prevalence and risk factors. *Crit Care.* (2019) 23:395. doi: 10.1186/s13054-019-2682-4

Dres M, Goligher EC, Dubé B-P, Morawiec E, Dangers L, Reuter D, et al. Diaphragm function and weaning from mechanical ventilation: an ultrasound and phrenic nerve stimulation clinical study. *Ann Intensive Care.* (2018) 8:53. doi: 10.1186/s13613-018-0401-y

Simpson JA, Labugger R, Hesketh GG, D'Arsigny C, O'Donnell D, Matsumoto N, et al. Differential detection of skeletal troponin I isoforms in serum of a patient with rhabdomyolysis: markers of muscle injury? *Clin Chem.* (2002) 48:1112–4. doi: 10.1093/clinchem/48.7.1112

Sorichter S, Mair J, Koller A, Gebert W, Rama D, Calzolari C, et al. Skeletal troponin I as a marker of exercise-induced muscle damage. *J Appl Physiol.* (1997) 83:1076–82. doi: 10.1152/jappl.1997.83.4.1076

Chapman DW, Simpson JA, Iscoe S, Robins T, Nosaka K. Changes in serum fast and slow skeletal troponin I concentration following maximal eccentric contractions. *J Sci Med Sport.* (2013) 16:82–5. doi: 10.1016/j.jsams.2012. 05.006

Foster GE, Nakano J, Sheel AW, Simpson JA, Road JD, Reid WD. Serum skeletal troponin I following inspiratory threshold loading in healthy young and middle-aged men. *Eur J Appl Physiol.* (2012) 112:3547–58. doi: 10.1007/s00421-012-2337-5

Trentini A, Spadaro S, Rosta V, Manfrinato MC, Cervellati C, Dalla Corte F, et al. Fast skeletal troponin I, but not the slow isoform, is increased in patients under statin therapy: a pilot study. *Biochem Med.* (2019) 29:010703. doi: 10.11613/BM.2019.010703

Kellum JA, Lameire N, KDIGO AKI Guideline Work Group. Diagnosis, evaluation, and management of acute kidney injury: a KDIGO summary (Part 1). *Crit Care.* (2013) 17:204. doi: 10.1186/cc11454

Spadaro S, Grasso S, Dres M, Fogagnolo A, Dalla Corte F, Tamburini N, et al. Point of care ultrasound to identify diaphragmatic dysfunction after thoracic surgery. *Anesthesiology.* (2019) 131:266–78. doi: 10.1097/ALN.0000000000002774

Goligher EC, Laghi F, Detsky ME, Farias P, Murray A, Brace D, et al. Measuring diaphragm thickness with ultrasound in mechanically ventilated patients: feasibility, reproducibility and validity. *Intensive Care Med.* (2015) 41:642–9. doi: 10.1007/s00134-015-3687-3

Umbrello M, Formenti P, Longhi D, Galimberti A, Piva I, Pezzi A, et al. Diaphragm ultrasound as indicator of respiratory effort in critically ill patients undergoing assisted mechanical ventilation: a pilot clinical study. *Crit Care.* (2015) 19:161. doi: 10.1186/s13054-015-0894-9

Vivier E, Mekontso Dessap A, Dimassi S, Vargas F, Lyazidi A, Thille AW, et al. Diaphragm ultrasonography to estimate the work of breathing during non-invasive ventilation. *Intensive Care Med.* (2012) 38:796–803. doi: 10.1007/s00134-012-2547-7

Kim WY, Suh HJ, Hong S-B, Koh Y, Lim CM. Diaphragm dysfunction assessed by ultrasonography: influence on weaning from mechanical ventilation. *Crit Care Med.* (2011) 39:2627–30. doi: 10.1097/CCM.0b013e3182266408

DiNino E, Gartman EJ, Sethi JM, McCool FD. Diaphragm ultrasound as a predictor of successful extubation from mechanical ventilation. *Thorax.* (2014) 69:423–7. doi: 10.1136/thoraxjnl-2013-204111

Schepens T, Verbrugghe W, Dams K, Corthouts B, Parizel PM, Jorens PG. The course of diaphragm atrophy in ventilated patients assessed with ultrasound: a longitudinal cohort study. *Crit Care.* (2015) 19:422. doi: 10.1186/s13054-015-1141-0

Hoffman L. *Longitudinal Analysis: Modeling Within-Person Fluctuation and Change.* Routledge (2015).

Demoule A, Jung B, Prodanovic H, Molinari N, Chanques G, Coirault C, et al. Diaphragm dysfunction on admission to the intensive care unit. Prevalence, risk factors, and prognostic impact-a prospective study. *Am J Respir Crit Care Med.* (2013) 188:213–9. doi: 10.1164/rccm.201209-1668OC

Supinski GS, Callahan LA. Diaphragm weakness in mechanically ventilated critically ill patients. *Crit Care.* (2013) 17:R120. doi: 10.1186/cc12792

Sax H, Contesse J, Dubach P, Reinhart WH. Creatine kinase MB during myocardial infarction: relationship to preexisting coronary heart disease and medication. *Acta Cardiol.* (1997) 52:423–30.

Barthel BL, Cox D, Barbieri M, Ziemba M, Straub V, Hoffman EP, et al. Elevation of fast but not slow troponin I in the circulation of patients with Becker and

Duchenne muscular dystrophy. *Muscle Nerve.* (2021) 64:43–9. doi: 10.1002/mus.27222

Simpson JA, Labugger R, Collier C, Brison RJ, Iscoe S, Van Eyk JE. Fast and slow skeletal troponin I in serum from patients with various skeletal muscle disorders: a pilot study. *Clin Chem.* (2005) 51:966–72. doi: 10.1373/clinchem.2004.042671

Dres M, Dubé B-P, Goligher E, Vorona S, Demiri S, Morawiec E, et al. Usefulness of parasternal intercostal muscle ultrasound during weaning from mechanical ventilation. *Anesthesiology.* (2020) 132:1114–25. doi: 10.1097/ALN.0000000000003191

Guttmann J, Eberhard L, Fabry B, Bertschmann W, Zeravik J, Adolph M, et al. Time constant/volume relationship of passive expiration in mechanically ventilated ARDS patients. *Eur Respir J.* (1995) 8:114–20. doi: 10.1183/09031936.95.08010114

Schepens T, Goligher EC. Lung- and diaphragm-protective ventilation in acute respiratory distress syndrome: rationale and challenges. *Anesthesiology.* (2019) 130:620–33. doi: 10.1097/ALN.00000000000 02605

Bertoni M, Spadaro S, Goligher EC. Monitoring patient respiratory effort during mechanical ventilation: lung and diaphragm-protective ventilation. *Crit Care.* (2020) 24:106. doi: 10.1186/s13054-020-2777-y

Spadaro S, Scaramuzzo G, Volta CA. Can abdominal muscle ultrasonography during spontaneous breathing and cough predict reintubation in mechanically ventilated patients? *Chest.* (2021) 160:1163–4. doi: 10.1016/j.chest.2021.07.006

2

Pulmonary Interstitial Matrix and Lung Fluid Balance from Normal to the Acutely Injured Lung

*Egidio Beretta[1], Francesco Romanò[2], Giulio Sancini[1], James B. Grotberg[3], Gary F. Nieman[4] and Giuseppe Miserocchi[1]**

[1] Department of Medicine and Surgery, School of Medicine and Surgery, Università degli Studi di Milano-Bicocca, Monza, Italy, [2] Univ. Lille, CNRS, ONERA, Arts et Métiers, Centrale Lille, FRE 2017-LMFL-Laboratoire de Mécanique des Fluides de Lille – Kampé de Fériet, Lille, France, [3] Department of Biomedical Engineering, University of Michigan, Ann Arbor, MI, United States, [4] Department of Surgery, State University of New York Upstate Medical University, Syracuse, NY, United States

***Correspondence:**
Giuseppe Miserocchi
giuseppe.miserocchi@unimib.it

This review analyses the mechanisms by which lung fluid balance is strictly controlled in the air-blood barrier (ABB). Relatively large trans-endothelial and trans-epithelial Starling pressure gradients result in a minimal flow across the ABB thanks to low microvascular permeability aided by the macromolecular structure of the interstitial matrix. These edema safety factors are lost when the integrity of the interstitial matrix is damaged. The result is that small Starling pressure gradients, acting on a progressively expanding alveolar barrier with high permeability, generate a high transvascular flow that causes alveolar flooding in minutes. We modeled the trans-endothelial and trans-epithelial Starling pressure gradients under control conditions, as well as under increasing alveolar pressure (Palv) conditions of up to 25 cmH_2O. We referred to the wet-to-dry weight (W/D) ratio, a specific index of lung water balance, to be correlated with the functional state of the interstitial structure. W/D averages $\sim$5 in control and might increase by up to $\sim$9 in severe edema, corresponding to $\sim$70% loss in the integrity of the native matrix. Factors buffering edemagenic conditions include: (i) an interstitial capacity for fluid accumulation located in the thick portion of ABB, (ii) the increase in interstitial pressure due to water binding by hyaluronan (the "safety factor" opposing the filtration gradient), and (iii) increased lymphatic flow. Inflammatory factors causing lung tissue damage include those of bacterial/viral and those of sterile nature. Production of reactive oxygen species (ROS) during hypoxia or hyperoxia, or excessive parenchymal stress/strain [lung overdistension caused by patient self-induced lung injury (P-SILI)] can all cause excessive inflammation. We discuss the heterogeneity of intrapulmonary distribution of W/D ratios. A W/D $\sim$6.5 has been identified as being critical for the transition to severe edema formation. Increasing Palv for W/D > 6.5, both trans-endothelial and trans-epithelial gradients favor filtration leading to alveolar flooding. Neither CT scan nor ultrasound can identify this initial level of lung fluid balance perturbation. A suggestion is put forward to identify a non-invasive tool to detect the earliest stages of perturbation of lung fluid balance before the condition becomes life-threatening.

Keywords: SARS-CoV-2, ARDS, edema, alveolar pressure, P-SILI, computational model

INTRODUCTION

Efficient gas diffusion in the air-blood barrier is only possible by strict control of extravascular water volume to prevent edema-induced tissue swelling and alveolar flooding. In normal lungs, the thickness of the air-blood barrier does not exceed ~0.2 μm. Edema is prevented by an extremely low microvascular permeability and dynamic remodeling of the interstitial matrix (Miserocchi and Rivolta, 2012). The physiologic parameters controlling lung fluid balance are dynamic and change over the life span of individuals to ensure a healthy match of regional ventilation to the metabolic requirement.

This study merges the understanding of normal physiologic fluid balance control with the ramifications of what can occur when this control is lost. We will first review how a healthy lung can tightly control extravascular lung water by specific mechanical alterations to parenchymal structure that will efficiently minimize edema. Next, we will investigate how progressive loss of this anti-edemagenic control inevitably leads to severe edema. We present a detailed analysis of Starling pressure gradients sustaining flows across the endothelial and epithelial barriers. We stress the point that the heterogeneity in edema distribution allows us to distinguish between lung regions that can still provide control of fluid balance to allow gas exchanges and other regions that have lost this capacity because of breakage of the interstitial matrix. We correlate the Starling pressure gradients with the specific regional edema formation measured as the lung tissue wet-to-dry weight ratio (W/D). This study provides contribution to the understanding of acute lung injury pathophysiology and the role of mechanical ventilation in edema formation. In particular, this study is one of the first to discuss trans-endothelial and trans-epithelial flows as distinct events for a given lung distension pressure. It is hoped that this review might provide indications aimed at avoiding an unintentional ventilator-induced lung injury (VILI).

THE AIR-BLOOD BARRIER AND THE MOLECULAR STRUCTURE OF THE INTERSTITIAL COMPARTMENT

The air–blood barrier (ABB) represents the interface for gas exchanges; the capillary endothelium is in close apposition with the alveolar epithelium so that the thickness of ABB is as low as 0.3 μm and its surface is in the range of 100 m^2 in the human lung (Weibel, 2015).

The ABB includes two portions: a thin side (**Figure 1A**) that accounts for more than 50% of alveolar surface that contains minimal interstitial space (Weibel, 2017), and a thick side (**Figure 1B**) that includes most of the parenchymal extra cellular matrix (ECM) and lymphatics. It has been suggested that the thick portion acts as a reservoir capacity where fluid filtered at the level of the thin portion might accumulate to be drained down a pressure gradient generated by lymphatics (Unruh et al., 1984; Conforti et al., 2002).

The special arrangement of the endothelial and epithelial cells is seen in **Figure 2**. Type-1 epithelial (Epi1) cells cover about 95% of the surface of each alveolus, with the rest being covered by globular Epi2 cells.

The body of Epi1 cells forms a series of interconnected structures that envelop, through several stalks, approximately 40 capillaries. There are only about 40 Epi1 cells lining a single alveolus facing about 170 endothelial cells, so any Epi1 cell covers about four endothelial cells. An average volume of ~1,700 μm^3 of an Epi1 cell spreads over a surface area of ~5,000 μm^2, and allows for a thickness of as low as 0.3 μm. Such a low number results from the combination of low number of Epi1 cells and extended plasma membrane surface. On the whole, the overall surfaces of Epi1 and endothelial cells are comparable.

Two important functional features of ABB are the following: very strict control of water balance by minimizing fluid exchanges across the endothelial and epithelial barriers, and remarkable mechanical resistance to the increase in tension related to change in lung volumes. These two important features rely on the structure-function relationship between the epithelial and endothelial cells and the macromolecular structure of the interstitial compartment separating the epithelial and endothelial layers.

The structure of the interstitial compartment includes a mesh of collagen and elastic fibers whose main role is to provide mechanical support and elasticity (Miserocchi and Rivolta, 2012). These molecules are chemically very stable and resistant to proteolysis. Within the space between these molecules, there is a dense mesh of molecules, belonging to the proteoglycan family, whose main role is to exert a strict control on the amount of extravascular water that must be kept to a minimum. Microvascular permeability is controlled by the low molecular weight heparan-sulfate proteoglycan (HS-PG, 300–500 kDa) of the basement membrane and by small peptidoglycans of the glycocalyx (PDGL), normally assuring high resistivity of the paracellular route (Reitsma et al., 2007). Large molecular weight chondroitin-sulfate proteoglycans (CS-PG > 1,000 kDa) bound to hyaluronan act as link proteins through low energy non-covalent bonds with other molecules and cells providing rigidity to the parenchymal mesh.

THE CONTROL OF EXTRAVASCULAR WATER UNDER PHYSIOLOGICAL CONDITIONS

The hydraulic pressure (Pint) in lung interstitial compartment is in the sub-atmospheric range, averaging ~10 cmH_2O (Miserocchi et al., 1990), and a negative Pint value represents the fluid dynamic equilibrium between capillary filtration down a high resistance pathway (low microvascular permeability) and a lower resistance pathway represented by lymphatic drainage. The equilibrium is also favored by the transcapillary oncotic pressure gradient (favoring absorption) that exceeds the hydraulic gradient (favoring filtration) (Parker et al., 1978).

Figure 3 presents the fluid exchange models for the thin the thick portions of the ABB, and the parameters defining the pressure gradients that sustain potential water and solute fluxes

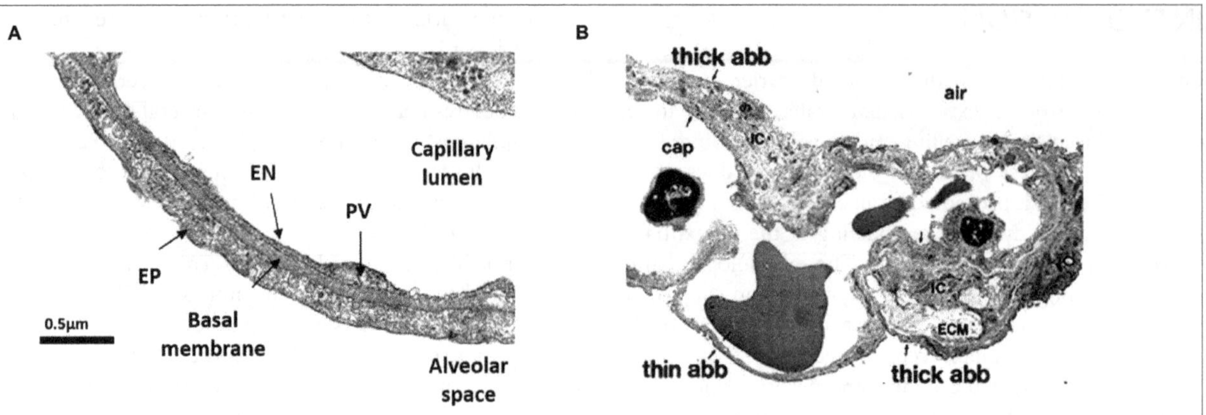

FIGURE 1 | Morphology of the air-blood barrier (ABB). **(A)** Thin portion of ABB showing the close apposition between alveolar epithelium (EP) and capillary endothelium (EN). PV is plasmalemmal vesicle (from Botto et al., 2006). **(B)** Microscopy image showing the ABB and its thin and thick portions. ECM, extra cellular matrix; cap, lung capillary; ic, interstitial cell (from Conforti et al., 2002).

across the endothelium and the epithelium. Note that lymphatics are only present in the thick portion of the ABB.

Transcapillary and transepithelial water exchanges are governed by the Starling law where P and Π are the hydraulic and the colloid osmotic pressures across any two compartments. Water flow (J_v) is defined as:

$$J_v = Kf \cdot [(P_1 - P_2) - \sigma(\Pi_1 - \Pi_2)] \quad (1)$$

where Kf (*filtration coefficient*) $= Lp \cdot A$, with Lp being the hydraulic conductance, A the surface area available for flow, and $[(P_1 - P_2) - \sigma(\Pi_1 - \Pi_2)]$ the Starling pressure gradient generating flow.

In this study, we will focus on the Starling pressure gradients, and based on experimentally measured values, will analyze how they are modified to cause severe perturbation in lung fluid balance. Relevance will also be given to the estimate of the effect of increasing alveolar pressure on these gradients, a point that, so far, has remained unexplored but of utmost importance in mechanical ventilation. In a companion study, the Starling pressure gradients presented in this study will be used to model the transcapillary, transepithelial, and lymphatic flows in physiological condition as well as in developing severe lung edema.

Our whole analysis considers W/D as the more precise and reliable index of the lung fluid balance that has been related to experimentally measured values of variables and coefficients appearing in Eq. 1. The validity of W/D as an index of water balance was confirmed by Parker and Townsley (2004) who reported its excellent correlation with albumin and total proteins collected from the bronchoalveolar lavage fluid, an index of derangement of fluid balance in experimental models of graded lung injury.

Table 1 reports the Starling pressure gradients in a healthy lung at end-expiration and at end- inspiration. End-expiration corresponds to functional residual capacity (FRC) ~22% TLC in supine position, while end-inspiration corresponds to ~32% TLC (Agostoni and Mead, 1964). Water balance under physiological condition is defined by a lung wet weight/dry weight ratio (W/D) of ~5 (Conforti et al., 2002). In **Table 1** and from here on, positive values of a Starling gradient across the endothelium and the epithelium indicate fluid filtration into the interstitial space and the alveolar compartment, respectively; negative values of a Starling gradient indicate fluid clearance from these compartments.

Table 1 reports the expected values of hydraulic pressure for the capillary, interstitial, and alveolar fluids (Pcap, Pint, and $Pliq_{alv}$, respectively) as well as those of oncotic pressure (Πcap, Πint, and Πliq_{alv}, respectively). The value of $Pliq_{alv}$, the pressure of the liquid phase coating the alveolar surface, was estimated from the equation $Pliq_{alv} = Palv - \frac{2\gamma}{R}$, (Beck and Lai-Fook, 1983). We considered Palv = 0 at end-inspiration and at end-expiration (FRC) during spontaneous breathing, and we assumed a physiological value for $\gamma = 1$ dynes/cm substantially unchanged up to 70% TLC (Bachofen et al., 1970). We assumed an alveolar radius of ~ 50 μm at TLC (Beck and Lai-Fook, 1983) and its decrease at FRC being proportional to $(FRC/TLC)^{1/3}$ (equal to 0.6). Accordingly, given the low value of γ, the ratio $2\gamma/R = Pliq_{alv}$ is ~ 0 cmH_2O. Clearly, the large change in trans-epithelial Starling gradient reflects the remarkable change in Pint.

Endothelial and epithelial protein reflection coefficients (σ_{endo} and σ_{epi}, respectively) are also reported. Hydraulic (ΔP) and oncotic ($\sigma\Pi$P) pressure gradients and the total Starling pressure gradient are reported in bold. Concerning σ, it was experimentally derived at high flow rates as $\sigma = 1 - \phi$ (ϕ being the lymph/plasma protein partition coefficient). However, this condition might not provide a σ value corresponding to the physiological condition of very low flow rates. For both endothelium and epithelium, we assumed $\sigma = 0.85$ (Parker et al., 2006), a higher value compared to those previously provided by Parker et al. (1978). Furthermore, under healthy conditions, the epithelium is almost totally impermeable to proteins (Gorin and Stewart, 1979), and water transport can only occur *via* coupled Na^+ active absorption (Matthay et al., 1982). One report showed that epithelial monolayers generally have an electrical resistance that is an order of magnitude higher than

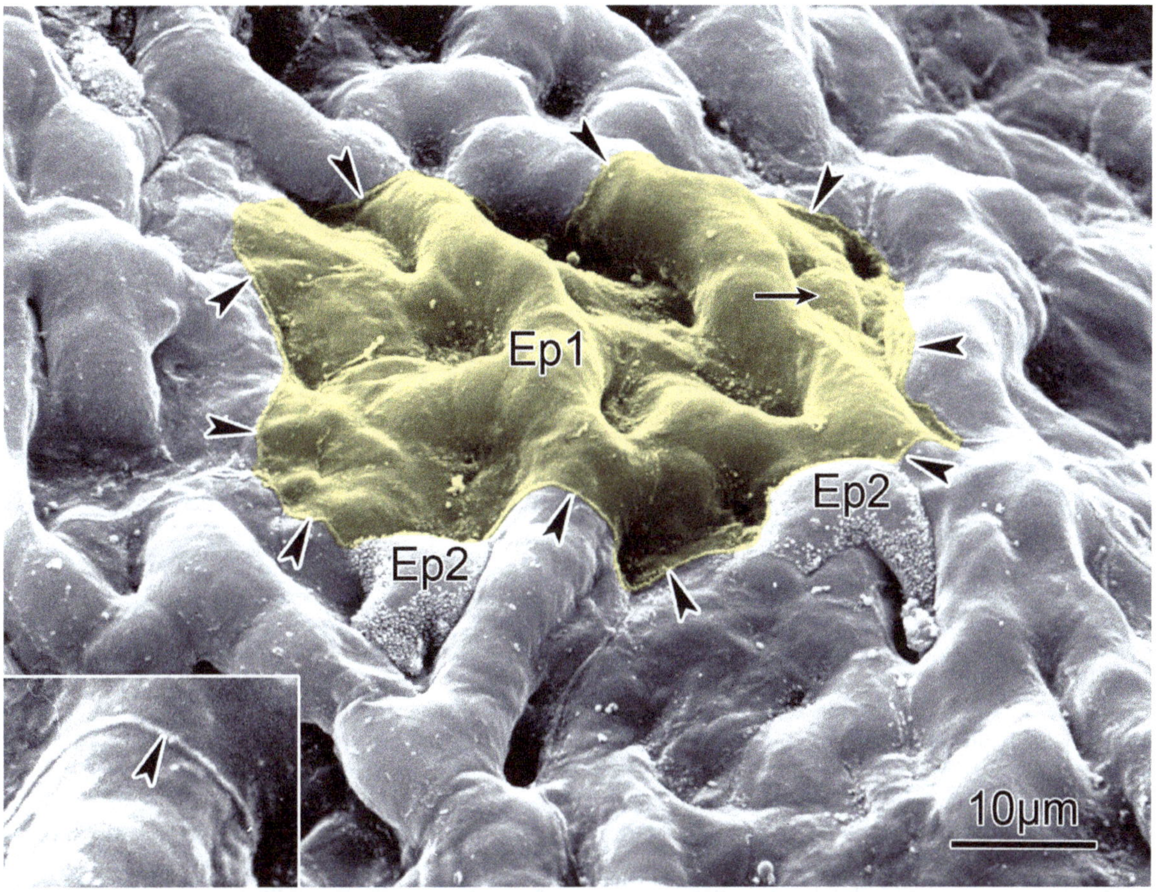

FIGURE 2 | Scanning electron micrograph of the alveolar surface of a human lung showing protruding capillaries and two type II cells (Ep2) sitting in niches and characterized by a rim of microvilli. Small arrow points to cell body of a type I cell (Ep1) that covers several capillary meshes (yellow); the boundary of its cytoplasmic leaflet is marked by arrowheads outlining a small lip of the cell junction between adjoining cells (inset, compare **Figure 1B**). The surface area covered by this cytoplasmic leaflet is 1,300 mm^2. Scale bar = 10 μm (from Weibel, 2015); reprinted with permission of the American Thoracic Society.

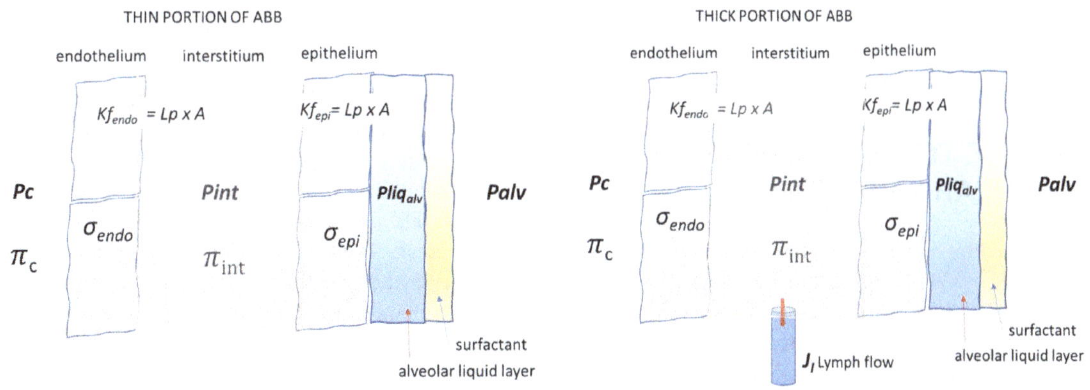

FIGURE 3 | Lung fluid compartments of the ABB and parameters governing fluid exchanges. Pc, Pint, and $Pliq_{alv}$ are capillary, interstitial, and alveolar liquid hydraulic pressure, respectively; Πc and Πint are capillary and interstitial oncotic pressure, respectively; σ_{endo} and σ_{epi} are the protein reflection coefficient of endothelium and epithelium, respectively; Palv is the alveolar pressure; Lp, A, Kf_{endo}, and Kf_{epi} are the hydraulic conductance, overall filtration surface, and endothelial and epithelial filtration coefficient, respectively. Lymphatic drainage (Jl) occurs from the thick portion of ABB where lymphatics are located.

TABLE 1 | Trans-endothelial and trans-epithelial Starling pressure gradients at end-expiration (functional residual capacity, FRC) and end-inspiration under physiological conditions (referring to Point A in **Figure 4**).

	Trans-endothelial			Trans-epithelial	
	End-expiration	End-inspiration		End-expiration	End-inspiration
Pcap*	9	9	Pint**	−10	−24
Pint**	−10	−24	Pliq alv#	~0	~0
σ end##	0.85	0.85	σ epi##	0.85	0.85
Πcap**	26.8	26.8	Πint**	13.8	13.8
Πint**	13.8	13.8	Πliq alv	0	0
			γ	1	1
ΔP	**19**	**33**	**ΔP**	**−10**	**−24**
σ·ΔΠ	**−11.0**	**−11.0**	**σ·ΔΠ**	**−11.7**	**−11.7**
Starling gradient	**8.0**	**22.0**	**Starling gradient**	**−21.7**	**−35.7**

Table reports the expected values for capillary, interstitial and alveolar liquid hydraulic pressure (Pcap, Pint and Pliq alv, respectively) as well as for capillary, interstitial and alveolar liquid oncotic pressure (Πcap, Πint and Πliq alv, respectively). Endothelial (σ endo) and epithelial (σ epi) protein reflection coefficients are also reported. In bold, hydraulic (ΔP) and oncotic (σΠP) pressure gradients and total Starling pressure gradient. Positive values of the Starling gradient at endothelial level indicate filtration into interstitium; negative value at epithelial level indicate alveolar reabsorption.

*Pressure values are expressed in cmH_2O; σ is a pure number. *From Hakim et al., 1993; **from Miserocchi et al., 1993; #calculated from Beck and Lai-Fook, 1983; ##from Parker et al., 2006. Surface tension γ = 1 dyne/cm.*

that of endothelial monolayers and much lower solute diffusion permeability (Parker et al., 2006).

Concerning the microvascular district, one should add the important notion that functional compartmentation has been described considering a "true" alveolar compartment and an extra-alveolar capillary compartment. The latter has higher Lp and lower surface area compared to the "true" alveolar district, which has a much lower Lp but an incredibly much higher surface. Definitely, the "true" alveolar compartment only contributes about 6% of total convective albumin flux recovered in the lung lymph (Parker, 2007). Therefore, under physiological conditions, despite the existence of trans-endothelial and trans-epithelial pressure gradients shown in **Table 1** (referring specifically to the "true" alveolar district), minimal fluxes occur thanks to low permeability coefficients. One shall consider that capillary surface area (A) might differ among humans, reflecting the individual extension of the alveolar capillary network that was found to vary by ~3 fold based on the estimate of the capillary blood volume (Vc) (Miserocchi et al., 2008).

THE RESPONSE TO THE INCREASE IN MICROVASCULAR FILTRATION

Figure 4 shows how Pint varies with increasing water balance as expressed by the W/D ratio. Point A corresponds to the physiological condition, while Point B corresponds to the physiological response acting to buffer an increase in microvascular filtration in response to an edemagenic condition.

The latter may occur because of a variety of reasons, such as hyperventilation and increase in cardiac output on sustained exercise (e.g., marathon running) (Zavorsky et al., 2014). The lung is well-equipped to respond to increased microvascular filtration due to specific morpho-functional features of the interstitial tissue structure. Indeed, increased free water filtered in the interstitium is captured by hyaluronan to form gel, whose increase in steric hindrance causes a remarkable increase in Pint from -10 cmH_2O (**Figure 5**, point A) to ~ +5 cmH_2O (point B) (Miserocchi et al., 1993). At point B, the W/D ratio does not exceed 5.5 (10% increase relative to the control value), reflecting low tissue compliance (~0.5 $ml.mmHg^{-1}\cdot 100$ g of wet $weight^{-1}$) (Miserocchi et al., 1993). As long as the filtration coefficient and the protein reflection coefficient remain within physiological values, interstitial gel formation provides a "safety factor" against edema formation to face an increase in microvascular filtration. Indeed, the increase in interstitial pressure (see Eq. 1) prevents further filtration and may actually favor fluid re-absorption (see Paragraph 8 for estimate of actual Starling pressure gradients). The correlation between rigidity of the extracellular matrix and low microvascular permeability was confirmed in a micro-nano biomimetic system by growing endothelial and epithelial cell layers on opposite sides of a porous mesh mimicking the extracellular structure of the basal lamina in the lung. Varying the rigidity of the mesh, and using different concentrations of polycaprolactone with gelatine, it was found that effective barrier properties were actually increased by increasing the stiffness of the matrix (Higuita-Castro et al., 2017).

Respiratory mechanics was monitored by low-frequency forced oscillation technique (FOT) in closed-chest mechanically ventilated rats under conditions referring to points A and B (Dellacà et al., 2008). The results suggested that the changes in reactance and resistance when shifting from A to B could reflect the changes in viscoelastic properties of the lung tissue, in the absence of the accumulation of extravascular fluid into the alveoli. It was, therefore, proposed that the estimate of lung mechanics with FOT might represent a non-invasive, potentially clinically useful tool to detect the earliest stages of perturbation of lung fluid balance before the condition becomes life-threatening. The next paragraph describes how the loss of safety factor (**Figure 4**, point C), due to fragmentation of the interstitial matrix structure, leads to a decrease in Pint to 0 cmH_2O and to a critical increase in W/D ratio.

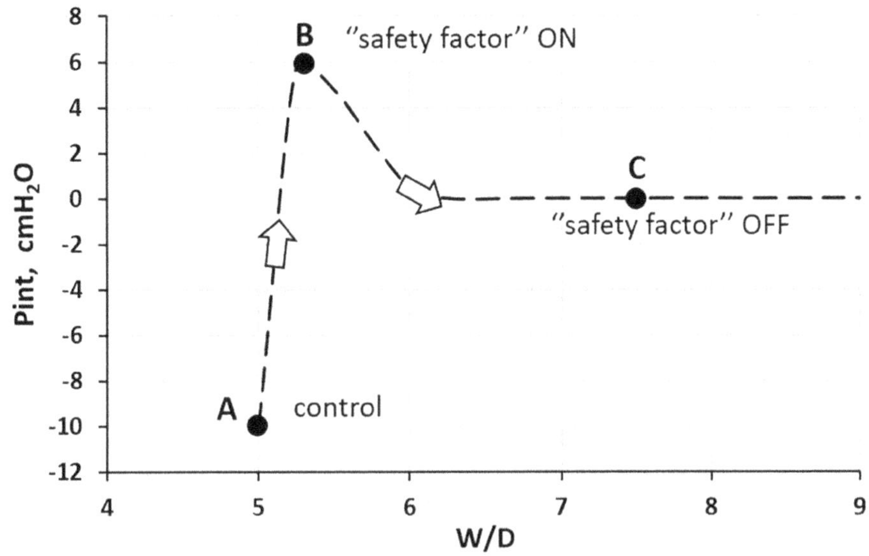

FIGURE 4 | Relationship between interstitial hydraulic pressure (Pint) and wet-to-dry weight (W/D) ratio at end-expiration. Point A corresponds to physiological condition; point B to the "safety factor" (see text for explanation); point C corresponds to the absence of the "safety factor" reflecting the remarkable loss of integrity of the interstitial matrix (Miserocchi et al., 1990, 1993).

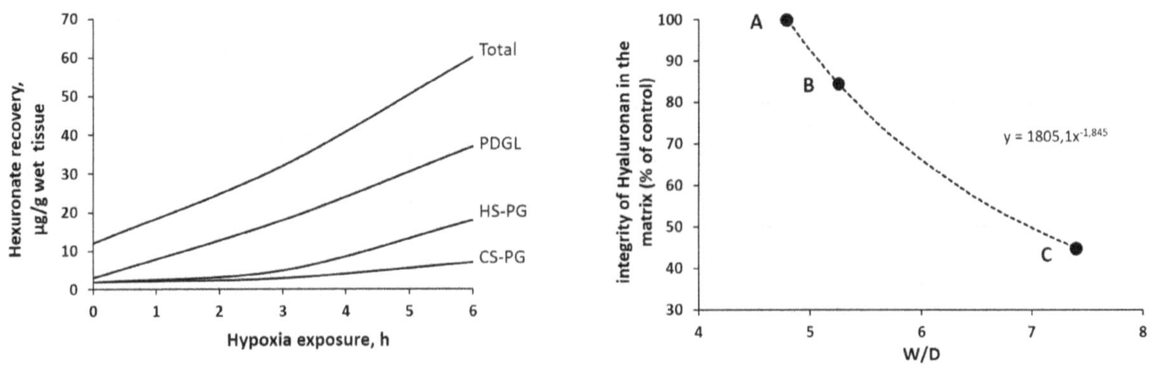

FIGURE 5 | Left: time course of the recovery of fragments of proteoglycan families upon 12% O_2 exposure (redrawn from Miserocchi et al., 2001). Peptidoglycans (PDGLs) control the permeability of the glycocalyx; heparin-sulfate proteoglycans (HS-PGs) control the permeability of endothelial and epithelial cells; chondroitin-sulfate proteoglycans (CS-PGs) provide rigidity to the interstitial matrix. **Right:** relationship between loss of integrity of interstitial hyaluronan (a hydrophilic non-sulfated glycosaminoglycan) and increase in W/D ratio. Points A, B, and C correspond to those reported in **Figure 4**.

THE TISSUE DAMAGE AND THE CRITICAL INCREASE IN W/D RATIO

The inflammation caused by a sterile (e.g., severe hypoxia, hyperoxia, surgery, excessive parenchymal stress/strain) or bacterial/viral mechanism may trigger the fragmentation of the macromolecular architecture of the interstitial compartment, involving the whole proteoglycan family. **Figure 5** (left) shows, as an example, the time course of the recovery of fragments of proteoglycan families on 12% O_2 exposure (Miserocchi et al., 2001). Over time, fragment recovery occurs at a greater rate for PDGL and HS-PG, compared to CS-PG. The loss of integrity of the native architecture of the proteoglycan family of the interstitial matrix leads to a combination of two effects: (i) increase in microvascular permeability, which weakens the restriction to fluid leak, and (ii) increase in tissue compliance that brings Pint back to 0 cmH_2O (**Figure 4**, point C, W/D ~7.5). As a consequence, the "safety factor" is abolished and the corresponding increase in W/D ratio reflects the increase in filtration rate leading to the development of edema. The right panel of **Figure 5** shows the negative correlation between the loss of integrity of the interstitial matrix and the increase in W/D. With 50% fragmentation of native hyaluronan, W/D increases by up to ~ 7.5, a frankly edematous state (Negrini et al., 1996; Miserocchi et al., 2001).

Differences in the sequence of a fragmentation of proteoglycans may be demonstrated among various models of experimental pulmonary edema (Negrini et al., 1996; Miserocchi et al., 1999). Thus, there may be a variable time-dependent contribution to edema formation due to the increase in microvascular permeability (due to the fragmentation of HS-PG and PGDL) and/or increase in tissue compliance (reflecting the fragmentation of CS-PG). The inflammatory-dependent activation of proteases (MMP-2 and MMP-9) contributes to proteoglycan fragmentation (Passi et al., 1999). Heparan-sulfate disassembly has been reported by recent findings of HA exudates in the alveolar spaces of the lungs of patients with coronavirus disease-2019 (COVID-19) (Hellman et al., 2020).

It is noteworthy to consider the difference in timing between the phase of fragmentation of the interstitial mesh (3–6 h) and the immunity response reported for patients with COVID-19 that develops with a much slower kinetics during the first week after infection (Hou et al., 2020; Long et al., 2020).

CAUSES OF LESION OF THE AIR-BLOOD BARRIER

Severe Acute Respiratory Syndrome Coronavirus-2

Sepsis is due to lung lesions (Bachofen and Weibel, 1977). Concerning the kinetics of severe acute respiratory syndrome coronavirus-2 (SARS-CoV-2), a tempting hypothesis is that the entrance of virus into the ABB might resemble that of engineered nanoparticles (NPs) delivered through the airways for therapy. Findings highlight the intimate connections between viruses and NP with host lipid interactions. Both viruses and NPs could exploit dual entry, namely, crossing the plasma membrane or uptake *via* endosomes. Human ACE2-binding interface tends to have a predominantly negative electrostatic potential, allowing interaction with the SARS-CoV-2 S protein (Hassanzadeh et al., 2020). It takes less than 1 h for NPs to move into the lung interstitial space and reach the circulatory system (Dal Magro et al., 2017). Recent data suggest that heparan-sulfate proteoglycan on cell surface facilitates the attachment of SARS-CoV-2 particles to the cell surface to promote cell entry (Zhang et al., 2020). In particular, it was shown that SARS-CoV-2 spike protein interacts with both heparan-sulfate and the binding domain of ACE2 (Clausen et al., 2020). Vascular and thrombotic complications, such as symptomatic acute pulmonary embolism, deep-vein thrombosis, ischaemic stroke, myocardial infarction, and systemic arterial embolism, have been reported in severe COVID-19 cases (Farhangrazi et al., 2020).

Reactive Oxygen Species

Molecular oxygen is activated in either hyperoxia or hypoxia into reactive oxygen species (ROS). Effective antioxidant defenses counteract the reactivity of ROS. However, the overwhelming production of ROS coupled with their insufficient scavenging by endogenous antioxidants will lead to tissue damage and cell death (Kulkarni et al., 2007). ROS are implicated in the increase in alveolar permeability (Waxman and Kolliputi, 2009; Kolliputi et al., 2010). It was found that exposure to 100% O_2 increased alveolar epithelium permeability similar to that caused by the alloxan model of lung edema, and that this occurred before the onset of interstitial or alveolar edema (Matalon and Egan, 1981, 1984).

Hyperoxia also causes damage to endothelial cells (Kistler et al., 1967) and tissue structure (Chow et al., 2003; Kallet and Matthay, 2013) because of increased production of reactive oxygen species (ROS) at mitochondrial level (Freeman and Crapo, 1981).

The risk of ROS-dependent lung injury is reported to occur at $FIO_2 > 0.7$, and may worsen at $FIO_2 > 0.8$ for prolonged exposure. To limit the exposure to high levels of FIO_2, there is a recommendation by ARDS Network to target PaO_2 levels between 55 and 80 mmHg in mechanically ventilated patients. Milder levels of hyperoxemia would be supported by data suggesting that $PaO_2 > 80$ mmHg is associated with worse clinical outcomes at all levels of acute respiratory distress syndrome severity (Aggarwal et al., 2018).

Type-1 epithelial (Epi1) cells could be completely destroyed by hyperoxia (Weibel, 1971), so, after a few days of hyperoxia exposure, the whole alveolar surface would be found to be lined only by cuboidal Epi2 cells (Kapanci et al., 1969; Kaplan et al., 1969), a finding also reported for oxygen poisoning in human lung (Nash et al., 1967). The role of Epi2 cells was interpreted as that of regeneration of new Epi1 cells (Adamson and Bowden, 1974; Bachofen and Weibel, 1974; Evans et al., 1975). Neo-formed Epi1 cells appear able to branch and form at least four or even more lining units on endothelial cells (so called "epithelial plate") (Weibel, 2015). Ischemia-reperfusion injury (a primary graft dysfunction) is a form of high-permeability pulmonary edema due to endothelial lesion (Liang et al., 2019).

Lung Overdistension

Lung overdistension is a major cause of tissue lesion. Going from low to high transpulmonary pressure causes an increase in fluid filtration rate (Bo et al., 1977). Inflating the lungs to total capacity is found to cause free solute movement across the lung epithelium because of larger pore radii. Furthermore, decreasing lung volume does not produce a smaller pore radius that either remains the same or becomes larger. This phenomenon is interpreted as depending on permanent lung lesion (Egan, 1980). Furthermore, data by Egan (1982) suggest that acute lung distension at Palv = 40 may cause epithelial albumin leak but not alveolar flooding: the interpretation of this result is that, upon short exposure to considerable lung distension, no time is given for remarkable matrix fragmentation. A 5-fold increase in Jv over 6 h with step change of Palv from 10 to 20 cmH_2O (Tarbell et al., 1999; Tarbell, 2010). W/D was found to increase from 6.63 to 7.45 over 2 h with Palv up at 48 cmH_2O (Yoshikawa et al., 2004); this same study reported an increase in albumin concentration in bronchoalveolar lavage fluid by up to 250 mg/ml.

Other data report a significant increase in endothelial Kf for alveolar pressure exceeding 42 cmH_2O (Parker et al., 1984). A remarkable increase in Lp was found over 8h due to increased size of pores, and thus increase in filtration surface area, for only 10% increase in strain (lung-on-a-chip microdevice model, Huh et al., 2012). Experimental models of an injurious ventilatory strategy were found to predispose to subsequent bacteremia and associated impaired host defense (Lin et al., 2003).

The Alveolar Folding/Unfolding Zone

The specific topology of EpiI cells is such that they are far from being flat (see **Figure 2**; Weibel, 2015). Furthermore, these cells present numerous pleats on their surface, as deduced by following the profile of the basement membrane, that are subjected to the cyclic folding/unfolding process on changing lung volume (Bachofen et al., 1987). Based on data from electron microscopy, unfolding was found to be completed in healthy lung upon reaching a transpulmonary pressure ~ 15 cmH_2O, corresponding to ~75–80% Vital Capacity (VC), (with a surface tension not exceeding 5-7 dynes/cm, Bachofen et al., 1987). The folding-unfolding process was confirmed also for the human lung by estimating the increase in lung diffusion capacity on increasing lung volumes from FRC up to 100% VC. It was found that the increase in diffusion capacity could be modeled according to the increase of the ratio between the alveolar surface and thickness of the air-blood barrier (Salv/τ) (Miserocchi et al., 2008).

The result was that the increase in diffusion capacity was proportional to the increase of Salv up to a lung volume of ~80% VC, at which the "reserve" surface of the unfolding pleats was completed. Above this volume, the diffusion capacity was proportional to the decrease in τ. It was, therefore, concluded that above ~80% VC, thinning of septa occurred because of direct tissue stretching. Further data confirm that in the healthy lung, increasing volume might occur without much strain of the EpiI cell surface thanks to the "reserve" surface of the pleats, and that direct stretching of the septa occurs with increasing strain above 75–80% VC (Knudsen and Ochs, 2018). **Figure 6** shows the volume-pressure curve of the lung, chest wall, and respiratory system in a healthy subject to show: (i) the FRC (red dot) and (ii) the percent of lung distention (65–80% of VC) and corresponding alveolar pressure (15–25 cmH_2O) upon approaching the saturation of the alveolar unfolding process (shaded area).

In the supine subject, FRC is decreased down to about 22% (Agostoni and Mead, 1964) so, assuming that the saturation of the unfolding process also occurs at about 80% of lung distension, the range of the folding/unfolding process is increased.

One may attempt to comment on the clinical outcome from mechanically ventilated patients with ARDS considering the ventilatory strategy with specific relation to the folding/unfolding zone. One can, therefore, pose the question of how a ventilatory strategy implying a cycling involvement of the folding/unfolding zone might have an impact on lung function. Protti et al. (2013) reported 50% increase of death when oscillating lung volume across 70% lung distension, compared to a strategy

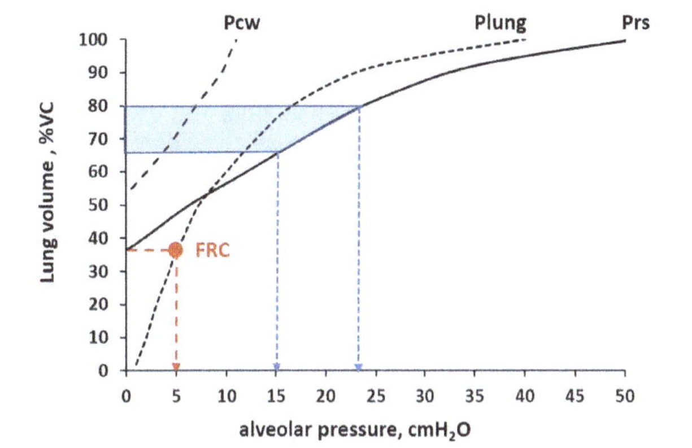

FIGURE 6 | Volume-pressure curve of the lung, chest wall, and total respiratory system (Plung, Pcw, Prs, respectively) to identify the relative lung distention at functional residual capacity (FRC) (Palv = 5 cmH_2O, red arrow) and completion of the alveolar unfolding process occurring in the range Palv 15–25 cmH_2O (blue arrows), corresponding to ~65–80% Vital Capacity (VC, shaded area).

of ventilation set either above or kept below 70% VC. The occurrence of repetitive recruitment and de-recruitment during mechanical ventilation of a diseased lung (bleomycin treatment or surfactant deactivation by Tween 20 detergent) was shown to cause remarkable alveolar instability with atelectasis in some alveoli and overdistention of adjacent ones, referred to as atelectrauma and volutrauma, respectively (Perlman et al., 2011; Rausch et al., 2011; Cressoni et al., 2014; Makiyama et al., 2014; Bates and Smith, 2018; Knudsen and Ochs, 2018; Retamal et al., 2018; Bates et al., 2020; Gaver et al., 2020). Accordingly, it was hypothesized that these maneuvers set a vicious cycle by which the alveolar damage progresses within the lung from atelectatic to adjacent non-atelectatic lung regions through mechanical interdependence. Data from Hamlington et al. (2018) also prove that the sequence of cyclic folding/unfolding leads to a remarkable increase in microvascular permeability due to progressive increase in endothelial lesions (rich-get-richer scheme). It appears, therefore, that a ventilatory strategy implying a cyclic folding/unfolding process favors tissue damage.

The Rest Lung Approach (RLA) (Acute Respiratory Distress Syndrome Network et al., 2000) and Open Lung Approach (OLA) (Writing Group for the Alveolar Recruitment for Acute Respiratory Distress Syndrome Trial (ART) Investigators, 2017) are the two main protective ventilation strategies being used currently. The RLA assumes the two-compartment ARDS model with collapsed, edematous, and unstable tissue in the dependent portion of the lung and small volume of normal tissue in the non-dependent portion of the lung (Gattinoni and Pesenti, 2005). Using a low tidal volume and plateau pressure, the RLA is designed to "Rest" the dependent injured lung tissue by keeping it completely out of the ventilation cycle and "Protect" the small amount of normal lung tissue from overdistension. The OLA assumes that lung protection is better afforded by completely opening the collapsed and edema-filled tissue using higher PEEP with and without recruitment maneuvers. Unfortunately, these protective ventilation strategies have not been effective in further lowering mortality over the last 20 years, suggesting the need for novel protective ventilation strategies to be tested (Caser et al., 2014; Fan et al., 2018).

Airway pressure release ventilation (APRV), set and adjusted using the Time-Controlled Adaptive Ventilation (TCAV^{TM}) method[1], sets ventilator pressure above the folding/unfolding zone and uses a very brief release phase, personalized to changes in lung collapse time constants, that does not give the tissue sufficient time to fold. The TCAV^{TM} method has been reported to be protective as compared to cyclic ventilation crossing the folding/unfolding zone (Roy et al., 2012, 2013a,b; Kollisch-Singule et al., 2014a,b, 2015). A reduced microstrain has been reported for a ventilation implying alveolar pressure above the folding/unfolding zone (PEEP 16–24 cmH_2O) and a short time at low pressure (Kollisch-Singule et al., 2014a) using the TCAV^{TM} method. Data from Yoshida et al. (2009) indicated that APRV with Palv 21 cmH_2O was more efficient than Pressure Support Ventilation (PSV) set at PEEP 10 with Ppeak 23 cmH_2O that implies cycling crossing of the folding/unfolding zone. In a bleomycin injury lung model, tissue damage could be moderated by ventilation at PEEP = 20 cmH_2O, where unfolding is almost completed (Knudsen and Ochs, 2018). Finally, a multilevel analysis of data from 3,562 patients with ARDS revealed that the least risk of death in the hospital correlated with a ventilatory strategy at alveolar pressure high enough to avoid a wide range of cycling crossing of the folding/unfolding zone (Amato et al., 2015). It has also been shown that in preterm infants ($\leq$32 weeks of gestation), alveolar recruitment is more efficient with continuous than with discontinuous CPAP ($\sim$5 cmH_2O), which normalizes the FRC volume (Lam et al., 2020).

The TCAV^{TM} method, which is a novel Stabilizing the Lung Approach (SLA), was developed based on the fact that cyclic recruitment-derecruitment in surfactant-deprived lungs leads to a significant degree of alveolar instability (Nieman et al., 2020b). The goals of the SLA are to very quickly stabilize alveoli and prevent folding/unfolding injury. Once stable, the collapsed tissue can be gradually reopened over an extended period of time (hours or days). Using a very brief release phase, directed by changes in lung collapse time constants, has been shown to very quickly stabilize alveoli. The extended inspiratory time, known as the continuous positive airway pressure (CPAP) phase, gradually opens the collapsed lung tissue over an extended period of time (Roy et al., 2012, 2013a,b; Kollisch-Singule et al., 2014a, 2015). The SLA may facilitate edema re-adsorption and reduce mechanical damage to endothelial and epithelial cells, as compared with the RLA and RLA methods (Nieman et al., 2020a,b). The possible mechanisms for the efficacy the TCAV^{TM}s methods in reducing edema accumulation and expediting edema removal are based on the following: (i) very quickly avoiding the cycling folding/unfolding of alveolar walls using a very brief release phase, (ii) the rapid lung inspiration at the end of the release phase gradually recruits alveoli *via* a "ratchet" mechanism similar to the way the newborn opens their collapsed fluid-filled lungs at birth (Tingay et al., 2021), (iii) stabilizing and then progressively opening alveoli will maintain normal surfactant protein concentration.

Patient-Self-Inflicted Lung Injury

The case of the patient-self-inflicted lung injury (*P-SILI*) deserves a particular consideration. Evidence has been provided for high tidal volumes developed by patients receiving non-invasive respiratory support based on increasing alveolar pressure. Furthermore, a correlation was found between diaphragmatic swings and risk for P-SILI due to lung overdistension (Carteaux et al., 2016; Brochard et al., 2017). The correlation between lung overdistension and lung lesion can be easily accepted (Cruces et al., 2020). However, the understanding of potential "exaggerated" diaphragm contractions has remained elusive. Perturbation in respiratory drive has been invoked by reviewing some possible reflex mechanisms of neural control of breathing (Brochard et al., 2017; Telias et al., 2018). We wish to consider a so far overlooked physiological feature of the diaphragm as a pressure generator. For a given neural drive, diaphragmatic contraction appears to be quite stable and cannot be modified once started, as the diaphragm is almost void of proprioceptors (Corda et al., 1965). From a mechanical standpoint, the question is: what is the outcome of diaphragmatic contraction when the diaphragm is facing a change in mechanical load? If the load is increased (e.g., adding external respiratory elastance), the inspired volume will decrease (Pengelly et al., 1971). In fact, no "load compensating reflex" is present, as no proprioceptor afferent input is present. The opposite case is now that of removing part of the elastance that the diaphragm faces during its contraction. This case occurs by increasing alveolar pressure; in fact, increasing alveolar pressure might remove part or all of lung elastance. The result is an increase in lung volume, since the first breath gives rise to over distension and lung injury (Pengelly et al., 1971). One could estimate that by removing the elastance roughly equivalent to that of the lung, the increase in inspiratory volume would amount to $\sim$150–200% of the control value. Such increase is expected to vary among patients, as lung elastance is related with the number of ventilated units, being higher with increasing alveolar flooding. Neuromuscular blockers obviously contrast this phenomenon (Forel et al., 2006; Papazian et al., 2010). External (inspiratory) intercostal muscles do exhibit proprioceptors innervation: accordingly, they might increase their contraction on adding external elastance ("load compensating reflex") but would be silent on increasing alveolar pressure (thus, the decrease in elastance remains unopposed). One could consider that a patient exposed to increased alveolar pressure has to perform active expiration that is normally passively relying on the elastic recoil of the respiratory system. If the above interpretation is valid, it would not be paradoxical to retain the P-SILI acronym, but the expansion should read Patient-Strategy Induced Lung Injury!

[1] tcavnetwork.org

FACTORS PREVENTING THE DEVELOPMENT OF EDEMA: INTERSTITIAL CAPACITANCE, LYMPHATIC FLOW, AND VASOMOTION

The first line of defense against increased microvascular filtration is fluid accumulation in the thick portion of the air blood barrier. Up to W/D ~5.5, some fluid accumulates in the endothelial cells whose swelling may account for ~45% of their control volume, while ~85% of filtered fluid accumulates in the thick portion of the air-blood barrier (Conforti et al., 2002) where lymphatics are present. This morphological arrangement corresponds to a model of a relatively rigid initial compartment (the thin portion of the ABB) that communicates by a relatively high-resistance pathway to a larger downstream capacity (the thick portion of the ABB) (Unruh et al., 1984).

Human lymphatics extend deep inside the pulmonary lobule; indeed, a peripheral distribution of lymphatics (defined as interstitial lymphatics) was described down to the peri-microvascular district near the alveolar, the alveolar ducts, and the interalveolar septa (Schraufnagel, 1992; Hainis et al., 1994; Schraufnagel et al., 1994; Weber et al., 2018). These lymphatics converge into a central compartment, becoming large conducting vessels associated with the broncho-vascular bundle (Weber et al., 2018).

Under baseline conditions, lymph flow rate is 0.063 ml/min/100 g (Effros and Parker, 2009), and only about 4% of this value corresponds to alveolar fluid clearance. The latter corresponds to the transepithelial active sodium transport. If the "safety factor" is intact, most fluid clearance occurs *via* Starling-depended fluid re-absorption (Miserocchi, 2009) back into the capillaries, with only a minor fraction (~18%) *via* lymphatics (Pearse et al., 1993).

Lymphatics can increase flow, and thus, provide a passive negative-feedback control loop to offset an increase in extravascular volume (Miserocchi, 2009). Interestingly, lymph flow was found to be proportional to the rate of increase in lung weight that is directly related to the microvascular filtration rate (Mitzner and Sylvester, 1986). Interstitial fluid ought to percolate through the interstitium down a pressure gradient generated by lymphatics themselves that were shown to generate a subatmospheric pressure compatible with the measured value of Pint (Miserocchi et al., 1989). Redistribution of fluid downstream from filtration sites was modeled by relating the increase in lymphatic flow in response to increase in filtration rate as a function of interstitial fluid resistance (Roselli et al., 1984). These authors found that, for interstitial compliance in the physiological range (intact matrix), a 3-fold increase in lymphatic flow could balance the increased filtration rate by holding interstitial pressure at about 2 cmH_2O. When interstitial hydration increases, matrix fragmentation would actually decrease tissue resistance for fluid flux toward lymphatics, in line with the model developed by Unruh et al. (1984). In case of experimental lung lesion, lung lymph flow was found to increase by ~8- to 10-fold (Rutili et al., 1982).

A recent microfluidic study revealed considerable differences among lung regions concerning interstitial fluid dynamics from capillary filtration sites, through the porosity of the interstitium, and into the lymphatic network. This conclusion came about by combining specific lymphatic immunohistochemistry with high-resolution X-ray computed tomography and finite-element mathematical modeling that identified differences related to the functional interaction between tissue mechanical properties and the action of the lymphatic pump (Robinson et al., 2019). Lymphatic clearance of alveolar fluid can only occur with an epithelial barrier lesion, as confirmed by data from hyperoxia (Hainis et al., 1994; Schraufnagel et al., 1994) and ventilator-induced lung injury lesion models (Schraufnagel et al., 2003).

Mechanical ventilation and positive end-expiratory pressure (PEEP) impede lung lymph flow by increased intrathoracic pressure and increased central venous pressure. PEEP may, thus, enhance edema formation of the lung (Hedenstierna and Lattuada, 2008). Obviously, when lung W/D increases, the lymphatic flow cannot balance the flow of filtration. This occurs in case of severe endothelial and epithelial lesions. Alveolar flooding occurs when the increase in lung W/D exceeds 35% of baseline (Taylor and Parker, 1985), corresponding to ~6.25.

Figure 7A shows the distribution of extravascular interstitial and alveolar water upon increasing W/D by up to 10, normalized to 1 kg lung (Cressoni et al., 2013) and assuming ~35% increase in interstitial water (Negrini et al., 2001b). **Figure 7B** provides images of the morphological changes of the lung from control (left) to a transition phase implying fluid accumulation in the interstitial space (center) and alveolar flooding (right). On mechanical ground, alveolar flooding implies a progressive loss of alveolar expandable units, and correspondingly, a decrease in lung compliance.

Based on the pressure generating a trans-endothelial flow, a morphological-based model was developed to describe the interaction between control of extravascular lung water and capillary perfusion under edemagenic conditions (Mazzuca et al., 2016). The model focused in particular on the fact that the increase in Pint, besides buffering and even reversing the transcapillary Starling gradient, leads to capillary de-recruitment because of the compressive effect of positive interstitial pressure; the resultant decrease in exchange surface area is a potent factor to decrease Kf. Data on humans confirmed blood flow limitation in edemagenic lung regions, despite the administration of a vasodilator agent (Scherrer et al., 1996).

Precapillary vasoconstriction is a further strong anti-edemagenic mechanism (Negrini et al., 2001a; Mazzuca et al., 2019). In fact, redirection of blood flow from edematous to normal lung regions has been correlated with the increase in Pint in the former as well as with the corresponding precapillary vasoconstriction and vasodilation in the two regions, respectively (Rivolta et al., 2011). Interestingly, inter-individual differences have been documented concerning capillary recruitment/de-recruitment under edemagenic conditions, such as exercise or exposure to hypoxia; in particular, capillary de-recruitment has been interpreted as individual proneness to develop lung edema (Bartesaghi et al., 2014; Beretta et al., 2017a,b). In general, a greater density of pulmonary capillaries favors

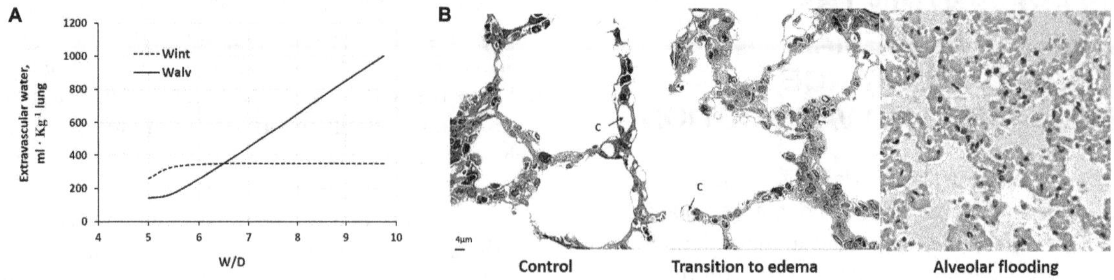

FIGURE 7 | (A) Distribution of extravascular lung water to the interstitial (Wint) and alveolar (Walv) compartment on increasing W/D. **(B)** Morphological changes of the lung from control (left) to a transition phase with fluid accumulation in the interstitial space (center) and alveolar flooding (right). c, pulmonary capillary (redrawn from Miserocchi, 2007).

oxygen diffusion-transport at the alveolar level (Beretta et al., 2017a,b); however, it involves a greater risk factor of developing lung edema because of greater capillary surface for microvascular filtration (Mazzuca et al., 2016). It is tempting to consider pulmonary hypertension, as observed under strong edemagenic conditions (hypoxia), as the consequence of precapillary vasoconstriction represents a powerful means to limit microvascular filtration (Negrini et al., 2001a; Mazzuca et al., 2019).

There is an interesting report concerning the preventive effect of gadolinium in models of lung lesions caused by Palv at ~30 cmH_2O that induces a ~2-fold increase in Kf. The data suggest that gadolinium prevents increased microvascular permeability caused by stretch-activated cation channel-induced increases in intracellular calcium concentration (Parker et al., 1998). Another potentially edema-preventive strategy considers the role of NADPH oxidase type 2 (NOX2) that is a major source of ROS in the lung. Pre-treatment with an inhibitor of NOX2 (Fisher et al., 2021) was hypothesized as preventive of the secondary inflammatory component. A further study suggests that dietary antioxidants could represent a potential treatment for oxidative stress lung injury in patients on mechanical ventilation (Patel et al., 2020).

MODELING THE STARLING GRADIENTS IN THE PROGRESSION TOWARD SEVERE LUNG EDEMA

Table 2 summarizes the database to compare the Starling gradients as edema progresses from point B ("safety factor") to point C. When the "safety factor" is on, trans-endothelial Starling gradients are decreased; in particular some fluid reabsorption may actually occur across the capillary wall at end-expiration. This last point is confirmed by Pearse et al. (1993) who, adopting an experimental model that limited the increase of W/D at ~6, found that ~42% of water filtered into the interstitium was cleared by reabsorption into the pulmonary capillaries. At point B, considering γ is still equal to 1 dynes/cm, negative values of Starling gradients across the epithelium prevent any risk of alveolar flooding.

We ignore the value of surface tension at point C (W/D ~7.5), as well as the corresponding value of $Pliq_{alv}$. Assuming that γ value increased by up to 25 dyne/cm at point C (due to both surfactant dilution and de-activation), $Pliq_{alv}$ would decrease to −17 cmH_2O, so the resultant Starling trans-epithelial pressure gradient would potentially cause alveolar flooding. Modeling the increase in γ between 20 and 40 dynes/cm would only slightly change the result confirming that a W/D in the range 6.5–7 represents the critical threshold for alveolar flooding.

In **Figure 8**, we modeled the (A) trans-endothelial and (B) trans-epithelial Starling gradients on increasing W/D, in relation to the corresponding values of interstitial pressure (Pint), with Palv = 0 cmH_2O.

With the "safety factor" on (point B), both trans-endothelial and trans-epithelial Starling gradients promote fluid reabsorption, in line with data from Egan et al. (1976, 1977). The critical factor leading to alveolar flooding is the development of a remarkably increasing negativity of $Pliq_{alv}$ as a consequence of the progressive increase in surface tension (γ) due to surfactant de-activation. We assumed an increase in γ from 1 to 25 dynes/cm for W/D > 6.5 (see **Table 2**).

Changes in Starling gradients and permeability parameters may be combined differently within the whole lung. In fact, the available experimental evidence confirms the heterogeneity in both regional lung fluid accumulation and perfusion under edemagenic conditions (Bachofen et al., 1993). Basal lung regions are, in general, more exposed to edema because of greater blood perfusion, implying higher capillary Kf (Rivolta et al., 2011). Alveolar flooding was found to occur in a quite non-homogeneous fashion revealing considerable regional differences (Wu et al., 1995).

Figure 9 reports the estimated Starling pressure gradients at the (A) endothelial and (B) epithelial levels with increasing alveolar pressure of up to 25 cmH_2O, as a function of W/D. We modeled the Starling pressure gradients on increasing W/D by increasing surface tension values from 1 to 40 dynes/cm. For W/D in the physiological range (5–6.5), the increase in Palv shifts the trans-endothelial gradients toward filtration, and on the opposite, the trans-epithelial toward alveolar re-absorption. Both effects tend to wane as W/D increases. Thus, in the W/D range of 5–6.5, the increase in Palv causes capillary filtration and alveolar clearance; accordingly, lymphatics have to cope

TABLE 2 | Trans-endothelial and trans-epithelial Starling pressure gradients at end-expiration, with "safety factor" (point B in **Figure 4**) and after some degree of matrix fragmentation (point C in **Figure 4**).

	Trans-endothelial			Trans-epithelial	
	Point B (W/D = 5.5)	Point C (W/D~7.5)		Point B (W/D = 5.5)	Point C (W/D~7.5)
Pcap*	9	9	Pint**	5.7	0
Pint**	5.7	0	Pliq alv#	~0	−17
σ end##	0.85	0.5	σ epi##	0.85	0.5
Πcap**	26.8	14.7	Πint**	13.8	9.3
Πint**	13.8	9.3	Πliq alv	0	5
			γ	1	25
ΔP	**4**	**9**	**ΔP**	**5.7**	**17**
σΔΠ	**−11.0**	**0.0**	**σΔΠ**	**−11.7**	**−2.15**
Starling gradient	**−7.0**	**6.3**	**Starling gradient**	**−6.0**	**14.85**

This table reports the expected values for capillary, interstitial, and alveolar liquid hydraulic pressures (Pcap, Pint, and Pliq alv, respectively) as well as for capillary, interstitial, and alveolar liquid oncotic pressures (Πcap, Πint, and Πliq alv, respectively). Endothelial (σ endo) and epithelial (σ epi) protein reflection coefficients are also reported. In bold, hydraulic (ΔP) and oncotic (σΠP) pressure gradients and total Starling pressure gradient. Positive values of the Starling gradient at endothelial level indicate filtration into interstitium; negative values at epithelial level indicate alveolar reabsorption. From B to C (the phase corresponding to progressive fragmentation of the matrix), Pint returned to zero, suggesting loss of the physiological alveolar mechanical tethering interaction (Mead et al., 1970). Accordingly, from point C on, we considered Pint = Palv, as suggested by Glucksberg and Bhattacharya (1991).

*Pressure values are expressed in cmH_2O; σ is a pure number. *From Hakim et al., 1993; **from Miserocchi et al., 1993; #calculated from Beck and Lai-Fook, 1983; ##from Parker et al., 2006. Surface tension (γ), dyne/cm.*

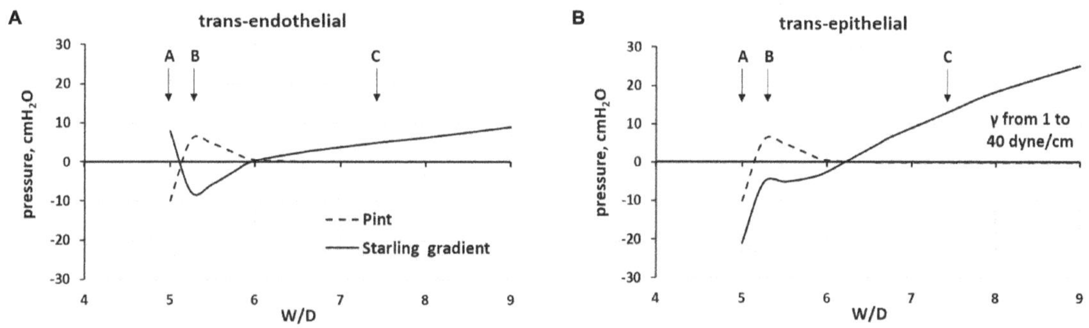

FIGURE 8 | Modeling of **(A)** trans-endothelial and **(B)** trans-epithelial Starling pressure gradients (solid line) on increasing W/D, based on experimentally measured values of interstitial pressure (Pint, dashed line), with Palv = 0 cmH_2O. Points A, B, and C as from **Figure 4**.

with both flows. For W/D > 6.5, both trans-endothelial and trans-epithelial gradients favor filtration, leading to alveolar flooding. Note that for W/D > 6.5, the Starling pressure gradients, referring to different Palv, overlap, reflecting the fact that when the proteoglycan matrix is disrupted, the increase in Palv impacts equally on the increase in capillary pressure, interstitial pressure (Glucksberg and Bhattacharya, 1991), and $Pliq_{alv}$ (Beck and Lai-Fook, 1983).

The graphs in **Figure 9** may be considered either as representing the Starling pressure-dependent course of developing edema, and as representing the regional differences in water balance within the lung. Indeed, novel CT imaging methods (Cereda et al., 2016, 2017) showed that aerated and non-aerated lung regions were diffusely intermingled. The erratic distribution of edema can be justified by the heterogeneous susceptibility to edema formation at alveolar level that was attributed to local differences in microvascular permeability possibly dependent upon alveolar morphology, as suggested by a novel lung imaging technique under experimental edemagenic conditions (Mazzuca et al., 2019). Heterogeneity in alveolar mechanics and fluid dynamics is confirmed by data from Smith et al. (2020) who generated VILI in mice ventilated with 50 cycles/min from FRC up to a plateau pressure of 37.5 cmH_2O. Studying the alveolar de-recruitability on decreasing Palv, three alveolar phenotypes were described as a consequence of VILI: (1) flooded alveoli that cannot be recruited at any pressure, (2) unstable alveoli that are open at high pressures but readily collapse as pressure is reduced, and (3) relatively normal alveoli that remain open at low pressures.

An important relationship exists during cyclic mechanical ventilation between peak airway pressure (Ppeak) and positive end-expiratory pressure (PEEP). The data in **Figure 9** suggest that the trans-endothelial filtration gradient increases with increasing Ppeak and PEEP. Conversely, no risk of alveolar flooding occurs for W/D < ~6.5, as trans-epithelial gradients are in favor of fluid absorption. This may be partially balanced by a decrease in filtration surface as a consequence of a decrease in overall capillary blood volume (Miserocchi et al., 2008). Blood flow is also temporarily reduced, being proportional to the decrease in the difference between pulmonary artery and alveolar pressure.

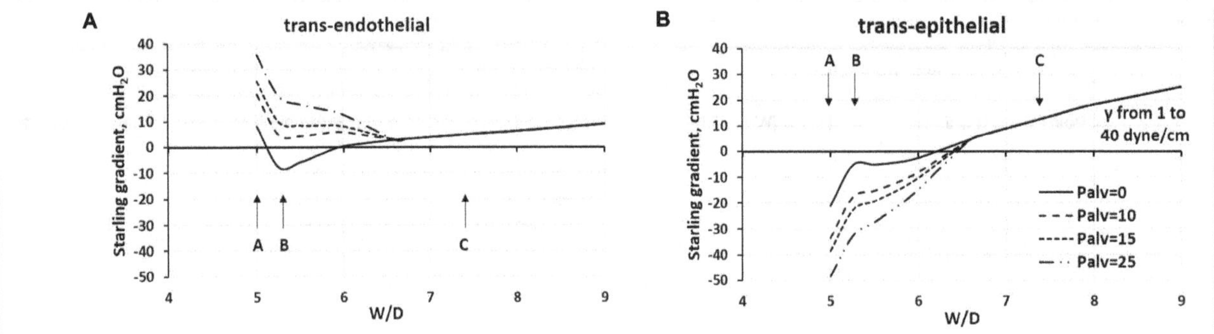

FIGURE 9 | Estimated Starling pressure gradients at **(A)** endothelial and **(B)** epithelial levels on increasing alveolar pressure by up to 25 cmH_2O, and on varying W/D from 5 to 9. Points A, B, and C refer to those in **Figure 4**.

Lymphatic drainage can increase in this situation to maintain lung fluid balance. However, the time evolution of this situation should be regarded in terms of increase in W/D ratio as related to the progression of the fragmentation of the interstitial matrix (**Figure 5**).

The TCAV^{TM} method, if applied pre-emptively before the development of severe lung injury, has been shown to prevent collapse of the acutely injury lung, maintaining a fully open lung, and if applied following the development of severe lung injury, will rapidly stabilize alveoli even with fast collapse time constants. If the ventilation strategy can put a "cast" within the acutely injured lung, much like putting a cast on a broken arm, the mechanisms of VILI-induced edema generation would be eliminated (Nieman et al., 2018).

One shall note that edema clearance in experimental models of ARDS can only occur in lung regions where W/D ratio does not exceed 6.5–7, as only in these regions the Starling gradients allow fluid reabsorption (see **Figure 9**). The presence of these regions can justify the observed average decrease in W/D ratio for the whole lung from about from ~9 to ~7; the latter value still corresponds to severe edema (Habashi, 2005; Matsuzawa et al., 2010; Roy et al., 2013a,b; Kollisch-Singule et al., 2014a,b, 2015).

TIME CONSTANT OF DEVELOPING SEVERE ALVEOLAR EDEMA

The development of lung edema depends upon various combination of an increase in Lp and in A as well as a decrease in σ, involving both the endothelium and the epithelium. Increase in capillary pressure and lung overdistension were shown to cause damage to the endothelial and epithelial barriers (Wu et al., 1995). The critical phase of edema pivots around a W/D of ~ 6–6.25. We hypothesize that for W/D to exceed 6, capillary filtration should occur down this still low-pressure gradient *via* increase in Lp and decrease in σ acting over a progressively larger portion of the alveolar compartment surface area, which may cause matrix fragmentation. Consider that the Lp of the "true" alveolar compartment is physiologically 20 times lower than that of the extra-alveolar compartment (Parker et al., 2006) while the capillary surface area is in the order of 70 m^2 on a morphological basis. We suggest that a W/D ~ 6.5 is the likely threshold, above which fluid will seep from capillary to alveoli down a small driving pressure gradient acting over a large surface of damaged air-blood barrier.

An exponential increase in lung weight (above a W/D of ~ 6) has been modeled with a relatively short time constant (~4 min) by moderate increase in either Lp or decrease in σ (Mazzuca et al., 2016). Similar time constants were found for the exponential increase in lung weight in response to a step increase in venous pressure (Parker and Townsley, 2004). The above hypothesis is strengthened by the finding that a >3-fold increase in microvascular filtration already causes an increase in trans-capillary convective transport of proteins compared to either diffusive or vesicular transport, suggesting lowering of the σ value (Egan et al., 1977). Other data predict that a 50% increase in lung water may occur within 45 min after a step increase in left atrial pressure (2–14 cmH_2O) and pulmonary artery pressure (13–22 cmH_2O) (Rutili et al., 1982).

THE WAY TO RECOVERY

A good model to explain the clearance of alveolar edema is the one proposed in full-term newborns (Miserocchi et al., 1994). Alveolar fluid clearance occurs down a two-step coupled mechanism: (1) epithelial water absorption *via* Na^+-dependent transport and (2) Starling-dependent capillary re-absorption. Note that fluid reabsorption into lung capillaries is a self-limited mechanism due to increase in the colloid osmotic pressure at the interstitial end of the glycocalyx generated by protein accumulation preventing further absorption (Curry, 2005; Levick and Michel, 2010; Mazzuca et al., 2019). A recent report (Tingay et al., 2021) shows that the transition from fluid-filled to aerated lungs in full-term newborns is accomplished using ventilation patterns characterized by a rapid high-peak inspiratory flow to "ratchet" open collapsed and flooded airway. The collapse of these newly recruited airways during expiration was minimized by partially closing the glottis to keep the lung pressurized. Thus, the inspiratory phase allows for rapid lung aeration extending from the central to distal lung portions; the expiratory phase maintains alveolar pressure allowing for fluid clearance.

Maintaining a pressurized lung during expiration in a lung with low permeability of the epithelium and low compliance of the interstitial matrix results in an increase in interstitial pressure (as at point B) generating a trans-endothelial absorption *via* the Starling gradient. These two features are incompletely developed in preterm lung, and therefore, hinder alveolar fluid reabsorption (Miserocchi et al., 1995). An intact epithelial barrier allows Na^+-dependent alveolar fluid reabsorption. Matthay and Wiener-Kronish (1990) provided the first evidence in humans to support the hypothesis that active ion transport across the alveolar epithelial barrier is the primary mechanism for the clearance of edema fluid. Na^+ transport across the distal airway epithelium is the main determinant of alveolar fluid clearance, as demonstrated in several different species, such as the human lung (Berthiaume and Matthay, 2007). With an intact epithelium, the clearance of alveolar fluid is rapid in patients with severe hydrostatic edema (Verghese et al., 1999). In contrast, in the majority of patients with acute lung injury, alveolar fluid clearance is impaired by reduced Na^+ absorption (Ware and Matthay, 2001).

Controversies regarding the optimal mechanical ventilation strategy in patients with severe edema centers around the maintenance of alveolar pressure that favors fluid clearance and avoids the complication of volutrauma and atelectrauma. To favor alveolar fluid re-absorption in experimental edema models, the ventilatory strategy should allow to decrease W/D below 6.5, a cut-off suggesting restoration of control of lung fluid balance (**Figures 8, 9**).

The re-deposition of an interstitial macromolecular matrix assuring low microvascular permeability and low interstitial tissue compliance appears critical for the control of lung fluid balance, since this would re-establish a "safety factor." Most endothelial but not epithelial cells appear to be involved in the mechano-transduction signaling process in response to edemagenic conditions (Botto et al., 2006) that influence a specific cascade of cellular events aiming at remodeling of matrix macromolecules (Palestini et al., 2002, 2011; Daffara et al., 2004). There are indications that post-infection activation of fibroblast does not allow the re-establishment of a matrix composition similar to the native composition (Li et al., 2016). In particular, the activation of fibroblast impacts hyaluronan synthase that controls the deposition of bundles of hyaluronan that actually represents the fibrotic response to recovery. In the presence of hyaluronan fragments during the early phase of lung injury, the balance between hyaluronan synthase isoforms and hyaluronidases plays an important role in the pathogenesis of lung fibrosis (Li et al., 2000). Recent data suggest that hyaluronan synthesis occurs in a matter of days (Bell et al., 2019).

CONCLUSION

Although the sequence of events leading to severe lung edema have been delineated, at this point, there remains a wide gap in our knowledge of how to prevent the loss of lung fluid balance when W/D $>$ 6 and the critical role of properly set mechanical ventilation. The data from this analysis support the contention that in diseased portions of the lungs (W/D $> >$6.5) the mechanisms necessary to clear edema fluid have been lost. Since the distribution of edema is heterogeneous by nature, in the lung portions where W/D $<$ 6.5, the control of lung fluid balance is only possible when the built-in safety factors, intact matrix, interstitial capacity, and lymphatics not yet saturated, are still functional. Once both barriers (endothelium and epithelium) are breeched, and built-in safety components (capacity reservoirs and lymph flow) are saturated, massive flooding occurs. These considerations may help to "debug" the controversies concerning the outcome of various experimental models of lung lesion or clinical outcome in patients. Comparing data from different ventilatory strategies appears difficult, as these are highly influenced by the number of alveolar units allowing fluid clearance that cannot be directly measured. Reported values for W/D of the whole lung to validate ventilatory strategies aimed at facilitating edema re-adsorption, reducing mechanical damage, and preventing further increase in permeability never fell below 6.8 (see Paragraph 8). So far, neither CT scan nor ultrasound has been correlated to the corresponding regional values of W/D ratios. It would be useful to identify a non-invasive tool to detect the earliest stages of perturbation in lung fluid balance before the condition becomes life-threatening. Ventilatory support strategies, during either spontaneous breathing or mechanical ventilation, should carefully balance factors that can harm functioning alveolar units. Aiming at high oxygen saturation at the expense of alveolar hyperoxia should also be considered (see Paragraph 6.2). The clinical problem appears to be that of avoiding damage to the alveolar units that still retain gas diffusion-transport function. This certainly represents a critical question considering the severe complication of alveolar instability generated by cyclic recruitment-derecruitment in edematous lung regions (Bates and Smith, 2018; Bates et al., 2020; Gaver et al., 2020). The impact of positive airway pressure is complex for many reasons, considering in particular that an opposite flow may occur, depending on alveolar pressure, across the endothelium and the epithelium. A ventilation strategy that would keep the acutely injured lung open and stable would theoretically be optimal at minimizing pulmonary edema accumulation. The critical issue remains to be minimizing tissue damage caused by lung overdistension, and at the same time, avoiding tissue injury by cyclic folding/unfolding.

AUTHOR CONTRIBUTIONS

EB, JG, GN, and GM joined their competences to complete the study. GM and EB conceived the work. FR and GS contributed to the computational part. All authors contributed to the article and approved the submitted version.

REFERENCES

Acute Respiratory Distress Syndrome Network, Brower, R. G., Matthay, M. A., Morris, A., Schoenfeld, D., Thompson, B. T., et al. (2000). Ventilation with lower tidal volumes as compared with traditional tidal volumes for acute lung injury and the acute respiratory distress syndrome. *N. Engl. J. Med.* 342, 1301–1308. doi: 10.1056/NEJM200005043421801

Adamson, I. Y., and Bowden, D. H. (1974). The type 2 cell as progenitor of alveolar epithelial regeneration. A cytodynamic study in mice after exposure to oxygen. *Lab. Invest.* 30, 35–42.

Aggarwal, N. R., Brower, R. G., Hager, D. N., Thompson, B. T., Netzer, G., Shanholtz, C., et al. (2018). Oxygen exposure resulting in arterial oxygen tensions above the protocol goal was associated with worse clinical outcomes in acute respiratory distress syndrome. *Crit. Care Med.* 46, 517–524. doi: 10. 1097/CCM.0000000000002886

Agostoni, E., and Mead, J. (1964). "Statics of the respiratory system," in *Handbook of Physiology Respiration*, eds W. O. Fenn and H. Rahn (Washington DC: American Physiological Society), 387–409.

Amato, M. B., Meade, M. O., Slutsky, A. S., Brochard, L., Costa, E. L., Schoenfeld, D. A., et al. (2015). Driving pressure and survival in the acute respiratory distress syndrome. *N. Engl. J. Med.* 372, 747–755. doi: 10.1056/NEJMsa1410639

Bachofen, H., Hildebrandt, J., and Bachofen, M. (1970). Pressure-volume curves of air- and liquid-filled excised lungs-surface tension *in situ*. *J. Appl. Physiol.* 29, 422–431. doi: 10.1152/jappl.1970.29.4.422

Bachofen, H., Schürch, S., Michel, R. P., and Weibel, E. R. (1993). Experimental hydrostatic pulmonary edema in rabbit lungs. Barrier lesions. *Am. Rev. Respir. Dis.* 147, 989–996. doi: 10.1164/ajrccm/147.4.989

Bachofen, H., Schürch, S., Urbinelli, M., and Weibel, E. R. (1987). Relations among alveolar surface tension, surface area, volume, and recoil pressure. *J. Appl. Physiol.* 62, 1878–1887. doi: 10.1152/jappl.1987.62.5.1878

Bachofen, M., and Weibel, E. R. (1974). Basic pattern of tissue repair in human lungs following unspecific injury. *Chest* 65, 14S–19S.

Bachofen, M., and Weibel, E. R. (1977). Alterations of the gas exchange apparatus in adult respiratory insufficiency associated with septicemia. *Am. Rev. Respir. Dis.* 116, 589–615. doi: 10.1164/arrd.1977.116.4.589

Bartesaghi, M., Beretta, E., Pollastri, L., Scotti, V., Mandolesi, G., Lanfranconi, F., et al. (2014). Inter-individual differences in control of alveolar capillary blood volume in exercise and hypoxia. *Respir. Physiol. Neurobiol.* 190, 96–104. doi: 10.1016/j.resp.2013.08.021

Bates, J., Gaver, D. P., Habashi, N. M., and Nieman, G. F. (2020). Atelectrauma Versus volutrauma: a tale of two time-constants. *Crit. Care Explor.* 2:e0299. doi: 10.1097/CCE.0000000000000299

Bates, J., and Smith, B. J. (2018). Ventilator-induced lung injury and lung mechanics. *Ann Transl Med.* 6, 378. doi: 10.21037/atm.2018.06.29

Beck, K. C., and Lai-Fook, S. J. (1983). Alveolar liquid pressure in excised edematous dog lung with increased static recoil. *J. Appl. Physiol. Respir. Environ. Exerc. Physiol.* 55, 1277–1283. doi: 10.1152/jappl.1983.55.4.1277

Bell, T. J., Brand, O. J., Morgan, D. J., Salek-Ardakani, S., Jagger, C., Fujimori, T., et al. (2019). Defective lung function following influenza virus is due to prolonged, reversible hyaluronan synthesis. *Matrix Biol.* 80, 14–28. doi: 10. 1016/j.matbio.2018.06.006

Beretta, E., Lanfranconi, F., Grasso, G. S., Bartesaghi, M., Alemayehu, H. K., Pratali, L., et al. (2017a). Air blood barrier phenotype correlates with alveolo-capillary O2 equilibration in hypobaric hypoxia. *Respir. Physiol. Neurobiol.* 246, 53–58. doi: 10.1016/j.resp.2017.08.006

Beretta, E., Lanfranconi, F., Grasso, G. S., Bartesaghi, M., Alemayehu, H. K., and Miserocchi, G. (2017b). Reappraisal of DLCO adjustment to interpret the adaptive response of the air-blood barrier to hypoxia. *Respir. Physiol. Neurobiol.* 238, 59–65. doi: 10.1016/j.resp.2016.08.009

Berthiaume, Y., and Matthay, M. A. (2007). Alveolar edema fluid clearance and acute lung injury. *Respir. Physiol. Neurobiol.* 159, 350–359. doi: 10.1016/j.resp. 2007.05.010

Bo, G., Hauge, A., and Nicolaysen, G. (1977). Alveolar pressure and lung volume as determinants of net transvascular fluid filtration. *J. Appl. Physiol. Respir. Environ. Exerc. Physiol.* 42, 476–482. doi: 10.1152/jappl.1977.42.4.476

Botto, L., Beretta, E., Daffara, R., Miserocchi, G., and Palestini, P. (2006). Biochemical and morphological changes in endothelial cells in response to hypoxic interstitial edema. *Respir. Res.* 7:7. doi: 10.1186/1465-9921-7-7

Brochard, L., Slutsky, A., and Pesenti, A. (2017). Mechanical ventilation to minimize progression of lung injury in acute respiratory failure. *Am. J. Respir. Crit. Care Med.* 195, 438–442. doi: 10.1164/rccm.201605-1081CP

Carteaux, G., Millán-Guilarte, T., De Prost, N., et al. (2016). Failure of noninvasive ventilation for *de novo* acute hypoxemic respiratory failure: role of tidal volume. *Crit. Care Med.* 44, 282–290. doi: 10.1097/CCM.000000000000 1379

Caser, E. B., Zandonade, E., Pereira, E., Gama, A. M., and Barbas, C. S. (2014). Impact of distinct definitions of acute lung injury on its incidence and outcomes in Brazilian ICUs: prospective evaluation of 7,133 patients*. *Crit. Care Med.* 42, 574–582. doi: 10.1097/01.ccm.0000435676.68435.56

Cereda, M., Xin, Y., Hamedani, H., Bellani, G., Kadlecek, S., Clapp, J., et al. (2017). Tidal changes on CT and progression of ARDS. *Thorax* 72, 981–989. doi: 10.1136/thoraxjnl-2016-209833

Cereda, M., Xin, Y., Meeder, N., Zeng, J., Jiang, Y., Hamedani, H., et al. (2016). Visualizing the propagation of acute lung injury. *Anesthesiology* 124, 121–131. doi: 10.1097/ALN.0000000000000916

Chow, C. W., Herrera Abreu, M. T., Suzuki, T., and Downey, G. P. (2003). Oxidative stress and acute lung injury. *Am. J. Respir. Cell Mol. Biol.* 29, 427–431.

Clausen, T. M., Sandoval, D. R., Spliid, C. B., Pihl, J., Perrett, H. R., Painter, C. D., et al. (2020). SARS-CoV-2 infection depends on cellular Heparan Sulfate and ACE2. *Cell* 183, 1043–1057.e15. doi: 10.1016/j.cell.2020.09.033

Conforti, E., Fenoglio, C., Bernocchi, G., Bruschi, O., and Miserocchi, G. A. (2002). Morpho-functional analysis of lung tissue in mild interstitial edema. *Am. J. Physiol. Lung Cell. Mol. Physiol.* 282, L766–L774. doi: 10.1152/ajplung.00313. 2001

Corda, M., Voneuler, C., and Lennerstrand, G. (1965). Proprioceptive innervation of the diaphragm. *J. Physiol.* 178, 161–177. doi: 10.1113/jphysiol.1965.sp007621

Cressoni, M., Cadringher, P., Chiurazzi, C., Amini, M., Gallazzi, E., Marino, A., et al. (2014). Lung inhomogeneity in patients with acute respiratory distress syndrome. *Am. J. Respir. Crit. Care Med.* 189, 149–158. doi: 10.1164/rccm. 201308-1567OC

Cressoni, M., Gallazzi, E., Chiurazzi, C., Marino, A., Brioni, M., Menga, F., et al. (2013). Limits of normality of quantitative thoracic CT analysis. *Crit. Care* 17:R93. doi: 10.1186/cc12738

Cruces, P., Retamal, J., Hurtado, D. E., Erranz, B., Iturrieta, P., González, C., et al. (2020). A physiological approach to understand the role of respiratory effort in the progression of lung injury in SARS-CoV-2 infection. *Crit. Care* 24:494. doi: 10.1186/s13054-020-03197-7

Curry, F. R. (2005). Microvascular solute and water transport. *Microcirculation* 12, 17–31. doi: 10.1080/10739680590894993

Daffara, R., Botto, L., Beretta, E., Conforti, E., Faini, A., Palestini, P., et al. (2004). Endothelial cells as early sensors of pulmonary interstitial edema. *J. Appl. Physiol.* 97, 1575–1583. doi: 10.1152/japplphysiol.00236.200

Dal Magro, R., Ornaghi, F., Cambianica, I., Beretta, S., Re, F., Musicanti, C., et al. (2017). ApoE-modified solid lipid nanoparticles: a feasible strategy to cross the blood-brain barrier. *J. Control. Release* 10, 103–110. doi: 10.1016/j.jconrel.2017. 01.039

Dellacà, R. L., Zannin, E., Sancini, G., Rivolta, I., Leone, B. E., Pedotti, A., et al. (2008). Changes in the mechanical properties of the respiratory system during the development of interstitial lung edema. *Respir. Res.* 9:51. doi: 10.1186/1465-9921-9-51

Effros, R. M., and Parker, J. C. (2009). Pulmonary vascular heterogeneity and the Starling hypothesis. *Microvasc. Res.* 78, 71–77. doi: 10.1016/j.mvr.2009. 03.004

Egan, E. A. (1980). Response of alveolar epithelial solute permeability to changes in lung inflation. *J. Appl. Physiol. Respir. Environ. Exerc. Physiol.* 49, 1032–1036. doi: 10.1152/jappl.1980.49.6.1032

Egan E. A. (1982). Lung inflation, lung solute permeability, and alveolar edema. *J. Appl. Physiol. Respir. Environ. Exerc. Physiol.* 53, 121–125. doi: 10.1152/jappl. 1982.53.1.121

Egan, E. A., Nelson, R. M., and Gessner, I. H. (1977). Solute permeability of the alveolar epithelium in acute hemodynamic pulmonary edema in dogs. *Am. J. Physiol.* 233, H80–H86. doi: 10.1152/ajpheart.1977.233. 1.H80

Egan, E. A., Nelson, R. M., and Olver, R. E. (1976). Lung inflation and alveolar permeability to non-electrolytes in the adult sheep *in vivo*. *J. Physiol.* 260, 409–424. doi: 10.1113/jphysiol.1976.sp011522

Evans, M. J., Cabral, L. J., Stephens, R. J., and Freeman, G. (1975). Transformation of alveolar type 2 cells to type 1 cells following exposure to NO2. *Exp. Mol. Pathol.* 22, 142–150. doi: 10.1016/0014-4800(75)90059-3

Fan, E., Brodie, D., and Slutsky, A. S. (2018). Acute respiratory distress syndrome: advances in diagnosis and treatment. *JAMA* 319, 698–710. doi: 10.1001/jama.2017.21907

Farhangrazi, Z. S., Sancini, G., Hunter, A. C., and Moghimi, S. M. (2020). Airborne Particulate Matter and SARS-CoV-2 partnership: virus hitchhiking, stabilization and immune cell targeting - a hypothesis. *Front. Immunol.* 11:579352. doi: 10.3389/fimmu.2020.579352

Fisher, A. B., Dodia, C., and Chatterjee, S. (2021). A peptide inhibitor of peroxiredoxin 6 phospholipase A_2 activity significantly protects against lung injury in a mouse model of ventilator induced lung injury (VILI). *Antioxidants* 10:925. doi: 10.3390/antiox10060925

Forel, J., Roch, A., Marin, V., Michelet, P., Demory, D., Blache, J., et al. (2006). Neuromuscular blocking agents decrease inflammatory response in patients presenting with acute respiratory distress syndrome. *Crit. Care Med.* 34:10.

Freeman, B. A., and Crapo, J. D. (1981). Hyperoxia increases oxygen radical production in rat lungs and lung mitochondria. *J. Biol. Chem.* 256, 10986–10992.

Gattinoni, L., and Pesenti, A. (2005). The concept of "baby lung". *Intensive Care Med.* 31, 776–784. doi: 10.1007/s00134-005-2627-z

Gaver, D. P. III, Nieman, G. F., Gatto, L. A., Cereda, M., Habashi, N. M., and Bates, J. (2020). The POOR Get POORer: a hypothesis for the pathogenesis of ventilator-induced lung injury. *Am. J. Respir. Crit. Care Med.* 202, 1081–1087. doi: 10.1164/rccm.202002-0453CP

Glucksberg, M. R., and Bhattacharya, J. (1991). Effect of alveolar and pleural pressures on interstitial pressures in isolated dog lungs. *J. Appl. Physiol.* 70, 914–918. doi: 10.1152/jappl.1991.70.2.914

Gorin, A. B., and Stewart, P. A. (1979). Differential permeability of endothelial and epithelial barriers to albumin flux. *J. Appl. Physiol. Respir. Environ. Exerc. Physiol.* 47, 1315–1324. doi: 10.1152/jappl.1979.47.6.1315

Habashi, N. M. (2005). Other approaches to open-lung ventilation: airway pressure release ventilation. *Crit. Care Med.* 33, S228–S240. doi: 10.1097/01.ccm.0000155920.11893.37

Hainis, K. D., Sznajder, J. I., and Schraufnagel, D. E. (1994). Lung lymphatics cast from the airspace. *Am. J. Physiol.* 267(2 Pt 1), L199–L205. doi: 10.1152/ajplung.1994.267.2.L199

Hakim, T. S., Gilbert, E., and Camporesi, E. (1993). Positive end-expiratory pressure increases capillary pressure relative to wedge pressure in the closed and open chest. *J. Crit. Care* 8, 80–86. doi: 10.1016/0883-9441(93)90011-9

Hamlington, K. L., Bates, J., Roy, G. S., Julianelle, A. J., Charlebois, C., Suki, B., et al. (2018). Alveolar leak develops by a rich-get-richer process in ventilator-induced lung injury. *PLoS One* 13:e0193934. doi: 10.1371/journal.pone.0193934

Hassanzadeh, K., Perez Pena, H., Dragotto, J., Buccarello, L., Iorio, F., Pieraccini, S., et al. (2020). Considerations around the SARS-CoV-2 spike protein with particular attention to COVID-19 brain infection and neurological symptoms. *ACS Chem. Neurosci.* 11, 2361–2369. doi: 10.1021/acschemneuro.0c00373

Hedenstierna, G., and Lattuada, M. (2008). Lymphatics and lymph in acute lung injury. *Curr. Opin. Crit. Care* 14, 31–36. doi: 10.1097/MCC.0b013e3282f2f4b5

Hellman, U., Karlsson, M. G., Engström-Laurent, A., Cajander, S., Dorofte, L., Ahlm, C., et al. (2020). Presence of hyaluronan in lung alveoli in severe Covid-19: An opening for new treatment options? *J. Biol. Chem.* 295, 15418–15422. doi: 10.1074/jbc.AC120.015967

Higuita-Castro, N., Nelson, M. T., Shukla, V., Agudelo-Garcia, P. A., Zhang, W., Duarte-Sanmiguel, S. M., et al. (2017). Using a novel microfabricated model of the alveolar-capillary barrier to investigate the effect of matrix structure on Atelectrauma. *Sci. Rep.* 7:11623.

Hou, H., Wang, T., Zhang, B., Luo, Y., Mao, L., Wang, F., et al. (2020). Detection of IgM and IgG antibodies in patients with coronavirus disease 2019. *Clin. Transl. Immunol.* 9:e01136. doi: 10.1002/cti2.1136

Huh, D., Leslie, D. C., Matthews, B. D., Fraser, J. P., Jurek, S., Hamilton, G. A., et al. (2012). A human disease model of drug toxicity-induced pulmonary edema in a lung-on-a-chip microdevice. *Sci. Transl. Med.* 4:159ra147. doi: 10.1126/scitranslmed.3004249

Kallet, R. H., and Matthay, M. A. (2013). Hyperoxic acute lung injury. *Respir. Care* 58, 123–141. doi: 10.4187/respcare.01963

Kapanci, Y., Weibel, E. R., Kaplan, H. P., and Robinson, F. R. (1969). Pathogenesis and reversibility of the pulmonary lesions of oxygen toxicity in monkeys. II. Ultrastructural and morphometric studies. *Lab. Invest.* 20, 101–118.

Kaplan, H. P., Robinson, F. R., Kapanci, Y., and Weibel, E. R. (1969). Pathogenesis and reversibility of the pulmonary lesions of oxygen toxicity in monkeys. I. Clinical and light microscopic studies. *Lab. Invest.* 20, 94–100.

Kistler, G. S., Caldwell, P. R., and Weibel, E. R. (1967). Development of fine structural damage to alveolar and capillary lining cells in oxygen-poisoned rat lungs. *J. Cell Biol.* 32, 605–628. doi: 10.1083/jcb.32.3.605

Knudsen, L., and Ochs, M. (2018). The micromechanics of lung alveoli: structure and function of surfactant and tissue components. *Histochem. Cell Biol.* 150, 661–676. doi: 10.1007/s00418-018-1747-9

Kolliputi, N., Shaik, R. S., and Waxman, A. B. (2010). The inflammasome mediates hyperoxia-induced alveolar cell permeability. *J. Immunol.* 184, 5819–5826. doi: 10.4049/jimmunol.0902766

Kollisch-Singule, M., Emr, B., Jain, S. V., Andrews, P., Satalin, J., Liu, J., et al. (2015). The effects of airway pressure release ventilation on respiratory mechanics in extrapulmonary lung injury. *Intensive Care Med. Exp.* 3:35. doi: 10.1186/s40635-015-0071-0

Kollisch-Singule, M., Emr, B., Smith, B., Roy, S., Jain, S., Satalin, J., et al. (2014a). Mechanical breath profile of airway pressure release ventilation: the effect on alveolar recruitment and microstrain in acute lung injury. *JAMA Surg.* 149, 1138–1145. doi: 10.1001/jamasurg.2014.1829

Kollisch-Singule, M., Emr, B., Smith, B., Ruiz, C., Roy, S., Meng, Q., et al. (2014b). Airway pressure release ventilation reduces conducting airway micro-strain in lung injury. *J. Am. Coll. Surg.* 219, 968–976. doi: 10.1016/j.jamcollsurg.2014.09.011

Kulkarni, A. C., Kuppusamy, P., and Parinandi, N. (2007). Oxygen, the lead actor in the pathophysiologic drama: enactment of the trinity of normoxia, hypoxia, and hyperoxia in disease and therapy. *Antioxid. Redox Signal.* 9, 1717–1730. doi: 10.1089/ars.2007.1724

Lam, R., Schilling, D., Scottoline, B., Platteau, A., Niederhausen, M., Lund, K. C., et al. (2020). The effect of extended continuous positive airway pressure on changes in lung volumes in stable premature infants: a randomized controlled trial. *J. Pediatr.* 217, 66–72.e1. doi: 10.1016/j.jpeds.2019.07.074

Levick, J. R., and Michel, C. C. (2010). Microvascular fluid exchange and the revised Starling principle. *Cardiovasc. Res.* 87, 198–210. doi: 10.1093/cvr/cvq062

Li, Y., Liang, J., Yang, T., Monterrosa Mena, J., Huan, C., Xie, T., et al. (2016). Hyaluronan synthase 2 regulates fibroblast senescence in pulmonary fibrosis. *Matrix Biol.* 55, 35–48. doi: 10.1016/j.matbio.2016.03.004

Li, Y., Rahmanian, M., Widström, C., Lepperdinger, G., Frost, G. I., and Heldin, P. (2000). Irradiation-induced expression of hyaluronan (HA) synthase 2 and hyaluronidase 2 genes in rat lung tissue accompanies active turnover of HA and induction of types I and III collagen gene expression. *Am. J. Respir. Cell Mol. Biol.* 23, 411–418. doi: 10.1165/ajrcmb.23.3.4102

Liang, S., Wang, Y., and Liu, Y. (2019). Dexmedetomidine alleviates lung ischemia-reperfusion injury in rats by activating PI3K/Akt pathway. *Eur. Rev. Med. Pharmacol. Sci.* 23, 370–377. doi: 10.26355/eurrev_201901_16785

Lin, C. Y., Zhang, H., Cheng, K. C., and Slutsky, A. S. (2003). Mechanical ventilation may increase susceptibility to the development of bacteremia. *Crit. Care Med.* 31, 1429–1434. doi: 10.1097/01.CCM.0000063449.58029.81

Long, Q. X., Liu, B. Z., Deng, H. J., Wu, G. C., Deng, K., Chen, Y. K., et al. (2020). Antibody responses to SARS-CoV-2 in patients with COVID-19. *Nat. Med.* 26, 845–848. doi: 10.1038/s41591-020-0897-1

Makiyama, A. M., Gibson, L. J., Harris, R. S., and Venegas, J. G. (2014). Stress concentration around an atelectatic region: a finite element model. *Respir. Physiol. Neurobiol.* 201, 101–110. doi: 10.1016/j.resp.2014.06.017

Matalon, S., and Egan, E. A. (1981). Effects of 100% O2 breathing on permeability of alveolar epithelium to solute. *J. Appl. Physiol. Respir. Environ. Exerc. Physiol.* 50, 859–863. doi: 10.1152/jappl.1981.50.4.859

Matalon, S., and Egan, E. A. (1984). Interstitial fluid volumes and albumin spaces in pulmonary oxygen toxicity. *J. Appl. Physiol. Respir. Environ. Exerc. Physiol.* 57, 1767–1772. doi: 10.1152/jappl.1984.57.6.1767

Matsuzawa, Y., Nakazawa, K., Yamamura, A., Akashi, T., Kitagaki, K., Eishi, Y., et al. (2010). Airway pressure release ventilation reduces the increase in bronchoalveolar lavage fluid high-mobility group box-1 levels and lung water in experimental acute respiratory distress syndrome induced by lung lavage. *Eur. J. Anaesthesiol.* 27, 726–733. doi: 10.1097/EJA.0b013e328333c2b0

Matthay, M. A., and Wiener-Kronish, J. P. (1990). Intact epithelial barrier function is critical for the resolution of alveolar edema in humans. *Am. Rev. Respir. Dis.* 142(6 Pt 1), 1250–1257. doi: 10.1164/ajrccm/142.6_Pt_1.1250

Matthay, M. A., Landolt, C. C., and Staub, N. C. (1982). Differential liquid and protein clearance from the alveoli of anesthetized sheep. *J. Appl. Physiol. Respir. Environ. Exerc. Physiol.* 53, 96–104. doi: 10.1152/jappl.1982.53.1.96

Mazzuca, E., Aliverti, A., and Miserocchi, G. (2019). Understanding vasomotion of lung microcirculation by *in vivo* imaging. *J. Imaging* 5:22. doi: 10.3390/jimaging5020022

Mazzuca, E., Aliverti, A., and Miserocchi, G. (2016). Computational micro-scale model of control of extravascular water and capillary perfusion in the air blood barrier. *J. Theor. Biol.* 400, 42–51. doi: 10.1016/j.jtbi.2016.03.036

Mead, J., Takishima, T., and Leith, D. (1970). Stress distribution in lungs: a model of pulmonary elasticity. *J. Appl. Physiol.* 28, 596–608. doi: 10.1152/jappl.1970.28.5.596

Miserocchi, G. (2007). "Lung interstitial pressure and structure in acute hypoxia," in *Hypoxia and the Circulation*, eds R. C. Roach, P. D. Wagner and P. H. Hackett (New York, NY: Springer).

Miserocchi, G., Poskurica, B. H., del Fabbro, M., and Crisafulli, B. (1995). Pulmonary interstitial pressure in premature rabbits. *Respir. Physiol.* 102, 239–249. doi: 10.1016/0034-5687(95)00070-4

Miserocchi, G., and Rivolta, I. (2012). Mechanistic considerations on the development of lung edema: vascular, perivascular and molecular aspects from early stage to tissue and vascular remodeling. *Curr. Respir. Med. Rev.* 8, 82–89.

Miserocchi, G. (2009). Mechanisms controlling the volume of pleural fluid and extravascular lung water. *Eur. Respir. Rev.* 18, 244–252. doi: 10.1183/09059180.00002709

Miserocchi, G., Messinesi, G., Tana, F., Passoni, E., Adamo, S., Romano, R., et al. (2008). Mechanisms behind inter-individual differences in lung diffusing capacity. *Eur. J. Appl. Physiol.* 102, 561–568. doi: 10.1007/s00421-007-0625-2

Miserocchi, G., Negrini, D., and Gonano, C. (1990). Direct measurement of interstitial pulmonary pressure in *in situ* lung with intact pleural space. *J. Appl. Physiol.* 69, 2168–2174. doi: 10.1152/jappl.1990.69.6.2168

Miserocchi, G., Negrini, D., Del Fabbro, M., and Venturoli, D. (1993). Pulmonary interstitial pressure in intact *in situ* lung: transition to interstitial edema. *J. Appl. Physiol.* 74, 1171–1177. doi: 10.1152/jappl.1993.74.3.1171

Miserocchi, G., Negrini, D., Mukenge, S., Turconi, P., and Del Fabbro, M. (1989). Liquid drainage through the peritoneal diaphragmatic surface. *J. Appl. Physiol.* 66, 1579–1585. doi: 10.1152/jappl.1989.66.4.1579

Miserocchi, G., Passi, A., Albertini, R., Negrini, D., and De Luca, G. (1999). Interstitial pressure and proteoglycan degradation in hydraulic- and elastase-induced lung edema. *Chest* 116(1 Suppl.):31S. doi: 10.1378/chest.116.suppl_1.31s

Miserocchi, G., Passi, A., Negrini, D., Del Fabbro, M., and De Luca, G. (2001). Pulmonary interstitial pressure and tissue matrix structure in acute hypoxia. *Am. J. Physiol. Lung Cell. Mol. Physiol.* 280, L881–L887. doi: 10.1152/ajplung.2001.280.5.L881

Miserocchi, G., Poskurica, B. H., and Del Fabbro, M. (1994). Pulmonary interstitial pressure in anesthetized paralyzed newborn rabbits. *J. Appl. Physiol.* 77, 2260–2268. doi: 10.1152/jappl.1994.77.5.2260

Mitzner, W., and Sylvester, J. T. (1986). Lymph flow and lung weight in isolated sheep lungs. *J. Appl. Physiol.* 61, 1830–1835. doi: 10.1152/jappl.1986.61.5.1830

Nash, G., Blennerhassett, J. B., and Pontoppidan, H. (1967). Pulmonary lesions associated with oxygen therapy and artifical ventilation. *N. Engl. J. Med.* 276, 368–374. doi: 10.1056/NEJM196702162760702

Negrini, D., Passi, A., Bertin, K., Bosi, F., and Wiig, H. (2001b). Isolation of pulmonary interstitial fluid in rabbits by a modified wick technique. *Am. J. Physiol. Lung Cell. Mol. Physiol.* 280, L1057–L1065. doi: 10.1152/ajplung.2001.280.5.L1057

Negrini, D., Candiani, A., Boschetti, F., Crisafulli, B., Del Fabbro, M., Bettinelli, D., et al. (2001a). Pulmonary microvascular and perivascular interstitial geometry during development of mild hydraulic edema. *Am. J. Physiol. Lung Cell. Mol. Physiol.* 281, L1464–L1471. doi: 10.1152/ajplung.2001.281.6.L1464

Negrini, D., Passi, A., de Luca, G., and Miserocchi, G. (1996). Pulmonary interstitial pressure and proteoglycans during development of pulmonary edema. *Am. J. Physiol.* 270(6 Pt 2), H2000–H2007. doi: 10.1152/ajpheart.1996.270.6.H2000

Nieman, G. F., Andrews, P., Satalin, J., Wilcox, K., Kollisch-Singule, M., Madden, M., et al. (2018). Acute lung injury: how to stabilize a broken lung. *Crit. Care* 22:136. doi: 10.1186/s13054-018-2051-8

Nieman, G. F., Gatto, L. A., Andrews, P., Satalin, J., Camporota, L., Daxon, B., et al. (2020b). Prevention and treatment of acute lung injury with time-controlled adaptive ventilation: physiologically informed modification of airway pressure release ventilation. *Ann. Intensive Care* 10:3. doi: 10.1186/s13613-019-0619-3

Nieman, G. F., Al-Khalisy, H., Kollisch-Singule, M., Satalin, J., Blair, S., Trikha, G., et al. (2020a). A physiologically informed strategy to effectively open, stabilize, and protect the acutely injured lung. *Front. Physiol.* 11:227. doi: 10.3389/fphys.2020.00227

Palestini, P., Botto, L., Rivolta, I., and Miserocchi, G. (2011). Remodelling of membrane rafts expression in lung cells as an early sign of mechanotransduction-signalling in pulmonary edema. *J. Lipids* 2011:695369. doi: 10.1155/2011/695369

Palestini, P., Calvi, C., Conforti, E., Botto, L., Fenoglio, C., and Miserocchi, G. (2002). Composition, biophysical properties, and morphometry of plasma membranes in pulmonary interstitial edema. *Am. J. Physiol. Lung Cell Mol. Physiol.* 282, L1382–L1390. doi: 10.1152/ajplung.00447.2001

Papazian, L., Forel, J. M., Gacouin, A., Penot-Ragon, C., Perrin, G., Loundou, A., et al. (2010). Neuromuscular blockers in early acute respiratory distress syndrome. *N. Engl. J. Med.* 363, 1107–1116.

Parker, J. C. (2007). Hydraulic conductance of lung endothelial phenotypes and Starling safety factors against edema. *Am. J. Physiol. Lung Cell. Mol. Physiol.* 292, L378–L380. doi: 10.1152/ajplung.00196.2006

Parker, J. C., Guyton, A. C., and Taylor, A. E. (1978). Pulmonary interstitial and capillary pressures estimated from intra-alveolar fluid pressures. *J. Appl. Physiol. Respir. Environ. Exerc. Physiol.* 44, 267–276. doi: 10.1152/jappl.1978.44.2.267

Parker, J. C., Ivey, C. L., and Tucker, J. A. (1998). Gadolinium prevents high airway pressure-induced permeability increases in isolated rat lungs. *J. Appl. Physiol.* 84, 1113–1118. doi: 10.1152/jappl.1998.84.4.1113

Parker, J. C., Stevens, T., Randall, J., Weber, D. S., and King, J. A. (2006). Hydraulic conductance of pulmonary microvascular and macrovascular endothelial cell monolayers. *Am. J. Physiol. Lung Cell. Mol. Physiol.* 291, L30–L37. doi: 10.1152/ajplung.00317.2005

Parker, J. C., and Townsley, M. I. (2004). Evaluation of lung injury in rats and mice. *Am. J. Physiol. Lung Cell. Mol. Physiol.* 286, L231–L246. doi: 10.1152/ajplung.00049.2003

Parker, J. C., Townsley, M. I., Rippe, B., Taylor, A. E., and Thigpen, J. (1984). Increased microvascular permeability in dog lungs due to high peak airway pressures. *J. Appl. Physiol. Respir. Environ. Exerc. Physiol.* 57, 1809–1816. doi: 10.1152/jappl.1984.57.6.1809

Passi, A., Negrini, D., Albertini, R., Miserocchi, G., and De Luca, G. (1999). The sensitivity of versican from rabbit lung to gelatinase A (MMP-2) and B (MMP-9) and its involvement in the development of hydraulic lung edema. *FEBS Lett.* 456, 93–96. doi: 10.1016/s0014-5793(99)00929-1

Patel, V., Dial, K., Wu, J., Gauthier, A. G., Wu, W., Lin, M., et al. (2020). Dietary antioxidants significantly attenuate Hyperoxia-induced acute inflammatory lung injury by enhancing macrophage function *via* reducing the accumulation of airway HMGB1. *Int. J. Mol. Sci.* 21:977. doi: 10.3390/ijms21030977

Pearse, D. B., Wagner, E. M., and Sylvester, J. T. (1993). Edema clearance in isolated sheep lungs. *J. Appl. Physiol.* 74, 126–132. doi: 10.1152/jappl.1993.74.1.126

Pengelly, L. D., Alderson, A. M., and Milic-Emili, J. (1971). Mechanics of the diaphragm. *J. Appl. Physiol.* 30, 797–805. doi: 10.1152/jappl.1971.30.6.797

Perlman, C. E., Lederer, D. J., and Bhattacharya, J. (2011). Micromechanics of alveolar edema. *Am. J. Respir. Cell. Mol. Biol.* 44, 34–39. doi: 10.1165/rcmb.2009-0005OC

Protti, A., Andreis, D. T., Monti, M., Santini, A., Sparacino, C. C., Langer, T., et al. (2013). Lung stress and strain during mechanical ventilation: Any difference between statics and dynamics? *Crit. Care Med.* 41, 1046–1055. doi: 10.1097/CCM.0b013e31827417a6

Rausch, S. M., Haberthür, D., Stampanoni, M., Schittny, J. C., and Wall, W. A. (2011). Local strain distribution in real three-dimensional alveolar geometries. *Ann. Biomed. Eng.* 39, 2835–2843. doi: 10.1007/s10439-011-0328-z

Reitsma, S., Slaaf, D. W., Vink, H., van Zandvoort, M. A., and oude Egbrink, M. G. (2007). The endothelial glycocalyx: composition, functions, and visualization. *Pflugers Arch.* 454, 345–359. doi: 10.1007/s00424-007-0212-8

Retamal, J., Hurtado, D., Villarroel, N., Bruhn, A., Bugedo, G., Amato, M., et al. (2018). Does regional lung strain correlate with regional inflammation in acute respiratory distress syndrome during nonprotective ventilation? An Experimental Porcine Study. *Crit. Care Med.* 46, e591–e599. doi: 10.1097/CCM.0000000000003072

Rivolta, I., Lucchini, V., Rocchetti, M., Kolar, F., Palazzo, F., Zaza, A., et al. (2011). Interstitial pressure and lung oedema in chronic hypoxia. *Eur. Respir. J.* 37, 943–949. doi: 10.1183/09031936.00066710

Robinson, S. K., Ramsden, J. J., Warner, J., Lackie, P. M., and Roose, T. (2019). Correlative 3D Imaging and Microfluidic Modelling of Human Pulmonary Lymphatics using Immunohistochemistry and High-resolution μCT. *Sci. Rep.* 9:6415. doi: 10.1038/s41598-019-42794-7

Roselli, R. J., Parker, R. E., and Harris, T. R. (1984). A model of unsteady-state transvascular fluid and protein transport in the lung. *J. Appl. Physiol. Respir. Environ. Exerc. Physiol.* 56, 1389–1402. doi: 10.1152/jappl.1984.56.5.1389

Roy, S. K., Emr, B., Sadowitz, B., Gatto, L. A., Ghosh, A., Satalin, J. M., et al. (2013a). Preemptive application of airway pressure release ventilation prevents development of acute respiratory distress syndrome in a rat traumatic hemorrhagic shock model. *Shock* 40, 210–216. doi: 10.1097/SHK.0b013e31829efb06

Roy, S., Habashi, N., Sadowitz, B., Andrews, P., Ge, L., Wang, G., et al. (2013b). Early airway pressure release ventilation prevents ARDS-a novel preventive approach to lung injury. *Shock* 39, 28–38. doi: 10.1097/SHK.0b013e31827b47bb

Roy, S., Sadowitz, B., Andrews, P., Gatto, L. A., Marx, W., Ge, L., et al. (2012). Early stabilizing alveolar ventilation prevents acute respiratory distress syndrome: a novel timing-based ventilatory intervention to avert lung injury. *J. Trauma Acute Care Surg.* 73, 391–400. doi: 10.1097/TA.0b013e31825c7a82

Rutili, G., Kvietys, P., Martin, D., Parker, J. C., and Taylor, A. E. (1982). Increased pulmonary microvasuclar permeability induced by alpha-naphthylthiourea. *J. Appl. Physiol. Respir. Environ. Exerc. Physiol.* 52, 1316–1323. doi: 10.1152/jappl.1982.52.5.1316

Scherrer, U., Vollenweider, L., Delabays, A., Savcic, M., Eichenberger, U., Kleger, G. R., et al. (1996). Inhaled nitric oxide for high-altitude pulmonary edema. *N. Engl. J. Med.* 334, 624–629. doi: 10.1056/NEJM199603073341003

Schraufnagel, D. E. (1992). Forms of lung lymphatics: a scanning electron microscopic study of casts. *Anat. Rec.* 233, 547–554. doi: 10.1002/ar.1092330409

Schraufnagel, D. E., Agaram, N. P., Faruqui, A., Jain, S., Jain, L., Ridge, K. M., et al. (2003). Pulmonary lymphatics and edema accumulation after brief lung injury. *Am. J. Physiol. Lung Cell. Mol. Physiol.* 284, L891–L897. doi: 10.1152/ajplung.00333.2002

Schraufnagel, D. E., Basterra, J. L., Hainis, K., and Sznajder, J. I. (1994). Lung lymphatics increase after hyperoxic injury. *Am. J. Pathol.* 144, 1393–1402.

Smith, B. J., Roy, G. S., Cleveland, A., Mattson, C., Okamura, K., Charlebois, C. M., et al. (2020). Three alveolar phenotypes govern lung function in murine ventilator-induced lung injury. *Front. Physiol.* 11:660. doi: 10.3389/fphys.2020.00660

Tarbell, J. M. (2010). Shear stress and the endothelial transport barrier. *Cardiovasc. Res.* 87, 320–330. doi: 10.1093/cvr/cvq146

Tarbell, J. M., Demaio, L., and Zaw, M. M. (1999). Effect of pressure on hydraulic conductivity of endothelial monolayers: role of endothelial cleft shear stress. *J. Appl. Physiol.* 87, 261–268. doi: 10.1152/jappl.1999.87.1.261

Taylor, A. E., and Parker, J. C. (1985). "Pulmonary interstitial spaces and lymphatics" in *Handbook of Physiology. The Respiratory System and Nonrespiratory Functions,* eds A. Fishman and A. Fisher (Bethesda, MD: American Physiological Society) 167–230.

Telias, I., Brochard, L., and Goligher, E. C. (2018). Is my patient's respiratory drive (too) high? *Intensive Care Med.* 44, 1936–1939. doi: 10.1007/s00134-018-5091-2

Tingay, D. G., Farrell, O., Thomson, J., Perkins, E. J., Pereira-Fantini, P. M., Waldmann, A. D., et al. (2021). Imaging the respiratory transition at birth: unraveling the complexities of the first breaths of life. *Am. J. Respir. Crit. Care Med.* 204, 82–91. doi: 10.1164/rccm.202007-2997OC

Unruh, H. W., Goldberg, H. S., and Oppenheimer, L. (1984). Pulmonary interstitial compartments and tissue resistance to fluid flux. *J. Appl. Physiol. Respir. Environ. Exerc. Physiol.* 57, 1512–1519. doi: 10.1152/jappl.1984.57.5.1512

Verghese, G. M., Ware, L. B., Matthay, B. A., and Matthay, M. A. (1999). Alveolar epithelial fluid transport and the resolution of clinically severe hydrostatic pulmonary edema. *J. Appl. Physiol.* 87, 1301–1312. doi: 10.1152/jappl.1999.87.4.1301

Ware, L. B., and Matthay, M. A. (2001). Alveolar fluid clearance is impaired in the majority of patients with acute lung injury and the acute respiratory distress syndrome. *Am. J. Respir. Crit. Care Med.* 163, 1376–1383. doi: 10.1164/ajrccm.163.6.2004035

Waxman, A. B., and Kolliputi, N. (2009). IL-6 protects against hyperoxia-induced mitochondrial damage *via* Bcl-2-induced Bak interactions with mitofusins. *Am. J. Respir. Cell Mol. Biol.* 41, 385–396. doi: 10.1165/rcmb.2008-0302OC

Weber, E., Sozio, F., Borghini, A., Sestini, P., and Renzoni, E. (2018). Pulmonary lymphatic vessel morphology: a review. *Ann. Anat.* 218, 110–117. doi: 10.1016/j.aanat.2018.02.011

Weibel, E. R. (1971). Oxygen effect on lung cells. *Arch. Intern. Med.* 128, 54–56.doi: 10.1001/archinte.1971.00310190058005

Weibel, E. R. (2015). On the tricks alveolar epithelial cells play to make a good lung. *Am. J. Respir. Crit. Care Med.* 191, 504–513. doi: 10.1164/rccm.201409-1663OE

Weibel, E. R. (2017). Lung morphometry: the link between structure and function. *Cell Tissue Res.* 367, 413–426. doi: 10.1007/s00441-016-2541-4

Writing Group for the Alveolar Recruitment for Acute Respiratory Distress Syndrome Trial (ART) Investigators, Cavalcanti, A. B., Suzumura, É. A., Laranjeira, L. N., Paisani, D. M., Damiani, L. P., et al. (2017). Effect of Lung Recruitment and Titrated Positive End-Expiratory Pressure (PEEP) vs Low PEEP on mortality in patients with acute respiratory distress syndrome: a randomized clinical trial. *JAMA* 318, 1335–1345. doi: 10.1001/jama.2017.14171

Wu, D. X., Weibel, E. R., Bachofen, H., and Schürch, S. (1995). Lung lesions in experimental hydrostatic pulmonary edema: an electron microscopic and morphometric study. Exp. *Lung Res.* 21, 711–730. doi: 10.3109/01902149509050838

Yoshida, T., Rinka, H., Kaji, A., Yoshimoto, A., Arimoto, H., Miyaichi, T., et al. (2009). The impact of spontaneous ventilation on distribution of lung aeration in patients with acute respiratory distress syndrome: airway pressure release ventilation versus pressure support ventilation. *Anesth. Analg.* 109, 1892–1900. doi: 10.1213/ANE.0b013e3181bbd918

Yoshikawa, S., King, J. A., Lausch, R. N., Penton, A. M., Eyal, F. G., and Parker, J. C. (2004). Acute ventilator-induced vascular permeability and cytokine responses in isolated and *in situ* mouse lungs. *J. Appl. Physiol.* 97, 2190–2199. doi: 10.1152/japplphysiol.00324.2004

Zavorsky, G. S., Milne, E. N., Lavorini, F., Rienzi, J. P., Lavin, K. M., Straub, A. M., et al. (2014). Interstitial lung edema triggered by marathon running. *Respir. Physiol. Neurobiol.* 190, 137–141. doi: 10.1016/j.resp.2013.10.007

Zhang, S., Liu, L., Yang, B., Li, R., Luo, J., Huang, J., et al. (2020). Clinical characteristics of 134 convalescent patients with COVID-19 in Guizhou, China. *Respir. Res.* 21:314. doi: 10.1186/s12931-020-01580-0

3

Right Ventricular Function in Acute Respiratory Distress Syndrome: Impact on Outcome, Respiratory Strategy and Use of Veno-Venous Extracorporeal Membrane Oxygenation

Matthieu Petit[1,2], Edouard Jullien[1,2] and Antoine Vieillard-Baron[1,2]*

[1] Medical Intensive Care Unit, University Hospital Ambroise Paré, APHP, Boulogne-Billancourt, France, [2] UFR des Sciences de la Santé Simone Veil, Université Paris-Saclay, Montigny-le-Bretonneux, France

***Correspondence:**
Antoine Vieillard-Baron
antoine.vieillard-baron@aphp.fr

Acute respiratory distress syndrome (ARDS) is characterized by protein-rich alveolar edema, reduced lung compliance and severe hypoxemia. Despite some evidence of improvements in mortality over recent decades, ARDS remains a major public health problem with 30% 28-day mortality in recent cohorts. Pulmonary vascular dysfunction is one of the pivot points of the pathophysiology of ARDS, resulting in a certain degree of pulmonary hypertension, higher levels of which are associated with morbidity and mortality. Pulmonary hypertension develops as a result of endothelial dysfunction, pulmonary vascular occlusion, increased vascular tone, extrinsic vessel occlusion, and vascular remodeling. This increase in right ventricular (RV) afterload causes uncoupling between the pulmonary circulation and RV function. Without any contractile reserve, the right ventricle has no adaptive reserve mechanism other than dilatation, which is responsible for left ventricular compression, leading to circulatory failure and worsening of oxygen delivery. This state, also called severe acute cor pulmonale (ACP), is responsible for excess mortality. Strategies designed to protect the pulmonary circulation and the right ventricle in ARDS should be the cornerstones of the care and support of patients with the severest disease, in order to improve prognosis, pending stronger evidence. Acute cor pulmonale is associated with higher driving pressure ($\geq$18 cmH_2O), hypercapnia ($PaCO_2 \geq 48$ mmHg), and hypoxemia ($PaO_2/FiO_2 < 150$ mmHg). RV protection should focus on these three preventable factors identified in the last decade. Prone positioning, the setting of positive end-expiratory pressure, and inhaled nitric oxide (INO) can also unload the right ventricle, restore better coupling between the right ventricle and the pulmonary circulation, and correct circulatory failure. When all these strategies are insufficient, extracorporeal membrane oxygenation (ECMO), which improves decarboxylation and oxygenation and enables ultra-protective ventilation by decreasing driving pressure, should be discussed in seeking better control of RV afterload. This review reports the pathophysiology of pulmonary hypertension in ARDS, describes right heart function, and proposes an RV protective approach, ranging from ventilatory settings and prone positioning to INO and selection of patients potentially eligible for veno-venous extracorporeal membrane oxygenation (VV ECMO).

Keywords: ARDS, right ventricle, VV ECMO, echocardiography, acute cor pulmonale (ACP)

INTRODUCTION

Acute respiratory distress syndrome (ARDS) is characterized by protein-rich alveolar edema, reduced lung compliance and severe hypoxemia (Thompson et al., 2017). Despite some evidence of improvements in mortality over recent decades (Brun-Buisson et al., 2004; Phua et al., 2009) due to better understanding of its pathophysiology and routine application of protective mechanical ventilation, ARDS remains a major public health problem with an approximately 30% 28-day mortality in recent cohorts (Bellani et al., 2016; Combes et al., 2018; Constantin et al., 2019). Pulmonary vascular dysfunction (Snow et al., 1982; Price et al., 2012) is one of the pivot points of the pathophysiology, resulting in a certain degree of pulmonary hypertension, higher levels of which are associated with morbidity and mortality (Bull et al., 2010). The hemodynamic consequences of such remodeling of the pulmonary circulation has led clinicians to pay attention to the right ventricle as the deleterious impact of right ventricular (RV) failure on prognosis is well demonstrated (Mekontso Dessap et al., 2016).

This review reports the pathophysiology of pulmonary hypertension and RV injury, describes RV function, and explains the interest of proposing a RV protective approach to manage ARDS patients, ranging from ventilatory settings and prone positioning to nitric oxide (NO) inhalation and selection of patients potentially eligible for veno-venous extracorporeal membrane oxygenation (VV ECMO) in this context. A few specificities of ARDS-related COVID-19, if any, will be mentioned.

PATHOPHYSIOLOGY OF RIGHT VENTRICULAR INJURY IN ACUTE RESPIRATORY DISTRESS SYNDROME

Right Ventricular Physiology

The right ventricle is composed of the filling chamber and the outflow chamber. Under normal conditions, the right ventricle ejects the blood into the pulmonary circulation, a system of low resistance and high compliance. In contrast to the left ventricle, its isovolumetric contraction pressure is very low and its isovolumetric relaxation is insignificant (Redington et al., 1990): it acts as a passive conduit. This is why its systolic function is sensitive to any increase in pulmonary vascular resistance (PVR) with no adaptation reserve, leading to dysfunction and ultimately to failure. However, the right ventricle is able to adapt to a certain degree of pulmonary hypertension by dilating, due to its high diastolic compliance (Laks et al., 1967).

Pulmonary Vascular Dysfunction

ARDS is characterized by acute onset hypoxemia (ARDS Definition Task Force et al., 2012) with increased pulmonary vascular permeability, leading to non-cardiogenic pulmonary edema (Ashbaugh et al., 1967). Along with alveolar damage, ARDS directly causes injury to the pulmonary circulation, through several pathophysiological mechanisms, involving endothelial dysfunction, distal pulmonary vascular occlusion at the level of the capillaries, pulmonary vasoconstriction, extrinsic vessel occlusion by alveoli distension and ultimately vascular remodeling (Price et al., 2012). All of these phenomena lead to elevation of PVR, pre-capillary pulmonary hypertension and increased RV afterload.

In COVID-19, a certain "protection" of the pulmonary circulation could occur with first the development of pulmonary angiogenesis (Ackermann et al., 2020) and second the virtual absence of hypoxic pulmonary vasoconstriction (Archer et al., 2020). Conversely, proximal obstruction of the pulmonary circulation has been reported to be frequent.

Focus on the Effect of Mechanical Ventilation

Inadequate mechanical ventilation may have a deleterious effect on RV function. During spontaneous breathing in a healthy subject, RV function is optimal with adequate venous return due to negative pleural pressure (Guyton et al., 1957), and RV afterload is limited because of a low transpulmonary pressure (TPP) as lung compliance is normal. In ARDS, a situation where lung compliance is decreased, positive pressure ventilation induces increased TPP at least during tidal ventilation and sometimes during expiration in the case when too high a positive end-expiratory pressure (PEEP) is applied. As a consequence, the pulmonary capillaries are stretched and their caliber reduced, resulting in an increase in PVR (Whittenberger et al., 1960; West et al., 1964). Cyclic increase in PVR during tidal ventilation is responsible for cyclic changes in RV afterload, and then in RV outflow (Vieillard-Baron et al., 1999) eventually leading to pulse pressure variations (**Figure 1**). At the same time, ventilator settings may indirectly impact the pulmonary circulation through changes in PaO_2 and $PaCO_2$, both of which strongly mediate pulmonary vasoconstriction (Yamamoto et al., 2001).

It was suggested at least at the beginning of the COVID-19 pandemic that lung compliance was less decreased than in classical ARDS (Gattinoni et al., 2020), thus potentially inducing less interaction with the pulmonary circulation. This is, however, still questionable.

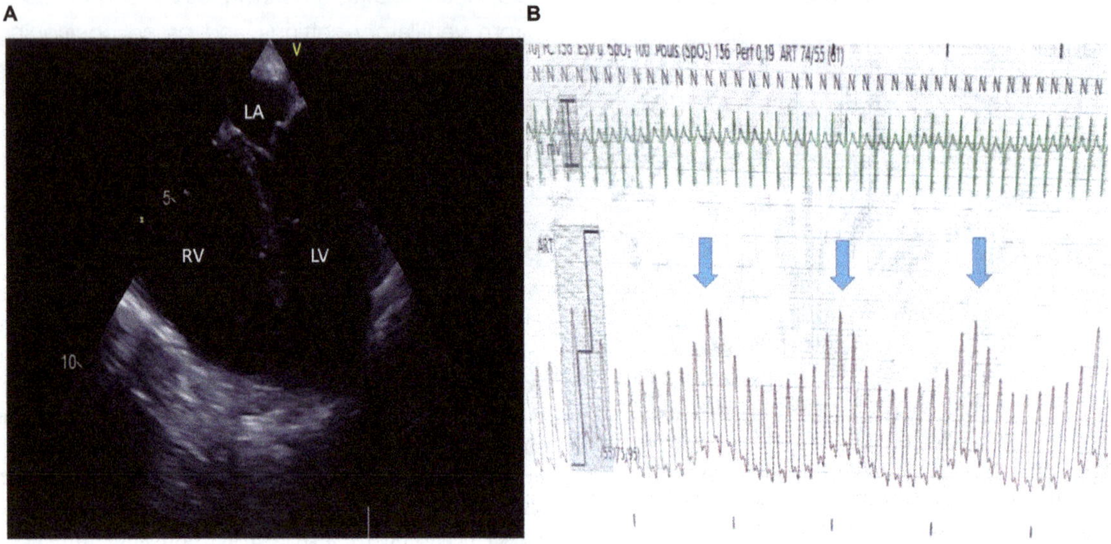

FIGURE 1 | Acute cor pulmonale in a patient ventilated for ARDS and in shock and completely adapted to the respirator. **(A)** A mid-esophageal 4-chamber view demonstrated severe RV dilatation with paradoxical septal motion. **(B)** Invasive low blood pressure with significant pulse pressure variation (blue arrows indicate insufflation) through a radial catheter. Central venous pressure was also elevated. LV, left ventricle; LA, left atrium; RV, right ventricle.

Right Ventricular Failure and Acute Cor Pulmonale

Acute cor pulmonale (ACP) is the last stage of the uncoupling between the right ventricle and the pulmonary circulation. It could be understood, especially in its most severe form, as an RV failure state. RV afterload is suddenly increased, and RV ejection is impaired. In consequence, the right ventricle increases in size. This RV dilatation participates in circulatory failure by compressing the left ventricle (LV) (Scharf et al., 1979). Moreover, in normal conditions, RV and LV systoles occur simultaneously, with the right and left ventricles starting and ending contraction almost at the same time. When RV systole is overloaded, RV contraction is prolonged, so that the right ventricle continues to push after the left ventricle has ended, and the pressure in the RV cavity is then higher than the pressure in the LV cavity during a short instant (Elzinga et al., 1980). This explains the paradoxical septal motion observed in ACP (**Figure 1A**).

ACUTE COR PULMONALE: INCIDENCE, RISK FACTORS, AND IMPACT ON OUTCOME

Prior to the widespread use of protective ventilation, ACP was reported in almost 60% of patients (Jardin et al., 1985). However, all patients were ventilated with high tidal volume and plateau pressure (Pplat) and all patients with severe RV dilatation finally died (Jardin et al., 1985). Since the era of protective ventilation, the incidence of ACP has declined to between 20 and 30% (Vieillard-Baron et al., 2001; Page et al., 2003; Mekontso Dessap et al., 2010, 2016), but may still be as high as 50% in the most severe ARDS (Vieillard-Baron et al., 2007). This leads physicians to take into consideration RV function in management strategies of patients with moderate to severe ARDS.

We still lack convincing data on the incidence of RV failure/ACP in ARDS related to COVID-19. One preliminary study in a very small series of patients reported an incidence of 17% (Evrard et al., 2020). Other studies not only including critically ill patients reported an RV dilatation in 35% of cases (Dweck et al., 2020) or an impact of RV dilatation on ICU transfer or death (Soulat-Dufour et al., 2021). In 90 COVID-19 patients, Bleakley et al. (2021) reported that radial RV dysfunction was common, while the longitudinal function was relatively spared. Micro-occlusive vasculopathy was also reported in COVID-19 by dual energy CT and was more clearly associated with RV dysfunction than the pulmonary embolism obstruction score (Ridge et al., 2020).

The largest study reporting risk factors for developing ACP was performed in 752 patients with moderate to severe ARDS submitted to protective ventilation (Mekontso Dessap et al., 2016). Driving pressure $\geq$ 18 cmH_2O, $PaCO_2 \geq$ 48 mmHg, $PaO_2/FiO_2 <$ 150 mmHg and pneumonia as causes of ARDS identified patients at risk of ACP. Incidence of ACP ranged from less than 10% when only one risk factor was present to close to 60% with 3–4 risk factors (Mekontso Dessap et al., 2016). Interestingly, neither Pplat nor PEEP was reported as a potential risk factor. An explanation could be that a low PEEP was homogenously applied (mean 8 cmH_2O) and Pplat was maintained below 27 cmH_2O in most patients. In other conditions, they both may affect pulmonary circulation and RV function. A high Pplat is associated with RV failure, especially when it reflects high TPP (Vieillard-Baron et al., 1999). The "safe Pplat" for the right ventricle was suggested to be below 27 cmH_2O (Jardin and Vieillard-Baron, 2007). Pplat is not always a surrogate of lung stress, because it reflects the compliance of the respiratory system (Gattinoni et al., 2004; Chiumello et al., 2008) and chest wall compliance must be taken into account, especially in obese patients. Monitoring of pleural pressure with an esophageal balloon could be of value in these patients, while data are missing. This could also be a specificity of COVID-19 patients who could tolerate higher Pplat, as many patients are obese and the association between Pplat and outcome in this subpopulation is unclear (De Jong et al., 2018).

The potential effect of PEEP on RV function is more questionable. Because of the opposite effect of lung distension on intra- and extra-alveolar pulmonary blood vessels, the relationship between lung distension and PVR is U-shaped (Whittenberger et al., 1960). Thus, the choice of the level of PEEP set by the clinician can directly affect the RV afterload because poor lung aeration on one side and alveolar overdistension on the other side can both raise PVR. In an experimental study, RV function was impaired when the lung was de-recruited and normalized after re-aeration (Duggan et al., 2003). As a matter of fact, lung CT-scan has shown a low amount of potentially recruitable lung (and so a high potential for overdistension) in most ARDS patients (Gattinoni et al., 2006) and a high PEEP was shown to induce hemodynamic instability more frequently in a randomized controlled trial, while no information was given on RV function, which was associated with worse outcome [Writing Group for the Alveolar Recruitment for Acute Respiratory Distress Syndrome Trial (ART) Investigators, 2017]. Despite a strict limitation of Pplat, a PEEP of 15 cmH_2O produced a significant increase in PVR associated with a decrease in cardiac output (Schmitt et al., 2001). The reasonable goal of PEEP is then to reach a balance between enough recruitment and no or minimal overdistension. In other words, the goal is to set the best PEEP to recruit the zones of the collapsed lung, which typically characterize ARDS (Puybasset et al., 2000), without inducing alveolar dead space. Nowadays, no definitive manner to determine the best PEEP is available, but RV function evaluation can be used as a monitoring parameter to avoid PEEP resulting in too much overdistension.

As briefly discussed above, hypercapnia induces pulmonary vasoconstriction (Kiely et al., 1996). Hypercapnia is the consequence of respiratory strategy, i.e., protective ventilation designed to reduce ventilator-induced lung injury, but which also reflects the severity of ARDS (Nuckton et al., 2002).

Finally, one of the prognostic factors in ARDS is hemodynamic instability. And RV failure is one of its mechanisms. While still debatable, many arguments suggest that pulmonary vascular dysfunction and RV failure/ACP could thus have a negative impact on in-hospital mortality (Bull et al., 2010; Mekontso Dessap et al., 2016). This leads to discussion of the potential interest of an RV protective ventilation strategy.

EVALUATION OF RIGHT VENTRICULAR FUNCTION AT THE BEDSIDE

Historically, a pulmonary arterial catheter has been used to evaluate RV function at the bedside. Some of the key elements of monitoring proposed were as follows: low cardiac output, right atrial pressure (RAP) higher than pulmonary artery occlusion pressure (PAOP), and pulmonary hypertension. Recently, the so-called transpulmonary gradient, i.e., the difference between mean pulmonary artery pressure and PAOP, was reported to be frequently abnormally increased and associated with outcome (Bull et al., 2010). However, use of a pulmonary arterial catheter has progressively declined and critical care echocardiography has been progressively implemented and performed in ARDS (Dres et al., 2018). Echocardiographic definition of RV injury is still challenging but in ARDS ACP or severe RV dilatation accurately reflects RV failure, especially when RAP is elevated (Vieillard-Baron et al., 2018). It is recommended by experts in the field to monitor RAP and invasive blood pressure and to perform echocardiography (Vieillard-Baron et al., 2016).

RIGHT VENTRICULAR PROTECTIVE STRATEGY

The main "rules" for protecting the RV in ARDS, by means of avoiding or correcting RV failure, are reported in **Figure 2**. While in our usual practice, we apply systematic daily evaluation of RV function by echocardiography in ARDS patient, **Figure 2** also allows to reemphasize that when echocardiography is not so easily available, pulse pressure variation should be understood as a marker of a deleterious interaction between the RV and the ventilator and then requires further hemodynamic evaluation by echocardiography.

Ventilatory Strategy

As largely discussed above in the physiological rationale, Pplat should be maintained below 27 cmH_2O, and permissive hypercapnia should be limited by careful increase in respiratory rate and by replacing the heat and moisture exchanger by a heated humidifier. Oxygenation should also be increased without too much PEEP (Vieillard-Baron et al., 2013), with a view to optimizing arterial oxygen delivery rather than PaO_2/FiO_2. Indeed, it has long been known that increased PEEP may improve oxygenation but reduce oxygen delivery because of its potential negative hemodynamic effect (Kumar et al., 1970).

Prone Positioning

In the most severe ARDS, it is unlikely that all of the predefined goals of an RV protective approach will be reached. In this situation, prone positioning has been reported to efficiently unload the right ventricle (Vieillard-Baron et al., 2007). It improves oxygenation without increasing PEEP and decreases hypercapnia and Pplat due to lung recruitment of the dependent areas of the lung without overdistension of the non-dependent areas (Guérin et al., 2020), rendering lung ventilation more homogeneous.

To optimize hemodynamic improvement, prone positioning should be performed without chest support, which may be responsible for a decrease in systemic venous return and cardiac output due to excessive elevation of intra-thoracic pressure (Chiumello et al., 2006; Brown et al., 2013).

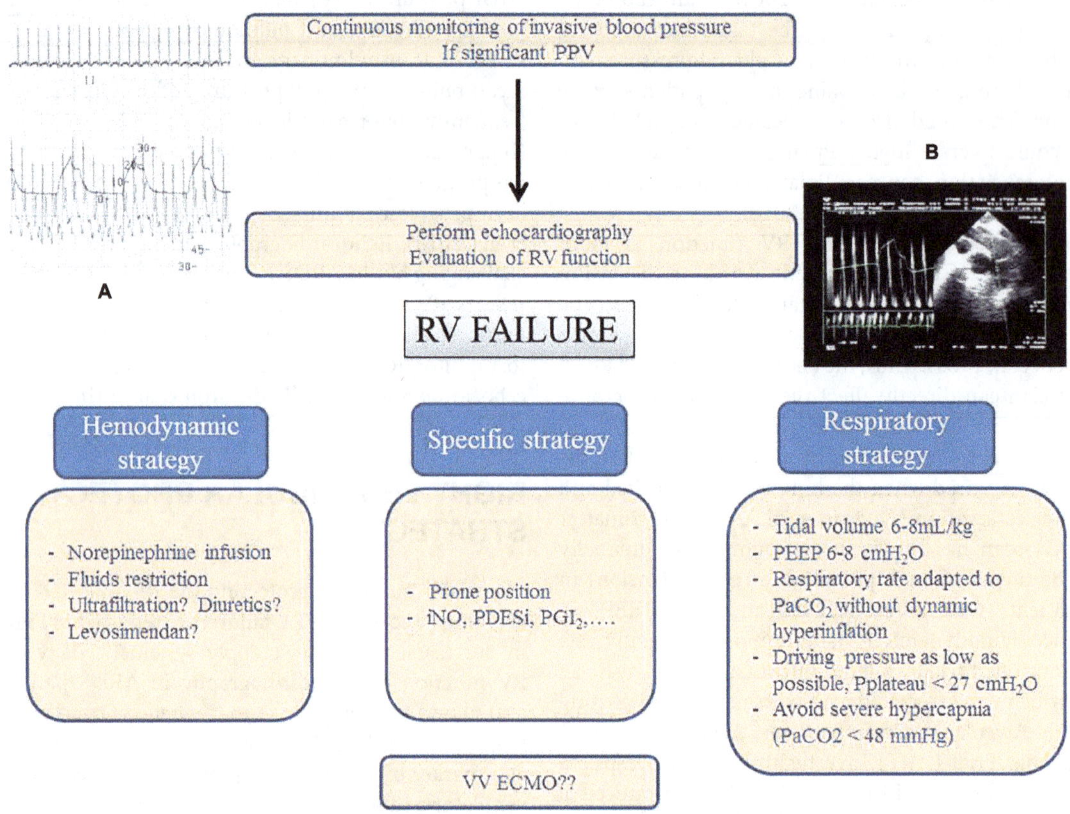

FIGURE 2 | Right ventricle protective strategy. Principles for detection and management of right ventricular (RV) failure in patients with ARDS. This should combine invasive blood pressure monitoring and echocardiography. In the case of significant pulse pressure variation (PPV, Panel **A**), critical care echocardiography must be performed. It usually demonstrates cyclic decrease in RV outflow at each insufflation (Panel **B** on an upper esophageal view with pulsed wave Doppler into the main pulmonary artery) with either isolated RV dilatation or acute cor pulmonale. Management is based on three different strategies: hemodynamic, respiratory, and specific. VV ECMO can be considered in the case of persistent RV failure. PEEP, positive end-expiratory pressure; iNO, inhaled nitric oxide; PDESi, phosphodiesterase type 5 inhibitor; PGI_2, prostaglandin I_2; VV ECMO, veno-venous extracorporeal membrane oxygenation.

Hemodynamic Support and Nitric Oxide Inhalation

When RV failure induces circulatory failure, hemodynamic support is based on two key principles: (i) strongly limit fluid expansion and (ii) restore blood pressure.

Fluid expansion may by itself induce RV failure (Patterson and Starling, 1914) and increase RAP and systemic congestion, leading to acute kidney injury (Chen et al., 2016, 2017). Moreover, it is very unlikely that fluid expansion increases cardiac output, even though significant pulse pressure variation, a marker of LV preload dependency, is observed (Vieillard-Baron et al., 2016; **Figure 1**). Correction of blood pressure by infusion of catecholamines helps improve RV function. In other experimental models of RV failure-related pulmonary circulation obstruction, norepinephrine decreases RV wall stress and RV end-diastolic pressure and improves RV stroke volume, unlike fluid expansion (Ghignone et al., 1984). One of supposed mechanisms is that norepinephrine corrects the functional RV ischemia induced by high RV wall stress combined with low blood pressure (Guyton et al., 1954; Vlahakes et al., 1981). The same observation was made in lung injury (Prewitt and Ghignone, 1983; Vieillard-Baron et al., 2003). In the case of associated LV systolic dysfunction, as observed in ARDS-related septic shock, dobutamine acting on both ventricles may be preferred, though there is no study supporting this approach.

Levosimendan is another inotropic drug called inodilator, acting *via* troponin C calcium binding. It was proposed when there is uncoupling between the right ventricle and the pulmonary circulation. This is strongly physiologically based in ARDS, but only one pilot study suggests an improvement in RV performance in ARDS patients (Morelli et al., 2006). Due to the potential side effects of levosimendan, more data are needed before making any recommendation.

Nitric oxide inhalation has nowadays been abandoned in ARDS after studies and meta-analyzes reported no beneficial effect on outcome (Gebistorf et al., 2016). However, the use of NO for a hemodynamic indication in a subgroup of patients with refractory RV failure despite respiratory optimization has never been evaluated. NO inhalation has been found to significantly decrease RV afterload in ARDS, especially in the case of hypercapnia (Puybasset et al., 2000).

In COVID-19-related ARDS, NO inhalation has been poorly studied, but the rationale is not strongly favored due to the virtual absence of hypoxic vasoconstriction. A few studies have reported an improvement in oxygenation (Longobardo et al., 2021; Robba et al., 2021), especially when cardiac biomarkers were elevated (Garfield et al., 2021), but no association was reported with RV function improvement (Bagate et al., 2020). However, the subgroup of patients with RV failure was not specially studied. In the absence of clear evidence, NO inhalation could be initiate when RV failure is persistent despite RV protective ventilator strategy or when prone position is contraindicated.

Veno-Venous Extracorporeal Membrane Oxygenation

The EOLIA trial suggested that ECMO could be effective in some of the most severe cases of ARDS, but failed to demonstrate a 20% increase in survival (Combes et al., 2018). One of the reasons, despite the non-negligible proportion of crossover between control patients and ECMO patients, could be that criteria for selecting eligible patients were mainly based on blood gas analysis, as proposed by the Berlin classification (Ferguson et al., 2012). By easily controlling blood oxygenation and decarboxylation (Schmidt et al., 2013), VV ECMO suppresses two of the major factors of raised PVR in ARDS and could then be sufficient to unload the right ventricle without the use of veno-arterial (VA) ECMO (Miranda et al., 2015). VV ECMO could also promote ultra-protective ventilation which could benefit the right ventricle by a more pronounced reduction of Pplat and driving pressure (Schmidt et al., 2019). Considering the inevitable complications of VV ECMO, including severe bleeding (Combes et al., 2018), better selection of patients is essential. How this subgroup of patients with severe ARDS and RV failure could be considered as the ideal target remains to be evaluated, while a recent pilot study showed in a non-selected echocardiographic cohort of severe ARDS patients fulfilling the EOLIA criteria that driving pressure and RV failure were the only two factors associated with ICU mortality, in contrast to classical severity markers in ARDS (Petit et al., 2021). Pre-ECMO implantation RV dysfunction is not rare and has an approximately 30% incidence of RV dilatation (Lazzeri et al., 2018).

Another potential technique to support the right ventricle is extracorporeal CO_2 removal. Data are too scarce for discussion of any recommendation (Papazian et al., 2019), but an experimental study in a porcine model of ARDS showed that CO_2 removal is able to decrease RV afterload and to improve coupling between the right ventricle and the pulmonary circulation (Morimont et al., 2015). Such a technique could be efficient and valuable in protecting the right ventricle in the case of severe ARDS with significant hypercapnia and RV failure despite application of an RV protective strategy, but probably does not promote ultraprotective ventilation in patients with moderate ARDS (McNamee et al., 2021).

CONCLUSION

Considering recent studies, RV failure in ARDS with its impact on outcome is now well recognized, as are its risk factors. Many studies suggest that to optimize respiratory settings it is essential to monitor RV function, while clinical impact of such a strategy on the outcome remains unclear. The RV protective approach should be prospectively evaluated in the future to improve the prognosis of the most seriously ill patients. ECMO could be part of this strategy in the most extreme situations.

AUTHOR CONTRIBUTIONS

MP, EJ, and AV-B wrote the manuscript. All authors contributed to the article and approved the submitted version.

REFERENCES

Ackermann, M., Verleden, S. E., Kuehnel, M., Haverich, A., Welte, T., Laenger, F., et al. (2020). Pulmonary vascular endothelialitis, thrombosis, and angiogenesis in Covid-19. *N. Engl. J. Med.* 383, 120–128. doi: 10.1056/NEJMoa2015432

Archer, S. L., Sharp, W. W., and Weir, E. K. (2020). Differentiating COVID-19 pneumonia from acute respiratory distress syndrome and high altitude pulmonary edema: therapeutic implications. *Circulation* 142, 101–104. doi: 10.1161/CIRCULATIONAHA.120.047915

ARDS Definition Task Force, Ranieri, V. M., Rubenfeld, G. D., Thompson, B. T., Ferguson, N. D., Caldwell, E., et al. (2012). Acute respiratory distress syndrome: the Berlin definition. *JAMA* 307, 2526–2533. doi: 10.1001/jama.2012.5669

Ashbaugh, D. G., Bigelow, D. B., Petty, T. L., and Levine, B. E. (1967). Acute respiratory distress in adults. *Lancet Lond. Engl.* 2, 319–323. doi: 10.1016/s0140-6736(67)90168-7

Bagate, F., Tuffet, S., Masi, P., Perier, F., Razazi, K., de Prost, N., et al. (2020). Rescue therapy with inhaled nitric oxide and almitrine in COVID-19 patients with severe acute respiratory distress syndrome. *Ann. Intensive Care* 10:151. doi: 10.1186/s13613-020-00769-2

Bellani, G., Laffey, J. G., Pham, T., Fan, E., Brochard, L., Esteban, A., et al. (2016). Epidemiology, patterns of care, and mortality for patients with acute respiratory distress syndrome in intensive care units in 50 countries. *JAMA* 315, 788–800. doi: 10.1001/jama.2016.0291

Bleakley, C., Singh, S., Garfield, B., Morosin, M., Surkova, E., Mandalia, M. S., et al. (2021). Right ventricular dysfunction in critically ill COVID-19 ARDS. *Int. J. Cardiol.* 327, 251–258. doi: 10.1016/j.ijcard.2020.11.043

Brown, Z. E., Görges, M., Cooke, E., Malherbe, S., Dumont, G. A., and Ansermino, J. M. (2013). Changes in cardiac index and blood pressure on positioning children prone for scoliosis surgery. *Anaesthesia* 68, 742–746. doi: 10.1111/anae.12310

Brun-Buisson, C., Minelli, C., Bertolini, G., Brazzi, L., Pimentel, J., Lewandowski, K., et al. (2004). Epidemiology and outcome of acute lung injury in European intensive care units. Results from the ALIVE study. *Intensive Care Med.* 30, 51–61. doi: 10.1007/s00134-003-2022-6

Bull, T. M., Clark, B., McFann, K., and Moss, M. (2010). Pulmonary vascular dysfunction is associated with poor outcomes in patients with acute lung injury. *Am. J. Respir. Crit. Care Med.* 182, 1123–1128. doi: 10.1164/rccm.201002-0250OC

Chen, C., Lee, J., Johnson, A. E., Mark, R. G., Celi, L. A., and Danziger, J. (2017). Right ventricular function, peripheral edema, and acute kidney injury in critical illness. *Kidney Int. Rep.* 2, 1059–1065. doi: 10.1016/j.ekir.2017.05.017

Chen, K. P., Cavender, S., Lee, J., Feng, M., Mark, R. G., Celi, L. A., et al. (2016). Peripheral edema, central venous pressure, and risk of AKI in critical illness. *Clin. J. Am. Soc. Nephrol.* 11, 602–608. doi: 10.2215/CJN.08080715

Chiumello, D., Carlesso, E., Cadringher, P., Caironi, P., Valenza, F., Polli, F., et al. (2008). Lung stress and strain during mechanical ventilation for acute respiratory distress syndrome. *Am. J. Respir. Crit. Care Med.* 178, 346–355. doi: 10.1164/rccm.200710-1589OC

Chiumello, D., Cressoni, M., Racagni, M., Landi, L., Li Bassi, G., Polli, F., et al. (2006). Effects of thoraco-pelvic supports during prone position in patients with acute lung injury/acute respiratory distress syndrome: a physiological study. *Crit. Care Lond. Engl.* 10:R87. doi: 10.1186/cc4933

Combes, A., Hajage, D., Capellier, G., Demoule, A., Lavoué, S., Guervilly, C., et al. (2018). Extracorporeal membrane oxygenation for severe acute respiratory distress syndrome. *N. Engl. J. Med.* 378, 1965–1975. doi: 10.1056/NEJMoa1800385

Constantin, J.-M., Jabaudon, M., Lefrant, J.-Y., Jaber, S., Quenot, J.-P., Langeron, O., et al. (2019). Personalised mechanical ventilation tailored to lung morphology versus low positive end-expiratory pressure for patients with acute respiratory distress syndrome in France (the LIVE study): a multicentre, single-blind, randomised controlled trial. *Lancet Respir. Med.* 7, 870–880. doi: 10.1016/S2213-2600(19)30138-9

De Jong, A., Cossic, J., Verzilli, D., Monet, C., Carr, J., Conseil, M., et al. (2018). Impact of the driving pressure on mortality in obese and non-obese ARDS patients: a retrospective study of 362 cases. *Intensive Care Med.* 44, 1106–1114. doi: 10.1007/s00134-018-5241-6

Dres, M., Austin, P. C., Pham, T., Aegerter, P., Guidet, B., Demoule, A., et al. (2018). Acute respiratory distress syndrome cases volume and ICU mortality in medical patients. *Crit. Care Med.* 46, e33–e40. doi: 10.1097/CCM.0000000000002816

Duggan, M., McCaul, C. L., McNamara, P. J., Engelberts, D., Ackerley, C., and Kavanagh, B. P. (2003). Atelectasis causes vascular leak and lethal right ventricular failure in uninjured rat lungs. *Am. J. Respir. Crit. Care Med.* 167, 1633–1640. doi: 10.1164/rccm.200210-1215OC

Dweck, M. R., Bularga, A., Hahn, R. T., Bing, R., Lee, K. K., Chapman, A. R., et al. (2020). Global evaluation of echocardiography in patients with COVID-19. *Eur. Heart J. Cardiovasc. Imaging* 21, 949–958. doi: 10.1093/ehjci/jeaa178

Elzinga, G., Piene, H., and de Jong, J. P. (1980). Left and right ventricular pump function and consequences of having two pumps in one heart. A study on the isolated cat heart. *Circ. Res.* 46, 564–574. doi: 10.1161/01.res.46.4.564

Evrard, B., Goudelin, M., Montmagnon, N., Fedou, A.-L., Lafon, T., and Vignon, P. (2020). Cardiovascular phenotypes in ventilated patients with COVID-19 acute respiratory distress syndrome. *Crit. Care* 24:236. doi: 10.1186/s13054-020-02958-8

Ferguson, N. D., Fan, E., Camporota, L., Antonelli, M., Anzueto, A., Beale, R., et al. (2012). The Berlin definition of ARDS: an expanded rationale, justification, and supplementary material. *Intensive Care Med.* 38, 1573–1582. doi: 10.1007/s00134-012-2682-1

Garfield, B., McFadyen, C., Briar, C., Bleakley, C., Vlachou, A., Baldwin, M., et al. (2021). Potential for personalised application of inhaled nitric oxide in COVID-19 pneumonia. *Br. J. Anaesth.* 126, e72–e75. doi: 10.1016/j.bja.2020.11.006

Gattinoni, L., Caironi, P., Cressoni, M., Chiumello, D., Ranieri, V. M., Quintel, M., et al. (2006). Lung recruitment in patients with the acute respiratory distress syndrome. *N. Engl. J. Med.* 354, 1775–1786. doi: 10.1056/NEJMoa052052

Gattinoni, L., Chiumello, D., Carlesso, E., and Valenza, F. (2004). Bench-to-bedside review: chest wall elastance in acute lung injury/acute respiratory distress syndrome patients. *Crit. Care Lond. Engl.* 8, 350–355. doi: 10.1186/cc2854

Gattinoni, L., Marini, J. J., and Camporota, L. (2020). The respiratory drive: an overlooked tile of COVID-19 pathophysiology. *Am. J. Respir. Crit. Care Med.* 202, 1079–1080. doi: 10.1164/rccm.202008-3142ED

Gebistorf, F., Karam, O., Wetterslev, J., and Afshari, A. (2016). Inhaled nitric oxide for acute respiratory distress syndrome (ARDS) in children and adults. *Cochrane Database Syst. Rev.* 2016:CD002787. doi: 10.1002/14651858.CD002787.pub3

Ghignone, M., Girling, L., and Prewitt, R. M. (1984). Volume expansion versus norepinephrine in treatment of a low cardiac output complicating an acute increase in right ventricular afterload in dogs. *Anesthesiology* 60, 132–135. doi: 10.1097/00000542-198402000-00009

Guérin, C., Albert, R. K., Beitler, J., Gattinoni, L., Jaber, S., Marini, J. J., et al. (2020). Prone position in ARDS patients: why, when, how and for whom. *Intensive Care Med.* 46, 2385–2396. doi: 10.1007/s00134-020-06306-w

Guyton, A. C., Lindsey, A. W., Abernathy, B., and Richardson, T. (1957). Venous return at various right atrial pressures and the normal venous return curve. *Am. J. Physiol.* 189, 609–615. doi: 10.1152/ajplegacy.1957.189.3.609

Guyton, A. C., Lindsey, A. W., and Gilluly, J. J. (1954). The limits of right ventricular compensation following acute increase in pulmonary circulatory resistance. *Circ. Res.* 2, 326–332. doi: 10.1161/01.res.2.4.326

Jardin, F., Gueret, P., Dubourg, O., Farcot, J. C., Margairaz, A., and Bourdarias, J. P. (1985). Two-dimensional echocardiographic evaluation of right ventricular size and contractility in acute respiratory failure. *Crit. Care Med.* 13, 952–956. doi: 10.1097/00003246-198511000-00035

Jardin, F., and Vieillard-Baron, A. (2007). Is there a safe plateau pressure in ARDS? The right heart only knows. *Intensive Care Med.* 33, 444–447. doi: 10.1007/s00134-007-0552-z

Kiely, D. G., Cargill, R. I., and Lipworth, B. J. (1996). Effects of hypercapnia on hemodynamic, inotropic, lusitropic, and electrophysiologic indices in humans. *Chest* 109, 1215–1221. doi: 10.1378/chest.109.5.1215

Kumar, A., Falke, K. J., Geffin, B., Aldredge, C. F., Laver, M. B., Lowenstein, E., et al. (1970). Continuous positive-pressure ventilation in acute respiratory failure: effects on hemodynamics and lung function. *N. Engl. J. Med.* 283, 1430–1436. doi: 10.1056/NEJM197012242832603

Laks, M. M., Garner, D., and Swan, H. J. (1967). Volumes and compliances measured simultaneously in the right and left ventricles of the dog. *Circ. Res.* 20, 565–569. doi: 10.1161/01.res.20.5.565

Lazzeri, C., Bonizzoli, M., Cianchi, G., Batacchi, S., Guetti, C., Cozzolino, M., et al. (2018). Right ventricular dysfunction and pre implantation vasopressors in refractory ARDS supported by VV-ECMO. *Heart Lung Circ.* 27, 1483–1488. doi: 10.1016/j.hlc.2017.10.011

Longobardo, A., Montanari, C., Shulman, R., Benhalim, S., Singer, M., and Arulkumaran, N. (2021). Inhaled nitric oxide minimally improves oxygenation in COVID-19 related acute respiratory distress syndrome. *Br. J. Anaesth.* 126, e44–e46. doi: 10.1016/j.bja.2020.10.011

McNamee, J. J., Gillies, M. A., Barrett, N. A., Perkins, G. D., Tunnicliffe, W., Young, D., et al. (2021). Effect of lower tidal volume ventilation facilitated by extracorporeal carbon dioxide removal vs standard care ventilation on 90-day mortality in patients with acute hypoxemic respiratory failure: the rest randomized clinical trial. *JAMA* 326:1013. doi: 10.1001/jama.2021.13374

Mekontso Dessap, A., Boissier, F., Charron, C., Bégot, E., Repessé, X., Legras, A., et al. (2016). Acute cor pulmonale during protective ventilation for acute respiratory distress syndrome: prevalence, predictors, and clinical impact. *Intensive Care Med.* 42, 862–870. doi: 10.1007/s00134-015-4141-2

Mekontso Dessap, A., Boissier, F., Leon, R., Carreira, S., Campo, F. R., Lemaire, F., et al. (2010). Prevalence and prognosis of shunting across patent foramen ovale during acute respiratory distress syndrome. *Crit. Care Med.* 38, 1786–1792. doi: 10.1097/CCM.0b013e3181eaa9c8

Miranda, D. R., van Thiel, R., Brodie, D., and Bakker, J. (2015). Right ventricular unloading after initiation of venovenous extracorporeal membrane oxygenation. *Am. J. Respir. Crit. Care Med.* 191, 346–348. doi: 10.1164/rccm.201408-1404LE

Morelli, A., Teboul, J.-L., Maggiore, S. M., Vieillard-Baron, A., Rocco, M., Conti, G., et al. (2006). Effects of levosimendan on right ventricular afterload in patients with acute respiratory distress syndrome: a pilot study. *Crit. Care Med.* 34, 2287–2293. doi: 10.1097/01.CCM.0000230244.17174.4F

Morimont, P., Guiot, J., Desaive, T., Tchana-Sato, V., Janssen, N., Cagnina, A., et al. (2015). Veno-venous extracorporeal CO2 removal improves pulmonary hemodynamics in a porcine ARDS model. *Acta Anaesthesiol. Scand.* 59, 448–456. doi: 10.1111/aas.12497

Nuckton, T. J., Alonso, J. A., Kallet, R. H., Daniel, B. M., Pittet, J.-F., Eisner, M. D., et al. (2002). Pulmonary dead-space fraction as a risk factor for death in the acute respiratory distress syndrome. *N. Engl. J. Med.* 346, 1281–1286. doi: 10.1056/NEJMoa012835

Page, B., Vieillard-Baron, A., Beauchet, A., Aegerter, P., Prin, S., and Jardin, F. (2003). Low stretch ventilation strategy in acute respiratory distress syndrome:

eight years of clinical experience in a single center. *Crit. Care Med.* 31, 765–769. doi: 10.1097/01.CCM.0000055402.68581.DC

Papazian, L., Aubron, C., Brochard, L., Chiche, J.-D., Combes, A., Dreyfuss, D., et al. (2019). Formal guidelines: management of acute respiratory distress syndrome. *Ann. Intensive Care* 9:69. doi: 10.1186/s13613-019-0540-9

Patterson, S. W., and Starling, E. H. (1914). On the mechanical factors which determine the output of the ventricles. *J. Physiol.* 48, 357–379. doi: 10.1113/jphysiol.1914.sp001669

Petit, M., Mekontso-Dessap, A., Masi, P., Legras, A., Vignon, P., and Vieillard-Baron, A. (2021). Evaluation of right ventricular function and driving pressure with blood gas analysis could better select patients eligible for VV ECMO in severe ARDS. *Crit. Care* 25:220. doi: 10.1186/s13054-021-03646-x

Phua, J., Badia, J. R., Adhikari, N. K. J., Friedrich, J. O., Fowler, R. A., Singh, J. M., et al. (2009). Has mortality from acute respiratory distress syndrome decreased over time?: a systematic review. *Am. J. Respir. Crit. Care Med.* 179, 220–227. doi: 10.1164/rccm.200805-722OC

Prewitt, R. M., and Ghignone, M. (1983). Treatment of right ventricular dysfunction in acute respiratory failure. *Crit. Care Med.* 11, 346–352. doi: 10.1097/00003246-198305000-00005

Price, L. C., McAuley, D. F., Marino, P. S., Finney, S. J., Griffiths, M. J., and Wort, S. J. (2012). Pathophysiology of pulmonary hypertension in acute lung injury. *Am. J. Physiol. Lung Cell. Mol. Physiol.* 302, L803–L815. doi: 10.1152/ajplung.00355.2011

Puybasset, L., Cluzel, P., Gusman, P., Grenier, P., Preteux, F., and Rouby, J. J. (2000). Regional distribution of gas and tissue in acute respiratory distress syndrome. I. Consequences for lung morphology. CT Scan ARDS Study group. *Intensive Care Med.* 26, 857–869. doi: 10.1007/s001340051274

Redington, A. N., Rigby, M. L., Shinebourne, E. A., and Oldershaw, P. J. (1990). Changes in the pressure-volume relation of the right ventricle when its loading conditions are modified. *Br. Heart J.* 63, 45–49. doi: 10.1136/hrt.63.1.45

Ridge, C. A., Desai, S. R., Jeyin, N., Mahon, C., Lother, D. L., Mirsadraee, S., et al. (2020). Dual-energy CT pulmonary angiography (DECTPA) quantifies vasculopathy in severe COVID-19 pneumonia. *Radiol. Cardiothorac. Imaging* 2:e200428. doi: 10.1148/ryct.2020200428

Robba, C., Ball, L., Battaglini, D., Cardim, D., Moncalvo, E., Brunetti, I., et al. (2021). Early effects of ventilatory rescue therapies on systemic and cerebral oxygenation in mechanically ventilated COVID-19 patients with acute respiratory distress syndrome: a prospective observational study. *Crit. Care* 25:111. doi: 10.1186/s13054-021-03537-1

Scharf, S. M., Brown, R., Saunders, N., Green, L. H., and Ingram, R. H. (1979). Changes in canine left ventricular size and configuration with positive end-expiratory pressure. *Circ. Res.* 44, 672–678. doi: 10.1161/01.RES.44.5.672

Schmidt, M., Pham, T., Arcadipane, A., Agerstrand, C., Ohshimo, S., Pellegrino, V., et al. (2019). Mechanical ventilation management during extracorporeal membrane oxygenation for acute respiratory distress syndrome. An International Multicenter Prospective Cohort. *Am. J. Respir. Crit. Care Med.* 200, 1002–1012. doi: 10.1164/rccm.201806-1094OC

Schmidt, M., Tachon, G., Devilliers, C., Muller, G., Hekimian, G., Bréchot, N., et al. (2013). Blood oxygenation and decarboxylation determinants during venovenous ECMO for respiratory failure in adults. *Intensive Care Med.* 39, 838–846. doi: 10.1007/s00134-012-2785-8

Schmitt, J.-M., Vieillard-Baron, A., Augarde, R., Prin, S., Page, B., and Jardin, F. (2001). Positive end-expiratory pressure titration in acute respiratory distress syndrome patients: impact on right ventricular outflow impedance evaluated by pulmonary artery Doppler flow velocity measurements. *Crit. Care Med.* 29, 1154–1158. doi: 10.1097/00003246-200106000-00012

Snow, R. L., Davies, P., Pontoppidan, H., Zapol, W. M., and Reid, L. (1982). Pulmonary vascular remodeling in adult respiratory distress syndrome. *Am. Rev. Respir. Dis.* 126, 887–892. doi: 10.1164/arrd.1982.126.5.887

Soulat-Dufour, L., Fauvel, C., Weizman, O., Barbe, T., Pezel, T., Mika, D., et al. (2021). Prognostic value of right ventricular dilatation in patients with COVID-19: a multicentre study. *Eur. Heart J. Cardiovasc. Imaging* [Epub ahead of print]. doi: 10.1093/ehjci/jeab067

Thompson, B. T., Chambers, R. C., and Liu, K. D. (2017). Acute respiratory distress syndrome. *N. Engl. J. Med.* 377, 562–572. doi: 10.1056/NEJMra1608077

Vieillard-Baron, A., Charron, C., Caille, V., Belliard, G., Page, B., and Jardin, F. (2007). Prone positioning unloads the right ventricle in severe ARDS. *Chest* 132, 1440–1446. doi: 10.1378/chest.07-1013

Vieillard-Baron, A., Loubieres, Y., Schmitt, J. M., Page, B., Dubourg, O., and Jardin, F. (1999). Cyclic changes in right ventricular output impedance during mechanical ventilation. *J. Appl. Physiol. Bethesda Md* 87, 1644–1650. doi: 10.1152/jappl.1999.87.5.1644

Vieillard-Baron, A., Matthay, M., Teboul, J. L., Bein, T., Schultz, M., Magder, S., et al. (2016). Experts' opinion on management of hemodynamics in ARDS patients: focus on the effects of mechanical ventilation. *Intensive Care Med.* 42, 739–749. doi: 10.1007/s00134-016-4326-3

Vieillard-Baron, A., Naeije, R., Haddad, F., Bogaard, H. J., Bull, T. M., Fletcher, N., et al. (2018). Diagnostic workup, etiologies and management of acute right ventricle failure: a state-of-the-art paper. *Intensive Care Med.* 44, 774–790. doi: 10.1007/s00134-018-5172-2

Vieillard-Baron, A., Price, L. C., and Matthay, M. A. (2013). Acute cor pulmonale in ARDS. *Intensive Care Med.* 39, 1836–1838. doi: 10.1007/s00134-013-3045-2

Vieillard-Baron, A., Prin, S., Chergui, K., Dubourg, O., and Jardin, F. (2003). Hemodynamic instability in sepsis: bedside assessment by Doppler echocardiography. *Am. J. Respir. Crit. Care Med.* 168, 1270–1276. doi: 10.1164/rccm.200306-816CC

Vieillard-Baron, A., Schmitt, J. M., Augarde, R., Fellahi, J. L., Prin, S., Page, B., et al. (2001). Acute cor pulmonale in acute respiratory distress syndrome submitted to protective ventilation: incidence, clinical implications, and prognosis. *Crit. Care Med.* 29, 1551–1555. doi: 10.1097/00003246-200108000-00009

Vlahakes, G. J., Turley, K., and Hoffman, J. I. (1981). The pathophysiology of failure in acute right ventricular hypertension: hemodynamic and biochemical correlations. *Circulation* 63, 87–95. doi: 10.1161/01.CIR.63.1.87

West, J. B., Dollery, C. T., and Naimark, A. (1964). Distribution of blood flow in isolated lung; relation to vascular and alveolar pressures. *J. Appl. Physiol.* 19, 713–724. doi: 10.1152/jappl.1964.19.4.713

Whittenberger, J. L., McGREGOR, M., Berglund, E., and Borst, H. G. (1960). Influence of state of inflation of the lung on pulmonary vascular resistance. *J. Appl. Physiol.* 15, 878–882. doi: 10.1152/jappl.1960.15.5.878

Writing Group for the Alveolar Recruitment for Acute Respiratory Distress Syndrome Trial (ART) Investigators (2017). Effect of lung recruitment and titrated positive end-expiratory pressure (PEEP) vs low PEEP on mortality in patients with acute respiratory distress syndrome: a randomized clinical trial. *JAMA* 318, 1335–1345. doi: 10.1001/jama.2017.14171

Yamamoto, Y., Nakano, H., Ide, H., Ogasa, T., Takahashi, T., Osanai, S., et al. (2001). Role of airway nitric oxide on the regulation of pulmonary circulation by carbon dioxide. *J. Appl. Physiol.* 91, 1121–1130. doi: 10.1152/jappl.2001.91.3.1121

4

Effects of Different Levels of Variability and Pressure Support Ventilation on Lung Function in Patients with Mild–Moderate Acute Respiratory Distress Syndrome

Lorenzo Ball [1,2], Yuda Sutherasan [3], Martina Fiorito [1], Antonella Dall'Orto [1], Lorenzo Maiello [1], Maria Vargas [4], Chiara Robba [1,2], Iole Brunetti [2], Davide D'Antini [1,5], Pasquale Raimondo [1,5], Robert Huhle [6], Marcus J. Schultz [6,7,8†], Patricia R. M. Rocco [9†], Marcelo Gama de Abreu [10†] and Paolo Pelosi [1,2†]*

[1] Department of Surgical Sciences and Integrated Diagnostics, University of Genoa, Genoa, Italy, [2] Anesthesia and Intensive Care, Ospedale Policlinico San Martino Istituto di Ricerca e Cura a Carattere Scientifico (IRCCS) for Oncology and Neurosciences, Genova, Italy, [3] Division of Pulmonary and Pulmonary Critical Care Medicine, Department of Medicine, Ramathibodi Hospital, Mahidol University, Bangkok, Thailand, [4] Department of Neurosciences, Reproductive and Odonthostomatological Sciences, University of Naples Federico II, Naples, Italy, [5] Department of Anaesthesia and Intensive Care, University of Foggia, Foggia, Italy, [6] Mahidol Oxford Tropical Medicine Research Unit (MORU), Mahidol University, Bangkok, Thailand, [7] Department of Intensive Care, Laboratory of Experimental Intensive Care and Anesthesiology (LEICA), Amsterdam University Medical Centers, Location Academic Medical Center (AMC), Amsterdam, Netherlands, [8] Nuffield Department of Medicine, Oxford University, Oxford, United Kingdom, [9] Laboratory of Pulmonary Investigation, Carlos Chagas Filho Institute of Biophysics, Federal University of Rio de Janeiro, Rio de Janeiro, Brazil, [10] Pulmonary Engineering Group, Department of Anaesthesiology and Intensive Care Medicine, University Hospital Carl Gustav Carus, Technische Universität Dresden, Dresden, Germany

***Correspondence:**
Lorenzo Ball
lorenzo.ball@unige.it

† These authors share senior authorship

Background: Variable pressure support ventilation (vPSV) is an assisted ventilation mode that varies the level of pressure support on a breath-by-breath basis to restore the physiological variability of breathing activity. We aimed to compare the effects of vPSV at different levels of variability and pressure support (ΔP_S) in patients with acute respiratory distress syndrome (ARDS).

Methods: This study was a crossover randomized clinical trial. We included patients with mild to moderate ARDS already ventilated in conventional pressure support ventilation (PSV). The study consisted of two blocks of interventions, and variability during vPSV was set as the coefficient of variation of the ΔP_S level. In the first block, the effects of three levels of variability were tested at constant ΔP_S: 0% ($PSV_{0\%}$, conventional PSV), 15% ($vPSV_{15\%}$), and 30% ($vPSV_{30\%}$). In the second block, two levels of variability (0% and variability set to achieve ±5 cmH_2O variability) were tested at two ΔP_S levels (baseline ΔP_S and ΔP_S reduced by 5 cmH_2O from baseline). The following four ventilation strategies were tested in the second block: PSV with baseline ΔP_S and 0% variability (PSV_{BL}) or ±5 cmH_2O variability ($vPSV_{BL}$), PSV with ΔP_S reduced by 5 cmH_2O and 0% variability (PSV_{-5}) or ±5 cmH_2O variability ($vPSV_{-5}$). Outcomes included gas exchange, respiratory mechanics, and patient-ventilator asynchronies.

Results: The study enrolled 20 patients. In the first block of interventions, oxygenation and respiratory mechanics parameters did not differ between $vPSV_{15\%}$ and $vPSV_{30\%}$

compared with $PSV_{0\%}$. The variability of tidal volume (V_T) was higher with $vPSV_{15\%}$ and $vPSV_{30\%}$ compared with $PSV_{0\%}$. The incidence of asynchronies and the variability of transpulmonary pressure (P_L) were higher with $vPSV_{30\%}$ compared with $PSV_{0\%}$. In the second block of interventions, different levels of pressure support with and without variability did not change oxygenation. The variability of V_T and P_L was higher with $vPSV_{-5}$ compared with PSV_{-5}, but not with $vPSV_{BL}$ compared with PSV_{BL}.

Conclusion: In patients with mild-moderate ARDS, the addition of variability did not improve oxygenation at different pressure support levels. Moreover, high variability levels were associated with worse patient-ventilator synchrony.

Keywords: variable pressure support ventilation, acute respiratory distress (ARDS), asynchronies, respiratory mechanic, assisted ventilation

INTRODUCTION

Pressure support ventilation (PSV) is an assisted ventilation mode commonly used in critically ill patients (Esteban et al., 2013). The maintenance of spontaneous respiratory activity in acute respiratory distress syndrome (ARDS) patients improves respiratory function and decreases the need for vasopressor and sedative drugs (Putensen et al., 2001). Assisted ventilation modes have been commonly used in the management of patients with ARDS, in particular those with mild to moderate hypoxemic respiratory failure (Bellani et al., 2016).

In the last years, researchers have proposed to vary the level of pressure support on a breath-by-breath basis to restore the physiological variability of breathing activity (Tobin et al., 1988). Variable pressure support ventilation (vPSV), compared with conventional PSV, improved oxygenation in the experimental models of ARDS (Gama de Abreu et al., 2008) and ventilator-patient synchrony in a small pilot study in critically ill patients with acute respiratory failure (Spieth et al., 2013). These effects could be mediated by an amelioration of the ventilation-perfusion matching (Huhle et al., 2016), as well as a recruitment effect due to the repetitive delivery of breaths with a higher tidal volume, which might also result in a reduction of lung inhomogeneity (Mauri et al., 2017). However, so far, the only clinical study published has used only one variability level at fixed pressure support (ΔP_S) (Spieth et al., 2013). Therefore, the effects of different levels of variability and the impact of variability at different ΔP_S levels remain unknown. Different levels of variability might modify differently the ventilation perfusion-matching and might affect differently gas exchange and respiratory mechanics.

The aim of this study was to evaluate the effects of vPSV, at different levels of variability and pressure support, on short-term lung function parameters in patients with mild to moderate ARDS. We tested the hypothesis that vPSV would improve gas exchange, respiratory mechanics, and patient-ventilator asynchrony. We also hypothesized that the degree of variability and the level of ΔP_S would influence the effects of vPSV.

METHODS

Study Design

This was a prospective, crossover, randomized clinical trial conducted in a single university hospital intensive care unit (ICU).

Inclusion and Exclusion Criteria

Patients aged >18 years with mild to moderate ARDS (PaO_2/FIO_2 ratio between 100 and 300 mmHg with a positive end-expiratory pressure, PEEP $\geq$5 cmH_2O) already receiving PSV per clinical indication were screened for inclusion. Exclusion criteria were pregnancy, chronic obstructive pulmonary disease, presence of pneumothorax or chest tubes, and unavailability of research staff.

Interventions

According to the local clinical practice, conventional PSV was delivered by an Evita Infinity V500 ventilator (Dräger Medical AG, Lübeck, Germany) targeting a V_T of 6–8 ml/kg of predicted body weight, respiratory rate $\leq$25 min^{-1} with PEEP and FIO_2 titrated to achieve a peripheral oxygen saturation $\geq$92%. This ventilator can operate in vPSV mode setting the variability of the ΔP_S and delivers breaths with an approximately Gaussian distribution, truncated at 3 SDs from the mean ΔP_S. The parameter "variability" of this ventilator refers to the range of ΔP_S, e.g., 90% "variability" results in a 30% coefficient

---

Abbreviations: PSV, pressure support ventilation; ARDS, acute respiratory distress syndrome; vPSV, variable pressure support ventilation; ΔP_S, pressure support level; ICU, intensive care unit; PEEP, positive end-expiratory pressure; PBW, predicted body weight; SAPS, simplified acute physiology score; SOFA, sequential organ failure assessment score; RASS, richmond agitation-sedation scale; $PSV_{0\%}$, pressure support ventilation with no variability; $vPSV_{15\%}$, variable pressure support ventilation with 15% CV variability; $vPSV_{30\%}$, variable pressure support ventilation with 30% CV variability; V_T, tidal volume; PTP, esophageal pressure-time product; ΔP_{es}, esophageal pressure swings; P_L, peak transpulmonary pressure; PSV_{BL}, pressure support ventilation with no variability and baseline ΔP_S as per clinical indication; $vPSV_{BL}$, variable pressure support with variability set to achieve ±5 cmH_2O and baseline ΔP_S as per clinical indication; PSV_{-5}, pressure support ventilation with no variability and ΔP_S reduced by 5 cmH_2O from the baseline value; $vPSV_{-5}$, variable pressure support ventilation with variability set to achieve ±5 cmH_2O and ΔP_S reduced by 5 cmH_2O from the baseline value.

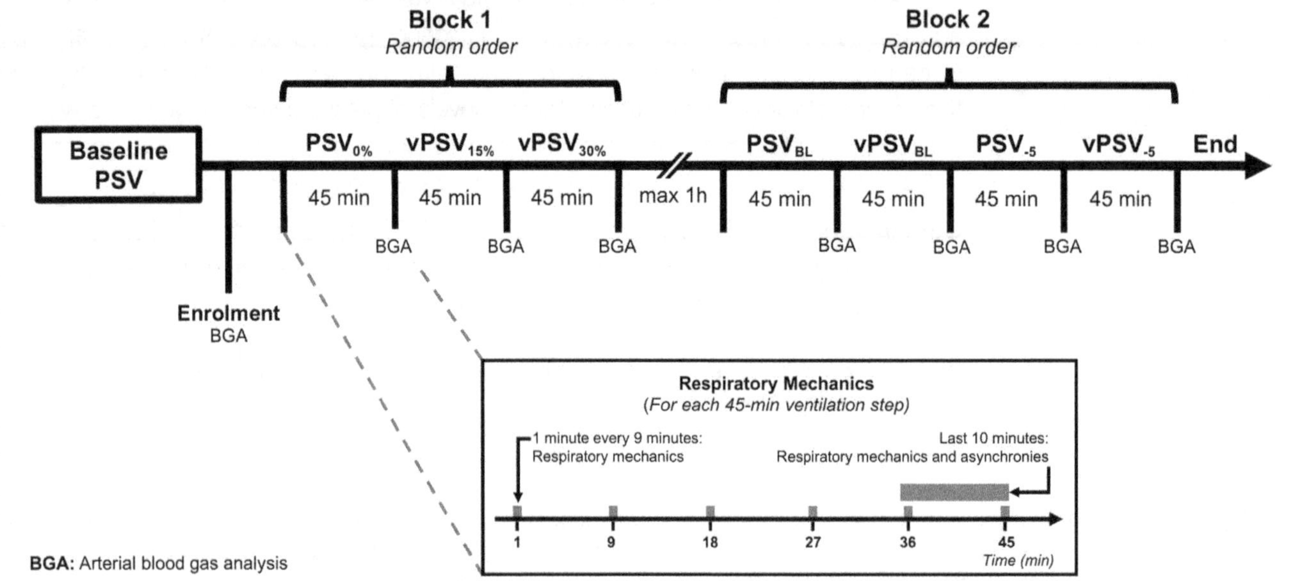

FIGURE 1 | Time course of interventions. Within each intervention block, different ventilation settings were delivered in random order. $PSV_{0\%}$, conventional PSV ventilation with no variability; $vPSV_{15\%}$, variable PSV with variability set to 15% CV; $vPSV_{30\%}$, variable PSV with variability set to 30% CV; PSV_{BL}, PSV with no variability and baseline ΔP_S as per clinical indication; $vPSV_{BL}$, variable pressure support with variability set to achieve ±5 cmH_2O and baseline ΔP_S as per clinical indication; PSV_{-5}, PSV with no variability and ΔP_S reduced by 5 cmH_2O from the baseline value; $vPSV_{-5}$, variable PSV with variability set to achieve ±5 cmH_2O and ΔP_S reduced by 5 cmH_2O from the baseline value; PSV, pressure support ventilation; CV, coefficient of variation.

of variation (CV). As illustrated in **Figure 1**, all patients underwent two blocks of interventions, receiving 45-min periods of ventilation with different settings. In the first block, the effects of three levels of variability were tested at constant ΔP_S to explore the effect of variability added to a fixed ΔP_S level, while in the second block, a variability of ±5 cmH_2O was added to ΔP_S set at either the baseline level or the baseline level minus 5 cmH_2O, to investigate the effects of variability at two ΔP_S levels. During the first block, the ΔP_S was set at a fixed value corresponding to the level chosen by the treating clinician before enrolment, and three different CV% levels were used: 0% ($PSV_{0\%}$), 15% ($vPSV_{15\%}$), and 30% ($vPSV_{30\%}$). During the second block, four ventilation settings were used: PSV with baseline ΔP_S (PSV_{BL}), baseline ΔP_S with variability set individually to ±5 cmH_2O ($vPSV_{BL}$), ΔP_S reduced by 5 cmH_2O compared with the baseline with either no variability (PSV_{-5}) or variability set to ±5 cmH_2O ($vPSV_{-5}$). The two blocks were performed sequentially, within 1 h from each other to allow for nursing assistance if required, and ventilation modes within each intervention block were assigned in random order with a Latin square design (as shown in **Figure 1**; **Supplementary Figures 1, 2**). The randomization sequence was generated with an online service, and a sealed envelope was opened at the moment of patient enrolment. Participants were blinded to the treatment assignment as were the operators involved in respiratory mechanics analysis.

Patient management procedures not related to mechanical ventilation, including sedation and fluid administration, were at the discretion of the treating clinician. When clinically feasible, we avoided changing FIO_2, PEEP, and ΔP_S during the study, and in case of desaturation below 92%, FIO_2 increase was prioritized over PEEP increase. After completion of the study protocol, ventilation was continued at the discretion of the treating physician.

Measurements

An esophageal balloon catheter (Compliance catheter, Microtek Medical B.V., Zutphen, The Netherlands) was inserted through the nose or mouth, filled with 1.5 ml, and correct positioning was verified with an occlusion maneuver (Akoumianaki et al., 2014). The flow was measured with a heated Fleisch-type pneumotachograph connected to a multi-channel transducer (ICU Lab, KleisTEK Engineering, Bari, Italy), while the tidal volume was measured as the integral of flow over time. Respiratory traces were recorded continuously throughout the study. An arterial blood gas analysis, heart rate, and invasive mean arterial pressure were recorded at baseline and the end of each ventilation step.

Pressure-time and flow-time curves were analyzed offline with a dedicated script written in MATLAB (MathWorks, MA, USA). The following parameters were computed breath by breath: V_T, PEEP, ΔP_S, mean airway pressure, inspiratory time to total time ratio (T_{insp}/T_{tot}), respiratory rate (RR), esophageal pressure swings (ΔP_{es}), and peak transpulmonary pressure (P_L). The respiratory muscle activity was quantified with the esophageal pressure-time product per min (PTP_{es}), calculated as follows (Mauri et al., 2016):

$$PTP_{es,min} = RR \cdot \int P_{mus}\, dt = RR \cdot \int (P_{cw,recoil} - P_{es})\, dt$$

where P_{mus} is the pressure generated by the respiratory muscles, and $P_{cw,recoil}$ is the chest wall recoil pressure, calculated assuming a fixed elastance of 5 cmH_2O/L. The asynchrony index was computed as the number of asynchronous events divided by the total number of ventilator cycles plus ineffective efforts during expiration multiplied by 100 (Blanch et al., 2015). Asynchronies were classified independently by two experienced operators (LB and MV), and discrepancies were resolved by consensus. The analysis of respiratory mechanics data was performed by three operators blinded to the ventilation settings (ADO, MF, and LM). Also, we measured the evolution of respiratory mechanics at min 1, 9, 18, 27, 36, and 45 from the start of each ventilation step. To allow sufficient time for patient adaptation, main analyses of respiratory mechanics and asynchronies were restricted to the last 10 min of each ventilation step.

Data Analysis and Sample Size Calculation

All variables are reported as medians [25th–75th percentile], if not otherwise specified. Measurements on multiple breaths were aggregated within-patients computing the median and the CV; then, between-patients medians [25th–75th percentile] were computed. Comparisons between continuous variables during the different ventilation steps were sought with Friedman's test and Dunn's *post-hoc* test. The primary endpoint was the partial pressure of arterial oxygen to FiO_2 ratio (PaO_2/FiO_2). From internal administrative data, we expected a baseline PaO_2/FiO_2 around 150 ± 50 mmHg. Using a Latin square crossover design, and assuming an intra-subject correlation of the PaO_2/FiO_2 between treatments with $\rho = 0.75$, we needed to enroll at least 16 patients to achieve 90% power (1-β) to detect a 20% relative increase in the PaO_2/FiO_2 ratio (Muller and Barton, 1989; Muller et al., 1992). To account for potential drop-off or missing respiratory mechanics data, we aimed to enroll 20 patients. Repeated measurement analysis of respiratory mechanics parameters at different timepoints within each ventilation block was performed using mixed-effects linear models using patients as random effects and timepoint, ventilation, and their interaction as fixed effects.

In one *post-hoc* analysis, associations were determined between the respiratory mechanics parameters of each breath and the ΔP_S received during the preceding breath in the $vPSV_{BL}$ and $vPSV_{-5}$ ventilation steps. For this purpose, mixed-effects linear models were used, using patients as random effects and the ΔP_S received during the preceding breath as the fixed effect.

All analyses were performed with R 3.2.3 (The R Foundation for Statistical Computing, www.r-project.org). Statistical significance was considered for two-tailed $p < 0.05$.

TABLE 1 | Baseline characteristics of patients.

Patient characteristics	
Number of patients	20
Age (years)	72 [59–79]
Female sex (N, %)	6/20 (30%)
Weight (kg)	80 [64–87]
Height (cm)	175 [165–180]
Body mass index (kg/m^2)	25.8 [22.7–29.5]
PBW (kg)	71 [58–75]
SAPS II	53 [38–60]
SOFA	7 [6–9]
RASS	−3 [−3 to −1]
Sedative drugs (N, %)	Propofol 5/20 (25%) Dexmedetomidine 3/20 (15%) Midazolam 4/20 (20%) None 8/20 (40%)
Analgesic drugs (N, %)	Fentanyl 8/20 (40%) Morphine 2/20 (10%) None 10/20 (50%)
Days of ventilation prior to inclusion	7 [5–9]
Primary reason for admission to the ICU	Acute respiratory failure: 10 (50%) Multiple trauma: 4 (20%) Brain hemorrhage: 3 (15%) Post-cardiac arrest: 3 (15%)
Risk factor for development of ARDS	Pneumonia: 11 (55%) Multiple fractures: 2 (10%) Sepsis: 4 (20%) Aspiration pneumonia: 3 (15%)
Blood gas analysis at enrolment PaO_2 (mmHg)	97 [79–120]
$PaCO_2$ (mmHg)	40 [36–46]
pHa	7.46 [7.44–7.51]
PaO_2/FIO_2 ratio (mmHg)	198 [154–250]
Ventilator settings at enrolment	
ΔP_S (cmH_2O)	15 [14–17]
PEEP (cmH_2O)	6 [5–8]
FIO_2 (%)	50 [43–58]
Tidal volume (mL/kg of PBW)	7.5 [7.0–8.5]
Respiratory rate (min^{-1})	15 [13–20]

PBW, predicted body weight; PEEP, positive end-expiratory pressure; ΔP_S, pressure support; SAPS, simplified acute physiology score; SOFA, sequential organ failure assessment score; RASS, richmond agitation-sedation scale; ICU, intensive care unit.

RESULTS

Twenty patients were enrolled and completed the study. Baseline characteristics are presented in **Table 1**. The FiO_2 and PEEP were kept constant during the study in all patients; one patient required ΔP_S reduction between ventilation block 1 and block 2 according to the treating clinician decision for reasons unrelated to the study procedures. **Tables 2, 3** show respiratory mechanics, hemodynamics, and arterial blood gas analysis in ventilation blocks 1 and 2, respectively. The distribution of key respiratory mechanics parameters in ventilation blocks 1 and 2 is illustrated in **Figures 2, 3**, respectively. **Supplementary Figures 3–11** report details the evolution over time of the respiratory mechanics parameters in the different ventilation steps.

Block 1: Physiological Effects of Different Variability Levels at Constant ΔP_S

The PaO_2/FiO_2 did not differ between ventilation steps in block 1 ($p = 0.62$, **Table 2**). Median respiratory mechanics variables, other gas exchange, and hemodynamic parameters did not

TABLE 2 | Gas exchange, hemodynamics, and respiratory mechanics in patients during pressure support ventilation at different levels of variability (Block 1).

	Ventilation modes			*p*-values		
	$PSV_{0\%}$	$vPSV_{15\%}$	$vPSV_{30\%}$	Overall	$vPSV_{15\%}$ vs. $PSV_{0\%}$	$vPSV_{30\%}$ vs. $PSV_{0\%}$
Ventilation settings						
$\Delta P_{S,set}$ (cmH_2O)	15.0 [13.0–16.0]	15.0 [13.0–16.0]	15.0 [13.0–16.0]	>0.99		
ΔP_S set variability (CV %)	0	15	30	<0.001		
Gas exchange						
PaO_2/FIO_2 (mmHg)	209 [157–242]	214 [160–256]	210 [179–252]	0.62		
PaO_2 (mmHg)	96 [79–118]	98 [85–116]	108 [82–123]	0.62		
$PaCO_2$ (mmHg)	44 [37–46]	43 [38–46]	43 [37–48]	0.95		
pH	7.45 [7.43–7.49]	7.49 [7.43–7.50]	7.47 [7.44–7.50]	0.64		
Hemodynamics						
Heart rate (min^{-1})	85 [72–92]	83 [75–90]	83 [73–91]	0.46		
Mean arterial pressure (mmHg)	78 [68–96]	79 [73–91]	82 [70–90]	0.37		
Respiratory mechanics						
$\Delta P_{S,measured}$ (cmH_2O)	14.6 [12.5–15.7]	14.6 [12.7–16.0]	14.7 [12.6–16.5]	0.39		
$PS_{measured}$ (CV, %)	1.2 [0.7–2.0]	15.6 [15.0–17.2][a]	29.7 [27.5–31.5][a]	<0.001	0.006	<0.001
Total PEEP (cmH_2O)	7.2 [6.1–8.5]	7.4 [6.2–8.6]	7.5 [6.2–8.4]	0.09		
Total PEEP (CV, %)	2.2 [1.1–3.1]	2.2 [1.2–3.8]	2.6 [1.7–3.3][a]	0.034	0.40	0.026
P_{mean} (cmH_2O)	11.6 [9.9–12.6]	12.1 [10.1–12.9]	11.6 [10.4–12.8]	0.16		
P_{mean} (CV, %)	3.7 [3.0–6.0]	8.1 [5.8–9.6][a]	13.2 [10.2–15.5][a]	<0.001	0.016	<0.001
Respiratory rate (min^{-1})	16.7 [13.7–21.4]	16.8 [13.9–21.4]	15.6 [13.8–19.7]	0.86		
Respiratory rate (CV, %)	11.6 [9.2–15.8]	12.5 [10.3–22.4]	17.9 [15.8–24.9][a]	0.002	0.17	<0.001
V_T (ml/kg of PBW)	8.1 [7.3–10.0]	8.8 [7.0–10.7]	8.9 [7.2–10.1]	0.95		
V_T (CV, %)	6.7 [4.5–9.1]	13.1 [10.7–14.4][a]	23.8 [17.8–28.1][a]	<0.001	0.006	<0.001
T_{insp}/T_{tot}	0.34 [0.29–0.41]	0.37 [0.32–0.41]	0.37 [0.30–0.43]	0.35		
T_{insp}/T_{tot} (CV, %)	11.1 [7.4–15.1]	10.9 [9.6–16.3]	14.6 [12.3–21.0]	0.08		
PTP_{es} (cmH_2O s min^{-1})	126 [102–226]	154 [103–194]	136 [121–208]	0.95		
PTP_{es} (CV, %)	26.8 [15.6–39.2]	30.1 [17.0–47.6]	36.2 [25.9–58.2][a]	0.029	0.71	0.026
ΔP_{es} (cmH_2O)	5.0 [2.1–7.6]	3.0 [1.3–7.4]	2.7 [1.6–5.4]	0.10		
ΔP_{es} (CV, %)	23.2 [18.0–34.2]	26.8 [19.7–40.9]	26.8 [24.3–47.5]	0.07		
P_L (cmH_2O)	18.0 [16.9–21.4]	17.8 [16.0–21.9]	17.4 [15.9–20.2]	0.27		
P_L (CV, %)	4.5 [2.7–11.7]	14.7 [13.2–15.9][a]	25.8 [21.4–27.3][a]	<0.001	0.025	<0.001
Asynchrony index (%)	1.6 [0.6–10.5]	2.2 [0.5–16.3]	5.1 [1.0–17.4][a]	0.031	0.21	0.019

Values are computed during the last 10 min of a 45-min ventilation period. Data are reported as inter-subject median [25th–75th percentile] of the intra-subject median values.
[a]Significantly different from $PSV_{0\%}$. $PSV_{0\%}$, pressure support ventilation with no variability; $vPSV_{15\%}$, variable pressure support ventilation with 15% CV variability; $vPSV_{30\%}$, variable pressure support ventilation with 30% CV variability.
CV, coefficient of variation; PEEP, positive end-expiratory pressure; PBW, predicted body weight; ΔP_S, pressure support; V_T, tidal volume; PTP, esophageal pressure-time product; ΔP_{es}, esophageal pressure swings; P_L, peak transpulmonary pressure.

change between $vPSV_{15\%}$ and $vPSV_{30\%}$ compared with $PSV_{0\%}$ (**Table 2**). However, the variability of ΔP_S, $PEEP_{tot}$, P_{mean}, and V_T was higher with $PSV_{15\%}$ and $PSV_{30\%}$ compared with $PSV_{0\%}$ (**Table 2**). The RR and $PTP_{es,min}$ had higher variability only with $vPSV_{30\%}$ (**Table 2**). Moreover, asynchronies were more frequent with $vPSV_{30\%}$ compared with $PSV_{0\%}$ ($p = 0.019$, **Table 2**).

Block 2: Physiological Effects of Variability at Two Levels of ΔP_S

The PaO_2/FiO_2, as well as other gas exchange and hemodynamic parameters, did not differ between ventilation steps in block 2 (**Table 3**). Ventilation modes with ΔP_S reduced by 5 cmH_2O (PSV_{-5} and $vPSV_{-5}$) had lower P_{mean}, V_T, P_L, and higher RR (**Table 3**). Adding ±5 cmH_2O variability ($vPSV_{BL}$ and $vPSV_{-5}$ steps) increased the variability of ΔP_S and P_{mean} compared to PSV without variability at the corresponding ΔP_S level. Adding ±5 cmH_2O variability increased the variability of V_T and P_L only when using the baseline ΔP_S, but not when the ΔP_S was reduced by 5 cmH_2O. The incidence of asynchronies was not different between ventilation steps in block 2 (**Table 3**).

Tables 2, 3 report extensive details on respiratory mechanics, hemodynamics, and arterial blood gas analysis in ventilation blocks 1 and 2, respectively. The distribution of key respiratory mechanics parameters in ventilation blocks 1 and 2 is illustrated in **Figures 3, 4**, respectively. **Supplemental Figures 3–11** report details the evolution over time of the respiratory mechanics parameters in the different ventilation steps.

TABLE 3 | Gas exchange, hemodynamics, and respiratory mechanics in patients during pressure support ventilation at different variability and pressure support level (Block 2).

	Ventilation modes				p-values			
	PSV_{BL}	$vPSV_{BL}$	PSV_{-5}	$vPSV_{-5}$	Overall	$vPSV_{BL}$ vs. PSV_{BL}	PSV_{-5} vs. PSV_{BL}	$vPSV_{-5}$ vs. PSV_{-5}
Ventilator Settings								
ΔP_S setting	Baseline		Baseline−5 cmH_2O					
$\Delta P_{S,set}$ (cmH_2O)	14.0 [12.0–16.0]	14.0 [12.0–16.0]	9.0 [7.0–11.0]	9.0 [7.0–11.0]	<0.001	0.99	<0.001	<0.001
Variability setting	None	± 5 cmH_2O	No variability	± 5 cmH_2O				
ΔP_S set variability (CV %)	0 [0–0]	11 [9–13]	0 [0–0]	15 [13–20]	<0.001	<0.001	0.99	<0.001
Gas exchange								
PaO_2/FIO_2 (mmHg)	213 [180–229]	194 [180–229]	215 [183–239]	197 [167–224]	0.61			
PaO_2 (mmHg)	95 [89–117]	99 [87–115]	99 [90–121]	98.8 [85–1112]	0.61			
$PaCO_2$ (mmHg)	42 [39–46]	43 [39–48]	44 [40–49]	44 [40–51]	0.18			
pH	7.47 [7.43–7.49]	7.48 [7.43–7.49]	7.47 [7.43–7.48]	7.47 [7.42–7.48]	0.21			
Hemodynamics								
Heart rate (min^{-1})	83 [77–93]	84 [77–92]	84 [77–92]	86 [76–92]	0.46			
Mean arterial pressure (mmHg)	88 [81–93]	82 [78–87]	80 [77–90]	86 [77–90]	0.37			
Respiratory mechanics								
$\Delta P_{S,measured}$ (cmH_2O)	13.2 [12.0–15.8]	13.6 [12.5–15.9]	8.4 [7.0–10.5][a]	8.5 [7.2–10.7]	<0.001	0.92	<0.001	0.67
$\Delta P_{Smeasured}$ (CV, %)	1.5 [0.9–4.8]	12.1 [11.1–14.3][a]	2.3 [1.7–6.6]	17.9 [15.2–18.6][b]	<0.001	0.001	0.99	<0.001
Total PEEP (cmH_2O)	7.6 [6.2–8.4]	7.5 [6.2–8.5]	7.7 [5.8–8.7][a]	7.7 [5.7–8.7]	0.001	0.99	0.009	0.92
Total PEEP (CV, %)	2.3 [1.4–4.9]	2.6 [1.8–8.0]	2.1 [1.6–4.3]	2.4 [1.4–5.9]	0.09			
P_{mean} (cmH_2O)	11.0 [9.7–12.6]	11.2 [9.7–13.1]	9.7 [8.4–11.9][a]	9.8 [8.4–11.8]	<0.001	0.67	<0.001	0.99
P_{mean} (CV, %)	5.4 [3.4–8.2]	8.1 [5.5–10.2][a]	2.5 [1.8–5.0]	6.0 [4.5–7.3][b]	<0.001	0.014	0.11	0.029
Respiratory rate (min^{-1})	14.7 [13.7–18.3]	17.6 [14.8–19.4]	22.9 [16.0–24.9][a]	20.1 [16.9–26.8]	0.022	0.96	0.041	0.95
Respiratory rate (CV, %)	18.8 [10.6–46.4]	32.0 [16.1–60.3]	13.1 [6.2–35.2]	14.6 [9.7–17.7]	0.003	0.43	0.43	0.99
V_T (ml/kg of PBW)	8.5 [7.2–9.4]	8.2 [7.0–9.1]	7.0 [5.9–7.6][a]	7.2 [6.0–7.7]	<0.001	0.92	<0.001	0.67
V_T (CV, %)	9.3 [5.1–15.7]	12.7 [11.1–15.3][a]	8.3 [4.2–13.6]	10.8 [9.4–14.6]	0.003	0.006	0.99	0.74
T_{insp}/T_{tot}	0.36 [0.30–0.37]	0.37 [0.30–0.39]	0.36 [0.32–0.39]	0.35 [0.32–0.38]	0.42			
T_{insp}/T_{tot} (CV, %)	9.3 [5.1–15.7]	12.7 [11.1–15.3][a]	8.3 [4.2–13.6]	10.8 [9.4–14.6]	0.058			
PTP_{es} (cmH_2O s min^{-1})	155.2 [118.4–262.8]	161.4 [87.1–248.3]	215.0 [128.1–357.9]	259.1 [151.1–422.8]	0.001	0.51	0.18	0.99
PTP_{es} (CV, %)	31.8 [20.6–52.3]	53.8 [23.9–71.1]	27.5 [16.0–40.5]	30.7 [18.5–44.7]	0.005	0.08	0.75	0.81
ΔP_{es} (cmH_2O)	4.4 [2.1–9.3]	5.3 [1.3–8.0]	5.6 [1.6–11.8]	10.4 [2.6–14.1]	<0.001	0.59	0.59	0.43
ΔP_{es} (CV, %)	32.7 [21.1–45.5]	40.9 [22.3–53.5]	22.8 [13.1–31.5]	20.6 [12.7–32.2]	<0.001	0.51	0.29	0.67
P_L (cmH_2O)	18.5 [15.9–23.2]	18.6 [16.1–23.4]	14.6 [11.5–20.8][a]	18.0 [14.0–21.6]	<0.001	0.99	<0.001	0.67
P_L (CV, %)	7.5 [3.8–12.6]	12.2 [11.1–17.0][a]	10.0 [4.2–13.1]	15.7 [12.4–17.3]	0.009	0.042	0.95	0.14
Asynchrony index (%)	1.5 [0.7–7.2]	2.4 [0.1–12.6]	0.9 [0.0–7.6]	1.3 [0–3.9]	0.21			

Values are computed during the last 10 min of a 45-min ventilation period. Data are reported as inter-subject median [25th–75th percentile] of the intra-subject median values.
[a]*Significant difference compared to PSV_{BL} ($p < 0.05$).*
[b]*Significant difference compared to PSV_{-5} ($p < 0.05$).*
PSV_{BL}, pressure support ventilation with no variability and baseline ΔP_S as per clinical indication; $vPSV_{BL}$, variable pressure support with variability set to achieve ±5 cmH_2O and baseline ΔP_S as per clinical indication; PSV_{-5}, pressure support ventilation with no variability and ΔP_S reduced by 5 cmH_2O from the baseline value; $vPSV_{-5}$, variable pressure support ventilation with variability set to achieve ±5 cmH_2O and ΔP_S reduced by 5 cmH_2O from the baseline value; CV, coefficient of variation; PEEP, positive end-expiratory pressure; PBW, predicted body weight; ΔP_S, pressure support; V_T, tidal volume; PTP, esophageal pressure-time product; ΔP_{es}, esophageal pressure swings; P_L, peak transpulmonary pressure.

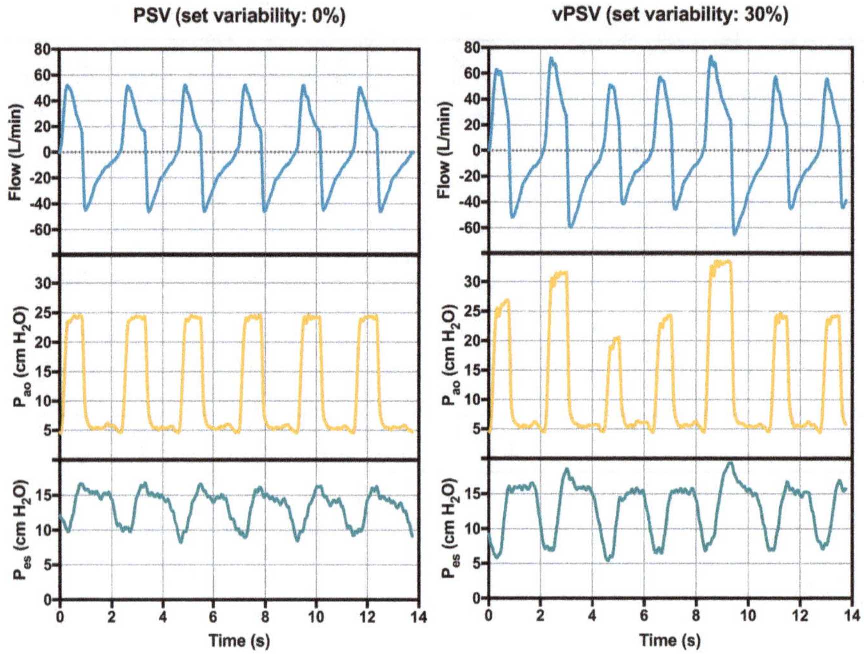

FIGURE 2 | Representative respiratory traces of a patient during conventional (left) and variable (right) pressure support ventilation. P_{ao}, pressure at the airway opening; P_{es}, esophageal pressure.

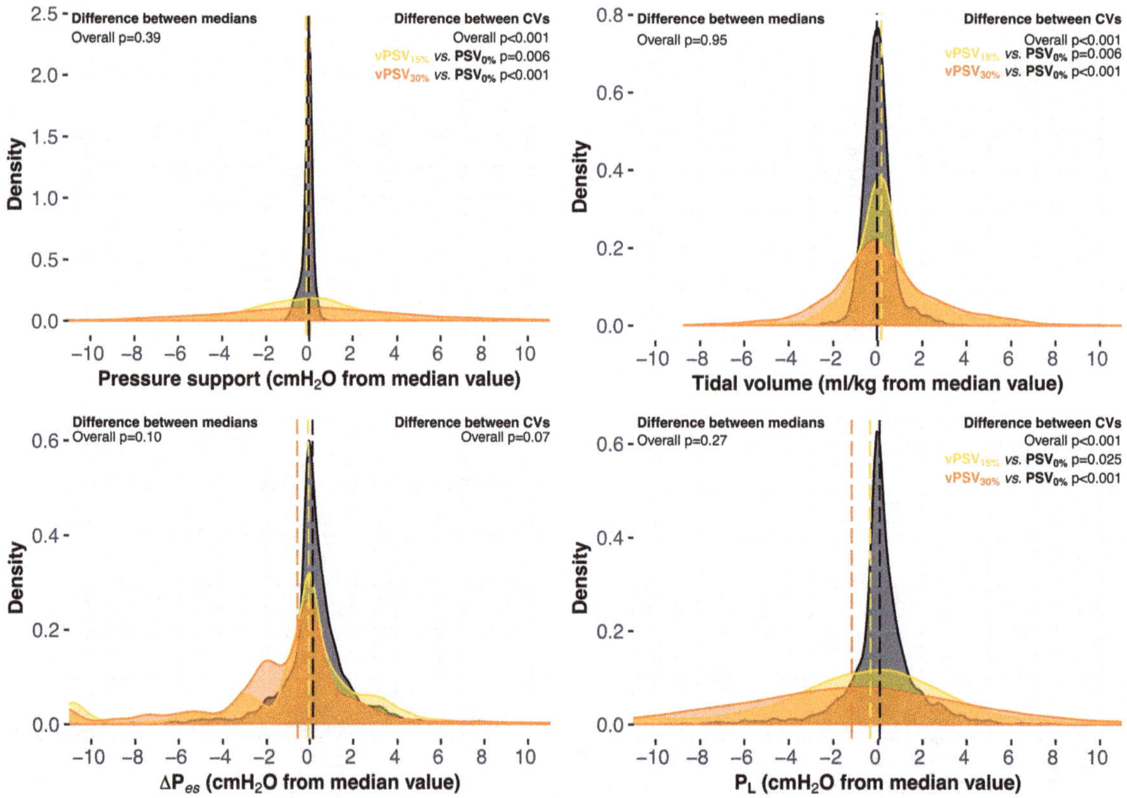

FIGURE 3 | Respiratory mechanics at different levels of variability (block 1). Variables are reported as the difference from the median value achieved during $PSV_{0\%}$ to allow between-patients visual comparisons. Dashed lines represent the medians of each ventilation step. $PSV_{0\%}$, conventional PSV ventilation with no variability; $vPSV_{15\%}$, variable PSV with variability set to 15% CV; $vPSV_{30\%}$, variable PSV with variability set to 30% CV; CV, coefficient of variation; ΔP_S, pressure support; ΔP_{es}, esophageal pressure swings; P_L, peak transpulmonary pressure.

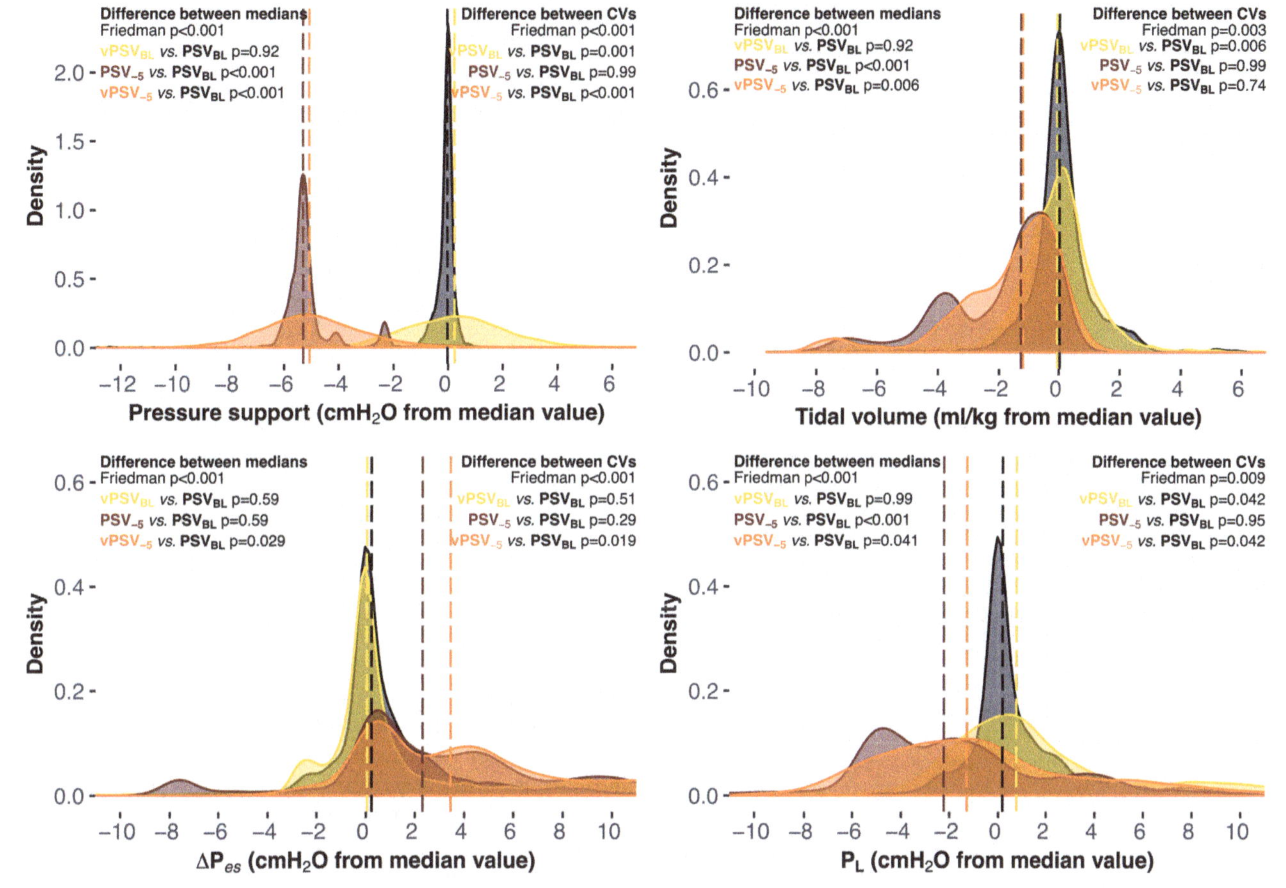

FIGURE 4 | Effects of variability on the distribution of respiratory mechanics parameters at different levels of pressure support (block 2). Variables are reported as the difference from the median value achieved during PSV_{BL} to allow between-patients visual comparisons. Dashed lines represent the medians of each ventilation step. PSV_{BL}, PSV with no variability and baseline ΔP_S as per clinical indication; $vPSV_{BL}$, variable pressure support with variability set to achieve ± 5 cmH_2O and baseline ΔP_S as per clinical indication; PSV_{-5}, PSV with no variability and ΔP_S reduced by 5 cmH_2O from the baseline value; $vPSV_{-5}$, variable PSV with variability set to achieve ± 5 cmH_2O and ΔP_S reduced by 5 cmH_2O from the baseline value; PSV, pressure support ventilation; CV, coefficient of variation; ΔP_S, pressure support; ΔP_{es}, esophageal pressure swings; P_L, peak transpulmonary pressure.

Post-hoc Analysis

Associations between respiratory mechanics parameters and the pressure level received in the preceding breath during $vPSV_{BL}$ and $vPSV_{-5}$ are reported in **Figure 5**. The ΔP_S received in the preceding breath was inversely associated with the magnitude of the inspiratory effort (ΔP_{es}) in the following breath, both during $vPSV_{BL}$ ($p = 0.003$) and $vPSV_{-5}$ ($p = 0.005$).

DISCUSSION

The main findings of this study are that in our mixed-ICU population of patients with mild to moderate ARDS: (1) vPSV with 15 or 30% variability did not influence gas exchange compared with conventional PSV; (2) at constant ΔP_S, vPSV increased the variability of V_T and P_L; (3) $vPSV_{30\%}$ increased the incidence of asynchronies; and (4) when the ΔP_S was reduced by 5 cmH_2O from the baseline value, adding variability did not increase the variability of V_T and P_L.

This is the first study comparing the short-term effects of vPSV at different levels of variability and ΔP_S in patients with ARDS. In previous studies, vPSV improved oxygenation in the experimental models of ARDS (Gama de Abreu et al., 2008; Spieth et al., 2011, 2012), but not in a cohort of hypoxemic critically ill patients (Spieth et al., 2013). However, that last study included mostly postoperative patients without a confirmed diagnosis of ARDS and investigated a single level of variability and pressure support. Opposite to what was found in preclinical studies in animals, vPSV had no effect on gas exchange, when the ΔP_S was set to the baseline value identified by the treating clinician and neither when it was reduced by 5 cmH_2O. This could be explained by several mechanisms; most importantly, the time investigated in each ventilation step was relatively short, and the fact that patients had an established diagnosis of ARDS mostly in their recovery phase and received mechanical ventilation for few days prior to the inclusion in this study. Under these conditions, patient lungs could have developed

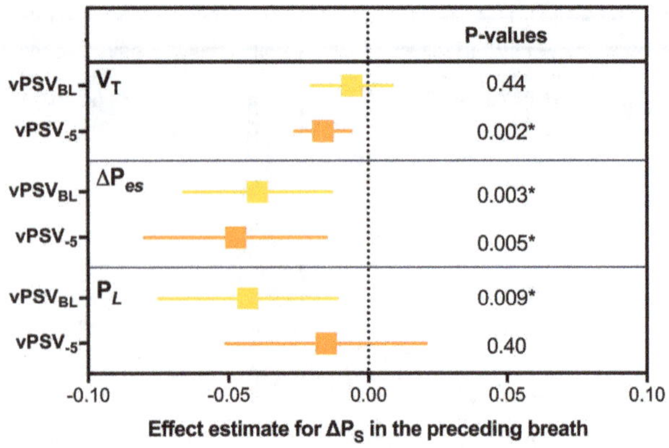

FIGURE 5 | Associations between respiratory mechanics parameters and the pressure level received in the preceding breath during variable PSV. Squares and confidence intervals refer to the effect estimate for ΔP_S in a mixed model comprising the ΔP_S received during the preceding breath as a fixed effect and the patient as a random effect with random intercept. The units of the estimates are expressed in the untransformed units of the variables, i.e., they represent the absolute change in V_T, ΔP_{es}, or P_L when the ΔP_S received during the preceding breath increases by 1 cmH_2O. vPSV$_{BL}$, variable PSV with variability set to achieve ±5 cmH_2O and baseline ΔP_S as per clinical indication; vPSV$_{-5}$, variable PSV ventilation with variability set to achieve ±5 cmH_2O and ΔP_S reduced by 5 cmH_2O from the baseline value; PBW, predicted body weight; PSV, pressure support ventilation; ΔP_S, pressure support; V_T, tidal volume; ΔP_{es}, esophageal pressure swings; P_L, peak transpulmonary pressure. *Significant association ($p < 0.05$).

consolidation, namely, the presence of lung regions scarcely responsive to recruitment (Cressoni et al., 2017). In this case, the breaths with higher ΔP_S received cyclically during variable pressure support might expose the patient to volutrauma in the aerated regions of the lung (Güldner et al., 2016; Pelosi et al., 2016) due to the reduced size of the lung aerated compartment. Another explanation for the possible lack of effect of variability on oxygenation might be that, different from what happens in PSV with a sigh, vPSV has no control over the time spent at higher pressure during tidal breathing. This might result in random breaths with higher P_S and short inspiratory time, both possibly insufficient to achieve recruitment. The tidal volume measured in this cohort was higher than the recommended targets, but this reflects the current clinical practice in patients with ARDS receiving assisted ventilation modes (Bellani et al., 2016; Writing Group for the PReVENT Investigators et al., 2018). During the second block of ventilations, the patients tolerated a ΔP_S reduction without worsening the gas exchange in the short term, at the price of a modest increase of the respiratory rate, suggesting that they were slightly over-assisted. This could have influenced patient-ventilator interaction (Kataoka et al., 2018) and the response to variability, as suggested by the finding that, during the second block of interventions, the variability of V_T was increased by vPSV compared with PSV only when the baseline ΔP_S was used. However, during ventilation steps with baseline ΔP_S, patients had a work of breathing estimated with the PTP_{es} of around 150 $cmH_2O \cdot s \cdot min^{-1}$, which is within the recommended range (Mauri et al., 2016). Interestingly, higher P_S resulted in a reduction in ΔP_{ES} in the following breath at both set ΔP_S levels, while the variability of V_T and P_L was increased by extrinsic variability only at higher ΔP_S. This seems to suggest that while a neural response to extrinsic variability is present independent of the level of assistance, its effects on the variability of V_T and P_L are influenced by the level of ΔP_S.

This study is underpowered to demonstrate the effects of vPSV on patient-centered outcomes like duration of ventilation. This is tested in another, yet ongoing clinical trial (Kiss et al., 2013). In the *post-hoc* analysis, the effects of vPSV on the response of patients in terms of inspiratory effort, transpulmonary pressure, and tidal volume developed in the following breath were studied. An inverse association between the ΔP_S received in the preceding breath and the inspiratory effort was observed. Different from other modified PSV modes such as the proportional assist ventilation (PAV) and the neurally adjusted ventilatory assist (NAVA), the variability of ΔP_S was random, i.e., is not related to the efforts of patients. This analysis suggests that there might be a complex interaction between the ventilator and a patient, in which the inspiratory effort and the adaptation of the patient to pressure support are influenced by the history of the previous breaths.

Limitations

This study has several limitations. The crossover design allowed the investigation of the effects of different levels of variability and ΔP_S in terms of gas exchange and respiratory mechanics in the short term but is intrinsically unable to investigate major clinical outcomes. The sample size is relatively low, no static measurements of respiratory mechanics were performed, and patients received heterogeneous sedation regimens that might have affected differently the respiratory drive. The population included in the study identifies a subgroup of critically ill patients meeting the criteria for mild to moderate ARDS who already received controlled or assisted mechanical ventilation for several days; however, the baseline patient characteristics were similar to those reported in a recent large observational study in patients with ARDS assisted non-invasively (Bellani et al., 2017). These patients with established respiratory failure, thus, possibly consolidated lung areas, might not benefit from the cyclic recruitment effect of vPSV, while patients with early ARDS might respond differently. However, the role of spontaneous breathing in the early management of ARDS is still unclear. This study could neither elucidate the mechanisms of the neural responses of the patients to variability nor the neuromuscular coupling of the respiratory muscles.

CONCLUSION

In our cohort of patients with mild to moderate ARDS, vPSV did not improve gas exchange at different levels of variability and pressure support. Compared with PSV, vPSV increased the variability of V_T, but not when low levels of variability were used in conjunction with lower pressure support. Moreover, vPSV did not exert a clinically relevant effect on the average inspiratory effort and work of breathing.

AUTHOR CONTRIBUTIONS

LB takes responsibility for the integrity of data. LB, PP, MV, and MG designed the study. LB, YS, MF, AD'O, DD'A, PRa, and IB conducted the study. LB, LM, MF, RH, AD'O, and CR analyzed the data. LB, MS, PP, PRo, and MG wrote the manuscript. All authors read and approved the final version of the manuscript.

REFERENCES

Akoumianaki, E., Maggiore, S. M., Valenza, F., Bellani, G., Jubran, A., Loring, S. H., et al. (2014). The application of esophageal pressure measurement in patients with respiratory failure. *Am. J. Respir. Crit. Care Med.* 189, 520–531. doi: 10.1164/rccm.201312-2193CI

Bellani, G., Laffey, J. G., Pham, T., Fan, E., Brochard, L., Esteban, A., et al. (2016). Epidemiology, patterns of care, and mortality for patients with acute respiratory distress syndrome in intensive care units in 50 countries. *JAMA* 315, 788–800. doi: 10.1001/jama.2016.0291

Bellani, G., Laffey, J. G., Pham, T., Madotto, F., Fan, E., Brochard, L., et al. (2017). Noninvasive ventilation of patients with acute respiratory distress syndrome. Insights from the LUNG SAFE study. *Am. J. Respir. Crit. Care Med.* 195, 67–77. doi: 10.1164/rccm.201606-1306OC

Blanch, L., Villagra, A., Sales, B., Montanya, J., Lucangelo, U., Luján, M., et al. (2015). Asynchronies during mechanical ventilation are associated with mortality. *Intensive Care Med.* 41, 633–641. doi: 10.1007/s00134-015-3692-6

Cressoni, M., Chiumello, D., Algieri, I., Brioni, M., Chiurazzi, C., Colombo, A., et al. (2017). Opening pressures and atelectrauma in acute respiratory distress syndrome. *Intensive Care Med.* 43, 603–611. doi: 10.1007/s00134-017-4754-8

Esteban, A., Frutos-Vivar, F., Muriel, A., Ferguson, N. D., Peñuelas, O., Abraira, V., et al. (2013). Evolution of mortality over time in patients receiving mechanical ventilation. *Am. J. Respir. Crit. Care Med.* 188, 220–230. doi: 10.1164/rccm.201212-2169OC

Gama de Abreu, M., Spieth, P. M., Pelosi, P., Carvalho, A. R., Walter, C., Schreiber-Ferstl, A., et al. (2008). Noisy pressure support ventilation: a pilot study on a new assisted ventilation mode in experimental lung injury. *Crit. Care Med.* 36, 818–827. doi: 10.1097/01.CCM.0000299736.55039.3A

Güldner, A., Braune, A., Ball, L., Silva, P. L., Samary, C., Insorsi, A., et al. (2016). Comparative effects of volutrauma and atelectrauma on lung inflammation in experimental acute respiratory distress syndrome. *Crit. Care Med.* doi: 10.1097/CCM.0000000000001721

Huhle, R., Pelosi, P., and de Abreu, M. G. (2016). Variable ventilation from bench to bedside. *Crit. Care Lond. Engl.* 20:62. doi: 10.1186/s13054-016-1216-6

Kataoka, J., Kuriyama, A., Norisue, Y., and Fujitani, S. (2018). Proportional modes versus pressure support ventilation: a systematic review and meta-analysis. *Ann. Intensive Care* 8:123. doi: 10.1186/s13613-018-0470-y

Kiss, T., Güldner, A., Bluth, T., Uhlig, C., Spieth, P. M., Markstaller, K., et al. (2013). Rationale and study design of ViPS - variable pressure support for weaning from mechanical ventilation: study protocol for an international multicenter randomized controlled open trial. *Trials* 14:363. doi: 10.1186/1745-6215-14-363

Mauri, T., Lazzeri, M., Bronco, A., Bellani, G., and Pesenti, A. (2017). Effects of variable pressure support ventilation on regional homogeneity and aeration. *Am. J. Respir. Crit. Care Med.* 195, e27–e28. doi: 10.1164/rccm.201609-1806IM

Mauri, T., Yoshida, T., Bellani, G., Goligher, E. C., Carteaux, G., Rittayamai, N., et al. (2016). Esophageal and transpulmonary pressure in the clinical setting: meaning, usefulness and perspectives. *Intensive Care Med.* 42, 1360–1373. doi: 10.1007/s00134-016-4400-x

Muller, K. E., and Barton, C. N. (1989). Approximate power for repeated-measures ANOVA lacking sphericity. *J. Am. Stat. Assoc.* 84, 549–555. doi: 10.1080/01621459.1989.10478802

Muller, K. E., Lavange, L. M., Ramey, S. L., and Ramey, C. T. (1992). Power calculations for general linear multivariate models including repeated measures applications. *J. Am. Stat. Assoc.* 87, 1209–1226. doi: 10.1080/01621459.1992.10476281

Pelosi, P., Ball, L., Abreu, M. G., de, and Rocco, P. R. M. (2016). General anesthesia closes the lungs: keep them resting. *Turk. J. Anesth. Reanim.* 44, 163–164. doi: 10.5152/TJAR.2016.002

Putensen, C., Zech, S., Wrigge, H., Zinserling, J., Stüber, F., Von Spiegel, T., et al. (2001). Long-term effects of spontaneous breathing during ventilatory support in patients with acute lung injury. *Am. J. Respir. Crit. Care Med.* 164, 43–49. doi: 10.1164/ajrccm.164.1.2001078

Spieth, P. M., Carvalho, A. R., Güldner, A., Kasper, M., Schubert, R., Carvalho, N. C., et al. (2011). Pressure support improves oxygenation and lung protection compared to pressure-controlled ventilation and is further improved by random variation of pressure support. *Crit. Care Med.* 39, 746–755. doi: 10.1097/CCM.0b013e318206bda6

Spieth, P. M., Güldner, A., Beda, A., Carvalho, N., Nowack, T., Krause, A., et al. (2012). Comparative effects of proportional assist and variable pressure support ventilation on lung function and damage in experimental lung injury. *Crit. Care Med.* 40, 2654–2661. doi: 10.1097/CCM.0b013e3182592021

Spieth, P. M., Güldner, A., Huhle, R., Beda, A., Bluth, T., Schreiter, D., et al. (2013). Short-term effects of noisy pressure support ventilation in patients with acute hypoxemic respiratory failure. *Crit. Care Lond. Engl.* 17:R261. doi: 10.1186/cc13091

Tobin, M. J., Mador, M. J., Guenther, S. M., Lodato, R. F., and Sackner, M. A. (1988). Variability of resting respiratory drive and timing in healthy subjects. *J. Appl. Physiol. (1985)* 65, 309–317. doi: 10.1152/jappl.1988.65.1.309

Writing Group for the PReVENT Investigators, Simonis, F. D., Serpa Neto, A., Binnekade, J. M., Braber, A., Bruin, K. C. M., et al. (2018). Effect of a low vs intermediate tidal volume strategy on ventilator-free days in intensive care unit patients without ARDS: a randomized clinical trial. *JAMA* 320, 1872–1880. doi: 10.1001/jama.2018.14280

5

Monitoring Expired CO_2 Kinetics to Individualize Lung-Protective Ventilation in Patients with the Acute Respiratory Distress Syndrome

Fernando Suárez-Sipmann[1,2,3†], Jesús Villar[1,4,5†], Carlos Ferrando[1,6,7†], Juan A. Sánchez-Giralt[2†] and Gerardo Tusman[8†]*

[1] CIBER de Enfermedades Respiratorias, Instituto de Salud Carlos III, Madrid, Spain, [2] Intensive Care Unit, Hospital Universitario La Princesa, Madrid, Spain, [3] Department of Surgical Sciences, Anesthesiology & Critical Care, Hedenstierna Laboratory, Uppsala University Hospital, Uppsala, Sweden, [4] Multidisciplinary Organ Dysfunction Evaluation Research Network (MODERN), Research Unit, Hospital Universitario Dr. Negrín, Las Palmas de Gran Canaria, Spain, [5] Keenan Research Center at the Li Ka Shing Knowledge Institute, St. Michael's Hospital, Toronto, ON, Canada, [6] Department of Anesthesiology and Critical Care, Hospital Clinic, Barcelona, Spain, [7] Hospital Clinic, Institut d'Investigacions Biomèdiques August Pi i Sunyer (IDIBAPS), Barcelona, Spain, [8] Department of Anesthesiology, Hospital Privado de Comunidad, Mar del Plata, Argentina

***Correspondence:**
Fernando Suárez-Sipmann
fsuarezsipmann@gmail.com

† These authors have contributed equally to this work

Mechanical ventilation (MV) is a lifesaving supportive intervention in the management of acute respiratory distress syndrome (ARDS), buying time while the primary precipitating cause is being corrected. However, MV can contribute to a worsening of the primary lung injury, known as ventilation-induced lung injury (VILI), which could have an important impact on outcome. The ARDS lung is characterized by diffuse and heterogeneous lung damage and is particularly prone to suffer the consequences of an excessive mechanical stress imposed by higher airway pressures and volumes during MV. Of major concern is cyclic overdistension, affecting those lung segments receiving a proportionally higher tidal volume in an overall reduced lung volume. Theoretically, healthier lung regions are submitted to a larger stress and cyclic deformation and thus at high risk for developing VILI. Clinicians have difficulties in detecting VILI, particularly cyclic overdistension at the bedside, since routine monitoring of gas exchange and lung mechanics are relatively insensitive to this mechanism of VILI. Expired CO_2 kinetics integrates relevant pathophysiological information of high interest for monitoring. CO_2 is produced by cell metabolism in large daily quantities. After diffusing to tissue capillaries, CO_2 is transported first by the venous and then by pulmonary circulation to the lung. Thereafter diffusing from capillaries to lung alveoli, it is finally convectively transported by lung ventilation for its elimination to the atmosphere. Modern readily clinically available sensor technology integrates information related to pulmonary ventilation, perfusion, and gas exchange from the single analysis of expired CO_2 kinetics measured at the airway opening. Current volumetric capnography (VCap), the representation of the volume of expired CO_2 in one single breath, informs about pulmonary perfusion, end-expiratory lung volume, dead space, and pulmonary ventilation inhomogeneities, all intimately related to cyclic overdistension during MV. Additionally, the recently described capnodynamic method provides the possibility to continuously measure the end-expiratory lung volume and effective pulmonary blood flow. All this information is accessed non-invasively and breath-by-breath helping clinicians to personalize ventilatory settings at the bedside and minimize overdistension and cyclic deformation of lung tissue.

Keywords: volumetric capnography, dead space, acute respiratory distress syndrome, ventilator-induced lung injury, mechanical ventilation

INTRODUCTION

The acute respiratory distress syndrome (ARDS) is the most severe form of acute respiratory failure that affects the lungs in a heterogeneous way, profoundly impairing their mechanical properties and gas-exchange functions. Diffuse lung pan-endothelial inflammation, the hallmark of the syndrome, leads to the invasion of alveolar spaces by edema and inflammation reducing effective pulmonary lung volume (i.e., functional residual capacity, FRC). The lung becomes heavier exerting a superimposed pressure on the dependent parts of the lung, critically decreasing regional transpulmonary pressure. This further reduces FRC by promoting lung collapse, a common pathophysiological feature of ARDS (Gattinoni et al., 2006).

Mechanical ventilation (MV) is the principal life-support intervention in the management of patients with ARDS but at the risk to perpetuate or aggravate lung damage. Ventilation-induced lung injury (VILI) results from the need to use high transpulmonary pressures and frequently higher tidal volumes (VT) to oxygenate and ventilate the heterogeneously ARDS lung. The delivered VT is distributed in a much smaller lung volume with important regional differences, with three important consequences: (1) less diseased lung regions will receive a larger fraction of the VT causing an increased cyclic tissue deformation or strain, a mechanism that triggers lung inflammation, (2) more diseased but ventilated regions will be submitted to a higher transpulmonary pressure for any given delivered VT increasing the local mechanical stress also known as cyclic overdistension, and (3) collapsed regions eventually re-open and close with each tidal inflation and deflation causing cyclic recruitment–de-recruitment, which can be considered an extreme form of regional strain. These are three of the most important mechanisms by which MV damages lung parenchyma. Lung imaging techniques, such as CT or intravital microscopy, have confirmed the heterogeneity of lung injury in ARDS at different scales, revealing the coexistence of normal, collapsed, and overdistended alveoli in different lungs regions. The resulting non-uniform distribution of tidal ventilation can be visualized in real time at the bedside by electrical impedance tomography (EIT), whereas more sophisticated techniques, such as PET and single-photon emission tomography (SPECT) imaging, have located the main inflammatory response in normally ventilated areas but not in collapsed ones (Bellani et al., 2009, 2011). Thus, lung collapse acts as a stress-raiser since it contributes to lung heterogeneity creating areas receiving an excessive VT in relation to their regional volume.

The introduction of lung-protective ventilation strategies aimed at reducing the mechanical stress imposed by the ventilator has contributed to reducing morbidity and mortality of patients with ARDS (ARDS Network, 2000). Ideally, these strategies should be individualized, but this requires useful and directed bedside clinical monitoring. However, routine monitoring only includes basic lung mechanics, gas exchange and intermittently, lung imaging techniques and thus, the clinical detection of overdistension or lung strain, and VILI remains difficult. The analysis of expired gases, in particular CO_2, is a well-established, robust, and clinically accessible monitoring option. Volumetric capnography (VCap), representing the volume of CO_2 expired in one breath, has specific features regarding the analysis of body CO_2 kinetics that can be of great value in detecting lung overdistension by providing continuous non-invasive information on lung perfusion, convective gas transport, lung diffusion, and dead space ventilation (VD), all intimately related and sensitive to the effects of lung overdistension. However, this source of highly relevant biological information is still largely underused in clinical practice. A progressive better understanding of the complex behavior and physiology of CO_2 kinetics have led to recent new developments for advanced analysis of the volumetric capnogram and a derived capnodynamic method that hold great promise in overcoming the difficulties in adopting the expired CO_2 monitoring in routine clinical practice.

The aim of this manuscript is to review the principles, uses, and physiological basis of expired CO_2 kinetics monitoring. We will review new developments and value of VD monitoring using VCap in patients with ARDS and describe the new capnodynamic method that continuously monitors effective lung volume and perfusion in a non-invasive way.

VOLUMETRIC CAPNOGRAPHY

The integration of an infrared CO_2 sensor and a flow sensor in a mainstream configuration allows for the reconstruction of the volumetric capnogram at the airway opening (**Figure 1**). As the cardiorespiratory system has an open arrangement, VCap contains implicit information regarding these systems expressed not only in their derived variables and indexes but also in its shape that helps the interpretation of normality and diseases throughout its derived-parameters. As mentioned above, CO_2 kinetics is context-sensitive, which means that VCap parameters must be interpreted when changes in metabolism, pulmonary perfusion, or ventilation occur one at a time

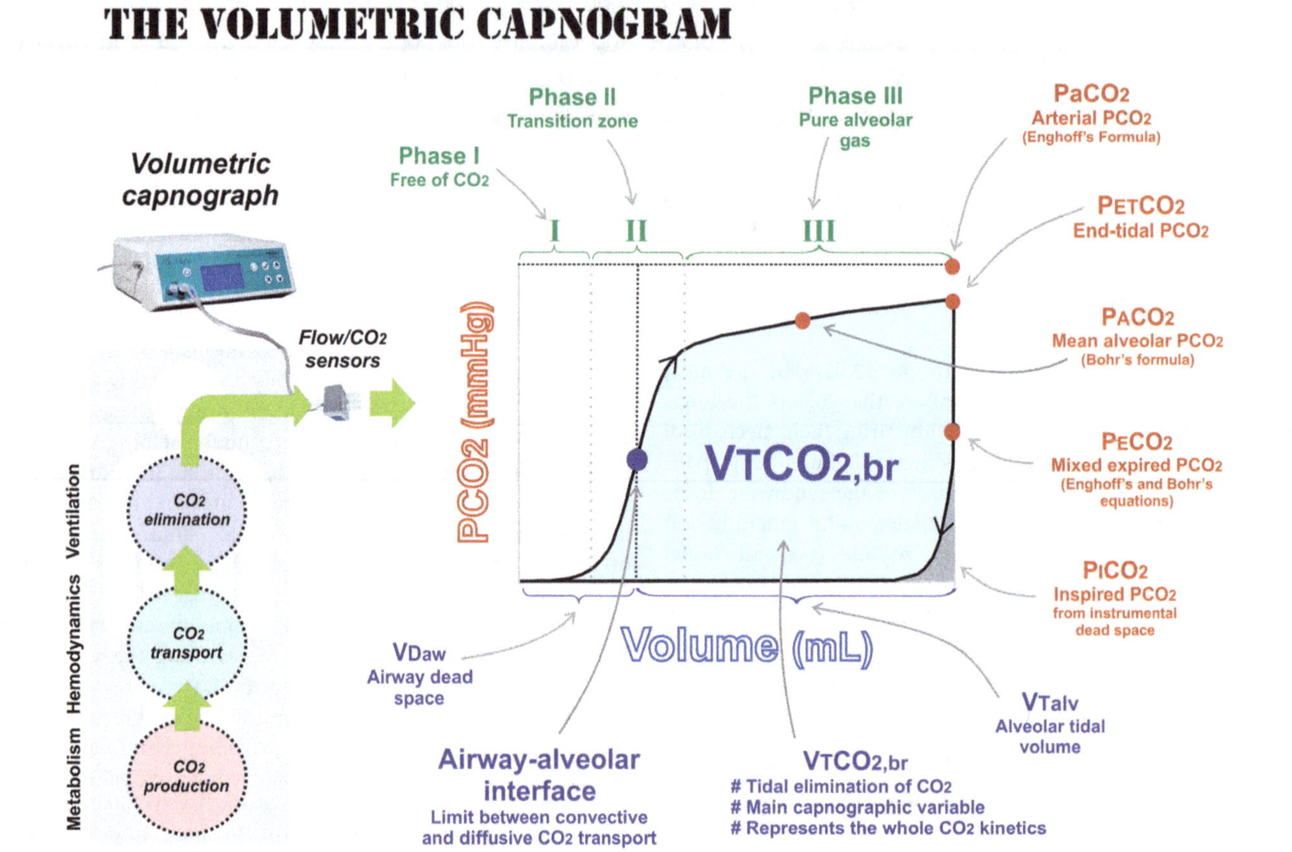

FIGURE 1 | Components of volumetric capnography. The volumetric capnogram is the plot of expired CO_2 in one tidal breath measured by mainstream flow and CO_2 sensors. The capnogram phases are shown in green: phase I is the portion of the expired gas without CO_2 that represents pure airway dead space; phase II is the transition zone composed by the progressive emptying of lung units with different time-constants and spatial distribution; and phase III is the pure alveolar gas expired once airway dead space (VD_{aw}) has been washed out. The relevant partial pressures of CO_2 measured by VCap are presented in red: end-tidal ($PETCO_2$), mean alveolar ($PACO_2$), mixed expired ($P\bar{E}CO_2$), and inspired ($PICO_2$) pressure. The arterial $PaCO_2$ is not directly measured, but it included for referencing of the other partial pressures. The volumes obtained by the VCap are presented in blue: volume of airway dead space (VD_{aw}), alveolar tidal volume (VT_{alv}), and volume of CO_2 eliminated per breath or area under the VCap curve ($VTCO_{2,br}$). The blue dot represents the airway–alveolar interface, the limit between convective and diffusive CO_2 transport close to the entrance of lung acini and, therefore, it also morphologically separates the conducting from the gas-exchanging lung compartment.

(Sipmann et al., 2014). For example, an increase in VT improves CO_2 elimination explained solely by a ventilatory change when metabolism and hemodynamics are constant.

Interpretation of CO_2 kinetics can be done during steady and non-steady state conditions, although the non-steady state is of particular interest in clinical monitoring as it allows to interpret and react to changes in pulmonary perfusion, end-expiratory lung volume, and/or alveolar ventilation after adjusting the ventilatory settings or to changing clinical conditions.

RATIONALE FOR THE MEASUREMENT OF DEAD SPACE AND ALVEOLAR CO_2 BY VOLUMETRIC CAPNOGRAPHY

Dead space ventilation is the wasted portion of ventilation not involved in gas exchange *per se*. It constitutes the evolutionary adaptive price paid by all mammals that depend on the bulk convective transport of ambient air to the gas–liquid gas-exchange interface, the alveolar–capillary membrane. By the end of the 19th century, Christian Bohr presented a method to estimate VD volume based on the mass balance of any gas breathed during the respiratory cycle (**Figure 2**) (Bohr, 1891). He brilliantly adapted his formula using CO_2 as the tracer gas, which still constitutes the basis of the clinical measurement of dead space. Aitken and Clark-Kennedy (1928) were the first to propose to represent CO_2 in relation to the expired volume, the VCap. Since then, the usefulness of this tool to calculate VD has been highlighted by many authors. Nowadays, major advances in CO_2 and flow sensing technology together with powerful hardware and computation capabilities have made real-time breath-by-breath VD calculations possible. The key feature to calculate VD using VCap relies on the precise measurement of mixed expired ($P\bar{E}CO_2$) and the mean alveolar ($PACO_2$) partial pressures of CO_2. The first necessary step was the simplification of the measurement of $P\bar{E}CO_2$, which represents the dilution of CO_2 within the lungs caused by the dead space effect. Initially, it could only be obtained by the cumbersome measurement using

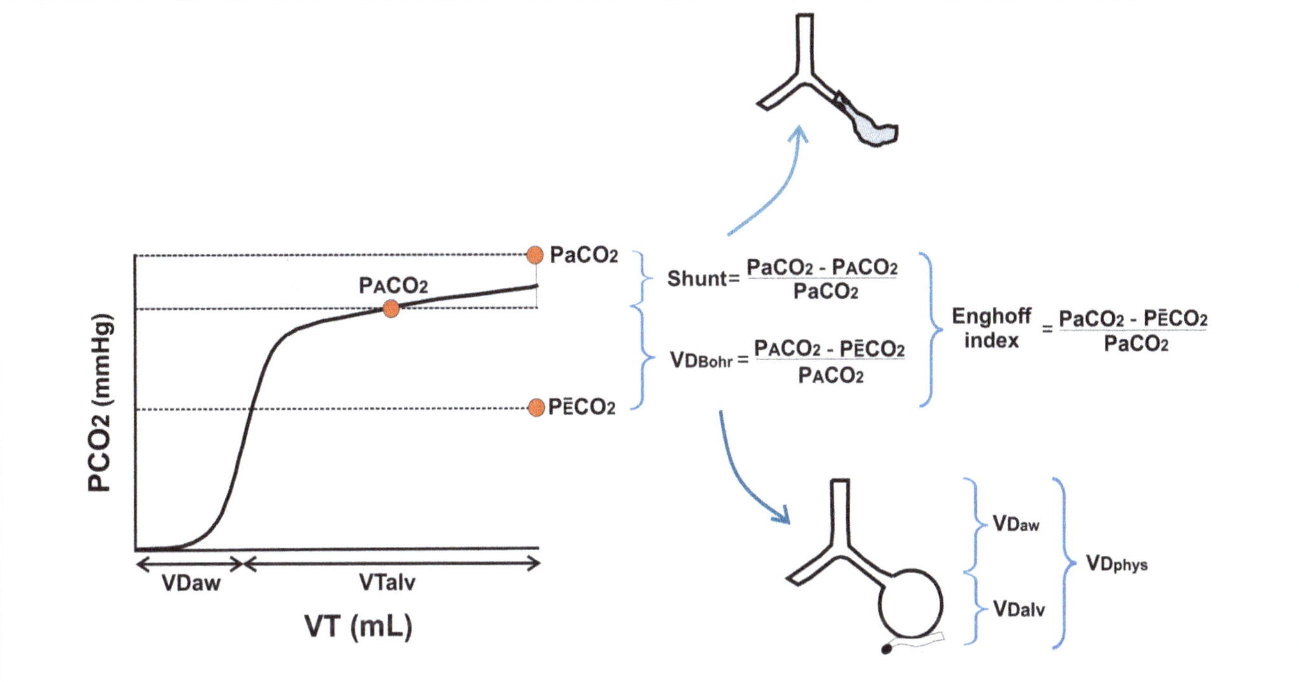

FIGURE 2 | Differences between Bohr's and Enghoff's approaches. The main physiological difference between Bohr's dead space (VD_{Bohr}) and Enghoff's index is visualized in one volumetric capnogram. While VD_{Bohr} represents true dead space in non-perfused alveoli and main conducted airways, the Enghoff's index includes also the effect of shunt and low V/Q in its calculation (gray area). $PaCO_2$, $PACO_2$, and $P\bar{E}CO_2$ are the arterial, alveolar, and mixed expired partial pressure of carbon dioxide, respectively. VD_{phys}, VD_{aw}, and VD_{alv} are physiological, airway, and alveolar dead spaces, respectively. VT is the tidal volume and VT_{alv} is the alveolar tidal volume.

the Douglas' bag. Currently, $P\bar{E}CO_2$ can be measured by VCap in one single breath by calculating the mixed expired fraction of CO_2 ($F\bar{E}CO_2$), which is then transformed to partial pressure and expressed in BTPS as follows:

$$F\bar{E}CO_2 = VTCO_{2,br}/VT$$

$$P\bar{E}CO_2 = F\bar{E}CO_2 \times (BP - PH_2O)$$

where $VTCO_{2,br}$ is the amount of CO_2 expired in one VT, P is barometric pressure, and PH_2O is water vapor pressure. The measurement of $P\bar{E}CO_2$ by VCap has been validated by different research groups, all showing good agreement with the Douglas bag method (Lum et al., 1998; Sinha and Soni, 2012) or a metabolic monitor (Kallet et al., 2005; Siobal et al., 2013) in children (Lum et al., 1998) and adults (Sinha and Soni, 2012) also with ARDS (Kallet et al., 2005; Siobal et al., 2013). More recently, using a more advanced analysis of VCap, Doorduin et al. (2016) compared $P\bar{E}CO_2$ measured by VCap versus the Douglas' bag in patients with ARDS and found a bias of 0.2 mmHg and limits of agreement of − 3.0 to 4.5 mmHg (Doorduin et al., 2016). Our data in an animal model of ARDS using the multiple inert gas elimination technique (MIGET), the gold standard method for gas-exchange analysis supported the above findings. Our group found a close correlation of $P\bar{E}CO_2$ measured by VCap with MIGET ($r = 0.92$; $p < 0.0001$), with a mean bias of −0.5 mmHg and limits of agreement between −2.5 and 1.5 mmHg (Tusman et al., 2011a).

The second, more recently introduced step, was the possibility to measure the mean alveolar partial pressure of CO_2 ($PACO_2$). This another essential component of the Bohr's formula is difficult to measure and is still controversial parameter because $PACO_2$ varies topographically and temporarily within inhomogeneous lungs along the respiratory cycle, even in healthy patients. This means that any single lung unit has its own $PACO_2$ according to its respective V/Q ratio. Therefore, many controversies arose about what the "alveolar gas" really means and what is the proper definition and representative value of $PACO_2$ (Rossier and Buhlmann, 1955). Two different approaches to describe the alveolar gas have been proposed in the past: the *ideal* and the *expired* alveolar gas. The *ideal alveolar gas* concept described by Riley and Cournand is based on the convenient and didactic assumption that the lung behaves as a perfect unit, where $PACO_2$ equals capillary PCO_2 (Riley and Cournand, 1949). However, this condition does not really exist even in healthy subjects due to the presence of airway dead space, anatomical shunt, stratified inhomogeneities, spatial and temporal V/Q mismatches, and incomplete gas mixing of inspired gases within the lungs (Fletcher et al., 1981; Crawford et al., 1985; Verbanck and Paiva, 2013). The impossibility to estimate $PACO_2$ in the past was solved by Henrik Enghoff who suggested to use PCO_2 in arterial blood ($PaCO_2$) in the Bohr's formula as a surrogate of $PACO_2$ (Enghoff, 1938). This solution to calculate VD is still used today although, strictly speaking, it calculates not only dead space but also all the spectrum of V/Q mismatch present in the lung (**Figure 2**). The *expired alveolar air* concept offers a better and more realistic approximation to $PACO_2$. Alveolar CO_2 fluctuates during the respiratory cycle changing ~4 mmHg between inspiration and expiration. DuBois described the "mean" $PACO_2$ as the absolute value representing the whole lung (Dubois et al., 1952). This concept was confirmed decades later using complex mathematical models that included other aspects that affect alveolar gas composition such as pulmonary capillary pulsatile blood flow, capillary recruitment, solubility of CO_2 in pulmonary tissue, and CO_2 chemical reactions in blood (Hlastala, 1972). The alveolar gas must necessarily be measured during expiration due to the location of the CO_2 sensor at the airway opening where inspiratory gases washes-out any remanent CO_2. Mean $PACO_2$ can conveniently be found at the midpoint of the phase III of the VCap. This phase is exclusively composed of alveolar gas where its slope represents the emptying of CO_2 from all alveoli at different rates during the expiratory time (Fletcher et al., 1981; Tusman et al., 2012). We tested this hypothesis in an animal model of ARDS by comparing the VCap-based $PACO_2$ with the one derived from the alveolar gas equation solved with data obtained from MIGET. We found a mean bias of − 0.1 mmHg with limits of agreement of −2.18 to 1.98 mmHg (Tusman et al., 2011a). This confirms the original DuBois' description of *mean* $PACO_2$, resolving the measurement of $PACO_2$ at the bedside and allowing the non-invasive calculation of Bohr's dead space breath by breath.

CURRENT INTERPRETATION OF BOHR'S AND ENGHOFF'S APPROACHES TO DEAD SPACE

According to the previous discussion, it is clear that Bohr's and Enghoff's approaches measure different but complementary aspects of gas exchange (**Figure 2**) (Tusman et al., 2012; Sipmann et al., 2014). The Bohr's equation measures "true" dead space because it uses parameters exclusively from the alveolar compartment, and thus is based on *the expired alveolar air concept*. The $PA\text{-}\bar{E}CO_2$ represents the degree of CO_2 dilution in naturally heterogeneous human lungs. This was confirmed in a model of ARDS where the Bohr's dead space calculated by VCap was in an excellent agreement (bias 0.01 and LoA −0.04 to 0.06) with the value obtained with the MIGET analysis (Tusman et al., 2011a). The Enghoff's approach measures not only dead space but also all the spectrum of V/Q mismatch present in the lung (**Figure 2**). This is because by using $PaCO_2$ as a surrogate of $PACO_2$ *(the ideal alveolar gas concept)*, the effects of low V/Q and shunt are included in its estimation. The true shunt and low V/Q zones let high venous blood PCO_2 pass through the alveoli increasing $PaCO_2$ much above $PACO_2$. Some authors called this effect "shunt" dead space (Fletcher et al., 1981), a misleading term as it mixes the two opposite extremes of V/Q mismatch. We observed a poor correlation between the Enghoff's approach with MIGET dead space ($r = 0.38$; $p = 0.0078$) but a good one with MIGET shunt ($r = 0.64$; $p < 0.0001$) (Tusman et al., 2011a). This is why we think that calling the result of the Enghoff's equation, a global index of gas exchange, as "dead space" is both physiologically and clinically incorrect!

DEAD SPACE SUBCOMPONENTS

The Bohr's equation calculates the whole *physiological* dead space. It can be expressed as an absolute volume in one breath (VD_{phys} in ml), as part of minute ventilation (VD in L) or, more commonly, as a fraction of VT (VD/VT) (Fletcher et al., 1981; Tusman et al., 2012). VCap is the only clinical monitoring tool that separates the volume of gas within conducting airways from the volume of gas in the alveolar compartment in one breath (**Figure 2**). The classical geometrical method to identify the midpoint of phase II of the capnogram, described by Fowler (1948), can be replaced by a more accurate mathematical analysis (Tusman et al., 2009). This is of great importance as the slope of phase II represents the emptying of lung units of different time constants and V/Q ratios and the midpoint the averaged interface between convective and diffusive intrapulmonary gas transport. We have named this point as the *airway-alveolar interface* (**Figure 1**), and it is needed to estimate airway dead space (VD_{aw}) and alveolar VT (VT_{alv}). Failure to correctly estimate this point can lead to interpretation errors of VCap and dead space components (Tusman et al., 2009). Finally, the alveolar dead space (VD_{alv}) is easily obtained by subtracting VD_{aw} from total VD_{phys} (Fletcher et al., 1981). VD_{aw} and VD_{alv} are commonly expressed as a fraction of VT to allow comparisons among different breaths and sizes of patients. The alveolar component is better expressed as a fraction of VT_{alv} (VD_{alv}/VT_{alv}) because it is an index that closely represents the inefficiency of gas exchange (Fletcher et al., 1981; Tusman et al., 2012).

VALUES OF DEAD SPACE IN PATIENTS WITH ACUTE RESPIRATORY DISTRESS SYNDROME

Table 1 shows a summary of published Bohr's and Enghoff's values from healthy volunteers to patients with ARDS (Nunn and Hill, 1960; Larsson and Severinghaus, 1962; Blanch et al., 1999; Åström et al., 2000; Beydon et al., 2002; Tusman et al., 2013; Doorduin et al., 2016; Gogniat et al., 2018). Mechanical ventilation *per se,* apart from pulmonary diseases, increases dead space. In patients with ARDS, VD is elevated by many other factors including instrumental dead space (HME, elbows, close-suction systems), using low VT ventilation, high respiratory rates, pulmonary vascular involvement, or high positive end-expiratory pressure (PEEP), among others. Instrumental dead space may be of major relevance in patients with ARDS because it is an easily modifiable factor and can sum up to 90 to 100 ml in some unfortunate configurations.

EVALUATION OF LUNG OVERDISTENSION BY VOLUMETRIC CAPNOGRAPHY

As discussed above, cyclic overdistension is one of the major mechanisms of VILI. It is referred to in different terms depending on whether it denotes functional (hyperdistension)

TABLE 1 | Published values of measured Bohr's and Enfhoff's approaches using capnography.

Kind of Patient	Authors	Ventilation	Enghoff's index	Bohr's VD/VT	VD_{aw}/VT	VD_{alv}/VT_{alv}
Healthy volunteers	Larsson and Severinghaus (1962) n = 11	Spontaneous mean VT ~ 630 mL	0.23 to 0.31	–	0.18 to 0.24	–
	Åström et al. (2000) n = 38	Spontaneous mean VT ~ 645 mL	Female = 0.23 Male = 0.31	Female = 0.20 Male = 0.26	Female = 0.16 Male = 0.21	–
	Tusman et al. (2013) n = 33	Spontaneous mean VT 546 mL	–	0.23 ± 0.08	0.17 ± 0.09	0.07 ± 0.06
Healthy anestetized	Nunn and Hill (1960) n = 12	Mandatory mean VT 474 mL	0.32	–	0.13	–
	Tusman et al. (2013) n = 33	Mandatory VT 6 mL/kg PEEP 6 cmH_2O	–	0.28 ± 0.07	0.18 ± 0.08	0.11 ± 0.05
Critically ill anestetized	Unpublished personal data n = 55	Mandatory VT 6 mL/kg PEEP 8 cmH_2O	–	0.41 ± 0.07	0.23 ± 0.07	0.23 ± 0.08
ARDS	Blanch et al. (1999) n = 17	Mandatory mean VT ~ 510 mL PEEP 5–10 cmH_2O	–	0.53 to 0.63	–	–
	Beydon et al. (2002) n = 10	Mandatory mean VT ~ 625 mL PEEP 5–10 cmH_2O	0.53 to 0.55	–	0.30 to 0.32	–
	Doorduin et al. (2016) n = 15	Mandatory VT 6.8 mL/kg PEEP 12 cmH_2O	0.68 ± 0.9	0.45 ± 0.7	–	–
	Gogniat et al. (2018) n = 14	Mandatory VT 6.5 mL/kg PEEP 10 cmH_2O	0.70 (0.58–0.74)	0.47 (0.45–0.56)	0.37 (0.31–0.45)	0.19 (0.15–0.23)

Data is presented as mean ± SD or median (1st–3rd quartiles). (–) data not available.

or morphological (hyperinflation) phenomena. Recently, a more conceptual and integrative framework adopted from bioengineering terminology has been introduced to describe the stress or lung deformation that the lung parenchyma suffers during inflation, especially at the end of inspiration when maximal airway pressures are reached. *Lung stress* is defined as the distribution of internal forces per area unit applied to an elastic material, and *lung strain* as the deformation or change in shape of an elastic material from a reference initial value when submitted to a force (Chiumello et al., 2008). Lung parenchyma is constituted by a network of elastic tissues that normally works within a certain range of normal stress and strain. The topographical distribution of stress and strain is heterogeneous due to the natural fractal configuration of the lungs and by the effects of gravity. Lung parenchyma is prone to damage if the normal limits of stress and strain for a particular lung region are exceeded (Protti et al., 2013; Hurtado et al., 2017).

Volumetric capnography informs about the occurrence of lung overdistension from a different but complementary perspective, as standard and transpulmonary lung mechanics. The Bohr's dead space increases with positive pressure ventilation, especially in the diseased lungs. The effects of PEEP on VD are well described in the literature (Blanch et al., 1999; Beydon et al., 2002). More importantly, PEEP and the resulting end-inspiratory pressure also increase VD_{alv} as it creates alveolar units with a high V/Q behavior. This is probably the most important parameter related to the risk of developing VILI as it reflects the phenomena occurring at the alveolar level, the most vulnerable part of the lung. Most reports describing the effects of PEEP or MV on VD and VD_{alv} use the Enghoff's approach, thereby introducing the confounder effect of low V/Q areas on its estimation. In their hallmark paper, Suter et al. (1975) defined the best PEEP as the one resulting in the highest compliance and the lowest VD_{alv}. This level also resulted in a reduced shunt, suggesting that the reduction in VD_{alv} could have been responsible in part to this effect. In an animal model of ARDS, we recently reproduced these results by applying 4 cmH_2O of PEEP below and above the "best" PEEP using the VCap analysis. The Bohr's derived VD_{alv}/VT_{alv} showed the lowest value at the open-lung PEEP and high values with 4 cmH_2O of PEEP below or above this value (**Figure 3**) (Tusman et al., 2011b). Of note, by measuring the Bohr's (i.e., true) dead space, we specifically analyzed the effects of PEEP on the high V/Q component, that is overdistension, eliminating the confounder of shunt or low V/Q regions, which is an important aspect to consider when aiming at monitoring overdistension.

Gogniat et al. (2018) analyzed the effects of PEEP on VD and VD_{alv} in 15 patients with ARDS. They found a similar behavior, i.e., increased overdistension when PEEP was not only above but also below the optimum level set according to the best lung compliance (**Table 2**) (Gogniat et al., 2018). The authors could identify two clear responses to PEEP when patients were split into two groups according to changes of driving pressure (DP) from baseline ventilation. Patients with DP $<$ 15% (i.e., with better compliance in response to PEEP) presented the lowest dead space and Enghoff's index values at any PEEP, whereas those with DP $>$ 15% responded exaggeratedly to an increased PEEP. **Table 2** shows that the Bohr's dead space increased proportional to PEEP, whereas Enghoff's index remained unchanged. As Enghoff's index includes all V/Q mismatches, it was affected by the opposite simultaneous effects of PEEP on true dead space (increased by overdistension) and shunt (decreased by alveolar recruitment), reducing the sensibility and specificity for detecting lung overdistension.

For examining the role of VD in detecting overdistension in more detail, the effects of increasing PEEP levels from 0 to

Variable		PEEP		
		<4-6 cmH$_2$O	"Best"	>4-6 cmH$_2$O
Suter et al., 1975	Shunt %	0.18 ± 0.03 *	0.15 ± 0.02	0.11 ± 0.02 *
	VD_{alv}/VT	0.27 ± 0.02 *	0.18 ± 0.01	0.22 ± 0.02*
Tusman et al., 2011	Shunt %	0.26 (0.20-0.36) *	0.08 (0.05-0.15)	0.06 (0.03-0.10) *
	VD_{alv}/VT_{alv}	0.28 (0.24-0.38) *	0.16 (0.12-0.18)	0.18 (0.16-0.25) *
	VD_{aw}/VT	0.43 (0.40-0.44) *	0.44 (0.42-0.47)	0.49 (0.45-0.50) *
	$VTCO_{2,br}$ (mL)	4.8 (4.1-5.9) *	5.1 (4.3-5.9)	4.8 (4.2-5.5) *

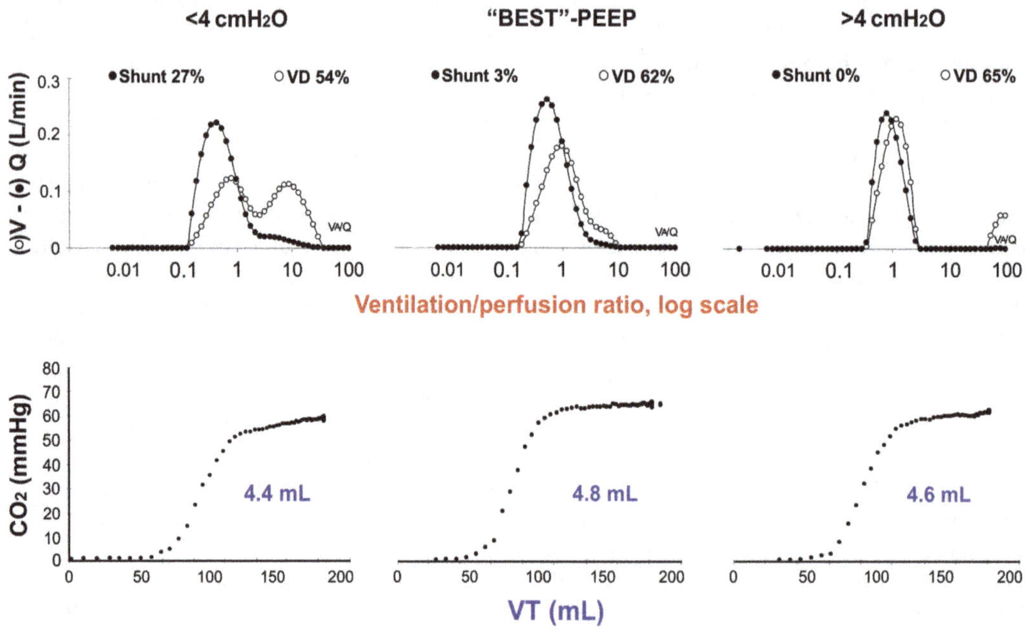

FIGURE 3 | Dead space at optimum PEEP. Comparison of the data obtained by Suter et al. (1975) using Enghoff's approach with our more recent data using VCap using Bohr's approach and multiple inert gas elimination technique (MIGET) (Tusman et al., 2011b). Physiological dead space measured by MIGET and VCap airway dead space increase proportional to PEEP, whereas shunt decreases with PEEP. An individualized level of PEEP ("Best" PEEP) corresponding to maximal respiratory system compliance, resulted in the lowest alveolar dead space and the highest elimination of CO_2 measured by VCap. PEEP above and below this optimum value results in an increased alveolar dead space and decreased the elimination of CO_2 per breath ($VTCO_{2,br}$). (*) $p < 0.05$ compared to best PEEP.

30 cmH$_2$O were analyzed in an experimental model of ARDS (Tusman et al., 2020). The Bohr's VD, with both its airway and alveolar components, increased in proportion when PEEP exceeded 15 cmH$_2$O, reflecting clear global lung overdistension that was confirmed by a parallel decrease in CO_2 elimination by the lungs, an increase in lung elastance, transpulmonary DP, and end-inspiratory transpulmonary pressure (**Figure 4**). However, at PEEP < 10 cmH$_2$O, VD_{aw} was minimal but VD_{alv} increased. This increase was associated to a low $VTCO_{2,br}$ and high lung elastance and transpulmonary DP.

TABLE 2 | Dead space and Enghoff's index in ARDS patients at different levels of PEEP.

Parameters	ΔP	Randomized PEEP (cmH_2O)			
		0	6	10	16
VDBohr/VT	All patients	0.44 (0.41–0.48)	0.45 (0.43–0.52)	0.47 (0.45–0.56)	0.51 (0.46–0.60)
	$\Delta P > 15\%$	0.50 (0.47–0.54)	0.55 (0.49–0.57)	0.59 (0.51–0.59)	0.61 (0.56–0.65)
	$\Delta P \leq 15\%$	0.41 (0.40–0.43)	0.44 (0.42–0.45)	0.45 (0.44–0.46)	0.47 (0.45–0.48)
		P = 0.012	*P* = 0.008	*P* = 0.006	*P* = 0.001
VDaw/VT	All patients	0.33 (0.29–0.36)	0.34 (0.30–0.40)	0.37 (0.31–0.45)	0.39 (0.34–0.47)
	$\Delta P > 15\%$	0.38 (0.31–0.40)	0.43 (0.33–0.45)	0.48 (0.36–0.50)	0.51 (0.41–0.55)
	$\Delta P \leq 15\%$	0.31 (0.29–0.33)	0.31 (0.29–0.34)	0.35 (0.29–0.37)	0.34 (0.30–0.38)
				P = 0.047	*P* = 0.018
VDalv/VTalv	All patients	0.18 (0.15–0.22)	0.19 (0.17–0.23)	0.19 (0.15–0.23)	0.22 (0.17–0.24)
	$\Delta P > 15\%$	0.20 (0.19–0.23)	0.22 (0.20–0.24)	0.21 (0.18–0.23)	0.25 (0.24–0.27)
	$\Delta P \leq 15\%$	0.16 (0.15–0.24)	0.17 (0.17–0.24)	0.16 (0.13–0.21)	0.16 (0.14–0.21)
			P = 0.047		*P* = 0.008
Enghoff's index	All patients	0.71 (0.60–0.73)	0.71 (0.58–0.74)	0.70 (0.63–0.75)	0.69 (0.59–0.77)
	$\Delta P > 15\%$	0.74 (0.73–0.74)	0.76 (0.74–0.77)	0.76 (0.75–0.76)	0.78 (0.77–0.79)
	$\Delta P \leq 15\%$	0.59 (0.56–0.70)	0.58 (0.55–0.69)	0.63 (0.54–0.69)	0.58 (0.53–0.63)
		P = 0.025	*P* = 0.008	*P* = 0.006	*P* = 0.002

VD_{Bohr}/VT = Bohr's dead space to tidal volume ratio, VD_{aw}/VT = airway dead space to tidal volume ratio, VD_{alv}/VT_{alv} = alveolar dead space to alveolar tidal volume ratio, and ΔP = driving pressure. Krustal-Wallis non-parametric test for ΔP inter-group comparison. Data is presented as median and 1st–3rd quartiles.

End-inspiratory transpulmonary pressure remained stable but high (~20 cmH_2O). These findings could be interpreted as an increase in stress and strain in the alveolar compartment of the aerated lung, despite lower levels of PEEP, caused by the stressor-raiser role of atelectasis (**Figures 4B,C**).

CAPNODYNAMICS FOR MONITORING LUNG STRAIN

Recently, a new method for monitoring lung overdistension by directly measuring lung strain based on expired CO_2 kinetics, the capnodynamic method, has been described (Suarez-Sipmann et al., 2019). Based on the principles of mass balance for CO_2 in the lung and the differential Fick principle for CO_2, the capnodynamic equation provides two highly relevant parameters for monitoring purposes: effective pulmonary blood flow ($EPBFCO_2$) (i.e., the non-shunted portion of cardiac output) and end-expiratory lung volume ($EELVCO_2$):

$$EELVCO_2 \cdot (FACO_2^n - FACO_2^{n-1}) = EPBFCO_2 \cdot \Delta t^n \cdot (CvCO_2 - CcCO_2^n) - VTCO_2^n$$

where $FACO_2{}^n$ refers to the alveolar fraction of CO_2 at the nth breath and $FACO_2{}^{n-1}$ for the preceding breath. Δt^n is the duration of the nth respiratory cycle, $CvCO_2$ and $CcCO_2{}^n$ is the mixed venous and capillary CO_2 content, $VTCO_2{}^n$ is the volume of CO_2 eliminated by the nth breath.

The mass balance occurs between the CO_2 content in the lung (represented on the left side of the equation) equals the difference between the CO_2 supplied to the lung by perfusion and the amount of CO_2 eliminated by the lung (on the right side of the equation). To solve the equation for its three unknowns: $EELVCO_2$, $EPBFCO_2$, and $CvCO_2$, a small modification in CO_2 alveolar concentration must occur under the assumption that $CvCO_2$ remains constant during the measurement cycle. All other parameters can be obtained non-invasively by VCap. The change in $FACO_2$ is obtained by a minimal modification of the breathing pattern (three consecutive respiratory cycles in which a short expiratory hold is added are repeatedly interspersed between six normal cycles) in a passively breathing patient under MV. Applying a repetitive sequence of six normal and three prolonged breaths, iterative mathematics can solve the capnodynamic equation after a set of nine equations is obtained. From then on, any new breath is added to the sequence providing a new solution (i.e., a new value of $EELVCO_2$ and $EPBFCO_2$, which can be monitored continuously). A more in-depth description of the method is beyond the scope of this manuscript. The method has been submitted to extensive experimental validation in challenging pulmonary and circulatory conditions (Sander et al., 2014, 2015). Recently, the first validations of $EPBFCO_2$ in patients on general anesthesia (Sigmundsson et al., 2021) and of $EELVCO_2$ (Öhman et al., 2020) have been published. Both performed well in good agreement with clinical reference methods and excellent trending abilities.

The decrease in FRC is one of the major contributors to VILI during MV. A way to quantify this risk is to determine lung strain, a measure of lung tissue deformation during inflation. To calculate lung strain, VT needs to be normalized to lung volume (strain = VT/FRC) (Chiumello et al., 2008), which during MV is referred to as end-expiratory lung volume as resting volume is influenced by the level of PEEP applied. When a certain threshold of strain is exceeded, the potential for mechanical damage to the ARDS lung increases (Bellani et al., 2011; González-López et al., 2012). The capnodynamic method offers the unprecedented possibility not only to measure EELV at the bedside, which has

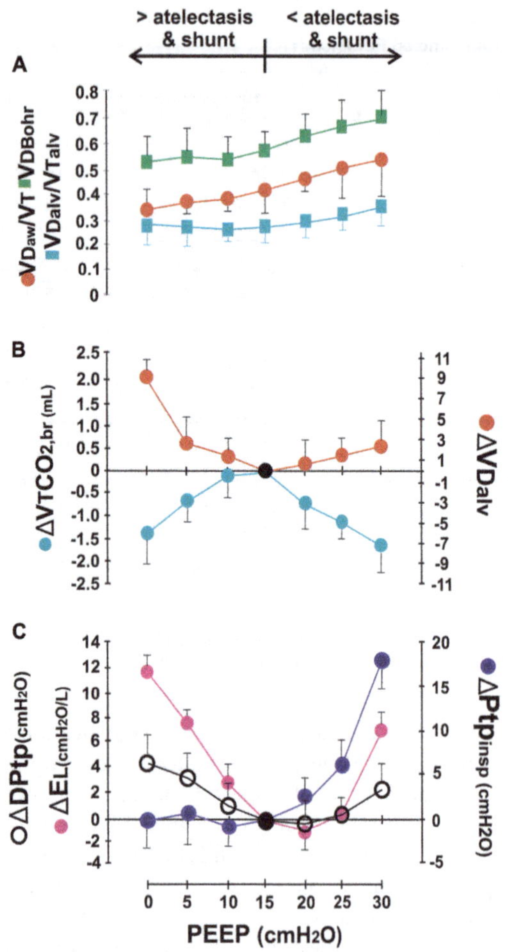

FIGURE 4 | Effects of PEEP in dead space and lung mechanics. Airway dead space increases in proportion to PEEP and has a direct impact on physiological Bohr's VD. Alveolar dead space (VDalv), on the contrary, changes according to the balance between recruitment and overdistension in the alveolar compartment. Panel **(A)** shows the effect of PEEP on absolute dead space values. Panels **(B,C)** present the differences in alveolar dead space (ΔVD_{alv}), elimination of CO_2 per breath ($\Delta VTCO_{2,br}$), transpulmonary driving pressure (ΔDPtp), transpulmonary end-inspiratory pressure (ΔPtp_{insp}), and lung elastance (ΔE_L) between certain PEEP level with the reference15-PEEP considered as the "Best" PEEP according to findings in gas exchange, lung ultrasound, and respiratory mechanics adapted from Tusman et al. (2020).

been very difficult to date, but also to do it in a non-invasive continuous way, extending and complementing the possibilities of VCap to measure lung overdistension and strain.

LUNG PERFUSION ESTIMATED BASED ON CO_2 KINETICS AND LUNG OVERDISTENSION

The hemodynamic consequence of lung overdistension is crucial information in mechanically ventilated patients with ARDS. Volumetric capnography has the unique ability to describe lung overdistension both from the ventilatory and hemodynamics perspective. Volumetric capnography assesses pulmonary perfusion *qualitatively* through the parameters $PETCO_2$ and VCO_2 (Tusman et al., 2010) and *quantitatively* by calculating the effective capillary pulmonary blood flow ($EPBF_{CO2}$) using equations based on the differential Fick's formula and the above-described capnodynamic method (Sander et al., 2014, 2015). Lung overdistension induced by high alveolar pressure can collapse pulmonary capillaries, decrease pulmonary blood flow, and increase right ventricle afterload. The association of high dead space with low VCO_2 or $EPBF_{CO2}$ has been observed during high PEEP ventilation, resulting in a *functional* overdistension because CO_2 exchange and elimination are impaired.

VCO_2 or $EPBF_{CO2}$ are decreased not only by lung overdistension but also by other hemodynamical causes like hypovolemia, embolism, arrhythmias, or heart failure. Therefore, physicians involved in the care of ventilated patients should first rule out any other hemodynamic problem when evaluating the hemodynamic consequence of lung overdistension. Again, the context-sensitive nature of CO_2 kinetics is relevant to make differential diagnoses. Many questions arise when the operator observes changes in pulmonary perfusion in ventilated patients. Is any acute hemodynamic problem of extra-pulmonary origin responsible for the low elimination of CO_2? Is the patient with normovolemia or has a preload-dependency? Have alveolar ventilation or body metabolism changed?

PREDICTION OF ACUTE RESPIRATORY DISTRESS SYNDROME OUTCOME

The role of VCap to determine the prognosis of patients with ARDS has been well established. Enghoff's index has been found to be strongly associated with mortality in the early and late course of ARDS (Nuckton et al., 2002; Kallet et al., 2014). The same research group showed that the risk to death increased by 22% for every 0.05 increase in Enghoff's index (OR = 1.22, 95% CI 1.11–1.35, $p < 0.001$) in patients with moderate and severe ARDS (Kallet et al., 2017). The magnitude of changes in the Enghoff's index varied according to ARDS etiology although, in each ARDS subgroup, this variable was always higher in non-survivors than in survivors. Recently, surrogates of VD, such as the ventilatory ratio—an index calculated by the quotient between measured and predicted minute ventilation and $PaCO_2$—was independently associated with mortality in patients with ARDS (Sinha et al., 2019). Why are these CO_2-based indexes, such good predictors of survival, better than the usual oxygen-based index in ARDS? When $PaCO_2$ is used to calculate dead space (according to the ideal alveolar gas concept) what it is measured is a global index of gas exchange including low V/Q and shunt. Lung physiology explains that shunt is represented not only by the $PA\text{-}aO_2$ but also by the $Pa\text{-}ACO_2$ difference. Therefore, these indexes based on $PaCO_2$ reflect the severity of ARDS by assessing shunt in combination with dead space. The prognostic value of Bohr's "true" dead space in a patient with ARDS is still unknown, but it is very likely that it also has an important role as a direct measure of lung ventilatory inefficiency and overdistension, both with likely strong influence on outcome.

CONCLUSION

Analysis of expired CO_2 kinetics by VCap provides important non-invasive cardiorespiratory information for clinical assessment, monitoring, and management of ARDS mechanically ventilated patients. Dead space and the Enghoff's index are calculated with high precision even in patients with very severe lung injury, as those with ARDS. The concept of VD is clinically useful not only to assess and adjust alveolar ventilation in the context of lung-protective MV but also to detect alveolar overdistension. Capnodynamic measurement of end-expiratory lung volume allows estimating strain that in combination with lung mechanics and lung perfusion can provide a more in-depth understanding of the lung condition and detect when this value exceeds safe limits. Real-time assessment of the elimination of CO_2 and effective pulmonary capillary blood flow provides information about the hemodynamic consequences of positive pressure ventilation. The combination of an increase in VD and a decrease in pulmonary capillary blood flow characterizes a situation of *functional* lung overdistension. Further studies are needed to explore the precise cutoff value to define harmful functional overdistension with VD and to determine its role as a screening tool to predict the evolution in patients with ARDS.

AUTHOR CONTRIBUTIONS

All authors listed have made a substantial, direct, and intellectual contribution to the work, and approved it for publication.

REFERENCES

Aitken, R. S., and Clark-Kennedy, A. E. (1928). On the fluctuation in the composition of the alveolar air during the respiratory cycle in muscular exercise. *J. Physiol.* 65, 389–411. doi: 10.1113/jphysiol.1928.sp002485

ARDS Network (2000). Ventilation with lower tidal volumes as compared with traditional tidal volumes for acute lung injury and the acute respiratory distress syndrome. *N. Engl. J. Med.* 342, 1301–1308. doi: 10.1056/nejm200005043421801

Åström, E., Niklason, L., Drefeldt, B., Bajc, M., and Jonson, B. (2000). Partitioning of dead space – a method and reference values in the awake human. *Eur. Respir. J.* 16, 659–664. doi: 10.1034/j.1399-3003.2000.16d16.x

Bellani, G., Guerra, L., Musch, G., Zanella, A., Patroniti, N., Mauri, T., et al. (2011). Lung regional metabolic activity and gas volume changes induced by tidal ventilation in patients with acute lung injury. *Am. J. Respir. Crit. Care Med.* 183, 1193–1199. doi: 10.1164/rccm.201008-1318oc

Bellani, G., Messa, C., Guerra, L., Spagnolli, E., Foti, G., Patroniti, N., et al. (2009). Lungs of patients with acute respiratory distress syndrome show diffuse inflammation in normally aerated regions: a [^{18}F]-fluoro-2-deoxy-D-glucose PET/CT study. *Crit. Care Med.* 37, 2216–2222. doi: 10.1097/ccm.0b013e3181aab31f

Beydon, L., Uttman, L., Rawal, R., and Jonson, B. (2002). Effects of positive end-expiratory pressure on dead space and its partitions in acute lung injury. *Intensive Care Med.* 28, 1239–1245. doi: 10.1007/s00134-002-1419-y

Blanch, L., Lucangelo, U., Aguilar, J. L., Fernandez, R., and Romero, P. V. (1999). Volumetric capnography in patients with acute lung injury: effects of positive end-expiratory pressure. *Eur. Respir. J.* 13, 1048–1054.

Bohr, C. (1891). Ueber die Lungenathmung. *Skan. Arch. Physiol.* 2, 236–268.

Chiumello, D., Carlesso, E., Cadringher, P., Caironi, P., Valenza, F., Polli, F., et al. (2008). Lung stress and strain during mechanical ventilation for acute respiratory distress syndrome. *Am. J. Respir. Crit. Care Med.* 178, 346–355. doi: 10.1164/rccm.200710-1589oc

Crawford, A. B., Makowska, M., Paiva, M., and Engel, L. A. (1985). Convection- and diffusion-dependent ventilation maldistribution in normal subjects. *J. Appl. Physiol.* 59, 838–846. doi: 10.1152/jappl.1985.59.3.838

Doorduin, J., Nollet, J. L., Vugts, M. P. A. J., Roesthuis, L. H., Akankan, F., Hoeven, J. G., et al. (2016). Assessment of dead-space ventilation in patients with acute respiratory distress syndrome: a prospective observational study. *Crit. Care* 20:121. doi: 10.1186/s13054-016-1311-8

Dubois, A. B., Britt, A., and Fenn, W. (1952). Alveolar CO2 during the respiratory cycle. *J. Appl. Physiol.* 4, 535–548. doi: 10.1152/jappl.1952.4.7.535

Enghoff, H. (1938). Volumen inefficax. Bemerkungen zur frage des schädlichen raumes. *Uppsala Läkareforen Forhandl* 44, 191–218.

Fletcher, R., Jonson, B., Cumming, G., and Brew, J. (1981). The concept of deadspace with special reference to the single breath test for carbon dioxide. *Br. J. Anaesth.* 53, 77–88. doi: 10.1093/bja/53.1.77

Fowler, W. S. (1948). Lung function studies. II. The respiratory dead space. *Am. J. Physiol. Leg.* 154, 405–410. doi: 10.1152/ajplegacy.1948.154.3.405

Gattinoni, L., Caironi, P., Cressoni, M., Chiumello, D., Ranieri, V. M., Quintel, M., et al. (2006). Lung recruitment in patients with the acute respiratory distress syndrome. *N. Engl. J. Med.* 354, 1775–1786. doi: 10.1056/nejmoa052052

Gogniat, E., Ducrey, M., Dianti, J., Madorno, M., Roux, N., Midley, A., et al. (2018). Dead space analysis at different levels of positive end-expiratory pressure in acute respiratory distress syndrome patients. *J. Crit. Care* 45, 231–238. doi: 10.1016/j.jcrc.2018.01.005

González-López, A., García-Prieto, E., Batalla-Solís, E., Amado-Rodríguez, L., Avello, N., Blanch, L., et al. (2012). Lung strain and biological response in mechanically ventilated patients. *Intensive Care Med.* 38, 240–247. doi: 10.1007/s00134-011-2403-1

Hlastala, M. P. (1972). A model of fluctuating alveolar gas exchange during the respiratory cycle. *Respir. Physiol.* 15, 214–232. doi: 10.1016/0034-5687(72)90099-0

Hurtado, D. E., Villarroel, N., Andrade, C., Retamal, J., Bugedo, G., and Bruhn, A. (2017). Spatial patterns and frequency distributions of regional deformation in the healthy human lung. *Biomech. Model. Mechanobiol.* 16, 1413–1423. doi: 10.1007/s10237-017-0895-5

Kallet, R. H., Daniel, B. M., Garcia, O., and Matthay, M. A. (2005). Accuracy of physiologic dead space measurements in patients with acute respiratory distress syndrome using volumetric capnography: comparison with the metabolic monitor method. *Respir. Care* 50, 462–467.

Kallet, R. H., Zhuo, H., Ho, K., Lipnick, M. S., Gomez, A., and Matthay, M. A. (2017). Lung injury. and other factors influencing the relationship between dead space fraction and mortality in ARDS. *Respir. Care* 62, 1241–1248. doi: 10.4187/respcare.05589

Kallet, R. H., Zhuo, H., Liu, K. D., Calfee, C. S., Matthay, M. A., and National Heart Lung and Blood Institute ARDS Network Investigators (2014). The association between physiologic dead-space fraction and mortality in subjects with ARDS enrolled in a prospective multi-center clinical trial. *Respir. Care* 59, 1611–1618. doi: 10.4187/respcare.02593

Larsson, C. P., and Severinghaus, J. W. (1962). Postural variations in dead space and CO_2 gradients breathing air and O2. *J. Appl. Physiol.* 17, 417–420. doi: 10.1152/jappl.1962.17.3.417

Lum, L., Saville, A., and Venkataraman, S. T. (1998). Accuracy of physiologic deadspace measurement in intubated pediatric patients using a metabolic monitor. *Crit. Care Med.* 26, 760–764. doi: 10.1097/00003246-199804000-00029

Nuckton, T. J., Alonso, J. A., Kallet, R. H., Daniel, B. M., Pittet, J.-F., Eisner, M. D., et al. (2002). Pulmonary dead-space fraction as a risk factor for death in the acute respiratory distress syndrome. *N. Engl. J. Med.* 346, 1281–1286. doi: 10.1056/nejmoa012835

Nunn, J. F., and Hill, D. W. (1960). Respiratory dead space and arterial to end-tidal CO_2 difference in anesthetized man. *J. Appl. Physiol.* 15, 383–389. doi: 10.1152/jappl.1960.15.3.383

Öhman, T., Sigmundsson, T. S., Hallbäck, M., Sipmann, F. S., Wallin, M., Oldner, A., et al. (2020). Clinical and experimental validation of a capnodynamic method for end-expiratory lung volume assessment. *Acta Anaesthesiol. Scand.* 64, 670–676. doi: 10.1111/aas.13552

Protti, A., Andreis, D. T., Monti, M., Santini, A., Sparacino, C. C., Langer, T., et al. (2013). Lung stress and strain during mechanical ventilation. *Crit. Care Med.* 41, 1046–1055. doi: 10.1097/ccm.0b013e31827417a6

Riley, R. L., and Cournand, A. (1949). "Ideal"; alveolar air and the analysis of ventilation-perfusion relationships in the lungs. *J. Appl. Physiol.* 1, 825–847.

Rossier, P., and Buhlmann, A. (1955). The respiratory dead space. *Physiol. Rev.* 35, 860–876. doi: 10.1152/physrev.1955.35.4.860

Sander, C. H., Hallback, M., Wallin, M., Emtell, P., Oldner, A., and Bjorne, H. (2014). Novel continuous capnodynamic method for cardiac output assessment during mechanical ventilation. *Br. J. Anaesth.* 112, 824–831. doi: 10.1093/bja/aet486

Sander, C. H., Lönnqvist, P.-A., Hallbäck, M., Sipmann, F. S., Wallin, M., Oldner, A., et al. (2015). Capnodynamic assessment of effective lung volume during cardiac output manipulations in a porcine model. *J. Clin. Monit. Comput.* 30, 761–769. doi: 10.1007/s10877-015-9767-7

Sigmundsson, T. S., Öhman, T., Hallbäck, M., Suarez-Sipmann, F., Wallin, M., Oldner, A., et al. (2021). Comparison between capnodynamic and thermodilution method for cardiac output monitoring during major abdominal surgery: an observational study. *Eur. J. Anaesth.* doi: 10.1097/eja.0000000000001566 [Epub online ahead of print].

Sinha, P., Calfee, C. S., Beitler, J. R., Soni, N., Ho, K., Matthay, M. A., et al. (2019). Physiologic analysis and clinical performance of the ventilatory ratio in acute respiratory distress syndrome. *Am. J. Respir. Crit. Care Med.* 199, 333–341. doi: 10.1164/rccm.201804-0692oc

Sinha, P., and Soni, N. (2012). Comparison of volumetric capnography and mixed expired gas methods to calculate physiological dead space in mechanically ventilated ICU patients. *Intensive Care Med.* 38, 1712–1717. doi: 10.1007/s00134-012-2670-5

Siobal, M. S., Ong, H., Valdes, J., and Tang, J. (2013). Calculation of physiologic dead space: comparison of ventilator volumetric capnography to measurements by metabolic analyzer and volumetric CO_2 monitor. *Respir. Care* 58, 1143–1151. doi: 10.4187/respcare.02116

Sipmann, F. S., Böhm, S. H., and Tusman, G. (2014). Volumetric capnography: the time has come. *Curr. Opin. Crit. Care* 20, 333–339. doi: 10.1097/mcc.0000000000000095

Suarez-Sipmann, F., Tusman, G., and Wallin, M. (2019). "Continuous non-invasive monitoring of cardiac output and lung volume based on CO_2 kinetics," in *Annual Update in Intensive Care and Emergency Medicine 2019*, ed. J.-L. Vincent (Cham: Springer), 215–229. doi: 10.1007/978-3-030-060 67-1_16

Suter, P. M., Fairley, B., and Isenberg, M. D. (1975). Optimum end-expiratory airway pressure in patients with acute pulmonary failure. *N. Engl. J. Med.* 292, 284–289. doi: 10.1056/nejm197502062920604

Tusman, G., Böhm, S. H., Sipmann, F. S., Scandurra, A., and Hedenstierna, G. (2010). Lung recruitment and positive end-expiratory pressure have different effects on CO_2 elimination in healthy and sick lungs. *Anes. Anal.* 111, 968–977. doi: 10.1213/ane.0b013e3181f0c2da

Tusman, G., Gogniat, E., Böhm, S. H., Scandurra, A., Sipmann, F. S., Torroba, A., et al. (2013). Reference values for volumetric capnography-derived non-invasive parameters in healthy individuals. *J. Clin. Monit. Comput.* 27, 281–288. doi: 10.1007/s10877-013-9433-x

Tusman, G., Gogniat, E., Madorno, M., Otero, P., Dianti, J., Ceballos, I. F., et al. (2020). Effect of PEEP on dead space in an experimental model of ARDS. *Respir. Care* 65, 11–20. doi: 10.4187/respcare.06843

Tusman, G., Scandurra, A., Böhm, S. H., Sipmann, F. S., and Clara, F. (2009). Model fitting of volumetric capnograms improves calculations of airway dead space and slope of phase III. *J. Clin. Monit. Comput.* 23, 197–206. doi: 10.1007/s10877-009-9182-z

Tusman, G., Sipmann, F. S., and Böhm, S. H. (2012). Rationale of dead space measurement by volumetric capnography. *Anesth. Analg.* 114, 866–874. doi: 10.1213/ane.0b013e318247f6cc

Tusman, G., Sipmann, F. S., Borges, J. B., Hedenstierna, G., and Böhm, S. H. (2011a). Validation of Bohr dead space measured by volumetric capnography. *Intensive Care Med.* 37, 870–874. doi: 10.1007/s00134-011-2164-x

Tusman, G., Suarez-Sipmann, F., Bohm, S. H., Borges, J. B., and Hedenstierna, G. (2011b). Capnography reflects ventilation/perfusion distribution in a model of acute lung injury. *Acta Anaesthesiol. Scand.* 55, 597–606. doi: 10.1111/j.1399-6576.2011.02404.x

Verbanck, S., and Paiva, M. (2013). Gas mixing in the airways and airspaces. *Compr. Physiol.* 1, 809–834. doi: 10.1002/cphy.c100018

6

The Renin-Angiotensin System as a Component of Biotrauma in Acute Respiratory Distress Syndrome

Katharina Krenn, Verena Tretter, Felix Kraft and Roman Ullrich*

Department of Anesthesia, General Intensive Care and Pain Medicine, Medical University of Vienna, Vienna, Austria

***Correspondence:**
Katharina Krenn
katharina.krenn@meduniwien.ac.at

Acute respiratory distress syndrome (ARDS) is a major concern in critical care medicine with a high mortality of over 30%. Injury to the lungs is caused not only by underlying pathological conditions such as pneumonia, sepsis, or trauma, but also by ventilator-induced lung injury (VILI) resulting from high positive pressure levels and a high inspiratory oxygen fraction. Apart from mechanical factors that stress the lungs with a specific physical power and cause volutrauma and barotrauma, it is increasingly recognized that lung injury is further aggravated by biological mediators. The COVID-19 pandemic has led to increased interest in the role of the renin-angiotensin system (RAS) in the context of ARDS, as the RAS enzyme angiotensin-converting enzyme 2 serves as the primary cell entry receptor for severe acute respiratory syndrome (SARS) coronavirus (CoV)-2. Even before this pandemic, studies have documented the involvement of the RAS in VILI and its dysregulation in clinical ARDS. In recent years, analytical tools for RAS investigation have made major advances based on the optimized precision and detail of mass spectrometry. Given that many clinical trials with pharmacological interventions in ARDS were negative, RAS-modifying drugs may represent an interesting starting point for novel therapeutic approaches. Results from animal models have highlighted the potential of RAS-modifying drugs to prevent VILI or treat ARDS. While these drugs have beneficial pulmonary effects, the best targets and application forms for intervention still have to be determined to avoid negative effects on the circulation in clinical settings.

Keywords: acute respiratory distress syndrome, ventilator-induced lung injury, renin-angiotensin system, biotrauma, mass spectrometry

INTRODUCTION

The renin-angiotensin system (RAS) plays a role in many cardiovascular, renal, and pulmonary processes. It is a network of peptides (**Figure 1**) that are enzymatically cleaved from the precursor protein angiotensinogen (56.8 kDa) that is mainly produced by the liver. The first step of RAS activation is the cleavage of angiotensinogen to angiotensin I (Ang I or Ang 1–10) by the protease renin, an enzyme produced by the kidney. In this context, "1–10" refers to the number of amino acid residues constituting the peptide. Ang I is subsequently cleaved to angiotensin II (Ang II or Ang 1–8) by angiotensin converting enzyme (ACE) (Skeggs et al., 1980; Corvol et al., 1995). Ang II-mediated effects are exerted through the Ang II type 1 (AT1) and 2 (AT2) receptors (Eckenstaler et al., 2021; Fatima et al., 2021). The production of Ang II by ACE is often called the "classical" activation of the RAS. Ang I and Ang II may also be enzymatically cleaved by other, "alternative" proteases including ACE2, resulting in a multitude of smaller peptides such as Ang 1–9 or Ang 1–7 (Imai et al., 2008; Santos et al., 2018). In addition to production of Ang 1–7 from Ang II by ACE2,

Ang 1–7 may be cleaved from Ang II by prolyl oligopeptidase (POP) in the circulation (Serfozo et al., 2020). Another enzyme, neprilysin, a neutral endopeptidase, cleaves Ang I to Ang 1–7 (Rice et al., 2004). The peptide Ang 1–7 in turn is a substrate for the N-domain of ACE and cleaved to the smaller peptide Ang 1-5 (Corradi et al., 2006). In a broader context, there is complex interaction between the RAS, the kinin–kallikrein system and the activity of chymase, which is expressed by mast cells and various tissues and may also cleave Ang I to Ang II (Abassi et al., 2021). Renin, ACE and AT1 receptors are important targets of anti-hypertensive and heart failure therapy (Aronson and Krum, 2012; Laurent et al., 2012). Recently, a neprilysin inhibitor/angiotensin receptor blocker combination was added to the spectrum of heart failure therapy (Gallo et al., 2021). ACE inhibitors most importantly block the production of Ang II from Ang I and therefore lead to an accumulation of Ang I and subsequently the peptide Ang 2–10 that is cleaved from Ang I by aminopeptidase A (Velez et al., 2009), and Ang 1–7 that is cleaved from Ang I by neprilysin. As ACE inhibitors also block the degradation of Ang 1–7 to Ang 1–5, this leads to a further increase in Ang 1-7 levels that is detectable in the plasma of patients treated with ACE inhibitors (Kovarik et al., 2015, 2017). Angiotensin receptor blockers lead to increased levels of Ang II (Vischer et al., 2021), whereas inhibition of renin downregulates the concentrations of all angiotensin peptides, since the production of Ang I is already inhibited. This review describes the involvement of the RAS in the biological reactions to mechanical ventilation and summarizes what is known about RAS regulation in critically ill and mechanically ventilated patients with ARDS and COVID-19 for the purpose of discovering new biomarkers and identifying new therapeutic targets.

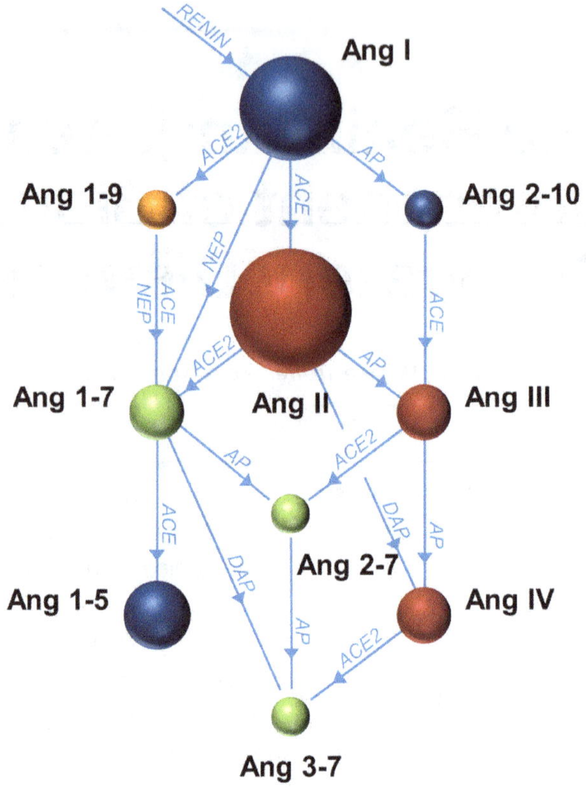

FIGURE 1 | The network of enzymes and peptides of the renin-angiotensin system in plasma. The enzymatic cascade is initiated by cleavage of angiotensinogen by renin to produce angiotensin (Ang) I. The network of enzymes that successively cleave the respective angiotensin metabolites is indicated in blue. ACE, angiotensin-converting enzyme; AP, aminopeptidase; NEP, neprilysin; DAP, diaminopeptidase.

CONCEPTS OF VENTILATOR-INDUCED LUNG INJURY

Mechanical ventilation is required in clinical conditions associated with acute pulmonary gas exchange deterioration, reduced vigilance, and loss of protective reflexes. The unphysiological state of positive pressure ventilation subsequently impacts the body further. The relevance of this impact increases with higher settings of mechanical power variables such as ventilation pressure, tidal volume and respiratory rate (Cressoni et al., 2016; Gattinoni et al., 2016). Components of ventilator-induced lung injury (VILI) include volutrauma and barotrauma, atelectrauma, and biotrauma (Gattinoni et al., 2010). Biotrauma involves upregulation of proinflammatory mediators and recruitment of neutrophils to the lungs which may augment pulmonary edema formation in VILI (Dreyfuss and Saumon, 1998). It is well established that experimental ventilation with high tidal volumes leads to increased levels of proinflammatory cytokines such as interleukin (IL)-6 and macrophage inhibitory protein (MIP)-2, a functional equivalent of IL-8 in rodents (Dreyfuss and Saumon, 1998; Halbertsma et al., 2005). This increase of proinflammatory mediators in the circulation caused by VILI may subsequently promote multiple system organ failure (Slutsky and Tremblay, 1998; Plotz et al., 2004). In a randomized controlled trial, Ranieri et al. (1999) showed that proinflammatory mediators in broncho-alveolar lavage fluid (BALF) and plasma were lower in a group of patients receiving lung-protective ventilation characterized by lower tidal volume and end-inspiratory plateau pressure as well as higher positive end-expiratory pressure (PEEP). The ARDS network study further underscored the clinical impact on ventilator-free days and survival of lung-protective ventilation with a reduced tidal volume of 6 ml/kg predicted body weight and an inspiratory plateau pressure of 30 cm of water at maximum (Acute Respiratory Distress Syndrome Network et al., 2000). At the interface of inflammatory activation and the fibroproliferative response that may occur following ARDS, scientists began to understand the relevance of Ang II as a mediator. Ang II is released from the lungs of patients suffering from ARDS (Wenz et al., 2000), and experimental data have shown its profibrotic effects in lung injury caused by bleomycin (Marshall et al., 2004). In the latter study, treatment with the ACE inhibitor ramipril or the AT1 receptor blocker losartan resulted in reduced pulmonary collagen deposition. Hypoxia as well as hyperoxia may occur in mechanically ventilated lungs – hypoxia for instance as a consequence of hypoventilated areas attributable to the primary lung disease, hyperoxia as a consequence of the high inspiratory fraction of oxygen needed for treatment of hypoxemic patients. Hypoxia as well as hyperoxia induce collagen production in human pulmonary fibroblasts (Lang et al., 2010; Liu et al., 2013), and may be involved in the development of fibrotic changes following ARDS.

EXPERIMENTAL EVIDENCE ABOUT THE ROLE OF THE RENIN-ANGIOTENSIN SYSTEM IN LUNG INJURY

The RAS and potential sites of intervention have been studied in various experimental settings, sometimes yielding conflicting results that depend on the exact parameters of the experimental models. Ventilation with a very high tidal volume of 40 ml/kg in rats led to increased protein content in BALF, pulmonary expression and serum levels of MIP-2, and lung tissue levels of Ang II after 4 h, while mRNA expression levels of ACE2 were decreased (Jerng et al., 2007). The effects on BALF protein levels, MIP-2 and ACE2 expression were absent in a group of rats ventilated with a low tidal volume (7 ml/kg) and were reversible with the ACE inhibitor captopril. Beneficial effects on BALF protein levels in the high tidal volume group were also achieved by AT1 or AT2 receptor blockers in this study. Furthermore, studies have shown protective effects of ACE and AT1 receptor inhibition in rodent models of lung injury (Lukkarinen et al., 2005; He et al., 2007; Shen et al., 2009). In addition to increased levels of proinflammatory markers, Ang II may lead to an imbalance in the expression of epithelial sodium channel (ENaC) subunits that inhibits alveolar fluid clearance and thereby promotes pulmonary edema (Deng et al., 2012a,b). ACE2 is a natural counterregulator of classical RAS activation and the subsequent increase in Ang II levels. This homolog of ACE protects from ARDS, whereas increased ACE activity and signaling through AT1 receptors further aggravate lung injury (Imai et al., 2007). ACE2 inactivates Ang II and thus counteracts the deleterious effects of Ang II-signaling through AT1 receptors such as increased vascular tone and permeability (Imai et al., 2005, 2008). Mice with genetic inactivation of ACE were protected from acid-induced lung injury and revealed decreased Ang II levels in plasma and lung tissue, while mice with an ACE2 knockout genetic background developed more severe lung injury (Imai et al., 2005). In another study, mice infected with H7N9 influenza virus were found to have increased Ang II levels accompanied by decreased ACE2 protein expression in the lung tissue after 3 days (Yang et al., 2014). The enzymatic cleavage of Ang II by ACE2 produces Ang 1–7, which is in itself biologically active and initiates protective effects through the Mas receptor (Santos et al., 2018). Ang 1–7 has been recognized as the principal mediator of the beneficial effects of recombinant ACE2 in a murine model of Ang II-mediated myocardial fibrosis (Patel et al., 2015) and as a protective treatment against ARDS induced by bronchial acid instillation and high stretch ventilation in rats (Zambelli et al., 2015).

The role of ACE activity in VILI is somewhat controversial and may depend on the exact parameters of the model system, the biological compartments that were investigated, and the analytic methods. In mechanically ventilated rats with tidal volumes of 18 ml/kg aiming at moderate alveolar hyperdistension, lung ACE activity was significantly decreased (Behnia et al., 1996). In a more recent study, an imbalance between ACE and ACE2 activity was found in ventilated rats exposed to lipopolysaccharide (LPS), resulting in increased Ang II and reduced Ang 1–7 levels in BALF (Wosten-van Asperen et al., 2011). In this model, the proinflammatory effects were attenuated by treatment with losartan or cyclic Ang 1–7. In another study using a lung injury model induced by instillation of hydrochloric acid and increased tidal volumes of 18 ml/kg in rats, infusion of Ang 1–7 improved oxygenation and reduced inflammation in the acute setting and led to reduced pulmonary collagen deposition after 2 weeks if it was continued through osmotic minipumps (Zambelli et al., 2015). Plasminogen activator inhibitor (PAI)-1 is a biomarker of ARDS (Bhargava and Wendt, 2012) and was increased in conjunction with Ang II in a rat model of VILI (Chen et al., 2008). Systemic PAI-1 levels and VILI were attenuated by treatment with the ACE inhibitor captopril, and, interestingly, also hepatic ischemia/reperfusion-induced lung injury in rats was ameliorated by treatment with captopril (El-Sayed et al., 2020).

Age is an important factor for interpreting the results of animal lung injury models. In a systematic review, Schouten et al. (2015) noted that older animals developed more edema, a higher degree of histological pulmonary damage, and were found to have higher mortality than juvenile/adult animals in studies of VILI, pneumonia, and lung injury induced by hyperoxia or LPS. In a study in rats, the same group found higher wet/dry lung weight ratio, BALF protein content, and proinflammatory cytokine levels in older animals exposed to VILI (tidal volume 15 mL/kg) and LPS (Schouten et al., 2016). The same study also investigated ACE and ACE2 and found that treatment with LPS alone or in combination with injurious mechanical ventilation led to an age-dependent decrease in membrane-bound ACE activity in lung tissue and to an increase in soluble ACE activity in BALF. Levels of soluble ACE activity correlated well with indicators of lung injury severity. The study also discussed a link between increased levels of tumor necrosis factor-α in BALF and subsequent activation of ADAM9, one of the enzymes responsible for ACE shedding. In addition to lung injury, Ang II promotes monocyte/macrophage infiltration in other tissues, reactive oxygen species production, and ageing-related neurodegeneration (Benigni et al., 2010).

Expression levels of RAS enzymes seem to depend on partial pressure of oxygen. Experimental models in mice (FiO_2 = 12%) as well as primary murine alveolar epithelial type II cells and human small airway epithelial cells exposed to 1% oxygen have demonstrated a hypoxia-induced increase in ACE2 mRNA expression (Sturrock et al., 2021). Furthermore, a cell culture study with primary murine pulmonary endothelial cells showed even higher ACE2 mRNA expression after exposure to hyperoxia (95% oxygen) and oscillating oxygen conditions between 0 and 95% than with hypoxia (5% oxygen) (Wohlrab et al., 2021). Both hypoxia and hyperoxia may occur in the lungs of patients with ARDS depending on regional ventilation.

CLINICAL EVIDENCE ABOUT THE ROLE OF THE RENIN-ANGIOTENSIN SYSTEM IN ACUTE RESPIRATORY DISTRESS SYNDROME

A beneficial effect of ACE inhibitor intake in patients was demonstrated for the first time by Mortensen et al. (2005) in hospitalized patients with community-acquired pneumonia. In this study, 30-day mortality was lower in patients with previous ACE inhibitor treatment. In a population-based study, the 90-day risk for hospitalization with pneumonia was also reduced in patients over 65 years of age with a new prescription of antihypertensive drugs if the prescribed drugs were ACE inhibitors of angiotensin receptor blockers (Shah et al., 2014). Another retrospective study addressed the impact of preexisting ACE inhibitor or angiotensin receptor blocker therapy during intensive care unit (ICU) admission on the course of ARDS (Kim et al., 2017). Although patients taking a RAS inhibitor required a longer duration of mechanical ventilation and a longer ICU stay, their survival was improved compared to patients who were not taking a RAS inhibitor. **Table 1** summarizes the literature on RAS-modifying drugs and risk and outcomes of pneumonia, ARDS and radiation pneumonitis, RAS activation in critical illness, ARDS and COVID-19, and randomized controlled clinical trials targeting the RAS in these conditions.

Actions of Ang II in ARDS are proinflammatory, profibrotic (Hrenak and Simko, 2020) and involved in regulation of alveolar fluid clearance in the lung (Deng et al., 2012a,b). It can therefore be speculated that RAS activation may be a relevant parameter in the pathogenesis and course of ARDS. Biomarker phenotyping of patients with ARDS has yielded at least two classes, including a "reactive" phenotype with higher proinflammatory activation associated with higher mortality (Calfee et al., 2014, 2015; Bos et al., 2017). Considering the association of increases in Ang II with proinflammatory activation in experimental lung injury (Jerng et al., 2007), it would be interesting to explore whether this phenotype is associated with higher RAS activation as well.

So far, few studies have systematically examined RAS activation in mechanically ventilated ICU patients. One study measured the plasma renin levels of 20 critically ill patients at multiple time points, and found an inverse correlation with urine output and mean arterial blood pressure (Gleeson et al., 2019). As a marker of tissue perfusion, renin outperformed lactate levels in prediction of prognosis in this study. Nearly two thirds of the included patients were in septic, hemorrhagic, or cardiogenic shock, but only two patients had a diagnosis of pneumonia, so that no conclusions about renin levels in ARDS can be drawn from this study. The angiotensin metabolite profile in mechanically ventilated patients with ARDS was investigated by Reddy et al. (2019) with mass spectrometry in protease-inhibited samples, and by Krenn et al. (2020) with RAS equilibrium analysis without protease inhibition. An analysis of plasma from blood samples that are immediately stabilized with a protease inhibitor cocktail yields the circulating concentrations of angiotensin metabolites. In contrast, RAS equilibrium analysis uses plasma or serum without protease inhibition. Before measurement with liquid chromatography tandem mass spectrometry (LC-MS/MS), the samples are incubated at 37°C to establish an equilibrium between production and cleavage of angiotensin metabolites. In serum or plasma, this is feasible due to the high molar surplus of angiotensinogen to renin that is physiologically present and the constant formation of the initial substrate Ang I of the RAS cascade during the 37°C incubation step. Nascent Ang I is immediately converted into downstream metabolites by soluble enzymes so that new equilibrium levels emerge. These levels arise from equal enzymatic formation and degradation rates of individual angiotensin metabolites in the sample and depend on all enzymes involved in the plasma angiotensin metabolism, so that ratios between product and precursor may be used as angiotensin-based markers of enzyme activities (Burrello et al., 2020; Zoufaly et al., 2020). Furthermore, it has been shown that the sum of Ang I and Ang II (PRA-S) is highly correlated with plasma renin activity (Goppner et al., 2019; Burrello et al., 2020; Krenn et al., 2020). A summary of angiotensin-based markers of RAS enzyme activities is presented in **Figure 2.** Overall, angiotensin metabolite concentrations in protease-inhibited samples show a strong correlation with their equilibrium levels (Basu et al., 2017). In the study by Reddy et al. (2019) Ang I (1–10) levels were higher in non-survivors than in survivors of ARDS, and the Ang II/Ang I ratio was lower in non-survivors than in survivors in both studies (Krenn et al., 2020). In comparison to postoperative patients, Ang I, Ang II, and Ang 1–7 plasma concentrations were increased in early ARDS, and the Ang II/Ang I ratio was inverted (Krenn et al., 2020). **Figure 3** illustrates the main changes in the plasmatic angiotensin metabolite profile associated with ARDS. These results pointed to endogenous ACE inhibition, as none of the patients with early ARDS were receiving RAS-blocking drugs, and active ACE concentrations measured in a mass spectrometry-based assay and ACE protein levels measured by ELISA were not changed. After 7 days of mechanical ventilation, RAS activation indicated by PRA-S as a marker of plasma renin activity correlated with driving pressure (Krenn et al., 2020), indicating that improvement of the respiratory situation with decreased driving pressure was associated with a larger decrease in RAS activation. The relatively low Ang II levels in contrast to Ang I concentrations may have been attributable to the following causes: Part of Ang II was metabolized to Ang 1–7 by ACE2, as our ACE2 inhibition experiments suggested (Krenn et al., 2020), but other proteases may have played a role as well. Annoni et al. (2019) actually found increased ACE protein levels in mechanically ventilated patients with early ARDS who did not survive, while ACE2 protein levels had not changed. This is at least further proof that the reduced Ang II/Ang I ratios in ARDS are more likely attributable to endogenous ACE inhibition, increased metabolization of Ang II by ACE2, or other, yet unknown, proteases than to reduced ACE expression. However, using another brand of ACE and ACE2 ELISAs, Gerard et al. (2021) found decreased ACE and increased ACE2 protein

TABLE 1 | Clinical data about effects of RAS-modifying drugs on outcome, characterization of RAS activation, and randomized clinical trials with RAS-modifying drugs in pneumonia, critical illness, ARDS, COVID-19 and radiation pneumonitis.

Authors and year	Type of study	Collective/cohort/eligibility for inclusion	No. of participants	Treatment groups/main outcomes
RAS modifying drugs and outcome				
Mortensen et al., 2005	Retrospective cohort study	Patients hospitalized with community acquired pneumonia	*n* = 787	ACEi therapy/30-day mortality ↓
Caldeira et al., 2012	Systematic review and meta-analysis	Studies including patients taking ACEi or ARB and analyzing risk and mortality of pneumonia	29 studies	ACEi or ARB therapy/Incidence of pneumonia ↓ with ACEi Pneumonia related mortality ↓ with ACEi and ARB
Shah et al., 2014	Population based study	New prescription of antihypertensive drugs in patients >65 years	*n* = 254.485	Drugs: ACEi, ARB, calcium channel blockers, beta blockers and thiazide diuretics/90-day risk of hospitalization with pneumonia ↓ with ACEi and ARB
Kim et al., 2017	Retrospective case control study	Patients admitted to the ICU with ARDS	*n* = 182	ACEi or ARB therapy/With RAS inhibitor: ICU mortality ↓ Duration of mechanical ventilation ↑ Length of ICU stay↑
Sun et al., 2018	Meta-analysis	Lung cancer patients with radiation therapy	*n* = 1.412	ACEi and ARB therapy/Incidence of symptomatic radiation pneumonitis ↓ with ACEi
RAS activation in critical illness and ARDS				
Gleeson et al., 2019	Prospective observational study	Patients admitted to the ICU	*n* = 20	Renin in plasma
Reddy et al., 2019	Pilot study, observational study	ICU patients with ARDS	*n* = 39	Angiotensin metabolite profile in plasma, protease inhibited
Annoni et al., 2019	Observational study	Mechanically ventilated ICU patients with ARDS	*n* = 96	ACE and ACE2 protein levels in plasma
Krenn et al., 2020	Observational study	Mechanically ventilated ICU patients with ARDS	*n* = 27	Angiotensin metabolite profile in RAS equilibrium analysis, active ACE levels, ACE and ACE2 protein levels in plasma
Gerard et al., 2021	Retrospective study	Patients with COVID-19 related/non-COVID ARDS	Tissue: COVID *n* = 15/non-COVID *n* = 13, Serum: COVID *n* = 35/non-COVID *n* = 24	ACE and ACE2 protein expression in lung tissue Ang II, Ang 1–7, ACE and ACE2 protein levels in serum
RAS activation in COVID-19				
Ozkan et al., 2021	Observational study	Hospitalized patients with COVID-19 and signs of pneumonia	*n* = 112	Ang II levels in serum
Kutz et al., 2021	Observational study with matched controls	Patients with COVID-19 admitted to the hospital and SARS-CoV-2 negative propensity-score matched controls	*n* = 43 in both groups	Angiotensin metabolite profile in RAS equilibrium analysis, angiotensin concentration-based markers of renin, ACE and ACE2 activities
Files et al., 2021	Observational study	Patients with moderate to severe acute respiratory failure due to COVID-19 and moderate acute respiratory failure negative for SARS-CoV-2	COVID-19: *n* = 22, SARS-COV-2 negative patients: *n* = 11	Ang II and Ang 1–7 plasma levels and ACE, ACE2 and POP activities in serum in fluorescent assays
Eleuteri et al., 2021	Observational study	Patients with COVID-19 related ARDS admitted to the ICU	*n* = 32	Renin, Ang I, Ang II, Ang 1–7 serum levels, Ang I/Ang II ratio as indicator of ACE activity
Reindl-Schwaighofer et al., 2021	Observational study	Patients hospitalized with COVID-19, and critically ill patients with influenza pneumonia	COVID-19: *n* = 126 Influenza: *n* = 27	Equilibrium plasma levels of Ang II, Ang 1–7 and active ACE2 levels
Wang et al., 2021	Observational study	Patients hospitalized with COVID-19	*n* = 242	Circulating Ang I, Ang II, Ang 1–7 and ACE2 levels
Osman et al., 2021	Observational study	Patients hospitalized with COVID-19 and healthy SARS-CoV-2 negative controls	COVID-19: *n* = 44 (16.6% male) Controls: *n* = 15 (46.7% male)	Ang I, Ang II, Ang 1–7 and ACE2 plasma levels, ACE2 mRNA expression and ACE2 and specific biomarker membrane protein expression in flow cytometry in peripheral blood mononuclear cells

(Continued)

TABLE 1 | (Continued)

Authors and year	Type of study	Collective/cohort/eligibility for inclusion	No. of participants	Treatment groups/main outcomes
RAS modifying drugs in randomized controlled clinical trials				
Boldt et al., 1995	RCT	Critically ill patients	$n = 45$	Enalapril/Hemodynamic and respiratory parameters
Khan et al., 2017	RCT	Patients with ARDS	$n = 46$	rhACE2/PaO_2/FiO_2 ratio, biomarkers, SOFA score
Small et al., 2018	RCT	Lung cancer patients with radiation therapy	$n = 33$	Captopril/Incidence of symptomatic radiation pneumonitis ↓
Sio et al., 2019	RCT	Lung cancer patients with chemo-radiation therapy	$n = 23$	Lisinopril/Incidence of chemo-radiation induced pulmonary distress ↓

ACE, angiotensin converting enzyme; ACEi, ACE inhibitor; Ang, angiotensin; ARB, angiotensin receptor blocker; ARDS, acute respiratory distress syndrome; ICU, intensive care unit; RAS, Renin-angiotensin system; RCT, randomized controlled trial; rhACE2, recombinant human ACE2; POP, prolyl oligopeptidase, SOFA score, sequential organ failure assessment score.

Angiotensin-based markers of enzyme activities

Renin activity Ang I + Ang II

ACE activity Ang II / Ang I

Alternative RAS activity

Ang 1-7 + Ang 1-5 / Ang I + Ang II + Ang 1-7 + Ang 1-5

FIGURE 2 | Definitions of angiotensin-based markers of renin-angiotensin system enzyme activities.

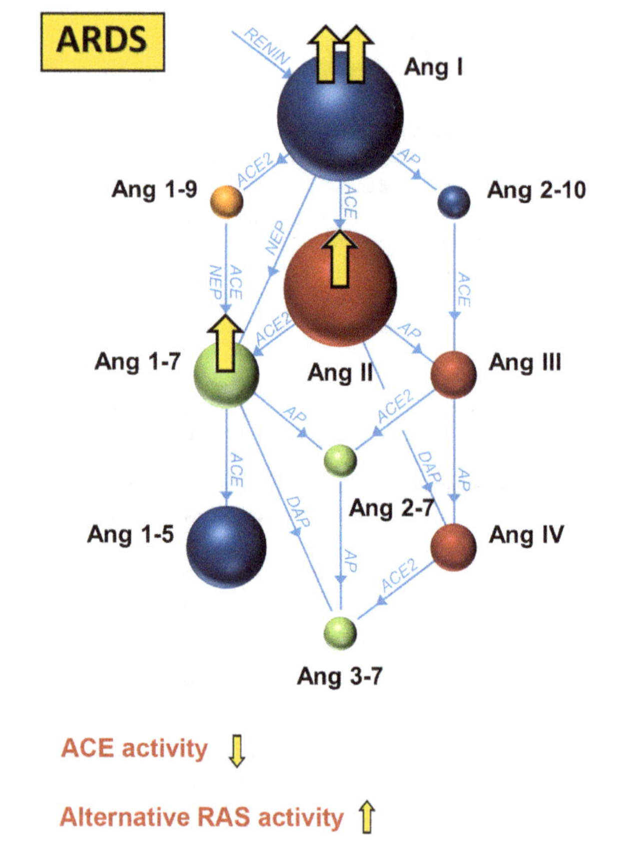

FIGURE 3 | Changes in the angiotensin metabolite profile in plasma of patients with ARDS. Studies in patients with ARDS revealed increased renin-angiotensin system (RAS) activation with higher Ang I than Ang II concentrations and increased Ang 1–7 levels. Decreased Ang II/Ang I ratios and increased alternative RAS activation may be caused be decreased ACE and increased ACE2 activities, or other, yet-to-be characterized, enzymes that process Ang II.

levels in the serum of patients with COVID-19-related and non-COVID ARDS. These seemingly conflicting results may be due to rather small sample sizes, a mix of underlying pathologies and biomarker phenotypes in patients with non-COVID ARDS and different specificities of ELISA kits.

Novel methods to measure active ACE and ACE2 concentrations offer new opportunities to study the role of these enzymes in a clinical context. These assays work by spiking the natural substrates to the samples to determine the specific product formation rate. For analysis of ACE activity, the samples are spiked with Ang I and incubated in the presence and absence of an ACE inhibitor, while the unspecific degradation of the substrate (Ang I) and product (Ang II) is prevented with protease inhibitors. Ang II is quantified by LC-MS/MS and the specific activity of ACE is calculated by determining the inhibitor-sensitive fraction of Ang II formation. The active ACE concentration is then calculated by relating the ACE activity in the sample to the activity of recombinant human ACE in plasma. The assay to determine active ACE2 follows an equivalent process, namely spiking Ang II, application of the ACE2-specific inhibitor MLN-4760, and quantification of Ang 1–7. The Ang 1–7 formation rate is calibrated to a standard curve of ACE2 from healthy human control plasma. With the help of this method, it was discovered that high concentrations of active ACE2 in the plasma of hospitalized patients with COVID-19 depend on disease severity (Reindl-Schwaighofer et al., 2021). Increased ACE2 protein expression in the lung tissue has recently been shown in patients with ARDS caused by COVID-19 as well as ARDS caused by other reasons and was primarily located in endothelial cells (Gerard et al., 2021). In this study, the pulmonary ACE protein expression was diminished in COVID-19-related and non-COVID ARDS. The same tendency of changes with increased ACE2 and decreased ACE protein levels, paired with increased Ang 1–7 levels, were found in the serum of patients with COVID-19-related and non-COVID ARDS. This is actually the opposite to findings of decreased ACE2 expression in rodent models of lung injury (Jerng et al., 2007; Wosten-van Asperen et al., 2011), but regulation of ACE2 expression appears to differ among species (Sajuthi et al., 2020; Ziegler et al., 2020). Another difference may be the prolonged course of COVID-19 and ARDS in critically ill patients, which may be accompanied by a dysregulated interferon response as a stimulus for ACE2 expression, as opposed to the relatively short duration of experiments modeling ARDS in animals (Gerard et al., 2021).

THE RENIN-ANGIOTENSIN SYSTEM IN COVID-19

In light of the COVID-19 pandemic, interest in the function of the RAS in the context of ARDS has grown, as ACE2 serves as the primary cell entry receptor for SARS-CoV-2 (Walls et al., 2020; Yan et al., 2020; Zhang et al., 2020). Increased plasma levels of Ang II were reported in a small group of patients with COVID-19 in the early phase of scientific description of COVID-19 (Liu et al., 2020). In patients with H7N9 avian influenza, higher Ang II plasma levels predicted a fatal outcome (Huang et al., 2014), and in a mouse study on H7N9 infection, Ang II levels were increased and lung tissue protein expression of ACE2 was decreased after 3 days (Yang et al., 2014). Based on cell culture and animal data on SARS-CoV and SARS-CoV-2 infection, and human data of ACE2 levels in conditions with increased susceptibility to severe COVID-19, multiple reviews arrived at the conclusion that Ang II levels should be increased and ACE2 should by downregulated by SARS-CoV-2 infection (Edmonston et al., 2020; Verdecchia et al., 2020; Iwasaki et al., 2021; Triposkiadis et al., 2021). Risk factors for mortality in patients with COVID-19 include older age, male gender, hypertension, type 2 diabetes mellitus, cardiovascular disease, chronic obstructive pulmonary disease, chronic kidney disease and asthma (Aktar et al., 2021). Obesity and type 2 diabetes, especially with poor glycemic control, lead to immune cell dysfunction and foster chronic inflammatory states (Fishkin et al., 2021; Rea and Alexander, 2021). It has also been reported that ACE2 expression diminishes in advanced age and in individuals with hypertension, cardiac hypertrophy, and heart failure (Rea and Alexander, 2021). Lower ACE2 serum levels were described in patients with type 2 diabetes despite increased ACE2 expression in the pancreas and lungs as well as correlation of ACE2 serum levels with HbA1c (Elemam et al., 2021). Rising soluble ACE2 levels correlated with worsening symptoms, B-type natriuretic peptide levels and mortality in patients with heart failure (Garcia-Escobar et al., 2021), and the sum of Ang 1–7 and Ang 1–5 concentrations as marker of alternative RAS activation predicted adverse events in patients with heart failure and preserved ejection fraction (Binder et al., 2019). In a large cohort of 497 patients from the Atherosclerosis Risk in Communities Study elevated soluble ACE2 levels were associated with increased cardiac biomarkers, left ventricular hypertrophy, as well as risk for hospitalization because of heart failure, risk for cardiovascular disease events and death (Hussain et al., 2021). A similar link between increased ACE2 plasma levels and male sex as well as biomarkers of ageing, cardiovascular disease and diabetes was established in even larger cohorts of elderly patients with atrial fibrillation (Wallentin et al., 2020). Although many patients with cardiovascular diseases are treated with ACE inhibitors or angiotensin receptor blockers, no negative impact of these drugs on the risk for severe COVID-19 was found (Hippisley-Cox et al., 2020). Therefore, these drugs should only be discontinued in COVID-19 patients with hemodynamic compromise (Alexandre et al., 2020). Increased expression of ACE2 and transmembrane serine protease (TMPRSS) 2 in lung tissue together with decreased soluble ACE2 levels were also observed in patients with chronic obstructive pulmonary disease (Fliesser et al., 2021). While several patient characteristics and conditions are associated with reduced soluble ACE levels, worsening of comorbidities such as heart failure or diabetes leads to rising soluble ACE2 levels. However, there is still controversy whether increased or decreased soluble ACE2 levels are indeed a susceptibility factor for severe COVID-19 (Leow, 2020; Rahman et al., 2021).

At first glance, results from studies measuring circulating angiotensin peptides and soluble ACE2 in patients with COVID-19 do not completely fit this theoretical model of increased Ang II and downregulated ACE2 levels. A study of Ang II serum levels in a cohort of 112 patients with COVID-19 reported a decrease in Ang II levels that was more pronounced in patients with ARDS and in non-survivors (Ozkan et al., 2021). Another study reported lower Ang II equilibrium levels in hospitalized patients with COVID-19 than in propensity score matched controls negative for SARS-CoV-2 (Kutz et al., 2021). ACE and ACE2 activities were unchanged in patients with COVID-19 in this study. Other studies showed slightly decreased ACE activity in the blood of patients with moderate to severe acute respiratory failure due to COVID-19 (Files et al., 2021) and higher Ang II levels in survivors than in non-survivors of COVID-related ARDS (Eleuteri et al., 2021). This is in line with the results from a study on severe sepsis that indicated low levels of Ang II and ACE on day 1 as predictors of mortality (Zhang et al., 2014). As discussed above for non-COVID ARDS, low Ang II plasma levels, especially if they are lower than the Ang I levels, may be caused by reduced ACE activity or by increased processing of Ang II into Ang 1–7 by ACE2 (Krenn et al., 2020) or POP (Triposkiadis et al., 2021). Increased ACE2 levels in the blood of patients with COVID-19 have already been described by several studies using ELISA as well as mass spectrometry-based assays (Fagyas et al., 2021; Gerard et al., 2021; Lundstrom et al., 2021; Patel et al., 2021; Reindl-Schwaighofer et al., 2021; Wang et al., 2021)., and were higher in more severely ill patients (Fagyas et al., 2021; Patel et al., 2021; Reindl-Schwaighofer et al., 2021). An increasing trend in ACE2 plasma levels within 7 days from hospital admission indicated a higher 90-day mortality (Wang et al., 2021). Differences in soluble ACE2 levels between sexes may also play a role, as a study involving only 16.6% men within the COVID-19 group found actually lower ACE2 and higher Ang I and Ang II plasma levels in patients with COVID-19 compared to SARS-CoV-2 negative controls (Osman et al., 2021). One explanation may be that ACE2 was shed from the lung tissue after infection with SARS-CoV-2 and therefore increasingly appeared in the circulation. However, the study by Gerard et al. (2021) showed that ACE2 protein expression in lung tissue was increased in patients who died from COVID-19-related ARDS, and that the pulmonary ACE2 expression was primarily localized to endothelial cells, while the number of alveolar type II cells was reduced. Whether the lung is indeed the source of circulating ACE2 is uncertain, but interestingly, the soluble ACE2 species found in the plasma of patients with COVID-19 had specific characteristics: There was less full-length ACE2, while the 70 kD species was increased (Garcia-Ayllon et al., 2021). It remains unknown whether this has functional implications for the pulmonary endothelium. Overall, the clinical findings at present contest the hypothesis of increased Ang II and decreased ACE2 in COVID-19 as a systemic phenomenon, while these changes might well play a role locally within the lung tissue (Gerard et al., 2021; Iwasaki et al., 2021). Furthermore, the above-mentioned clinical studies are difficult to compare to each other due to several limitations. The investigated patient cohorts differed in the severity of disease, grading of ventilatory support, and time points of sampling, so that differences may have been missed, for instance between patients requiring non-invasive versus invasive mechanical ventilation. The delay from the first positive test or onset of symptoms to sampling may also vary within and between studies. The studies offering information on circulating angiotensin metabolite concentrations in patients with COVID-19 are included in **Table 1**. In summary, RAS activation in severe COVID-19 may be the result of a variety of changes caused by COVID-19, ARDS, and critical illness with hemodynamic instability and acute kidney injury (Zarbock et al., 2021).

Angiotensin converting enzyme polymorphisms contribute to the relatively high standard deviation of Ang II plasma levels in patient cohorts and are associated with the severity of ARDS (Pabalan et al., 2021). From the beginning of the SARS-CoV-2 pandemic it has been obvious, that disease severity varies greatly between patients spanning a spectrum from no symptoms at all to critical illness with high mortality. A likely explanation for this phenomenon may be yet unknown genetic factors that predispose patients for one or the other outcome. Possible contributors may include the known polymorphisms in the genes of the RAS enzymes ACE and ACE2. The ACE gene is located on chromosome 17q23 and exhibits an insertion/deletion (I/D) polymorphism of a 287-base pair Alu repeat sequence in intron 16, giving rise to II and DD homozygotes, respectively, and ID heterozygotes. Different genotypes vary in the expression levels and plasma activities of ACE (Rigat et al., 1990; Gard, 2010), which can also influence the responsiveness to therapeutic ACE inhibitors (Haas et al., 1998). Several studies have shown considerable association between ACE genotype (as observed with variable prevalence in different ethnic populations) and various disease endpoints such as sepsis, ARDS (Pabalan et al., 2021), and risk of pneumonia (Nie et al., 2014). In the context of COVID-19, there may also be a connection between frequency of ACE genotypes in populations and severity and outcome of this disease (El-Arif et al., 2021). Furthermore, single-nucleotide polymorphisms in the ACE2 gene on chromosome Xp22.2 have been discussed as possible predetermining factors for COVID-19 severity. The best-characterized ACE2 polymorphism is the splice region variant (rs2285666, G > A, Intron 3/4), which has also been shown to be associated with hypertension, coronary heart disease and diabetes with cerebral stroke (Mohlendick et al., 2021). Other ACE2 polymorphisms may affect ACE2-spike protein binding affinity or binding of the co-factor TMPRSS2 that is needed for viral cell entry (El-Arif et al., 2021; Suryamohan et al., 2021). In a study including hospitalized patients with COVID-19 age, high soluble ACE2 levels, a low aldosterone to renin ratio and the TMPRSS2 rs2070788 non-AA genotype were factors that independently predicted disease severity (Akin et al., 2021). Allelic variants of ACE2 differ in serum levels of soluble ACE2, which also implies a possible altered susceptibility to SARS-CoV-2 infection (Mohlendick et al., 2021).

POTENTIAL FOR CLINICAL APPLICATION

An early randomized controlled trial on the hemodynamic and respiratory effects of enalapril in 45 critically ill patients was published in 1995 (Boldt et al., 1995). While enalapril dose-dependently decreased mean arterial pressure, the cardiac index and PaO_2/FiO_2 ratio were higher in patients treated with enalapril than in the control group.

After a successful phase I study of pharmacokinetics and pharmacodynamics of recombinant human (rh)ACE2 in healthy volunteers (Haschke et al., 2013), a clinical trial in patients with ARDS was terminated prematurely because the predefined effects on outcome were not achieved (Khan et al., 2017). In the phase I study, intravenous treatment with ACE2 decreased Ang II levels within 30 min of infusion. Ang 1–7 levels increased, decreased, or remained unchanged, and Ang 1–5 levels increased after all investigated doses of ACE2. Interestingly, the cardiovascular effects of ACE2 administration were absent in healthy individuals. In the phase II study, Ang II levels decreased within 12 h of rhACE2 (GSK2586881) infusion, whereas no change was observed in the placebo group. At the same time, Ang 1–7 and Ang 1–5 levels were increased in the treatment group. As in the phase I study, there were no episodes of hypotension associated with study treatment in the phase II trial. rhACE2 has also been applied in an international multicenter randomized controlled trial in hospitalized patients with COVID-19 (registered at clinicaltrials.gov as NCT04335136), but results are yet to be published. A case report on rhACE2 treatment in a patients with severe COVID-19 confirmed the intended effect of a reduction in Ang II levels during twice daily intravenous treatment with rhACE2 for 7 days (Zoufaly et al., 2020).

There is evidence that ACE inhibitors protect against radiation pneumonitis in lung cancer patients (**Table 1**). This includes two small randomized controlled trials (Small et al., 2018; Sio et al., 2019) and several studies analyzing the incidence of radiation pneumonitis in patients with or without ACE inhibitor or angiotensin receptor blocker therapy (Sun et al., 2018).

CURRENT RESEARCH GAPS AND PERSPECTIVES

Experimental and clinical evidence shows that the RAS is involved in VILI and other types of pulmonary inflammation where it may offer novel therapeutic targets. Despite the increasing precision and detail of describing RAS activation with mass spectrometry-based assays, many aspects of RAS enzyme activity remain elusive. ACE inhibitors, angiotensin receptor blockers and Ang 1–7 supplementation seem to protect from VILI in experimental studies in rodents, not only by affecting levels of RAS components but also by acting on proinflammatory cytokines such as IL-6 and MIP-2, and there is evidence of decreased histological lung injury (Jerng et al., 2007; Wosten-van Asperen et al., 2011; Zambelli et al., 2015). However, clinical data suggest that decreased ACE activity indicated by a low Ang II/Ang I ratio in early ARDS in mechanically ventilated patients is a poor prognostic sign, and that this decreased Ang II/Ang I ratio likely does not come from reduced circulating ACE protein levels. One may speculate that this is an endogenous protective mechanism in patients with ARDS to limit generation of potentially harmful Ang II that is not sufficient for improvement in non-survivors. However, hypoxia only causes death in a minority of patients with ARDS (Esan et al., 2010). Thus, non-survivors of ICU-stays also include patients with multi-organ failure or acute complications such as intracranial bleeding or myocardial infarction. Reasons for the diminished Ang II/Ang I ratio in ARDS may include the presence of a yet-to-be characterized endogenous ACE inhibitor, increased ACE2 activity (Krenn et al., 2020; Reindl-Schwaighofer et al., 2021), or increased activity of other, yet-to-be characterized proteases that process Ang II. Future mechanistic investigations will have to study which molecular mechanisms are really involved. In addition, the activity levels and concentrations of ACE and ACE2 in plasma are regulated by shedding of parts of the molecules from their cells of origin in various organs. This may be the primary reason why ACE2 increases in the systemic circulation in certain disease states. The mechanisms that lead to ACE2-shedding involve proteases, e.g., tumor necrosis factor-α convertase (TACE, ADAM17) (Lambert et al., 2005). Interestingly, ADAM17 activation may be enhanced by Ang II acting on AT 1 receptors and by bradykinin (Dey et al., 2010; Rahman et al., 2021), while ACE is the most important enzyme for inactivation of bradykinin (Schmaier, 2002). Based on this mechanism, ACE inhibition may also be involved in increased shedding of ACE2. Novel assays for calculating active ACE and ACE2 concentrations will help to further study the impact of these enzymes in ARDS, but a future goal will also be to further clarify from where the enzymes are shed and by which mechanisms.

Another broad field for future study is applying the findings about involvement of the RAS in ARDS in randomized controlled clinical trials. Various trials currently listed in *clinicaltrials.gov* aim to include patients with COVID-19 and to test a treatment with angiotensin receptor blockers, ACE inhibitors, or Ang 1–7. Apart from selecting the most suitable substances, the challenge is to establish the most effective form of application. Since the lungs can be reached by circulation, systemic application of RAS-modifying drugs has a substantial impact on angiotensin metabolite concentrations in plasma (Kovarik et al., 2015; Khan et al., 2017). Inhalation therapy is another option for treating ARDS. Depending on the molecule, this method may offer the benefit of positive local effects on the bronchial/alveolar epithelium without systemic toxicity. As another advantage, inhalation of RAS-modifying drugs can be expected to have fewer effects on systemic hemodynamics. As an example, inhaled Ang 1–7 has already been studied as an anti-inflammatory therapeutic agent in a mouse model of ovalbumin-induced chronic asthma (Magalhaes et al., 2020).

CONCLUSION

In summary, knowledge about RAS activation in experimental lung injury and clinical ARDS is increasing in quantity and detail. The mechanisms of regulating RAS enzyme activities and their shedding remain elusive, especially in the clinical setting, and require further study with innovative measurement tools. However, even with the current conception of RAS activation in ARDS, clinical studies can be designed to counteract primary and ventilator-induced lung injury. Several clinical trials with RAS-modifying drugs are currently underway for COVID-19, with most results still pending.

AUTHOR CONTRIBUTIONS

KK drafted the manuscript and prepared the figures. VT, FK, and RU assisted with literature search and revised the manuscript. FK drafted **Table 1**. All authors read and approved the submitted version of the manuscript.

ACKNOWLEDGMENTS

We thank Oliver Domenig, Ph.D., for assistance with preparation of **Figures 1, 2**.

REFERENCES

Abassi, Z., Skorecki, K., Hamo-Giladi, D. B., Kruzel-Davila, E., and Heyman, S. N. (2021). Kinins and chymase: the forgotten components of the renin-angiotensin system and their implications in COVID-19 disease. *Am. J. Physiol. Lung Cell Mol. Physiol.* 320, L422–L429. doi: 10.1152/ajplung.00548.2020

Acute Respiratory Distress Syndrome Network, Brower, R. G., Matthay, M. A., Morris, A., Schoenfeld, D., Thompson, B. T., et al. (2000). Ventilation with lower tidal volumes as compared with traditional tidal volumes for acute lung injury and the acute respiratory distress syndrome. *N. Engl. J. Med.* 342, 1301–1308. doi: 10.1056/NEJM200005043421801

Akin, S., Schriek, P., Van Nieuwkoop, C., Neuman, R. I., Meynaar, I., Van Helden, E. J., et al. (2021). A low aldosterone/renin ratio and high soluble ACE2 associate with COVID-19 severity. *J. Hypertens.* doi: 10.1097/HJH.0000000000003054 [Epub ahead of print].

Aktar, S., Talukder, A., Ahamad, M. M., Kamal, A. H. M., Khan, J. R., Protikuzzaman, M., et al. (2021). Machine learning approaches to identify patient comorbidities and symptoms that increased risk of mortality in COVID-19. *Diagnostics (Basel)* 11, 1383. doi: 10.3390/diagnostics11081383

Alexandre, J., Cracowski, J. L., Richard, V., Bouhanick, B., and Drugs, Covid-19' working group of the French Society of Pharmacology, Therapeutics (2020). Renin-angiotensin-aldosterone system and COVID-19 infection. *Ann. Endocrinol. (Paris)* 81, 63–67.

Annoni, F., Orbegozo, D., Rahmania, L., Irazabal, M., Mendoza, M., De Backer, D., et al. (2019). Angiotensin-converting enzymes in acute respiratory distress syndrome. *Intens. Care Med.* 45, 1159–1160. doi: 10.1007/s00134-019-05600-6

Aronson, D., and Krum, H. (2012). Novel therapies in acute and chronic heart failure. *Pharmacol. Ther.* 135, 1–17. doi: 10.1016/j.pharmthera.2012.03.002

Basu, R., Poglitsch, M., Yogasundaram, H., Thomas, J., Rowe, B. H., and Oudit, G. Y. (2017). Roles of angiotensin peptides and recombinant human ACE2 in heart failure. *J. Am. Coll. Cardiol.* 69, 805–819. doi: 10.1016/j.jacc.2016.11.064

Behnia, R., Molteni, A., Waters, C. M., Panos, R. J., Ward, W. F., Schnaper, H. W., et al. (1996). Early markers of ventilator-induced lung injury in rats. *Ann. Clin. Lab. Sci.* 26, 437–450. doi: 10.3109/9781420019261-20

Benigni, A., Cassis, P., and Remuzzi, G. (2010). Angiotensin II revisited: new roles in inflammation, immunology and aging. *EMBO Mol. Med.* 2, 247–257. doi: 10.1002/emmm.201000080

Bhargava, M., and Wendt, C. H. (2012). Biomarkers in acute lung injury. *Transl. Res.* 159, 205–217.

Binder, C., Poglitsch, M., Agibetov, A., Duca, F., Zotter-Tufaro, C., Nitsche, C., et al. (2019). Angs (Angiotensins) of the alternative renin-angiotensin system predict outcome in patients with heart failure and preserved ejection fraction. *Hypertension* 74, 285–294. doi: 10.1161/HYPERTENSIONAHA.119.12786

Boldt, J., Muller, M., Heesen, M., Harter, K., and Hempelmann, G. (1995). Cardiorespiratory effects of continuous i.v. administration of the ACE inhibitor enalaprilat in the critically ill. *Br. J. Clin. Pharmacol.* 40, 415–422. doi: 10.1111/j.1365-2125.1995.tb05790.x

Bos, L. D., Schouten, L. R., Van Vught, L. A., Wiewel, M. A., Ong, D. S. Y., Cremer, O., et al. (2017). Identification and validation of distinct biological phenotypes in patients with acute respiratory distress syndrome by cluster analysis. *Thorax* 72, 876–883. doi: 10.1136/thoraxjnl-2016-209719

Burrello, J., Buffolo, F., Domenig, O., Tetti, M., Pecori, A., Monticone, S., et al. (2020). Renin-angiotensin-aldosterone system triple-A analysis for the screening of primary aldosteronism. *Hypertension* 75, 163–172. doi: 10.1161/HYPERTENSIONAHA.119.13772

Caldeira, D., Alarcao, J., Vaz-Carneiro, A., and Costa, J. (2012). Risk of pneumonia associated with use of angiotensin converting enzyme inhibitors and angiotensin receptor blockers: systematic review and meta-analysis. *BMJ* 345:e4260. doi: 10.1136/bmj.e4260

Calfee, C. S., Delucchi, K., Parsons, P. E., Thompson, B. T., Ware, L. B., Matthay, M. A., et al. (2014). Subphenotypes in acute respiratory distress syndrome: latent class analysis of data from two randomised controlled trials. *Lancet Respir. Med.* 2, 611–620. doi: 10.1016/S2213-2600(14)70097-9

Calfee, C. S., Janz, D. R., Bernard, G. R., May, A. K., Kangelaris, K. N., Matthay, M. A., et al. (2015). Distinct molecular phenotypes of direct vs indirect ARDS in single-center and multicenter studies. *Chest* 147, 1539–1548. doi: 10.1378/chest.14-2454

Chen, C. M., Chou, H. C., Wang, L. F., and Lang, Y. D. (2008). Captopril decreases plasminogen activator inhibitor-1 in rats with ventilator-induced lung injury. *Crit. Care Med.* 36, 1880–1885. doi: 10.1097/CCM.0b013e31817c911d

Corradi, H. R., Schwager, S. L., Nchinda, A. T., Sturrock, E. D., and Acharya, K. R. (2006). Crystal structure of the N domain of human somatic angiotensin I-converting enzyme provides a structural basis for domain-specific inhibitor design. *J. Mol. Biol.* 357, 964–974. doi: 10.1016/j.jmb.2006.01.048

Corvol, P., Williams, T. A., and Soubrier, F. (1995). Peptidyl dipeptidase A: angiotensin I-converting enzyme. *Methods Enzymol.* 248, 283–305. doi: 10.1016/0076-6879(95)48020-x

Cressoni, M., Gotti, M., Chiurazzi, C., Massari, D., Algieri, I., Amini, M., et al. (2016). Mechanical power and development of ventilator-induced lung injury. *Anesthesiology* 124, 1100–1108. doi: 10.1097/ALN.0000000000001056

Deng, J., Wang, D. X., Deng, W., Li, C. Y., and Tong, J. (2012a). The effect of endogenous angiotensin II on alveolar fluid clearance in rats with acute lung injury. *Can. Respir. J.* 19, 311–318. doi: 10.1155/2012/951025

Deng, J., Wang, D. X., Deng, W., Li, C. Y., Tong, J., and Ma, H. (2012b). Regulation of alveolar fluid clearance and ENaC expression in lung by exogenous angiotensin II. *Respir. Physiol. Neurobiol.* 181, 53–61. doi: 10.1016/j.resp.2011.11.009

Dey, M., Baldys, A., Sumter, D. B., Gooz, P., Luttrell, L. M., Raymond, J. R., et al. (2010). Bradykinin decreases podocyte permeability through ADAM17-dependent epidermal growth factor receptor activation and zonula occludens-1 rearrangement. *J. Pharmacol. Exp. Ther.* 334, 775–783. doi: 10.1124/jpet.110.168054

Dreyfuss, D., and Saumon, G. (1998). Ventilator-induced lung injury: lessons from experimental studies. *Am. J. Respir. Crit. Care Med.* 157, 294–323. doi: 10.1164/ajrccm.157.1.9604014

Eckenstaler, R., Sandori, J., Gekle, M., and Benndorf, R. A. (2021). Angiotensin II receptor type 1 - An update on structure, expression and pathology. *Biochem. Pharmacol.* 192:114673. doi: 10.1016/j.bcp.2021.114673

Edmonston, D. L., South, A. M., Sparks, M. A., and Cohen, J. B. (2020). Coronavirus disease 2019 and hypertension: the role of angiotensin-converting enzyme 2 and the renin-angiotensin system. *Adv. Chronic Kidney Dis.* 27, 404–411. doi: 10.1053/j.ackd.2020.07.002

El-Arif, G., Farhat, A., Khazaal, S., Annweiler, C., Kovacic, H., Wu, Y., et al. (2021). The Renin-angiotensin system: a key role in SARS-CoV-2-induced COVID-19. *Molecules* 26:6945. doi: 10.3390/molecules26226945

Elemam, N. M., Hasswan, H., Aljaibeji, H., and Sulaiman, N. (2021). Circulating soluble ACE2 and upstream microRNA expressions in serum of type 2 diabetes mellitus patients. *Int. J. Mol. Sci.* 22:5263. doi: 10.3390/ijms22105263

Eleuteri, D., Montini, L., Cutuli, S. L., Rossi, C., Alcaro, F., and Antonelli, M. (2021). Renin-angiotensin system dysregulation in critically ill patients with acute respiratory distress syndrome due to COVID-19: a preliminary report. *Crit. Care* 25:91. doi: 10.1186/s13054-021-03507-7

El-Sayed, L. A., Osama, E., Mehesen, M. N., Rashed, L. A., Aboulkhair, A. G., Omar, A. I., et al. (2020). Contribution of angiotensin II in hepatic ischemia /reperfusion induced lung injury: acute versus chronic usage of captopril. *Pulm. Pharmacol. Ther.* 60:101888. doi: 10.1016/j.pupt.2020.101888

Esan, A., Hess, D. R., Raoof, S., George, L., and Sessler, C. N. (2010). Severe hypoxemic respiratory failure: part 1–ventilatory strategies. *Chest* 137, 1203–1216. doi: 10.1378/chest.09-2415

Fagyas, M., Fejes, Z., Suto, R., Nagy, Z., Szekely, B., Pocsi, M., et al. (2021). Circulating ACE2 activity predicts mortality and disease severity in hospitalized COVID-19 patients. *Int. J. Infect. Dis.* 115, 8–16. doi: 10.1016/j.ijid.2021.11.028

Fatima, N., Patel, S. N., and Hussain, T. (2021). Angiotensin II type 2 receptor: a target for protection against hypertension, metabolic dysfunction, and organ remodeling. *Hypertension* 77, 1845–1856. doi: 10.1161/HYPERTENSIONAHA.120.11941

Files, D. C., Gibbs, K. W., Schaich, C. L., Collins, S. P., Gwathmey, T. M., Casey, J. D., et al. (2021). A pilot study to assess the circulating renin-angiotensin-system in COVID-19 acute respiratory failure. *Am. J. Physiol. Lung Cell Mol. Physiol.* 321, L213–L218. doi: 10.1152/ajplung.00129.2021

Fishkin, T., Goldberg, M. D., and Frishman, W. H. (2021). Review of the metabolic risk factors for increased severity of coronavirus disease-2019. *Cardiol. Rev.* 29, 292–295. doi: 10.1097/CRD.0000000000000408

Fliesser, E., Birnhuber, A., Marsh, L. M., Gschwandtner, E., Klepetko, W., Olschewski, H., et al. (2021). Dysbalance of ACE2 levels - a possible cause for severe COVID-19 outcome in COPD. *J. Pathol. Clin. Res.* 7, 446–458. doi: 10.1002/cjp2.224

Gallo, G., Volpe, M., Battistoni, A., Russo, D., Tocci, G., and Musumeci, M. B. (2021). Sacubitril/valsartan as a therapeutic tool across the range of heart failure phenotypes and ejection fraction spectrum. *Front. Physiol.* 12:652163. doi: 10.3389/fphys.2021.652163

Garcia-Ayllon, M. S., Moreno-Perez, O., Garcia-Arriaza, J., Ramos-Rincon, J. M., Cortes-Gomez, M. A., Brinkmalm, G., et al. (2021). Plasma ACE2 species are differentially altered in COVID-19 patients. *FASEB J.* 35:e21745. doi: 10.1096/fj.202100051R

Garcia-Escobar, A., Jimenez-Valero, S., Galeote, G., Jurado-Roman, A., Garcia-Rodriguez, J., and Moreno, R. (2021). The soluble catalytic ectodomain of ACE2 a biomarker of cardiac remodelling: new insights for heart failure and COVID19. *Heart Fail Rev.* 26, 961–971. doi: 10.1007/s10741-020-10066-6

Gard, P. R. (2010). Implications of the angiotensin converting enzyme gene insertion/deletion polymorphism in health and disease: a snapshot review. *Int. J. Mol. Epidemiol. Genet.* 1, 145–157.

Gattinoni, L., Protti, A., Caironi, P., and Carlesso, E. (2010). Ventilator-induced lung injury: the anatomical and physiological framework. *Crit. Care Med.* 38, S539–S548. doi: 10.1097/CCM.0b013e3181f1fcf7

Gattinoni, L., Tonetti, T., Cressoni, M., Cadringher, P., Herrmann, P., Moerer, O., et al. (2016). Ventilator-related causes of lung injury: the mechanical power. *Intensive Care Med.* 42, 1567–1575. doi: 10.1007/s00134-016-4505-2

Gerard, L., Lecocq, M., Bouzin, C., Hoton, D., Schmit, G., Pereira, J. P., et al. (2021). Increased angiotensin-converting enzyme 2 and loss of alveolar type II cells in COVID-19 related ARDS. *Am. J. Respir. Crit. Care Med.* 204, 1024–1034. doi: 10.1164/rccm.202012-4461oc

Gleeson, P. J., Crippa, I. A., Mongkolpun, W., Cavicchi, F. Z., Van Meerhaeghe, T., Brimioulle, S., et al. (2019). Renin as a marker of tissue-perfusion and prognosis in critically Ill patients. *Crit. Care Med.* 47, 152–158. doi: 10.1097/CCM.0000000000003544

Goppner, C., Orozco, I. J., Hoegg-Beiler, M. B., Soria, A. H., Hubner, C. A., Fernandes-Rosa, F. L., et al. (2019). Pathogenesis of hypertension in a mouse model for human CLCN2 related hyperaldosteronism. *Nat. Commun.* 10:4678.

Haas, M., Yilmaz, N., Schmidt, A., Neyer, U., Arneitz, K., Stummvoll, H. K., et al. (1998). Angiotensin-converting enzyme gene polymorphism determines the antiproteinuric and systemic hemodynamic effect of enalapril in patients with proteinuric renal disease. Austrian study group of the effects of enalapril treatment in proteinuric renal disease. *Kidney Blood Press Res.* 21, 66–69. doi: 10.1159/000025845

Halbertsma, F. J., Vaneker, M., Scheffer, G. J., and Van Der Hoeven, J. G. (2005). Cytokines and biotrauma in ventilator-induced lung injury: a critical review of the literature. *Neth. J. Med.* 63, 382–392.

Haschke, M., Schuster, M., Poglitsch, M., Loibner, H., Salzberg, M., Bruggisser, M., et al. (2013). Pharmacokinetics and pharmacodynamics of recombinant human angiotensin-converting enzyme 2 in healthy human subjects. *Clin. Pharmacokinet.* 52, 783–792. doi: 10.1007/s40262-013-0072-7

He, X., Han, B., Mura, M., Xia, S., Wang, S., Ma, T., et al. (2007). Angiotensin-converting enzyme inhibitor captopril prevents oleic acid-induced severe acute lung injury in rats. *Shock* 28, 106–111. doi: 10.1097/SHK.0b013e3180310f3a

Hippisley-Cox, J., Young, D., Coupland, C., Channon, K. M., Tan, P. S., Harrison, D. A., et al. (2020). Risk of severe COVID-19 disease with ACE inhibitors and angiotensin receptor blockers: cohort study including 8.3 million people. *Heart* 106, 1503–1511. doi: 10.1136/heartjnl-2020-317393

Hrenak, J., and Simko, F. (2020). Renin-angiotensin system: an important player in the pathogenesis of acute respiratory distress syndrome. *Int. J. Mol. Sci.* 21:8038. doi: 10.3390/ijms21218038

Huang, F., Guo, J., Zou, Z., Liu, J., Cao, B., Zhang, S., et al. (2014). Angiotensin II plasma levels are linked to disease severity and predict fatal outcomes in H7N9-infected patients. *Nat. Commun.* 5:3595. doi: 10.1038/ncomms4595

Hussain, A., Tang, O., Sun, C., Jia, X., Selvin, E., Nambi, V., et al. (2021). Soluble angiotensin-converting enzyme 2, cardiac biomarkers, structure, and function, and cardiovascular events (from the atherosclerosis risk in communities study). *Am. J. Cardiol.* 146, 15–21. doi: 10.1016/j.amjcard.2021.01.017

Imai, Y., Kuba, K., and Penninger, J. M. (2007). Angiotensin-converting enzyme 2 in acute respiratory distress syndrome. *Cell Mol. Life Sci.* 64, 2006–2012.

Imai, Y., Kuba, K., and Penninger, J. M. (2008). The discovery of angiotensin-converting enzyme 2 and its role in acute lung injury in mice. *Exp. Physiol.* 93, 543–548. doi: 10.1113/expphysiol.2007.040048

Imai, Y., Kuba, K., Rao, S., Huan, Y., Guo, F., Guan, B., et al. (2005). Angiotensin-converting enzyme 2 protects from severe acute lung failure. *Nature* 436, 112–116. doi: 10.1038/nature03712

Iwasaki, M., Saito, J., Zhao, H., Sakamoto, A., Hirota, K., and Ma, D. (2021). Inflammation triggered by SARS-CoV-2 and ACE2 augment drives multiple organ failure of severe COVID-19: molecular mechanisms and implications. *Inflammation* 44, 13–34. doi: 10.1007/s10753-020-01337-3

Jerng, J. S., Hsu, Y. C., Wu, H. D., Pan, H. Z., Wang, H. C., Shun, C. T., et al. (2007). Role of the renin-angiotensin system in ventilator-induced lung injury: an *in vivo* study in a rat model. *Thorax* 62, 527–535. doi: 10.1136/thx.2006.061945

Khan, A., Benthin, C., Zeno, B., Albertson, T. E., Boyd, J., Christie, J. D., et al. (2017). A pilot clinical trial of recombinant human angiotensin-converting enzyme 2 in acute respiratory distress syndrome. *Crit. Care* 21:234. doi: 10.1186/s13054-017-1823-x

Kim, J., Choi, S. M., Lee, J., Park, Y. S., Lee, C. H., Yim, J. J., et al. (2017). Effect of renin-angiotensin system blockage in patients with acute respiratory distress syndrome: a retrospective case control study. *Korean J. Crit. Care Med.* 32, 154–163. doi: 10.4266/kjccm.2016.00976

Kovarik, J. J., Antlanger, M., Domenig, O., Kaltenecker, C. C., Hecking, M., Haidinger, M., et al. (2015). Molecular regulation of the renin-angiotensin system in haemodialysis patients. *Nephrol. Dial. Transplant.* 30, 115–123.

Kovarik, J. J., Kopecky, C., Antlanger, M., Domenig, O., Kaltenecker, C. C., Werzowa, J., et al. (2017). Effects of angiotensin-converting-enzyme inhibitor therapy on the regulation of the plasma and cardiac tissue renin-angiotensin system in heart transplant patients. *J. Heart Lung Transplant.* 36, 355–365. doi: 10.1016/j.healun.2016.08.022

Krenn, K., Hobart, P., Poglitsch, M., Croize, A., and Ullrich, R. (2020). Equilibrium angiotensin metabolite profiling in patients with acute respiratory distress syndrome indicates angiotensin converting enzyme inhibition. *Am J Respir. Crit. Care Med.* 202, 1468–1471. doi: 10.1164/rccm.201912-2504LE

Kutz, A., Conen, A., Gregoriano, C., Haubitz, S., Koch, D., Domenig, O., et al. (2021). Renin-angiotensin-aldosterone system peptide profiles in patients with COVID-19. *Eur. J. Endocrinol.* 184, 543–552. doi: 10.1530/EJE-20-1445

Lambert, D. W., Yarski, M., Warner, F. J., Thornhill, P., Parkin, E. T., Smith, A. I., et al. (2005). Tumor necrosis factor-alpha convertase (ADAM17) mediates regulated ectodomain shedding of the severe-acute respiratory syndrome-coronavirus (SARS-CoV) receptor, angiotensin-converting enzyme-2 (ACE2). *J. Biol. Chem.* 280, 30113–30119. doi: 10.1074/jbc.M505111200

Lang, Y. D., Hung, C. L., Wu, T. Y., Wang, L. F., and Chen, C. M. (2010). The renin-angiotensin system mediates hyperoxia-induced collagen production in human lung fibroblasts. *Free Radic. Biol. Med.* 49, 88–95. doi: 10.1016/j.freeradbiomed.2010.03.022

Laurent, S., Schlaich, M., and Esler, M. (2012). New drugs, procedures, and devices for hypertension. *Lancet* 380, 591–600. doi: 10.1016/S0140-6736(12)60825-3

Leow, M. K. S. (2020). Clarifying the controversial risk-benefit profile of soluble ACE2 in COVID-19. *Crit. Care* 24:396. doi: 10.1186/s13054-020-03097-w

Liu, S. S., Wang, H. Y., Tang, J. M., and Zhou, X. M. (2013). Hypoxia-induced collagen synthesis of human lung fibroblasts by activating the angiotensin system. *Int. J. Mol. Sci.* 14, 24029–24045. doi: 10.3390/ijms141224029

Liu, Y., Yang, Y., Zhang, C., Huang, F., Wang, F., Yuan, J., et al. (2020). Clinical and biochemical indexes from 2019-nCoV infected patients linked to viral loads and lung injury. *Sci. China Life Sci.* 63, 364–374. doi: 10.1007/s11427-020-1643-8

Lukkarinen, H. P., Laine, J., Aho, H., Zagariya, A., Vidyasagar, D., and Kaapa, P. O. (2005). Angiotensin II receptor inhibition prevents pneumocyte apoptosis in surfactant-depleted rat lungs. *Pediatr. Pulmonol.* 39, 349–358. doi: 10.1002/ppul.20187

Lundstrom, A., Ziegler, L., Havervall, S., Rudberg, A. S., Von Meijenfeldt, F., Lisman, T., et al. (2021). Soluble angiotensin-converting enzyme 2 is transiently elevated in COVID-19 and correlates with specific inflammatory and endothelial markers. *J. Med. Virol.* 93, 5908–5916. doi: 10.1002/jmv.27144

Magalhaes, G. S., Gregorio, J. F., Ramos, K. E., Cancado-Ribeiro, A. T. P., Baroni, I. F., Barcelos, L. S., et al. (2020). Treatment with inhaled formulation of angiotensin-(1-7) reverses inflammation and pulmonary remodeling in a model of chronic asthma. *Immunobiology* 225:151957. doi: 10.1016/j.imbio.2020.151957

Marshall, R. P., Gohlke, P., Chambers, R. C., Howell, D. C., Bottoms, S. E., Unger, T., et al. (2004). Angiotensin II and the fibroproliferative response to acute lung injury. *Am. J. Physiol. Lung Cell Mol. Physiol.* 286, L156–L164. doi: 10.1152/ajplung.00313.2002

Mohlendick, B., Schonfelder, K., Breuckmann, K., Elsner, C., Babel, N., Balfanz, P., et al. (2021). ACE2 polymorphism and susceptibility for SARS-CoV-2 infection and severity of COVID-19. *Pharmacogenet. Genomics* 31, 165–171. doi: 10.1097/FPC.0000000000000436

Mortensen, E. M., Restrepo, M. I., Anzueto, A., and Pugh, J. (2005). The impact of prior outpatient ACE inhibitor use on 30-day mortality for patients hospitalized with community-acquired pneumonia. *BMC Pulm. Med.* 5:12. doi: 10.1186/1471-2466-5-12

Nie, W., Zang, Y., Chen, J., Liu, T., Xiao, L., and Xiu, Q. (2014). Angiotensin-converting enzyme I/D polymorphism is associated with pneumonia risk: a meta-analysis. *J. Renin. Angiotensin Aldosterone Syst.* 15, 585–592. doi: 10.1177/1470320313507622

Osman, I. O., Melenotte, C., Brouqui, P., Million, M., Lagier, J. C., Parola, P., et al. (2021). Expression of ACE2, soluble ACE2, angiotensin I, angiotensin II and angiotensin-(1-7) is modulated in COVID-19 patients. *Front. Immunol.* 12:625732. doi: 10.3389/fimmu.2021.625732

Ozkan, S., Cakmak, F., Konukoglu, D., Biberoglu, S., Ipekci, A., Akdeniz, Y. S., et al. (2021). Efficacy of serum angiotensin II Levels in prognosis of patients with coronavirus disease 2019. *Crit. Care Med.* 49, e613–e623. doi: 10.1097/CCM.0000000000004967

Pabalan, N., Tharabenjasin, P., Suntornsaratoon, P., Jarjanazi, H., and Muanprasat, C. (2021). Ethnic and age-specific acute lung injury/acute respiratory distress syndrome risk associated with angiotensin-converting enzyme insertion/deletion polymorphisms, implications for COVID-19: A meta-analysis. *Infect. Genet. Evol.* 88:104682. doi: 10.1016/j.meegid.2020.104682

Patel, S. K., Juno, J. A., Lee, W. S., Wragg, K. M., Hogarth, P. M., Kent, S. J., et al. (2021). Plasma ACE2 activity is persistently elevated following SARS-CoV-2 infection: implications for COVID-19 pathogenesis and consequences. *Eur. Respir. J.* 57:2003730. doi: 10.1183/13993003.03730-2020

Patel, V. B., Takawale, A., Ramprasath, T., Das, S. K., Basu, R., Grant, M. B., et al. (2015). Antagonism of angiotensin 1-7 prevents the therapeutic effects of recombinant human ACE2. *J. Mol. Med. (Berl.).* 93, 1003–1013. doi: 10.1007/s00109-015-1285-z

Plotz, F. B., Slutsky, A. S., Van Vught, A. J., and Heijnen, C. J. (2004). Ventilator-induced lung injury and multiple system organ failure: a critical review of facts and hypotheses. *Intensive Care Med.* 30, 1865–1872. doi: 10.1007/s00134-004-2363-9

Rahman, M. M., Hasan, M., and Ahmed, A. (2021). Potential detrimental role of soluble ACE2 in severe COVID-19 comorbid patients. *Rev. Med. Virol.* 31, 1–12. doi: 10.1002/rmv.2213

Ranieri, V. M., Suter, P. M., Tortorella, C., De Tullio, R., Dayer, J. M., Brienza, A., et al. (1999). Effect of mechanical ventilation on inflammatory mediators in patients with acute respiratory distress syndrome: a randomized controlled trial. *JAMA* 282, 54–61. doi: 10.1001/jama.282.1.54

Rea, I. M., and Alexander, H. D. (2021). Triple jeopardy in ageing: COVID-19, co-morbidities and inflamm-ageing. *Ageing Res. Rev.* 73:101494. doi: 10.1016/j.arr.2021.101494

Reddy, R., Asante, I., Liu, S., Parikh, P., Liebler, J., Borok, Z., et al. (2019). Circulating angiotensin peptides levels in acute respiratory distress syndrome correlate with clinical outcomes: a pilot study. *PLoS One* 14:e0213096. doi: 10.1371/journal.pone.0213096

Reindl-Schwaighofer, R., Hodlmoser, S., Eskandary, F., Poglitsch, M., Bonderman, D., Strassl, R., et al. (2021). ACE2 elevation in severe COVID-19. *Am. J. Respir. Crit. Care Med.* 203, 1191–1196. doi: 10.1164/rccm.202101-0142LE

Rice, G. I., Thomas, D. A., Grant, P. J., Turner, A. J., and Hooper, N. M. (2004). Evaluation of angiotensin-converting enzyme (ACE), its homologue ACE2 and neprilysin in angiotensin peptide metabolism. *Biochem. J.* 383, 45–51. doi: 10.1042/BJ20040634

Rigat, B., Hubert, C., Alhenc-Gelas, F., Cambien, F., Corvol, P., and Soubrier, F. (1990). An insertion/deletion polymorphism in the angiotensin I-converting enzyme gene accounting for half the variance of serum enzyme levels. *J. Clin. Invest.* 86, 1343–1346. doi: 10.1172/JCI114844

Sajuthi, S. P., Deford, P., Li, Y., Jackson, N. D., Montgomery, M. T., Everman, J. L., et al. (2020). Type 2 and interferon inflammation regulate SARS-CoV-2 entry factor expression in the airway epithelium. *Nat. Commun.* 11:5139. doi: 10.1038/s41467-020-18781-2

Santos, R. A. S., Sampaio, W. O., Alzamora, A. C., Motta-Santos, D., Alenina, N., Bader, M., et al. (2018). The ACE2/angiotensin-(1-7)/MAS axis of the renin-angiotensin system: focus on angiotensin-(1-7. *Physiol. Rev.* 98, 505–553. doi: 10.1152/physrev.00023.2016

Schmaier, A. H. (2002). The plasma kallikrein-kinin system counterbalances the renin-angiotensin system. *J. Clin. Invest.* 109, 1007–1009. doi: 10.1172/JCI15490

Schouten, L. R., Helmerhorst, H. J., Wagenaar, G. T., Haltenhof, T., Lutter, R., Roelofs, J. J., et al. (2016). Age-dependent changes in the pulmonary renin-angiotensin system are associated with severity of lung injury in a model of acute lung injury in rats. *Crit. Care Med.* 44, e1226–e1235. doi: 10.1097/CCM.0000000000002008

Schouten, L. R., Schultz, M. J., Van Kaam, A. H., Juffermans, N. P., Bos, A. P., and Wosten-Van Asperen, R. M. (2015). Association between maturation and aging and pulmonary responses in animal models of lung injury: a systematic review. *Anesthesiology* 123, 389–408. doi: 10.1097/ALN.0000000000000687

Serfozo, P., Wysocki, J., Gulua, G., Schulze, A., Ye, M., Liu, P., et al. (2020). Ang II (Angiotensin II) conversion to angiotensin-(1-7) in the circulation is POP (Prolyloligopeptidase)-dependent and ACE2 (angiotensin-converting enzyme 2)-independent. *Hypertension* 75, 173–182. doi: 10.1161/HYPERTENSIONAHA.119.14071

Shah, S., Mcarthur, E., Farag, A., Nartey, M., Fleet, J. L., Knoll, G. A., et al. (2014). Risk of hospitalization for community acquired pneumonia with renin-angiotensin blockade in elderly patients: a population-based study. *PLoS One* 9:e110165. doi: 10.1371/journal.pone.0110165

Shen, L., Mo, H., Cai, L., Kong, T., Zheng, W., Ye, J., et al. (2009). Losartan prevents sepsis-induced acute lung injury and decreases activation of nuclear factor kappaB and mitogen-activated protein kinases. *Shock* 31, 500–506. doi: 10.1097/SHK.0b013e318189017a

Sio, T. T., Atherton, P. J., Pederson, L. D., Zhen, W. K., Mutter, R. W., Garces, Y. I., et al. (2019). Daily lisinopril vs placebo for prevention of chemoradiation-induced pulmonary distress in patients with lung cancer (Alliance MC1221): a pilot double-blind randomized trial. *Int. J. Radiat. Oncol. Biol. Phys.* 103, 686–696.

Skeggs, L. T., Dorer, F. E., Levine, M., Lentz, K. E., and Kahn, J. R. (1980). The biochemistry of the renin-angiotensin system. *Adv. Exp. Med. Biol.* 130, 1–27. doi: 10.1007/978-1-4615-9173-3_1

Slutsky, A. S., and Tremblay, L. N. (1998). Multiple system organ failure. Is mechanical ventilation a contributing factor? *Am. J. Respir. Crit. Care Med.* 157, 1721–1725. doi: 10.1164/ajrccm.157.6.9709092

Small, W. Jr., James, J. L., Moore, T. D., Fintel, D. J., Lutz, S. T., Movsas, B., et al. (2018). Utility of the ACE inhibitor captopril in mitigating radiation-associated pulmonary toxicity in lung cancer: results from NRG oncology RTOG 0123. *Am. J. Clin. Oncol.* 41, 396–401.

Sturrock, A., Zimmerman, E., Helms, M., Liou, T. G., and Paine, R. III (2021). Hypoxia induces expression of angiotensin-converting enzyme II in alveolar epithelial cells: implications for the pathogenesis of acute lung injury in COVID-19. *Physiol. Rep.* 9:e14854.

Sun, F., Sun, H., Zheng, X., Yang, G., Gong, N., Zhou, H., et al. (2018). Angiotensin-converting enzyme inhibitors decrease the incidence of radiation-induced pneumonitis among lung cancer patients: a systematic review and meta-analysis. *J. Cancer* 9, 2123–2131.

Suryamohan, K., Diwanji, D., Stawiski, E. W., Gupta, R., Miersch, S., Liu, J., et al. (2021). Human ACE2 receptor polymorphisms and altered susceptibility to SARS-CoV-2. *Commun. Biol.* 4:475. doi: 10.1038/s42003-021-02030-3

Triposkiadis, F., Starling, R. C., Xanthopoulos, A., Butler, J., and Boudoulas, H. (2021). The counter regulatory axis of the lung renin-angiotensin system in severe COVID-19: pathophysiology and clinical implications. *Heart Lung Circ.* 30, 786–794. doi: 10.1016/j.hlc.2020.11.008

Velez, J. C., Ryan, K. J., Harbeson, C. E., Bland, A. M., Budisavljevic, M. N., Arthur, J. M., et al. (2009). Angiotensin I is largely converted to angiotensin (1-7) and angiotensin (2-10) by isolated rat glomeruli. *Hypertension* 53, 790–797. doi: 10.1161/HYPERTENSIONAHA.109.128819

Verdecchia, P., Cavallini, C., Spanevello, A., and Angeli, F. (2020). The pivotal link between ACE2 deficiency and SARS-CoV-2 infection. *Eur. J. Intern. Med.* 76, 14–20. doi: 10.1016/j.ejim.2020.04.037

Vischer, A. S., Kuster, G. M., Twerenbold, R., Pfister, O., Zhou, Q., Villiger, A., et al. (2021). Influence of antihypertensive treatment on RAAS peptides in newly diagnosed hypertensive patients. *Cells* 10:534. doi: 10.3390/cells10030534

Wallentin, L., Lindback, J., Eriksson, N., Hijazi, Z., Eikelboom, J. W., Ezekowitz, M. D., et al. (2020). Angiotensin-converting enzyme 2 (ACE2) levels in relation to risk factors for COVID-19 in two large cohorts of patients with atrial fibrillation. *Eur. Heart J.* 41, 4037–4046. doi: 10.1093/eurheartj/ehaa697

Walls, A. C., Park, Y. J., Tortorici, M. A., Wall, A., Mcguire, A. T., and Veesler, D. (2020). Structure, function, and antigenicity of the SARS-CoV-2 spike glycoprotein. *Cell* 181, 281–292.e6.

Wang, K., Gheblawi, M., Nikhanj, A., Munan, M., Macintyre, E., O'neil, C., et al. (2021). Dysregulation of ACE (angiotensin-converting enzyme)-2 and renin-angiotensin peptides in SARS-CoV-2 mediated mortality and end-organ injuries. *Hypertension* HYERTENSIONAHA12118295. doi: 10.1161/HYPERTENSIONAHA.121.18295 [Epub ahead of print].

Wenz, M., Hoffmann, B., Bohlender, J., and Kaczmarczyk, G. (2000). Angiotensin II formation and endothelin clearance in ARDS patients in supine and prone positions. *Intensive Care Med.* 26, 292–298. doi: 10.1007/s001340051152

Wohlrab, P., Johann Danhofer, M., Schaubmayr, W., Tiboldi, A., Krenn, K., Markstaller, K., et al. (2021). Oxygen conditions oscillating between hypoxia and hyperoxia induce different effects in the pulmonary endothelium compared to constant oxygen conditions. *Physiol. Rep.* 9:e14590. doi: 10.14814/phy2.14590

Wosten-van Asperen, R. M., Lutter, R., Specht, P. A., Moll, G. N., Van Woensel, J. B., Van Der Loos, C. M., et al. (2011). Acute respiratory distress syndrome leads to reduced ratio of ACE/ACE2 activities and is prevented by angiotensin-(1-7) or an angiotensin II receptor antagonist. *J. Pathol.* 225, 618–627. doi: 10.1002/path.2987

Yan, R., Zhang, Y., Li, Y., Xia, L., Guo, Y., and Zhou, Q. (2020). Structural basis for the recognition of the SARS-CoV-2 by full-length human ACE2. *Science* 367, 1444–1448. doi: 10.1126/science.abb2762

Yang, P., Gu, H., Zhao, Z., Wang, W., Cao, B., Lai, C., et al. (2014). Angiotensin-converting enzyme 2 (ACE2) mediates influenza H7N9 virus-induced acute lung injury. *Sci. Rep.* 4:7027. doi: 10.1038/srep07027

Zambelli, V., Bellani, G., Borsa, R., Pozzi, F., Grassi, A., Scanziani, M., et al. (2015). Angiotensin-(1-7) improves oxygenation, while reducing cellular infiltrate and fibrosis in experimental acute respiratory distress syndrome. *Intensive Care Med. Exp.* 3:44. doi: 10.1186/s40635-015-0044-3

Zarbock, A., Chawla, L., and Bellomo, R. (2021). Why the renin-angiotensin-aldosterone system (RAAS) in critically ill patients can no longer be ignored. *Crit. Care* 25:389. doi: 10.1186/s13054-021-03816-x

Zhang, H., Penninger, J. M., Li, Y., Zhong, N., and Slutsky, A. S. (2020). Angiotensin-converting enzyme 2 (ACE2) as a SARS-CoV-2 receptor: molecular mechanisms and potential therapeutic target. *Intensive Care Med.* 46, 586–590. doi: 10.1007/s00134-020-05985-9

Zhang, W., Chen, X., Huang, L., Lu, N., Zhou, L., Wu, G., et al. (2014). Severe sepsis: low expression of the renin-angiotensin system is associated with poor prognosis. *Exp. Ther. Med.* 7, 1342–1348. doi: 10.3892/etm.2014.1566

Ziegler, C. G. K., Allon, S. J., Nyquist, S. K., Mbano, I. M., Miao, V. N., Tzouanas, C. N., et al. (2020). SARS-CoV-2 receptor ACE2 is an interferon-stimulated gene in human airway epithelial cells and is detected in specific cell subsets across tissues. *Cell* 181, 1016–1035 e19. doi: 10.1016/j.cell.2020.04.035

Zoufaly, A., Poglitsch, M., Aberle, J. H., Hoepler, W., Seitz, T., Traugott, M., et al. (2020). Human recombinant soluble ACE2 in severe COVID-19. *Lancet Respir. Med.* 8, 1154–1158.

7

Airway Pressure Release Ventilation with Time-Controlled Adaptive Ventilation (TCAV^{TM}) in COVID-19: A Community Hospital's Experience

Philippe Rola[1] and Benjamin Daxon[2]*

[1] *Intensive Care Unit, Santa Cabrini Hospital, Montreal, QC, Canada,* [2] *Mayo Clinic, Rochester, MN, United States*

***Correspondence:**
Philippe Rola
philipperola@gmail.com

Santa Cabrini Ospedale, a community hospital in Montreal, Canada, used the airway pressure release ventilation following a time-controlled adaptive ventilation (APRV-TCAV^{TM}) approach for several patients in the first wave of the coronavirus disease 2019 (COVID-19) outbreak in the spring of 2021. Based on favorable patient responses, it became the primary mode of invasive mechanical ventilation—from initiation through extubation—during the second and third waves of COVID-19. In this article, we describe our success with APRV-TCAV^{TM} over more conventional modes and protocols and look at three cases that aptly demonstrate our experience. We then outline several risks with our approach and the lessons learned from our experience. While we generally saw improvement in patients' clinical course with APRV-TCAV^{TM}, there are inherent risks with this approach that others must prepare for if they attempt to implement it in their practice.

Keywords: ARDS, COVID-19, APRV, TCAV, respiratory failure, critical care

INTRODUCTION

The coronavirus disease 2019 (COVID-19) pandemic hit the world in January of 2020 and reached Montreal, Canada, in March of that year. The harrowing reports of COVID-19's proclivity to develop acute respiratory failure with exceedingly high mortality were concerning to our critical care team. Of particular concern was the atypical nature of the COVID-19-associated acute respiratory distress syndrome (C-ARDS). Many patients displayed profound hypoxia with relatively little dyspnea—"happy hypoxics"—raising numerous questions about pathophysiology and treatment implications (Ferguson et al., 2020; Goligher et al., 2021). There were also early reports of dichotomized L and H phenotypes, which perhaps necessitated differing ventilatory strategies (Gattinoni et al., 2020; Marini and Gattinoni, 2020). While the optimum ventilator strategy for C-ARDS was unclear, a low tidal volume (LTV) or Acute Respiratory Distress Syndrome Network (ARDSnet) strategy was endorsed by most guidelines and widely applied (Alhazzani et al., 2020; Alqahtani et al., 2020; ANZICS, 2020). But the rapid multiorgan failure following intubation and high mortality rates belied confidence that this ventilatory approach was best suited to C-ARDS. The LTV approach utilizes a tidal volume based on the ideal body weight, but lung volume correlates poorly with this; furthermore, the pathologies causing C-ARDS do not affect the lung parenchyma according to a weight-based pattern.

One of the silver linings of the COVID-19 pandemic was the increased level of collaboration that occurred among medical professionals across the globe. While the online medical community has been gaining momentum in recent years through blogs, podcasts, Twitter, etc., under the rubric of Free Open-Access "Meducation" (FOAMed), the pandemic greatly accelerated this community's growth and impact. Through this collaboration, our critical care team at Santa Cabrini Ospedale explored the literature around airway pressure release ventilation (APRV) and posited that APRV following a time-controlled adaptive ventilation (TCAV) strategy (i.e., APRV-TCAV^{TM}) might provide ventilation better tailored to the diverse and unique pathologies of C-ARDS. And since our center did not have extracorporeal membrane oxygenation (ECMO) capabilities, we thought it all the more important to utilize a ventilatory strategy that could adequately support oxygenation.

Our hospital trialed the mode on select patients during the first wave and, in certain cases, achieved remarkable success. Given this success, we then transitioned to utilizing APRV-TCAV^{TM} as the primary mode for all intubated COVID-19 patients during the second and third waves and found our care markedly improved from what was expected using more traditional LTV approaches. This success came about through trial and error, however, and many lessons were learned that now inform a more thoughtful, safe, and effective way to use the mode and protocol.

THE AIRWAY PRESSURE RELEASE VENTILATION WITH TIME-CONTROLLED ADAPTIVE VENTILATION^{TM} APPROACH: A CURSORY REVIEW

In brief, APRV is a mode of ventilation that alternates between two levels of continuous positive airway pressure (CPAP) and allows for spontaneous breathing throughout the entirety of the respiratory cycle. It requires setting four parameters, namely, the pressure at each level of CPAP and the time spent at each—pressure high (P_{High}), pressure low (P_{Low}), time high (T_{High}), and time low (T_{Low}). These parameters are guided by a protocol referred to as time controlled adaptive ventilation (TCAV). TCAV^{TM} starts by setting the P_{High} at the prior mode's plateau pressure for a T_{High} that is based on the prior respiratory rate. A faster respiratory rate will result in a shorter T_{High} and a slower rate will result in a longer T_{High}. In general, most patients with severe ARDS require a P_{High} of 25–30 cm H_2O, and a T_{High} of 2.5–6 s. This time at a high level of CPAP is punctuated by infrequent, brief drops in pressure to zero, P_{Low}, and referred to as a "release." The duration of the releases, T_{Low}, is usually very short and depends upon the expiratory flow curves as described below. Put as succinctly as possible, TCAV^{TM} is a high CPAP with brief releases.

The extended time at a higher CPAP results in markedly increased mean airway pressures without concomitant increases in peak or plateau pressures. Over time, a lung subjected to these higher mean airway pressures is able to recruit and "open" (assuming the lung has not entered a fibroproliferative phase and all other clinical parameters being equal). The functional residual capacity can be regained, and more normal, homogenous lung architecture can be restored. In fact, APRV is sometimes described as simply a prolonged and judicious recruitment maneuver.

To maintain sufficient minute ventilation and to offload some of the ventilatory burden on the patient, releases are employed. While the release pressure, P_{Low}, is set to zero, some level of intrinsic positive end-expiratory pressure (iPEEP) is retained by terminating the release breath while there is still significant expiratory flow. This is performed by measuring the peak expiratory flow and adjusting the T_{Low} such that it cuts off expiration at or above 75% of peak flow (**Figure 1**). In some ventilators, it is carried out automatically, and once the expiratory flow decays by 25%, the T_{Low} terminates and pressure reverts back to P_{High}. In other words, the T_{Low} is set according to the time it takes the expiratory flow to decay to 75% of the peak expiratory flow. "Trapping" of air based on a time is the key element of this ventilatory strategy and results in an auto-peep that stabilizes the lung by minimizing the alveolar size variation during expiration. Initial *in vivo* animal experiments showed that with a cutoff of 75%, most of the exhaled air was from the conducting airways with a minimal change in the alveolar size (Nieman et al., 2018; Kollisch-Singule et al., 2019) thereby "splinting" the alveoli open. This air splint, in theory, minimizes atelectrauma and maximizes the maintenance of recruitment. While many misinterpret the settings as indicative of a driving pressure of P_{High}—P_{Low} (which would be excessively high in most cases) the driving pressure to the alveoli is in fact P_{High}—intrinsic PEEP. This intrinsic PEEP is easily confirmed with a brief expiratory hold, which always demonstrates a marked discrepancy between the set P_{Low} of zero and the measured airway pressure during a hold (**Figure 2**). Setting the P_{Low} and T_{Low} in this manner has been demonstrated in numerous animal studies to keep the alveoli stable, i.e., they do not collapse with each breath (Nieman et al., 2018).

As the lung recruits, the alveoli get a chance to heal, and if the patient's overall condition improves, the higher pressures can be gradually reduced and the number of releases spread out, a process referred to as "drop and stretch." With this, the patient takes on a larger share of the ventilatory burden, and support is slowly withdrawn until the patient reaches a point of breathing almost entirely on a lower level of CPAP.

Several points bear highlighting. First, the entirety of ventilation can be accounted for by the releases so that APRV can be used on paralyzed patients. In this case, any benefit from spontaneous breathing will be lost, but given the potential risks of patient self-inflicted lung injury (P-SILI), this may not necessarily be a bad thing. Second, nothing prevents APRV-TCAV from being used in a prone position. Third, restoration of lung volume and improvement in V/Q matching often result in improved oxygenation, an "apparent cure," before the previously injured alveoli have had a chance to heal. As a result, many clinicians often prematurely reduce the pressures, and as a result, alveoli quickly collapse again. Finally, tidal volume and traditional PEEP are not directly set. While P_{High}, P_{Low}, T_{High}, and T_{Low} can be adjusted to account for preferred tidal volumes and PEEP levels, their lack of direct control often results in clinicians adjusting the mode in ways that might be deleterious in the context of TCAV^{TM}, e.g., extending the T_{Low} to achieve more minute ventilation. Finally, not all APRV is TCAV^{TM}. While

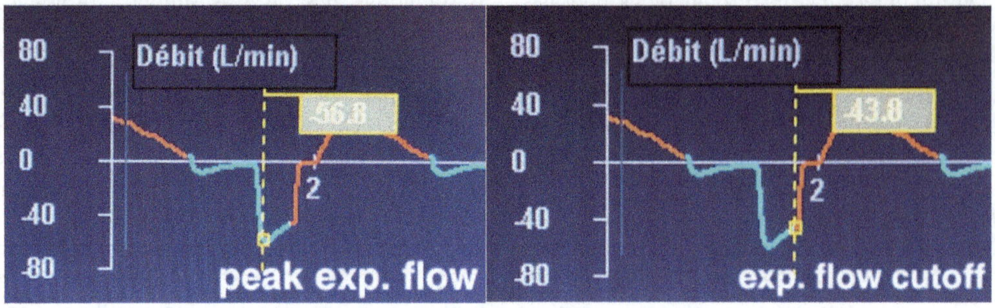

FIGURE 1 | Manual adjustment of TLow: peak expiratory flow is measured (left) and the TLow is set to obtain a cutoff at or above 75% of peak flow, in this case 77%.

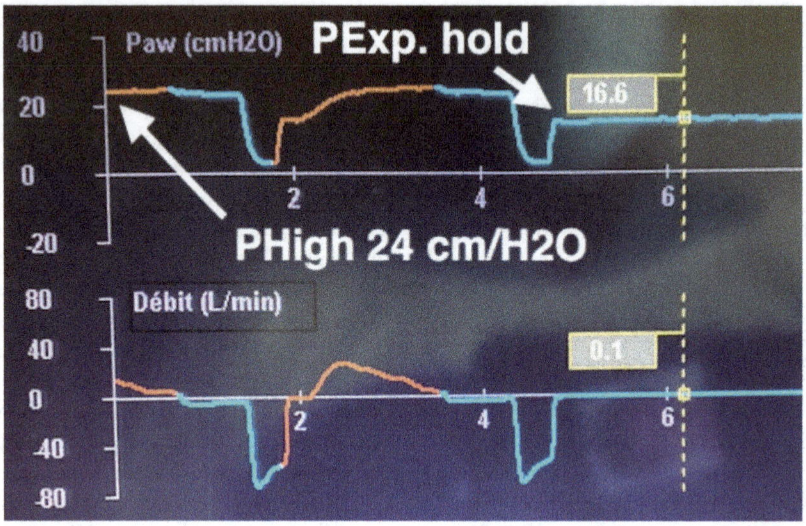

FIGURE 2 | Calculation of Effective PEEP/Driving pressure: an expiratory hold is performed and equilibration of pressure occurs. This is the effective PEEP. Driving pressure is PHigh – PExpiratory hold, in this case approximately 7–8 cmH2O.

many practitioners claim to practice a TCAV™ approach, the settings outlined above are precise and interlinked. Deviation from them in even small ways can result in profound harm. For a more extensive discourse on the mode and protocol, we refer readers to Kollisch-Singule et al. (2019) and Habashi et al. (2021).

OVERVIEW OF OUR EXPERIENCE THROUGH THE DIFFERENT WAVES

As one of the designated centers for COVID-19, our center was rapidly overwhelmed with deteriorating patients. Profound hypoxia was the rule, and we liberally used non-invasive ventilation and awake proning on the wards. Despite this, many deteriorated further, and our expanded-26-bed intensive care unit (ICU) had over 90% of its patients intubated, many requiring frequent proning cycles.

In the first wave, we saw a preponderance of elderly patients and an overall mortality rate of 67%, which is consistent with reports in the literature (Hyman et al., 2020; Luo et al., 2020). APRV-TCAV™ was mostly used as a rescue therapy since the medical and respiratory therapy teams were not familiar or comfortable with the APRV-TCAV™ approach. Despite this lack of experience, APRV-TCAV™ still rescued a few seemingly intractable cases, and we decided to leave those patients on the mode for the remainder of their course. They were among the few survivors of the ventilated cohort. While the numbers are too small to draw meaningful conclusions, they piqued our interest and established the mode as a viable alternative.

After reviewing our first-wave experience, delving into the literature, and discussing with colleagues at other institutions, we proceeded with APRV-TCAV™ as the primary mode of ventilation from intubation to liberation for the majority of cases during the second and third waves. Refractory hypoxia was limited to a few cases unresponsive to TCAV™, which usually ended up requiring transfer for ECMO. With a decreased incidence of refractory hypoxemia came a concurrent decrease in proning—a welcome relief from the nursing work intensity that was needed on other modes of ventilation during the first wave.

In most cases, the following would occur in, approximately, the first 24 h:

(a) Oxygen requirements would significantly decrease.
(b) Driving pressures would markedly decrease, often to less than 10 cm/20 h.
(c) Chest imaging would improve substantially.

All this would occur without substantial deterioration in other organ functions, e.g., there was no escalation of vasopressors, need to initiate continuous renal replacement therapy (CRRT), or worsening sedation needs. If anything, the patients' overall condition would improve in concert with improvement on the ventilator.

CHALLENGES AND CONSIDERATIONS WHEN USING AIRWAY PRESSURE RELEASE VENTILATION WITH TIME-CONTROLLED ADAPTIVE VENTILATION™

False Reassurance by Improved Oxygenation

These improvements were often misleading, however. Several consultants unfamiliar with APRV-TCAV™ were surprised that the patients were not being more aggressively weaned since they "clearly no longer had ARDS" based on their FiO_2 and chest X-ray (CXR). But while the lung may have been recruited and traditional parameters were improved, there was still an underlying pathology that required additional time to heal. If the P_{High} was decreased before the true alveolar stability was achieved, then the CXR would abruptly worsen and gas exchange would quickly regress. This phenomenon of needing to "stabilize" the lung after recruitment on APRV-TCAV™ has been reported elsewhere and likened to needing a cast for a period of time after setting a fracture (Nieman et al., 2018). Hence, clinicians will have to carefully observe patients' breathing patterns, ventilator curves, and gas exchange during weaning.

Risks With Changing Modes

The clinical improvement associated with the use of TCAV™ must be taken into account when considering a change of modes. While changing from a traditional pressure-control mode to an assist-control mode (given similar tidal volumes and PEEP) would not likely result in large swings in oxygenation, this does not always hold true for TCAV™. The clinician should clearly understand that there are several elements that will impact oxygenation in a potentially drastic way, especially if the change occurs before the alveolar stability is achieved as described above. First, TCAV™ is similar to the inverse ratio in that more time is spent at a higher pressure. Hence, switching to alternative modes with roughly the same high and low pressures but a substantially different time at those pressures can result in a significant drop in mean airway pressure. Second, if alveolar stability is not achieved, patients will likely derecruit. The rapidity and severity of deterioration are difficult to predict but can occur in minutes and likely correlate to the required P_{High} and the time spent there previously.

In our experience, these premature and/or inappropriate transitions occurred most often after hand-offs between treating physicians and during patient transport. When a physician is unfamiliar with TCAV™ and the clinical state requires a change to the settings, the clinician often changes to a mode that is more common and familiar. Transitioning to an alternative mode from APRV-TCAV™ before a lung has stabilized is fraught with complexities and nuance that is usually more difficult than making an adjustment to the APRV-TCAV™ settings. It is in this back-and-forth where patients are at most risk for harm and is one of the main reasons why a team buy-in is necessary. This holds true for patient transport as well where portable ventilators are often incapable of providing APRV-TCAV™. Hence, when deciding on, say, a CT scan, the risks of transporting with an alternative ventilatory mode must be weighed against the benefits of the scan. In our center, bedside ultrasound is used extensively, yet trips to CT scan were still required from time to time. This issue also applies to interhospital transfers.

One potential solution for transfers is to approximate TCAV™ by using inverse ratio ventilation with pressure control. The inspiratory pressure should match the P_{High}, and the PEEP should be zero. The inspiratory/expiratory (I:E) ratio will need to reflect the T_{High}:T_{Low}, often being set at the maximum ratio, and patients may need additional sedation and/or paralysis. APRV utilizes floating valves that allow patients to breathe *ad lib* as they would on CPAP. This is not possible on inverse ratio pressure control and will likely be too uncomfortable for spontaneously breathing patients. Utilizing this approach can often create a respiratory rate around 25 with a T_{Low} equivalent of 0.4 and may come close to matching the termination of expiratory flow at 75% (60/25 = 2.4 s cycle. At an I:E of 5:1 that is a "T_{High}" of 2 s and a "T_{Low}" of 0.4 s).

Bagging the Time-Controlled Adaptive Ventilation Patient

Personnel must understand that bagging is unlikely to help the hypoxic patient on TCAV™ and 100% FiO_2. Although a time-honored practice, hand-bagging will likely result in a much lower mean airway pressure—even when a PEEP valve is used—and may result in deterioration. Rapidly passing a suction catheter to rule out occlusion, analyzing the ventilator waveform and end-tidal CO_2 ($ETCO_2$), carefully observing the patient, and quickly scanning with point-of-care ultrasound (POCUS) or obtaining a CXR to rule out pneumothorax should be the initial reflexes. Bagging should only be considered after serious deliberation with the clear understanding that this may result in massive derecruitment.

Timing of Interhospital Transfer

In the escalation of ventilatory therapy, APRV usually sits just below veno-venous ECMO (VV-ECMO). In some cases, it may avoid the need for such escalation (Lim et al., 2016); however, when it is being used in a center that does not have VV-ECMO in-house, it is important for the treating team to realize that the inherent risks of transfers will be heightened if the patient is on maximal support with 100% FiO_2 and very high APRV-TCAV™

settings. Hence, the transfer should be considered when there is still some margin of safety as transferring may require coming off TCAV, which carries risks as described earlier. For those transfers we carried out, we kept the ventilator on for as much of the physical transfer to the ambulance stretcher and only switched to the transport ventilator when the whole team was ready to roll off with the patient.

CLINICAL VIGNETTES

In the following cases, we have illustrated some of these issues as well as showed the different ways in which APRV-TCAV™ was used.

Case 1—First Wave

A 55-year-old woman was admitted with severe COVID pneumonia initially managed with non-invasive ventilation but, on day 2, was intubated following severe desaturation to 21% SpO_2. She was initially put on pressure-controlled ventilation (PCV) with an inspired pressure (P_{insp}) of 24 cm H_2O, PEEP of 12 cm H_2O, and an FiO_2 of 80% (**Figure 3A**). On the ensuing days, there was little improvement, and she required serial proning. She continued needing an FiO_2 over 80% and her PCV settings increased to P_{insp} of 29 cm H_2O and PEEP of 15 cm H_2O with a driving pressure of 19 cm H_2O. She developed acute kidney injury (AKI) requiring renal replacement therapy. On day 9, PCV was set to inverse ratio ventilation of 2.7:1 with a slight improvement in oxygenation. Her oxygen requirements progressively worsened, and on day 14, while proned and paralyzed on CMV with a plateau pressure of 38 cm H_2O and FiO_2 100% for a PaO_2/FiO_2 (P/F) ratio of 58, APRV-TCAV™ was initiated at 34/2.5/0/0.4 (all APRV settings are referred to as $P_{High}/T_{High}/P_{Low}/T_{Low}$). In the next morning, her FiO_2 was down to 70% on 36/2.3/0/0.4 and later that day was further decreased to 55% with a P/F ratio of 100. Paralytics were discontinued. Over the next 5 days, her P/F ratio rose to 156, FiO_2 dropped to 45%, and a percutaneous tracheostomy was carried out on day 17 without complication (**Figure 3B**). There was no hemodynamic instability, and renal replacement therapy was ongoing. Following a changeover of the medical team, on day 23, while on APRV-TCAV with FiO_2 30%, a decision was made to switch to CMV. In the next few hours, her oxygen requirements rose progressively with concomitant hemodynamic instability requiring reinstitution of vasopressors. On the next day, with a P/F ratio of 83 on a PEEP of 10 cm H_2O, she would intermittently desaturate to 30–35% SpO_2. She was proned, but her SpO_2 remained in the 60's with a P/F ratio of 42. At this point, TCAV was reinstated at 42/2.4/0/0.3 in hopes to rerecruit the lungs. In the next 3 h, her SpO_2 climbed to 92%; however, her P/F ratios never rose above 100 thereafter, and she died suddenly on day 28, without any evidence of pneumothorax.

This case tragically illustrates the dangers of switching modes from APRV-TCAV™ without ensuring that alveoli have had sufficient time to heal and stabilize. It also demonstrates the need for teamwork and buy-in when using a mode with which all team members may not be comfortable. It also shows how excellent gas exchange can occur due to TCAV™ prior to achieving inherent alveolar stability.

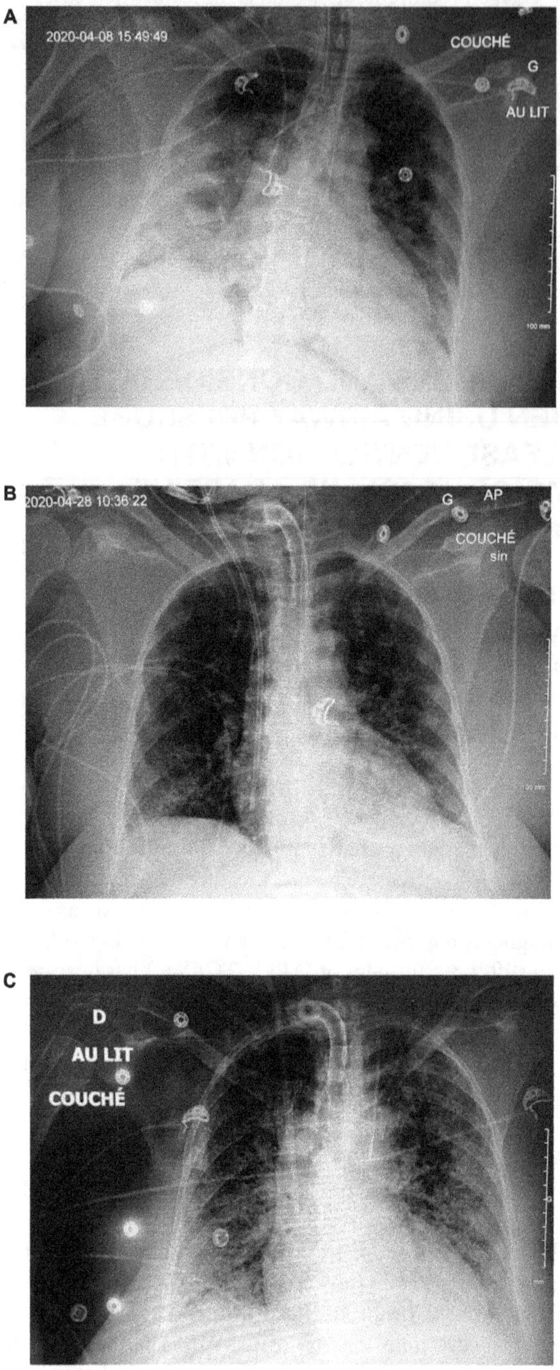

FIGURE 3 | Case 1: **(A)** CXR on ICU day 2 on PCV. **(B)** CXR on day 17 post-tracheostomy. **(C)** CXR following switch to CMV.

Case 2—Second Wave

A 32-year-old man presented to the ED with dyspnea and an SpO_2 of 60%. He was morbidly obese (150 kg) but with no other past medical history. His CXR showed severe volume loss

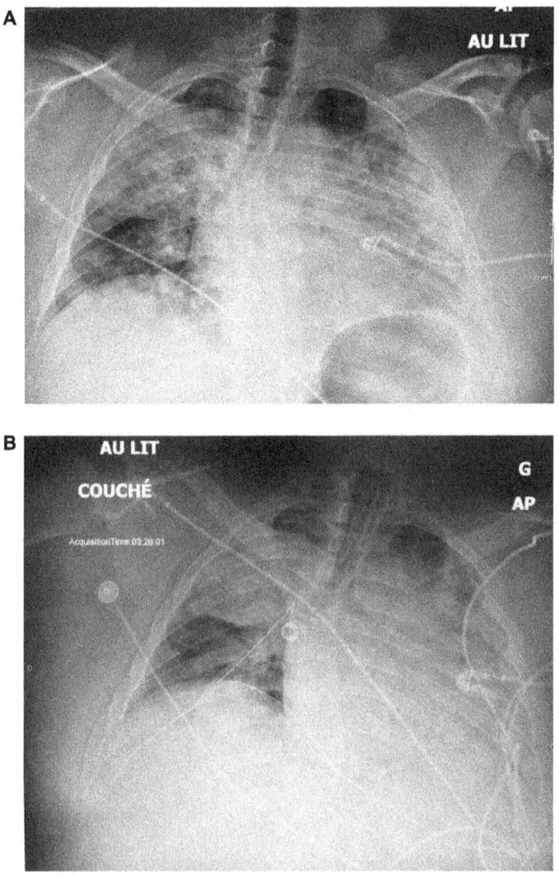

FIGURE 4 | Case 2: **(A)** Day 1 pre-intubation. **(B)** Day 1, 2 h post-intubation, on CMV.

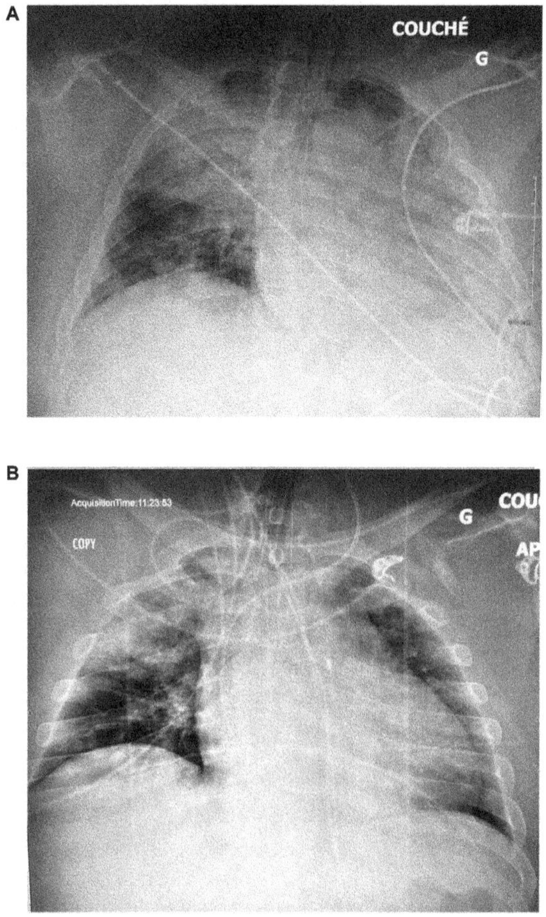

FIGURE 5 | Case 2: **(A)** Day 1, 1 h post APRV-TCAV. **(B)** Day 2, approximately 30 h after initiaition of TCAV(tm).

and bilateral infiltrates (**Figure 4**). Oxygenation only improved to 84% with high-flow nasal cannula (HFNC) and proning, and the decision was made to intubate him after he displayed respiratory fatigue. Following intubation, the patient suffered from profound desaturation to 20% with severe bradycardia to 18 bpm necessitating atropine, epinephrine, and 2 min of chest compressions. He was placed on CMV, and upon arrival of the critical care team, saturations had increased to 92% on FiO_2 of 100% and a PEEP of 14 cm H_2O, as well as an infusion of norepinephrine. With tidal volumes of 400 ml (approx 5 ml/kg ideal body weight), he had a driving pressure of 18 cm H_2O. His initial arterial blood gas (ABG) showed a pH of 7.28, a PCO_2 of 59 mmHg, and a PO_2 of 63 mmHg for a P/F ratio of 63. The CXR 2 hours post-intubation showed almost complete opacification of the left lung and significant infiltrate in the right upper lobe (**Figure 4B**). He was then put on APRV-TCAV^{TM} 35/1.8/0/0.3 and admitted to the ICU. Approximately, 1 hour after initiation of TCAV^{TM}, a second CXR showed slight recruitment of the lower left lobe with some appearance of the diaphragm (**Figure 5A**). To further augment recruitment, the P_{High} was increased by 2 cm H_2O to 37 cm H_2O. Mild hemodynamic instability persisted requiring continued norepinephrine infusion. POCUS revealed a moderately dilated right ventricle, relatively preserved left ventricular function with an ejection fraction of 50%, and a type 2 right ventricular outflow tract (RVOT) pattern indicative of mild pulmonary hypertension (López-Candales and Edelman, 2012). A pulmonary artery (PA) catheter was then inserted to monitor PA pressures, which were 35/25 cm H_2O at that time.

About 14 hours following TCAV^{TM} initiation, his FiO_2 was decreased from 100 to 35% and the P/F ratio rose to 300, while the driving pressure decreased from 18 to 11 cm H_2O. By the next morning, his CXR showed significant recruitment of the left lung (**Figure 5B**), and norepinephrine was weaned off. He developed some AKI, but given adequate cardiac output, moderately elevated CVP, and grade 1 venous excess ultrasound (VExUS) score, fluids were not deemed beneficial (Beaubien-Souligny et al., 2020). On day 5, the driving pressure had further decreased to 6 cm H_2O and the CXR showed further recruitment (**Figure 6A**). A small, probable pneumopericardium was noted and followed carefully but never required intervention. Over the next few days, his FiO_2 remained between 25 and 35% with driving pressures below 10 cm H_2O. His sedation was lightened, he was allowed to breathe more, and his AKI resolved, but his P_{High} could not be decreased below 33 cm H_2O without desaturation. On day 13, he was dropped to a P_{High} of

A

B

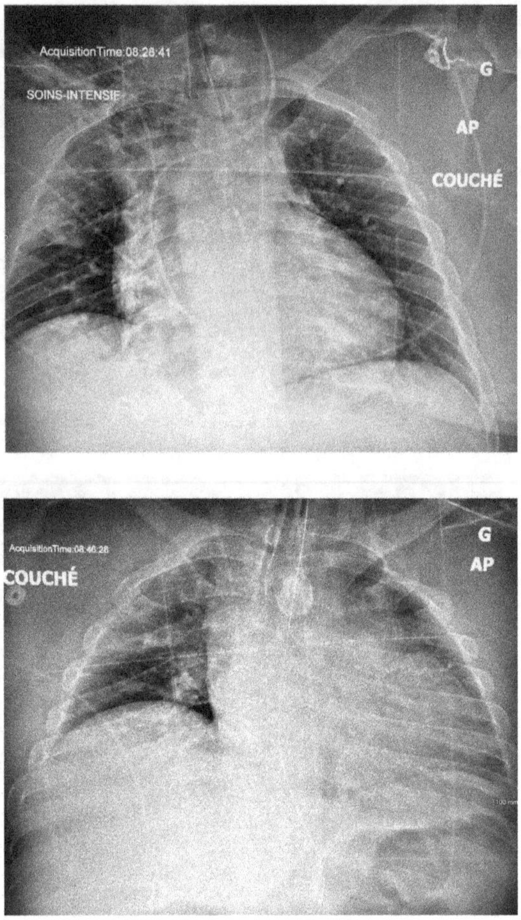

FIGURE 6 | Case 2: **(A)** ICU Day 5. **(B)** ICU Day 13.

A

B

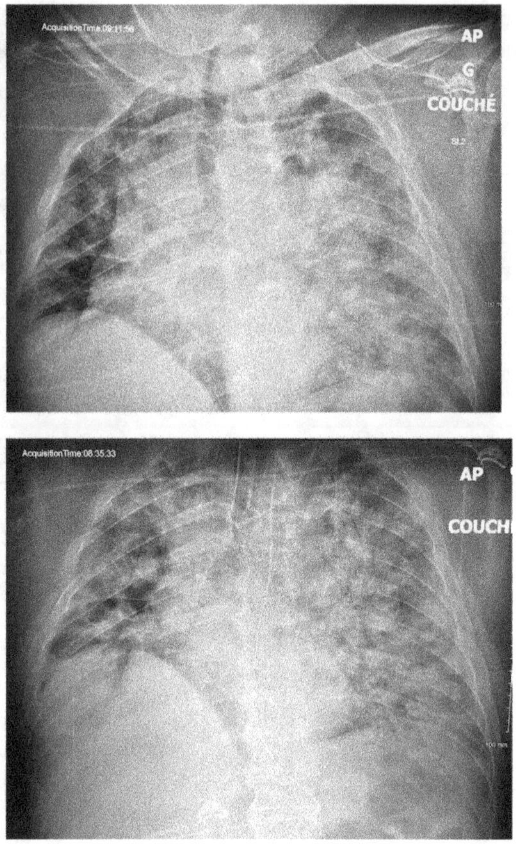

FIGURE 7 | Case 3: **(A)** CXR on Day 1 of admission to ICU, pre-intubation. **(B)** CXR on ICU Day 2, after 20 h of ventilation on PEEP 16cm/H_2O.

28 cm H_2O, but there was a clear loss of volume/derecruitment on CXR (**Figure 6B**) over 24 hours, despite PaO_2 remaining reasonable at 67 mmhg on 25% FiO_2. At this point, the P_{High} was increased to 33 cm H_2O as it was felt that alveolar stability had not been reached. Over the next few days, he remained stable and eventually tolerated dropping the P_{High}, and he finally was extubated on ICU day 18. This patient never required paralysis, nor proning, partly because of his body habitus, but also because once recruited, his P/F ratios never required it.

This case illustrates the concept of alveolar stability, which is not typically part of the daily assessment of most critically ill ventilated patients but is an inherent part of the TCAV^{TM} approach. It is likely that had the patient been rapidly weaned and extubated after his initial improvement in oxygenation, he would have required reintubation and regressed to a condition worse than after his initial intubation. His reassuring CXRs and persistent P/F ratios >200 nicely demonstrate the concept of "apparent cure" before the alveolar stability is achieved. It should also be noted that the patient had a profound drop in driving pressure, 18 to 6 cm H_2O, suggesting a significantly reduced level of mechanical power or energy delivered to the lung parenchyma (Costa et al., 2021).

Case 3—Third Wave

A 58-year-old man with obesity, hypertension, and dyslipidemia presented with a 1 week history of dyspnea and presented to a community hospital emergency room where he was put on high flow nasal cannulae and then transferred to our center for further management. On arrival, he was saturating 88% on 70% FiO_2, and his initial CXR showed extensive bilateral infiltrates and volume loss (**Figure 7A**). He developed agitation, and his saturation deteriorated to the low 80's despite increasing his FiO_2 to 100%. He was intubated and put on CMV with a tidal volume of 500 ml, respiratory rate of 26, and a PEEP of 16 cm H_2O with a resulting plateau pressure of 27 cm H_2O and a driving pressure of 11 cm H_20. Paralytics were not required. He required a norepinephrine infusion to maintain sufficient perfusion pressures. The FiO_2 was gradually reduced to 50%, but on day 2, his CXR showed no significant improvement (**Figure 7B**), and a transesophageal echocardiogram ruled out significant ventricular dysfunction and valvular disease. The decision was made to put him on APRV-TCAV^{TM} for recruitment purposes, and his initial settings were 29/1.5/0/0.4. An expiratory hold on these settings showed a driving pressure of 10. On the next day, his CXR showed significant recruitment (**Figure 8A**), and on day 4, his FiO_2 was down to 35% on settings of 29/1.5/0/0.4. An ABG showed pH of 7.48, PCO_2 of 51 mmHg, and PO_2 of 80 mmHg for a P/F ratio of 228. At this point, his norepinephrine drip

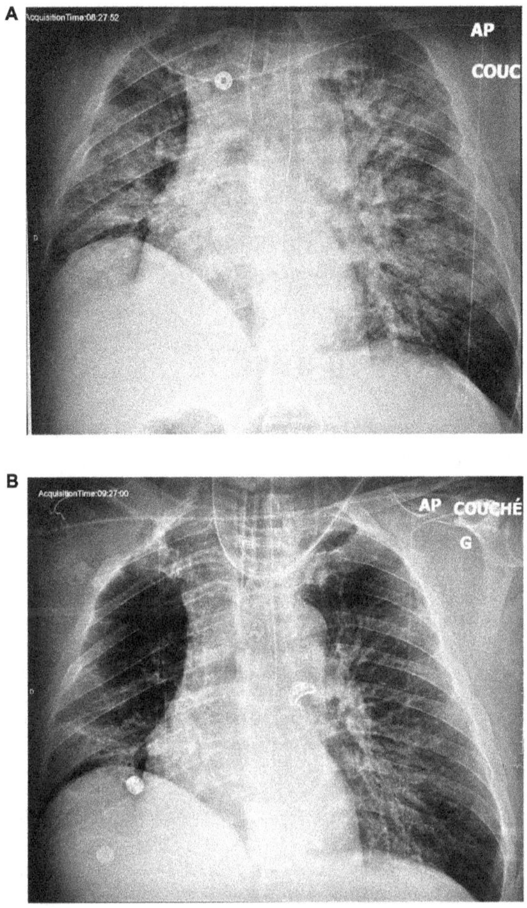

FIGURE 8 | Case 3: **(A)** CXR on ICU Day 3, after 24 h of APRV-TCAV(tm). **(B)** CXR on ICU Day 6.

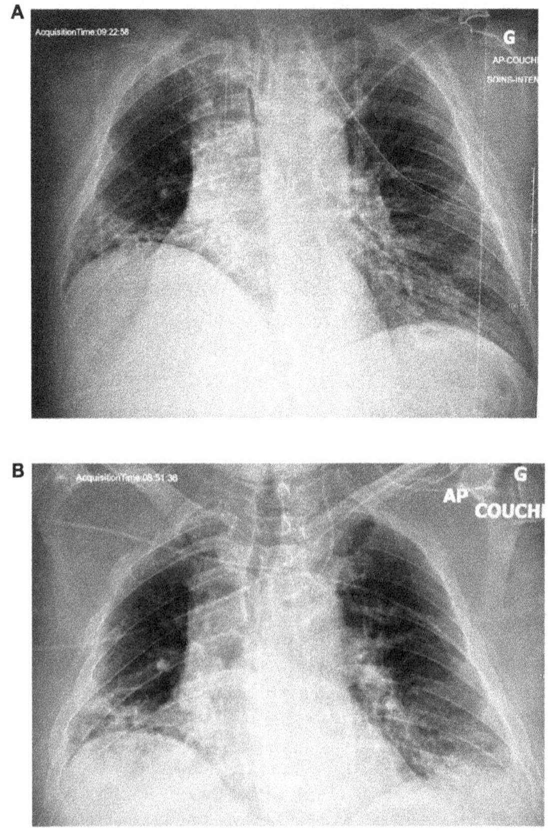

FIGURE 9 | Case 3: **(A)** ICU Day 11. **(B)** CXR on day 14, 24 h post-extubation.

had been weaned off, and the patient appeared stable. Several consultants suggested weaning, as the patient no longer met ARDS criteria; however, dropping the P_{High} transiently at the bedside resulted in significantly decreased release volumes with associated desaturations and an increase in the $EtCO_2$, suggesting derecruitment. Consequently, the treating team judged that alveolar stability had not been reached, and his settings were reverted back to their previous values. On day 10, he was successfully "dropped and stretched" to 18/10/0/0.4, which was essentially equivalent to a CPAP 18 cm H_2O. He was then extubated to HFNC and initially did reasonably well but 4 h later, desaturated and required reintubation. He was placed back on APRV-TCAV^{TM} with the setting of 28/2.5/0/0.4. On day 11, norepinephrine, which had been required post reintubation, was weaned off, and again his ventilatory settings were adjusted to 22/2.5/0/0.4, and FiO_2 was decreased to 25%. The CXR appeared well recruited (**Figure 8B**), and he was extubated on day 13 after several hours on a CPAP of 12 CmH_2O (**Figure 9A**) and subsequently remained stable (**Figure 9B**). This patient never required paralysis and subsequently did well and was eventually discharged.

This case illustrates several key elements of APRV-TCAV^{TM}. First, one can see how little recruitment happened in the first 24 h of CMV, whereas an impressive amount occurred in the first 24 h of TCAV^{TM}. Second, the time factor in alveolar stability was clear, as it took several hours before desaturation was noted, despite the patient having been on only 25% FiO_2 prior to the failed first extubation. While gas exchange was excellent, alveolar stability had not truly been achieved yet, which again illustrates the phenomenon of "apparent cure" when well-recruited patients may no longer fit the definition of ARDS but quickly decompensate with the desolation of ventilators support and pressures.

Time-Controlled Adaptive Ventilation in Clinical Practice Today

In general, different ventilatory modes are used in different phases or severity of illness. It is difficult to estimate the frequency of APRV-TCAV^{TM} use in the critical care community, but in our experience, while APRV as a mode is relatively well known, the TCAV^{TM} approach seems to be less so. However, recent studies and even meta-analyses have been published, indicating that, at least in some centers, experience with it is growing (Zhou et al., 2017; Ibarra-Estrada et al., 2021). Strategically, one may use CMV as a primary mode during acute illness and pressure support during weaning. Several modes or strategies may be used as rescues, such as inverse ratio ventilation, high-frequency oscillation, or APRV. APRV-TCAV™ can be used as a primary or as a rescue mode, but the authors would caution against inexperienced users attempting it without experienced supervision particularly in the most fragile rescue cases.

CONCLUSION

In the second wave onward, we had several patients who had an uneventful course with APRV-TCAV™ for the vast majority of their ventilation and were successfully extubated, a few who required ECMO, and some who passed away of non-pulmonary COVID complications, such as intracerebral hemorrhage and arterial thrombosis. Our experience is heterogeneous and uncontrolled, not one from which outcome data can be inferred, although it was clear in several cases that APRV-TCAV™ was able to oxygenate and rescue patients where a traditional lung-protective strategy had failed. Challenges abound with implementing TCAV™, the most critical ones being education and team buy-in. In inexperienced hands and minds, APRV-TCAV™ certainly has more challenges than a traditional LTV/ARDSnet approach, but in the authors' experience, APRV-TCAV offers substantial physiological advantages that are worth the investment to understand and implement. What is needed is well-designed comparative trials to see if the promising cases in our experience can translate into a survival benefit if APRV-TCAV™ is used as a primary mode.

AUTHOR CONTRIBUTIONS

PR was the clinician who managed and reported cases described. BD contributed extensive writing of the main text and review of the document. Both authors contributed to the article and approved the submitted version.

REFERENCES

Alhazzani, W., Møller, M. H., Arabi, Y. M., Loeb, M., Gong, M. N., Fan, E., et al. (2020). Surviving Sepsis Campaign: guidelines on the management of critically ill adults with Coronavirus Disease 2019 (COVID-19). *Intensive Care Med.* 46, 854–887.

Alqahtani, J. S., Mendes, R. G., Aldhahir, A., Rowley, D., AlAhmari, M. D., Ntoumenopoulos, G., et al. (2020). Global Current Practices of Ventilatory Support Management in COVID-19 Patients: an International Survey. *J. Multidiscip. Healthc.* 13, 1635–1648. doi: 10.2147/JMDH.S279031

ANZICS (2020). *The Australian and New Zealand Intensive Care Society (ANZICS) COVID-19 Guidelines.* Melbourne: ANZICS.

Beaubien-Souligny, W., Rola, P., Haycock, K., Bouchard, J., Lamarche, Y., Spiegel, R., et al. (2020). Quantifying systemic congestion with Point-Of-Care ultrasound: development of the venous excess ultrasound grading system. *Ultrasound. J.* 12:16. doi: 10.1186/s13089-020-00163-w

Costa, E. L. V., Slutsky, A. S., Brochard, L. J., Brower, R., Serpa-Neto, A., Cavalcanti, A. B., et al. (2021). Ventilatory variables and mechanical power in patients with acute respiratory distress syndrome. *Am. J. Respir. Crit. Care Med.* 204, 303–311. doi: 10.1164/rccm.202009-3467oc

Ferguson, N. D., Pham, T., and Gong, M. N. (2020). How severe COVID-19 infection is changing ARDS management. *Intensive Care Med.* 46, 2184–2186. doi: 10.1007/s00134-020-06245-6

Gattinoni, L., Chiumello, D., Caironi, P., Busana, M., Romitti, F., Brazzi, L., et al. (2020). COVID-19 pneumonia: Different respiratory treatment for different phenotypes? *Intensive Care Med.* 46, 1099–1102. doi: 10.1007/s00134-020-06033-2

Goligher, E. C., Ranieri, V. M., and Slutsky, A. S. (2021). Is severe COVID-19 pneumonia a typical or atypical form of ARDS? And does it matter? *Intensive Care Med.* 47, 83–85. doi: 10.1007/s00134-020-06320-y

Habashi, N. M., Camporota, L., Gatto, L. A., and Nieman, G. (2021). Functional Pathophysiology of SARS-CoV-2 Induced Acute Lung Injury and Clinical Implications. *J. Appl. Physiol.* 130, 877–891. doi: 10.1152/japplphysiol.00742.2020

Hyman, J. B., Leibner, E. S., Tandon, P., Egorova, N. N., Bassily-Marcus, A., Kohli-Seth, R., et al. (2020). Timing of Intubation and in-hospital mortality in patients with Coronavirus Disease 2019. *Crit. Care Explor.* 2:e0254. doi: 10.1097/CCE.0000000000000254

Ibarra-Estrada, M. Á., García-Salas, Y., Mireles-Cabodevila, E., López-Pulgarín, J. A., Chávez-Peña, Q., García-Salcido, R., et al. (2021). Use of airway pressure release ventilation in patients with acute respiratory failure due to coronavirus disease 2019: results of a single-center randomized controlled trial. *Crit. Care Med.* [Epub ahead of print]. doi: 10.1097/CCM.0000000000005312

Kollisch-Singule, M., Andrews, P., Satalin, J., Gatto, L. A., Nieman, G. F., and Habashi, N. M. (2019). The time-controlled adaptive ventilation protocol: mechanistic approach to reducing ventilator-induced lung injury. *Eur. Respir. Rev.* 28:180126. doi: 10.1183/16000617.0126-2018

Lim, J., Litton, E., Robinson, H., and Das Gupta, M. (2016). Characteristics and outcomes of patients treated with airway pressure release ventilation for acute respiratory distress syndrome: a retrospective observational study. *J. Crit. Care* 34, 154–159. doi: 10.1016/j.jcrc.2016.03.002

López-Candales, A., and Edelman, K. (2012). Shape of the right ventricular outflow Doppler envelope and severity of pulmonary hypertension. *Eur. Heart J. Cardiovasc. Imaging* 13, 309–316. doi: 10.1093/ejechocard/jer23

Luo, M., Cao, S., Wei, L., Zhao, X., Gao, F., Li, S., et al. (2020). Intubation, mortality, and risk factors in critically ill Covid-19 patients: a pilot study. *J. Clin. Anesth.* 67:110039. doi: 10.1016/j.jclinane.2020.110039

Marini, J. J., and Gattinoni, L. (2020). Management of COVID-19 respiratory distress. *JAMA* 323, 2329–2330. doi: 10.1001/jama.2020.6825

Nieman, G. F., Andrews, P., Satalin, J., Wilcox, K., Kollisch-Singule, M., Madden, M., et al. (2018). Acute lung injury: how to stabilize a broken lung. *Crit. Care* 22:136. doi: 10.1186/s13054-018-2051-8

Zhou, Y., Jin, X., Lv, Y., Wang, P., Yang, Y., Liang, G., et al. (2017). Early application of airway pressure release ventilation may reduce the duration of mechanical ventilation in acute respiratory distress syndrome. *Intensive Care Med.* 43, 1648–1659.

8

Astrocytes Downregulate Inflammation in Lipopolysaccharide-Induced Acute Respiratory Distress Syndrome: Applicability to COVID-19

Michal Izrael[1], Kfir Molakandov[1], Ariel Revel[1], Shalom Guy Slutsky[1], Tehila Sonnenfeld[1], Julia Miriam Weiss[1] and Michel Revel[1,2]*

[1] *Research and Development Department at Kadimastem Ltd, Nes-Ziona, Israel,* [2] *Department of Molecular Genetics, Weizmann Institute of Science, Rehovot, Israel*

***Correspondence:**
Michal Izrael
M.izrael@kadimastem.com;
michal.izrael@mail.huji.ac.il

Background: An acute respiratory distress syndrome (ARDS) is caused by the increased amounts of pro-inflammatory cytokines and neutrophil-mediated tissue injury. To date, there is no effective treatment for the ARDS available, while the need for one is growing due to the most severe complications of the current coronavirus disease-2019 (COVID-19) pandemic. The human astrocytes (AstroRx) have shown immunomodulatory properties in the central nervous system (CNS). This study aimed to evaluate the capacity of astrocytes to decrease lung inflammation and to be applied as a treatment therapy in ARDS.

Methods: First, we assessed the ability of clinical-grade AstroRx to suppress T-cell proliferation in a mixed lymphocyte reaction test. Next, we tested the therapeutical potential of AstroRx cells in a lipopolysaccharide (LPS)-based ARDS mouse model by injecting AstroRx intravenously (i.v). We determined the degree of lung injury by using a severity scoring scale of 0–2, based on the American Thoracic Society. The scoring measured the presence of neutrophils, fibrin deposits, and the thickening of alveolar walls. The state of inflammation was further assessed by quantifying the immune-cell infiltration to the bronchoalveolar lavage fluid (BALF) and by the presence of proinflammatory cytokines and chemokines in the BALF and serum.

Results: We detected that AstroRx cells were capable to suppress T-cell proliferation *in vitro* after exposure to the mitogen concanavalin A (ConA). *In vivo,* AstroRx cells were able to lower the degree of lung injury in LPS-treated animals compared with the sham injected animals ($P = 0.039$). In this study, 30% of AstroRx treated mice showed no lung lesions (responder mice), these mice presented a steady number of eosinophils, T cells, and neutrophils comparable with the level of naïve control mice. The inflammatory cytokines and chemokines, such as TNFα, IL1b, IL-6, and CXCL1, were also kept in check in responder AstroRx-treated mice and were not upregulated as in the sham-injected mice ($P < 0.05$). As a result, the LPS-treated ARDS mice had a higher survival rate when they were treated with AstroRx.

Conclusions: Our results demonstrate that the immunosuppressive activity of AstroRx cells support the application of AstroRx cells as a cell therapy treatment for ARDS. The immunoregulatory activity may also be a part of the mechanism of action of AstroRx reported in the amyotrophic lateral sclerosis (ALS) neurodegenerative disease.

Keywords: ARDS, astrocytes, immune-modulation, inflammation, embryonic stem cells

INTRODUCTION

An acute respiratory distress syndrome (ARDS) is a form of progressive hypoxemia respiratory failure and pulmonary edema in the absence of heart failure (1). The etiology of ARDS varies (e.g., pneumonia, sepsis, or acute pancreatitis) and great efforts have been made in intensive care medicine, but the overall mortality is still high (2, 3). Recently, a significant proportion of patients infected with coronavirus disease-2019 (COVID-19) developed viral pneumonia that caused an acute lung injury (ALI) capable of rapid progression to viral sepsis and ARDS with a high fatality rate especially in older and comorbidities populations (4–6). The phases in the development of ARDS include the exudation stage characterized by the inflammatory cell infiltration and pulmonary edema (stage 1), the proliferation of myofibroblasts (stage 2), and extracellular matrix (ECM) over-deposited (stage 3) (7). The fibrosis process (stages 2 and 3) is rapid and occurs within 1 week (8, 9). This inflammatory response process referred to as cytokine storm or cytokine release syndrome (CRS), contributes to the development of ARDS and often irreversible multi-organ dysfunction syndrome (MODS) associated with the severe-critical forms of COVID-19 (10, 11). Another key process in the development of ARDS is neutrophil accumulation in high abundance in the pulmonary microcirculation, lung interstitium, and alveolar airspace of the patients with ARDS (12). In addition, an ARDS is associated with systemic neutrophil priming, delayed neutrophil apoptosis, and clearance of neutrophils from the lungs. In animal models, lung injury could be ameliorated by reducing the number of circulating neutrophils (13).

Current management for COVID-19 (severe acute respiratory syndrome-coronavirus 2, SARS-CoV-2) infected patients with severe pneumonia and ARDS remains supportive, such as the use of anti-infection drugs, intubated ventilator-assisted breathing therapy, and extracorporeal membrane oxygenation (ECMO) (14–16). Since ARDS is associated with high mortality and morbidity, it is vital to develop new effective therapeutic approaches capable of immunomodulating the immune system and inflammatory response. This could be of great benefit in preventing the disease progression and reducing the case mortality rate in the high-risk patients with COVID-19. A growing body of evidence has shown that cell-based therapies hold therapeutic effects for ARDS. Most of the studies have focused on the therapeutic effects of mesenchymal stem cells (MSCs) (17, 18) and some studies have also investigated the possible applications of other cell types, such as pulmonary epithelial progenitors (19, 20).

Another approach using astrocytes is presented as they are the most abundant glial cell in the central nervous system (CNS). Astrocytes regulate the concentration of different neurotransmitters and ions, supply various metabolites and energy, regulate osmolarity, modulate synaptic activity, secrete neurotrophic and neuroprotective factors, promote neurogenesis (21–23), and remyelination (24). Moreover, the astrocytes are essential players in immune-modulation (25, 26). Astrocytes have a dual role as key immune modulators of the immune response of the CNS to infections, neurodegenerative disorders, and injuries (27). Following injury and in disease, their ability to respond to, and commence initial responses to injury/disease is increasingly apparent. Astrocytes serve as a contact between the CNS and the peripheral immune system. In many pathological conditions, astrocytes either secrete anti-inflammatory or pro-inflammatory factors which modulate the immune system (28–30). Astrocytes, take part in both the recruitment and restriction of leukocytes in the CNS (31, 32). Neuroinflammation is increasingly recognized as an important mediator of disease progression in patients with amyotrophic lateral sclerosis (ALS), and similar to ARDS, it is characterized by reactive tissue and infiltrating peripheral monocytes and lymphocytes (33). The astrocytes derived from the pluripotent stem cells (AstroRx) demonstrated neuroprotective A2-type characteristics, such as glutamate uptake capabilities, secretion of neuroprotective factors, promotion of axon outgrowth, and protection of motor neurons (MNs) from oxidative stress (34). Intrathecal injection of astrocytes (AstroRx) in an ALS animal model demonstrated a therapeutic benefit (34) and is being tested first in the human clinical trial in the patients with ALS (clinicaltrial.gov ID NCT03482050). The immune-modulatory effect of astrocytes outside the CNS, to the best of our knowledge, is not reported yet and can shed more light on its anti-inflammatory activity in ALS disease.

In this current study, the effect of astrocytes on ARDS is investigated for the first time. We deciphered the immunomodulatory effect of AstroRx first *in vitro* by evaluating T-cell proliferation in a mixed lymphocyte reaction test. Then, we assessed the effect of intravenous (i.v.) AstroRx injection on lung injury, lung inflammation, and survival in a lipopolysaccharide (LPS)-based ARDS mouse model. Altogether our results indicate that AstroRx has the potential to maintain immune homeostasis in the lung and thereby increase the chance of survival.

A

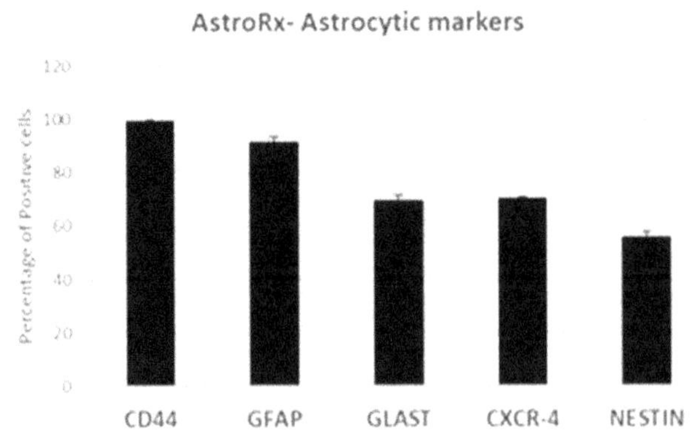

B

Pluripotent Markers	
EPCAM	0.0±0.0
SSEA_4	0.0±0.0
TRA-160	0.0±0.0

C

	Thy1.2+/ CD25+	Change from BL
LNC +ConA	26.3%	BL
LNC in AstroRx® media +ConA	26.4%	0.4%
LNC:AstroRx® 10:1 +ConA	22.4%	-14.8%
LNC:AstroRx® 5:1 +ConA	15.3%	-41.8%
LNC only	0.6%	-97.7%

D

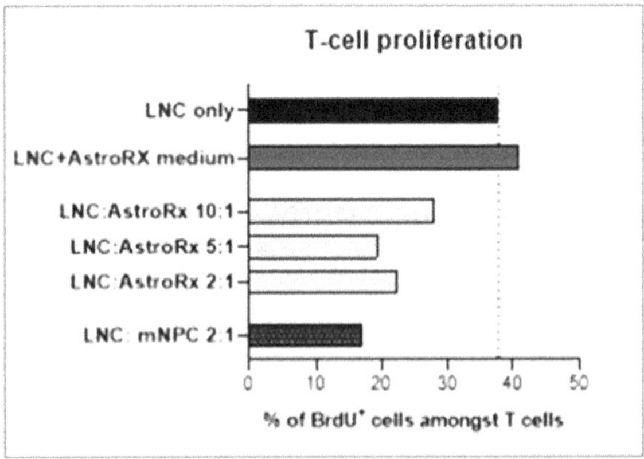

FIGURE 1 | Human astrocytes (AstroRx) demonstrate immunosuppressive capacities *in vitro*. **(A,B)** The AstroRx were analyzed by flow cytometry for astrocytic markers **(A)** and pluripotent stem cells markers **(B)**. **(C,D)** The immunosuppressive potential of AstroRx was assessed in a mixed lymphocyte reaction test. The AstroRx were co-cultured with murine lymph node cells (LNCs). **(C)** The LNCs were stained for T cell marker Thy1.2 and CD25 positive cells under ConA activation in the presence or absence of different amounts of AstroRx. **(D)** The proliferation state of T cells (CD3+) was determined by the proliferation marker BrdU in the presence of ConA. The LNCs only were used as negative control while the LNC with mouse neural precursor cells (mNPC) were used as a positive control. Average and ± SEM.

RESULTS

Suppression of T-cell Proliferation by AstroRx Cells

In a recent study, we have shown how human embryonic stem cell (hESC)-derived astrocytes (AstroRx) protect MNs *in vitro* and in the ALS animal models (34). In these studies, we demonstrated that AstroRx protected neurons by the secretion of neuroprotective and neurotrophic factors, uptake of glutamate, and regulation of oxidative stress. The immunomodulatory capacity of these human astrocytes (AstroRx) was not fully defined yet. To better understand if AstroRx can protect from inflammatory damage, we analyzed its immunosuppressive potential. For this, we used fully differentiated AstroRx, which expressed high levels of astrocytic markers (**Figure 1A**) and did not express pluripotent stem cells markers (**Figure 1B**). The AstroRx were co-cultured with murine lymph-node cells (LNC). The T-cell proliferation in this culture was induced by concanavalin A (ConA). When ConA was not added to the culture, the percentage of T cells in the culture was below 1%. The addition of either AstroRx cells or the conditioned medium of AstroRx cells did not affect the percentage of T cells in the culture (not shown).

In contrast, in the presence of ConA, the AstroRx cells profoundly influenced the T-cell population (Thy1.2^{+}/CD25^{+}), which decreased by about 15% in the LNC:AstroRx® (at a ratio of 10:1) co-culture. A greater inhibitory effect was achieved when using a ratio of 5:1 of LNC:AstroRx culture, which decreased T-cell population by 42%. This effect was not observed when only AstroRx-conditioned medium was added (**Figure 1C**), indicating that the effect was cell-contact dependent.

To evaluate the proliferation capacity of T cells in the presence of AstroRx, we performed a BrdU cell proliferation assay. The percentage of CD3^{+}/BrdU^{+} cells in a culture of LNC with ConA but without AstroRx was chosen to serve as a baseline (BL). Without ConA, the percentage of human proliferating cells among the T cells was below 1%, the addition of different amounts of AstroRx cells to LNCs in the absence of ConA did not affect the percentage of proliferating T cells (not shown). In the presence of ConA, 40% of T cells were BrdU+ and proliferating.

As a positive inhibitory control, we used mouse neural precursor cells (mNPCs), which were previously described for reducing T-cell proliferation (35). Co-culture with mNPCs had no effect on T-cell proliferation in the absence of ConA (not shown) but reduced the number of proliferating cells among the T cells by more than a half when T cells were exposed to ConA (**Figure 1D**). Interestingly, when T cells were co-cultured with AstroRx, the proliferation rate among the T cells decreased by more than a third in the LNC:AstroRx® 10:1 culture. Higher ratios of AstroRx® to LNC resulted in a greater inhibitory effect, similar to the range of co-cultures with mNPCs (decrease by 49 or 43% in LNC:AstroRx® 5:1 or LNC:AstroRx® 2:1 cultures, respectively).

The effect was not observed when AstroRx® conditioned media was added to the culture, again suggesting that the AstroRx suppression is mediated by a direct cell-contact or communication between the AstroRx cells and LNC. Altogether, these results show that AstroRx has the potential to suppress the T-cell proliferation in a dose-dependent manner.

AstroRx Cells Alleviate LPS-Induced Pulmonary Inflammation and Fibrosis

Next, we tested the immune suppressive features of AstroRx in an *in vivo* model for ARDS. Intratracheal administration of LPS in the BALB/c mice induces severe lung damage and is a prevalent ARDS animal model (36). To test whether the AstroRx was capable of limiting the lung inflammation and lung damage, we injected i.v. two different doses of AstroRx after LPS-induction ($n = 10$, 2×10^5 and $n = 10$, 5×10^5 cells). Naïve ($n = 4$), untreated mice and sham-injected LPS-treated mice ($n = 10$) served as the negative and positive controls, respectively. The treatment with AstroRx at both cell concentrations increased the survival of LPS-induced mice compared with the sham-injected animals (20% loss vs. 10% loss, **Figure 2A**). To assess the degree of lung injury in the mice that survived, we performed the histological analysis of the lung sections 72 h after an LPS treatment (**Figure 2B**). The sham-injected mice showed significant thickened alveolar walls and cell infiltration, while treatment with AstroRx cells at a concentration of 5×10^5 cells alleviated the LPS-induced damage. An analysis of ALI was performed according to a method described by Matute-Bello et al. using a severity scoring scale of 0–2, based on the American Thoracic Society Documents (37) assessing the alveolar wall thickness, fibrin presence, and neutrophil accumulation which sums together to a total severity score (**Figure 2C**). The treatment with AstroRx cells significantly lowered the total severity score as compared with the sham-injected ARDS animals with 3.22 compared with 4.6 (**Figure 2C**, $P = 0.039$). According to lung score, the animals within one group were categorized into the responders (lung score ≤ 2) and non-responders (lung score >2). The percentage of responders was higher among the AstroRx-treated mice compared with the sham injected mice (**Figures 2D,E**), and higher among the mice that received a high dose of AstroRx compared with the mice that received a low number of AstroRx.

AstroRx Attenuates LPS-Induced Cytokine and Chemokine Storm in Bronchoalveolar Lavage Fluid and Serum

To understand the factors that contributed to the reduced lung damage following the AstroRx treatment, we analyzed the infiltration of B and T lymphocytes, eosinophils, neutrophils, and macrophages into the bronchoalveolar lavage fluid (BALF).

In the sham-injected ARDS mice, most of the cells in the BALF consisted of neutrophils (>92%), while the immune profile of high-dose of AstroRx shift toward naïve mice the immune profile (**Figure 3**, **Supplementary Figure 1**, $p = 0.0274$ for neutrophils and macrophages and $p = 0.0206$ for T cells). The effect of AstroRx on the immune cells became even clearer when we analyzed the immune profile differentially in the responder and non-responder mice (**Figure 4**, **Supplementary Figure 2**, $P = 0.0286$). The responder mice (lung score ≤ 2) among the AstroRx-treated LPS-injected mice had an immune profile that was similar to one of the naïve non-LPS-injected mice in terms of cell proportion and a general low-level of absolute cell number. While the non-responder mice displayed an immune profile that resembled the sham-injected mice with a general heavy infiltration of immune cells and a specifically massive invasion of neutrophils.

As the immune profile is not only determined by the cells but also by molecules, we next analyzed the presence of cytokines and chemokines in the BALF and serum. At first sight, the expression of inflammatory cytokines and chemokines was quite heterogeneous within the group of AstroRx-treated animals (**Figure 5**, $P = 0.13$ and higher). But when we dissected the group again into responders and non-responders, it became clear, that the responders among the AstroRx treated mice showed low expression of TNFa, IL1b, IL-6, IL-5, CC2, and CXCL1 (**Figure 6** naïve vs. sham: $P = 0.0121$ (for all cytokines); 500k responders vs. non-responders: $P = 0.0091$ (for TNFa), $P = 0.0286$ for all other cytokines). Strikingly, their levels were similar to the levels in naïve, healthy mice. At the same time, the non-responder mice displayed cytokine/chemokine levels in the range of sham-injected mice. The same phenomenon was observed in blood serum as well (**Supplementary Figures 3**, **4** naïve vs. sham: $P = 0.0121$ (for TNFa and CXCL1); 500k responders vs. non-responders $P = 0.0235$ [for TNFa and CXCL1)]. Altogether, our data showed that AstroRx had the capability to reduce the infiltration of immune cells to the lungs and to prevent the rising of a cytokine storm in the responder mice. It is reasonable to assume that this capability contributed to the better survival rate among the AstroRx-treated mice.

MATERIALS AND METHODS

AstroRx Derived From Clinical Grade Human Embryonic Stem Cells (AstroRx®)

The protocol for manufacturing the human astrocytes (AstroRx®) from the embryonic stem cells was performed according to the protocol detailed in Izrael et al. (34). In brief, hESC line HADC100 was used as starting material for the derivation of AstroRx cells. The hESCs were grown

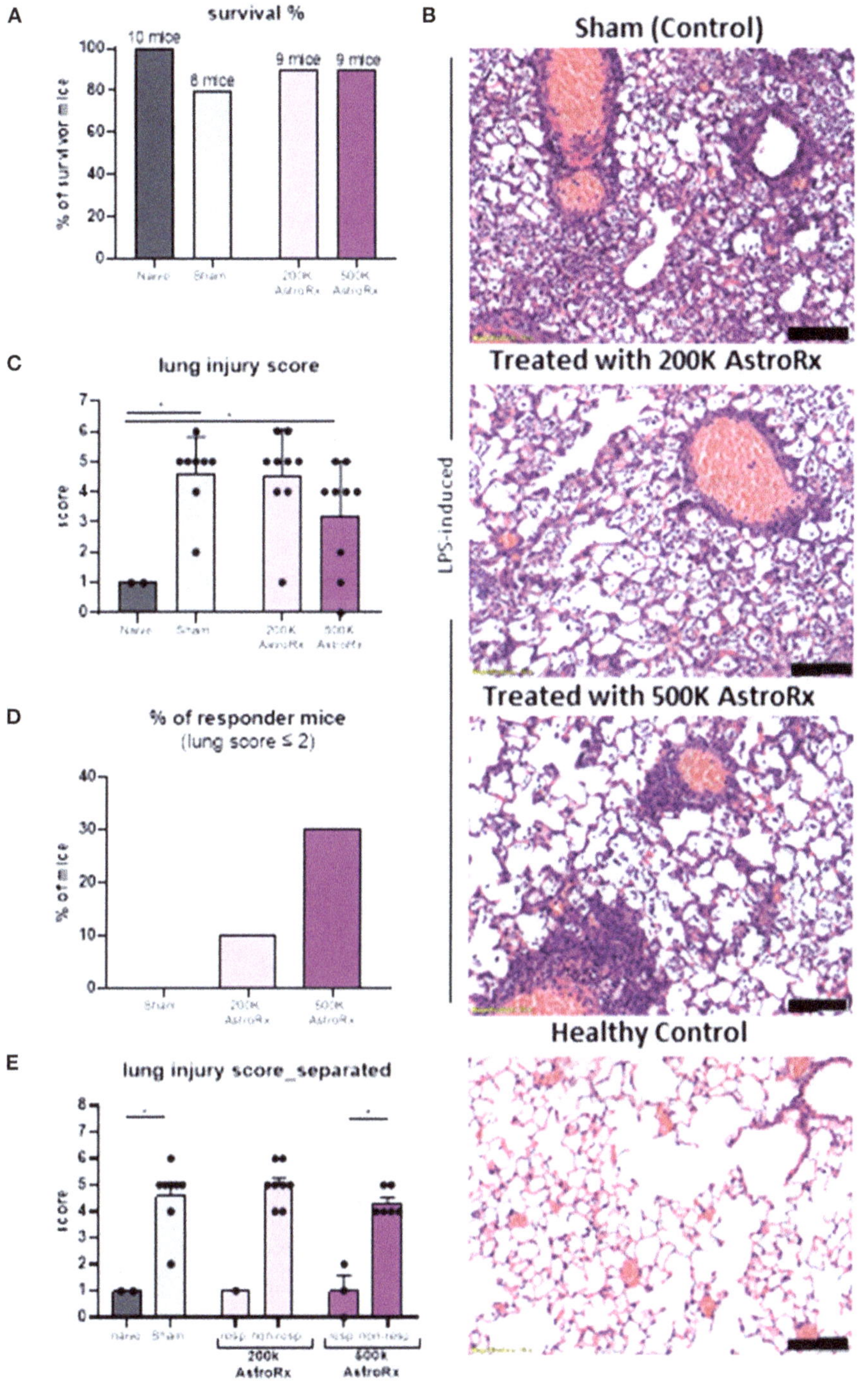

FIGURE 2 | The AstroRx cells alleviate lipopolysaccharide (LPS)-induced pulmonary inflammation and fibrosis. **(A)** The survival rate of animals treated with Plasmalyte (sham) and AstroRx cells (200K or 500K per animal). **(B)** H&E staining of lung sections from top to bottom: LPS-induced treated with vehicle (PlasmaLyte), LPS-induced treated with 200K AstroRx cells, LPS-induced treated with 500K AstroRx cells, or healthy controls (no-LPS). **(C)** An analysis for acute lung injury (ALI) was performed using a severity scoring scale of 0–2 (20 fields per animal were analyzed), based on the American Thoracic Society Documents, 2011 (37). **(D,E)** According to the lung score, the mice were categorized into responders (lung score ≤ 2) and non-responders (lung score >2), also considering the mice that had died from ARDS ($n = 10$), the results are expressed as mean ± SEM. Mann–Whitney comparison test. **(C,D)** Naïve vs. sham: $^{*}p = 0.0222$, **(C)** sham vs. 500k: $^{*}p = 0.0309$, **(E)** 500k responders vs. non-responders: $^{*}p = 0.0119$, $^{*}p < 0.05$. Scale bar: 100 μM.

in feeder free vitronectin coated flasks culture in essential 8^{TM} (E8) medium (Thermo Fischer Scientific, MA, USA). Once enough cells were grown, hESC were detached to generate neurospheres (NS) in suspension (3D) cultures. The harvested hESC colonies were transferred into the 100-mm ultralow attachment culture plates (Corning) containing

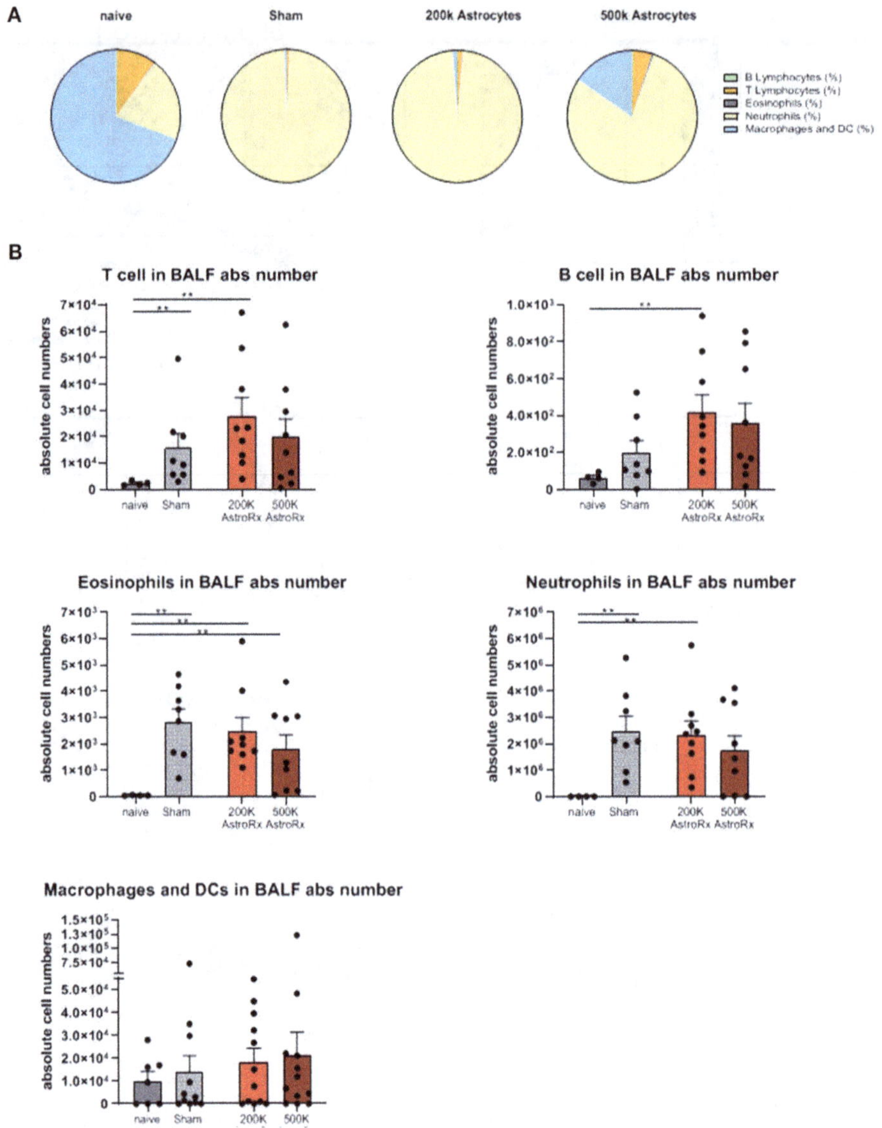

FIGURE 3 | Immune cells analyses of bronchoalveolar lavage. Bronchoalveolar lavage (BALF) was analyzed by flow cytometry for T cells, B cells, eosinophils, neutrophils, and macrophages/dendritic cells. **(A)** Proportions of each cell population by treatment. **(B)** An absolute number of each cell population in the BALF. The results are expressed as mean ± SEM. The Mann–Whitney comparison test. Naïve vs. sham: $^{**}p = 0.0081$, naïve vs. 200K astrocytes: $^{**}p = 0.0028$ (T cells, eosinophils, and neutrophils), $^{**}p = 0.0056$ (B cells), naïve vs. 500K astrocytes: $^{**}p = 0.0056$ (eosinophils), $^{**}p < 0.01$.

ITTSPP/B27 medium. The medium ITTSPP/B27 is a mixture of DMEM/F12 containing 1% B27 supplement, 1% glutamax, 1.5% HEPES at pH 7.4 (all from Thermo Fischer Scientific), 1% penicillin/streptomycin/amphotericin solution (Biological Industries, Israel), 25 µg/ml human insulin (ActRapid; Novo Nordisk, Denmark), 50 µg/ml human Apo-transferrin (Athens, GA, USA), 6.3 ng/ml progesterone, 10 µg/ml putrescine, 50 ng/ml sodium selenite, and 40 ng/ml triiodothyronine (T3) (all from Sigma, MO, USA). ITTSPP/B27 was supplemented with 20 ng/ml recombinant human epidermal growth factor (EGF) (R&D Systems, MN, USA). After 2 days, the medium was switched to ITTSPP/B27 supplemented with 20 ng/ml EGF and 10 µM all trans retinoic acid (Sigma, MO, USA). The culture was continued in suspension in the non-adherent plates for 7 days with daily replacement of the medium. During the last step, which allows for NS ripening, the culture was continued in ITTSPP/B27 medium supplemented with 20 ng/ml EGF for 18 days. The medium was replaced every other day. Then, round yellow NS were manually selected and transferred GMP-compliant laminin 521 (from Biolamina, Sweden) in ITTSPP/B27 supplemented with 20 ng/ml EGF. The medium was replaced every other day for 7–10 days (passage 0). To produce a monolayer of astrocyte progenitor cells (APC), the spheres were dissociated with TryplE (Thermo Fischer Scientific)

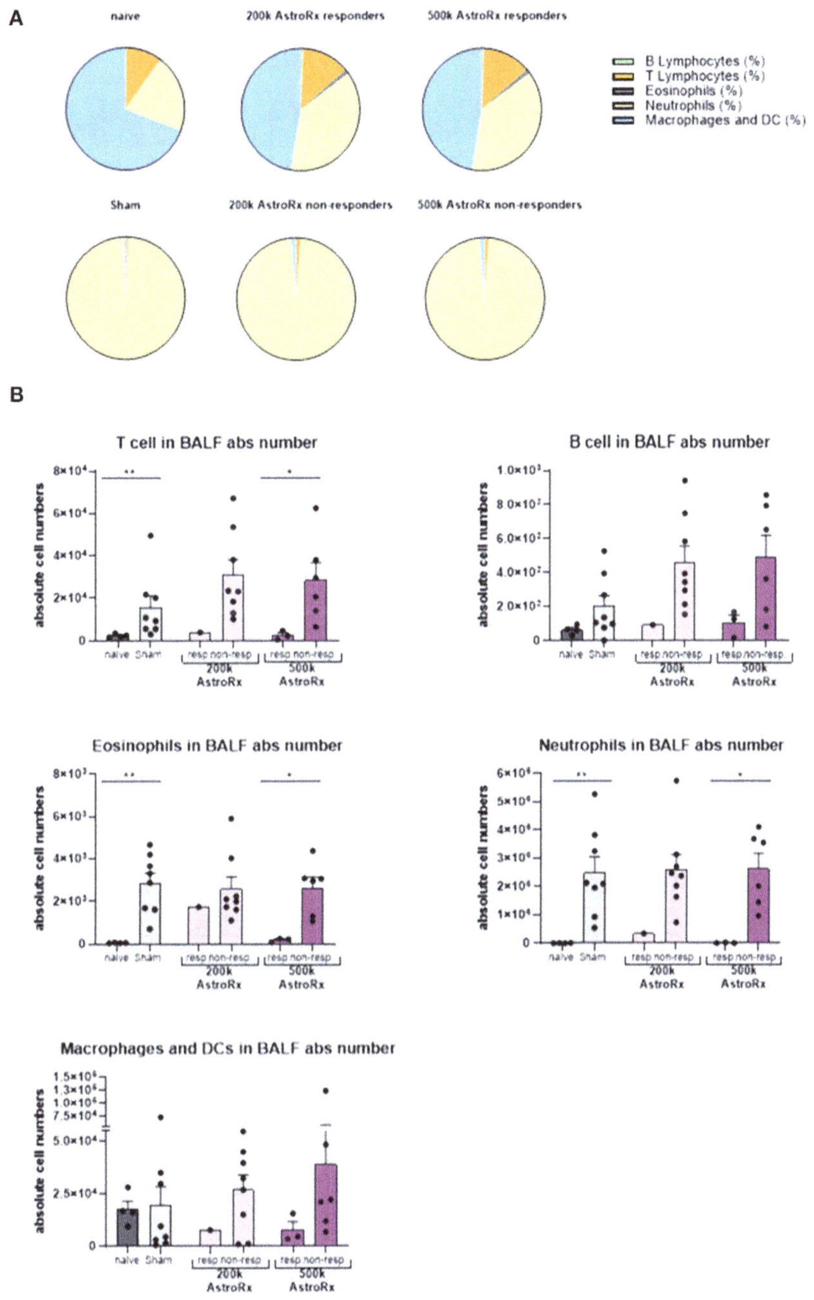

FIGURE 4 | Responder mice maintain immune homeostasis in the lungs after AstroRx treatment. Bronchoalveolar lavage was analyzed by flow cytometry for the immune cells. **(A)** The composition of cells in the BALF of responders and non-responders after AstroRx treatment. **(B)** An absolute number of immune cells in the BALF. The value of $n = 10$ mice for each experimental group (sham and both the groups of AstroRx treated mice) and $n = 4$ for naïve mice, the results are expressed as mean ± SEM. The Mann–Whitney comparison test. $^{*}p < 0.05$; $^{**}p < 0.01$; Naïve vs. sham: $^{**}p = 0.0081$ (T cells), $^{**}p = 0.0040$ (eosinophils and neutrophils), 500k responders vs. non-responders: $^{*}p = 0.0286$ (T cells, eosinophils, and neutrophils).

and reseeded on laminin coated flasks in N2/B27 medium consisting of DMEM/F12 with 0.5% (v/v) N_2 supplement, 1% (v/v) B27 supplement, 1% glutamax, and 1.5% HEPES (4-(2-hydroxyethyl)-1-piperazineethanesulfonic acid) at pH 7.4 (all from Thermo Fischer Scientific). The growth factors EGF and basic fibroblast growth factor (bFGF, R&D Systems) were added at 10 ng/ml each. The monolayer cells were further passaged weekly until enough cells were generated. The cells were then frozen in liquid nitrogen and stored as banks of APCs. Thawed APCs were further expanded and allowed to differentiate into the committed AstroRx cells by the removal of growth factors (EGF and bFGF), 50 µg/ml ascorbic acid (Sigma)

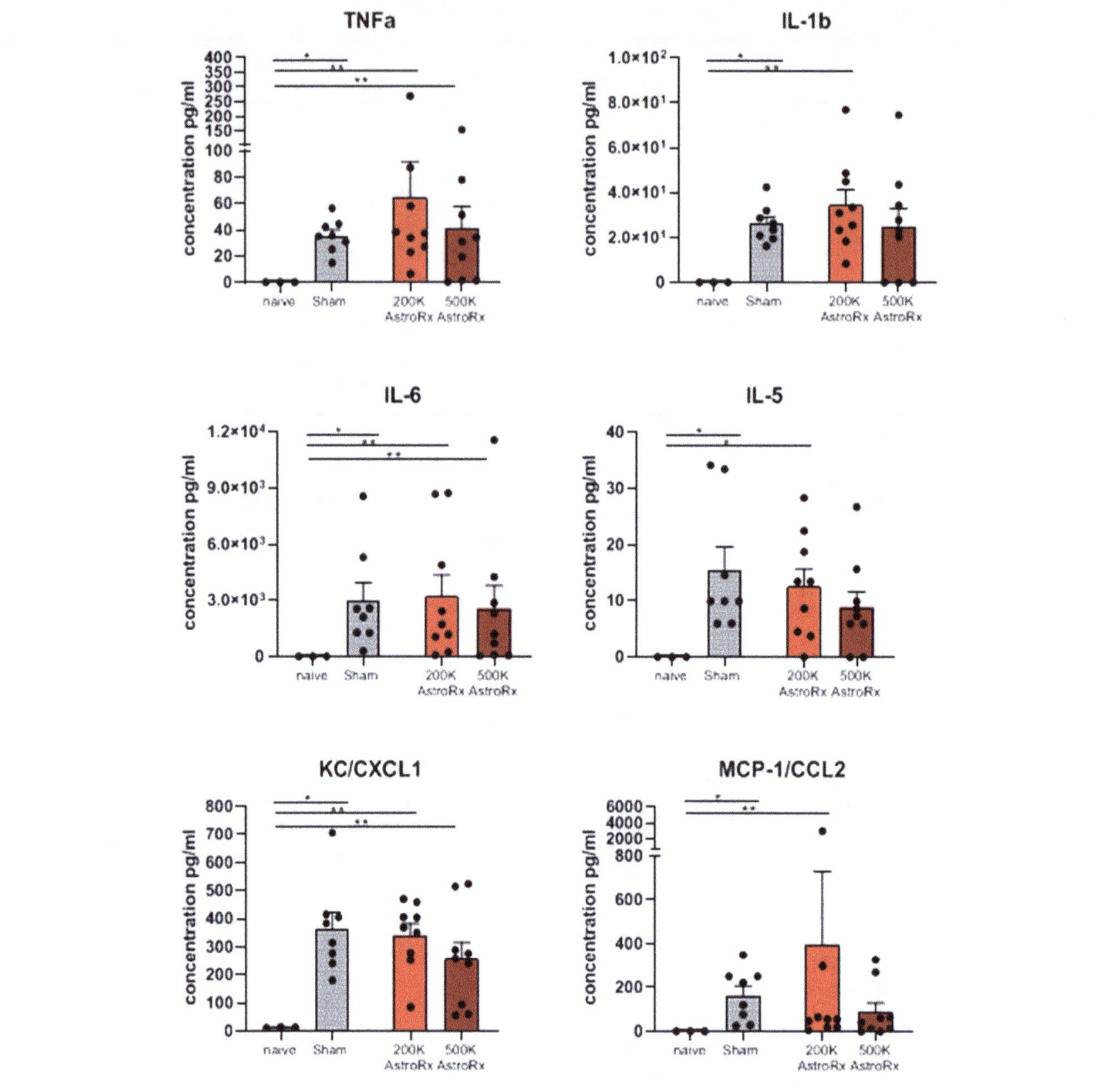

FIGURE 5 | Inflammatory cytokines/chemokines in lungs. The cytokines and chemokines in the BALF were quantified by ELISA (enzyme linked immunosorbent assay). The value of $n = 10$ mice for each experimental group (sham and both the groups of AstroRx treated mice) and $n = 4$ for naïve mice, the results are expressed as mean ± SEM. The Mann–Whitney comparison test. $^{*}p < 0.05$; $^{**}p < 0.01$; Naïve vs. sham: $^{*}p = 0.0121$, naïve vs. 200K or 500K astrocytes $p = 0.0091$ (TNFa, IL-6, CXCL1, and CCL2) and $^{*}p = 0.0318$ (IL-5).

was added, and the culture was continued for 7 days to yield AstroRx cells.

Animal Procedures

Female, 8 weeks old, BALB/C mice were obtained from Envigo (Israel) and maintained in SIA facility (Science in Action, Ness Ziona, Israel). Animal handling was performed according to the guidelines of the National Institute of Health (NIH) and the Association for Assessment and Accreditation of Laboratory Animal Care (AAALAC). The experiment was performed under the approval of "The Israel Board for Animal Experiments." A total of 30 BALB/C female mice were anesthetized using isoflurane and treated through intratracheal route of administration with LPS (IT, 800 μg of LPS—ChemCruz, The Netherlands, 055:B5) to induce ARDS, the animals were randomized to receive 200K, 500K AstroRx cells, or PlasmaLyte ($n = 10$ mice per experimental arm). Naive mice ($n = 4$, without LPS instillation) were used

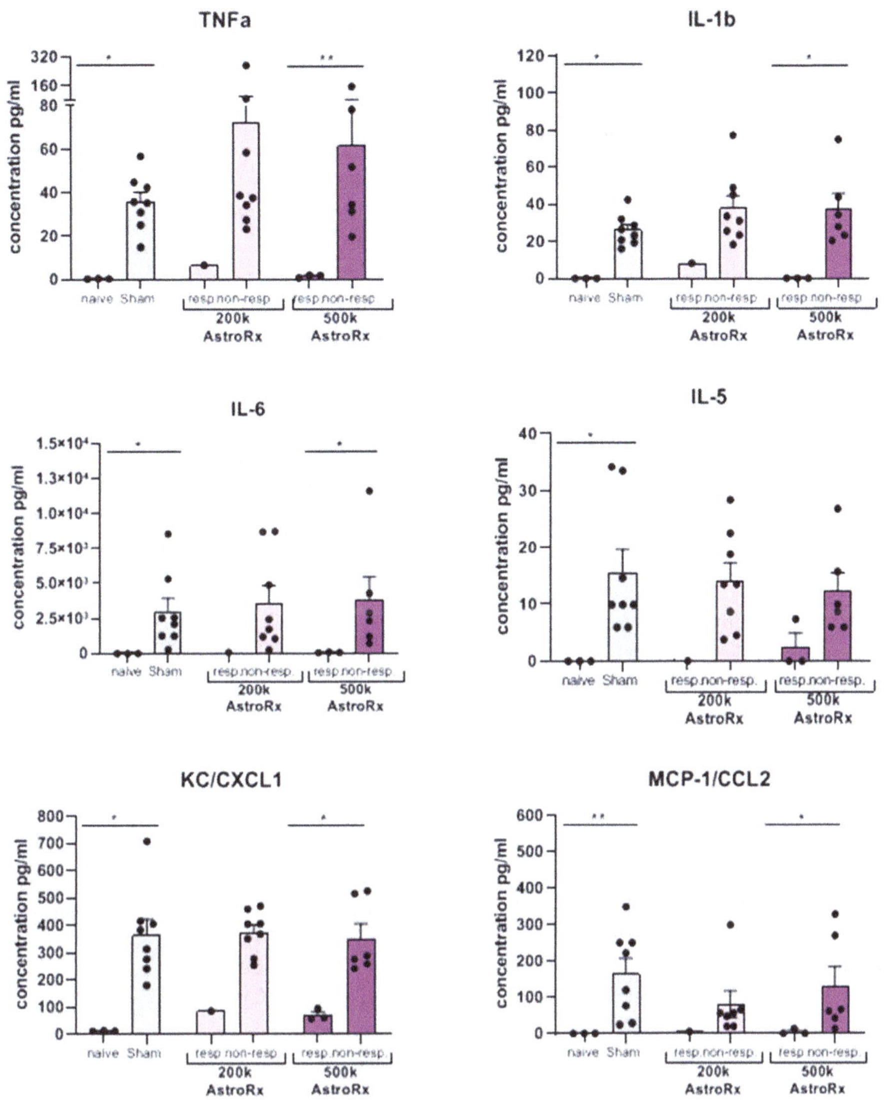

FIGURE 6 | Inflammatory cytokines/chemokines in the lungs are held in check in responder mice treated with AstroRx cells. The cytokines and chemokines in the BALF were quantified by ELISA. The value of $n = 10$ mice for each experimental group (sham and both the groups of AstroRx treated mice) and $n = 4$ for naïve mice, the results are expressed as mean ± SEM. The Mann–Whitney comparison test. $^{*}p < 0.05$; $^{**}p < 0.01$; naïve vs. sham: $^{*}p = 0.0121$ (for all cytokines/chemokines), 500K responders vs. non-responders: $^{**}p = 0.0091$ (TNFa), $^{*}p = 0.0286$ (IL-1b, IL-6, CXCL1, and CCL2).

as a control. Treated animals received i.v. injection of AstroRx cells or PlasmaLyte 6 h after LPS-induction. All the animals were sacrificed 72 h after the LPS instillation. The measurements of survival, body weight, hematology, lung histopathology, flow cytometry analysis of immune cells as well as cytokine and chemokines were collected from the BALF and serum. BALF was collected by intratracheal injection of 0.5 ml phosphate buffered saline (PBS) with 0.1 mM EDTA followed by a gentle aspiration three times. The recovered fluid was pooled and centrifuged. The BALF supernatant was preserved for the measurement of cytokines and chemokines. The sediment cells were resuspended and subjected to flow cytometry analysis.

Histology

Lungs were harvested and fixed in 4% formaldehyde. The tissues were then trimmed in a standard position and put in the embedding cassettes. One cassette per animal was prepared. The paraffin blocks were sectioned at ~ 4 μm thickness, put on the glass slides, and stained with H&E. Pictures were taken using an Olympus microscope (BX60, serial NO. 7D04032) at an objective magnification of × 4 and × 10 and microscope's Camera (Olympus DP73, serial NO. OH05504, Tokyo, Japan).

An analysis for ALI was performed according to the method described in Matute-Bello et al. using a severity scoring scale of 0–2, based on the American Thoracic Society Documents, 2011 (37). An analysis was performed by an independently certified veterinarian pathologist (Patho-logica Ltd., Ness Ziona, Israel) who was blinded to the experimental treatment.

Neutrophils

Not visible within the field—a score of 0; 1–5 neutrophils per field−1; more than 5 neutrophils per field−2.

Fibrin

Not visible within the field—a score of 0; a single well-formed band of fibrin within the airspace−1; multiple eosinophilic membranes−2.

Thickened Alveolar Walls

Due to technical artifacts, only septal thickening that is ≤two times the normal was considered. Less than ×2—score 0; ×2–×4—score 1; more than × 4—score 2.

The analysis was based on the measurements of 20 fields, using an objective magnification of ×4 and ×10 (high power fields, HPF).

Neutrophil cell count was performed using MATLAB color-based, brightness-based, and morphological-based segmentation. The cells were counted from a rectangle of 88,892 μm^2.

Cytokine and Chemokine Multiplex Measurements

The BALF cytokine concentrations were measured using the ProcartaPlex Luminex platform (Thermo Fischer Scientific, MA, USA). The measurements were performed two times (25 µl of each sample) with a custom multiplex panel detecting the following mouse cytokines: IFNγ, TNFα, RANTES, IL-6, IL-10, IL-1α, IL-1β, IP-10, MIP1α, and MCP-1/CCL2. The measurements were performed using the Luminex MAGPIX instrument, and results were analyzed with Xponent 4.2 software according to the instructions from the manufacturer.

Mixed lymphocyte Reaction Test

Three female C57/Bl6 mice at age of 6–8 weeks were euthanized by injection of a lethal dose of Pental (Pentobarbital Sodium). The lymph nodes were excised and drained to obtain lymph-node cells (LNCs). The LNCs from all the mice were pooled and then counted by a hemocytometer using trypan blue dye to exclude the dead cells. One million LNCs were seeded in RPMI-1640 medium (Biological Industries, 01-100-1A) supplemented with 2.5% fetal calf serum (Biological Industries, 04-121-1A), 1 mM L-glutamine (Biological Industries, 03-020-1C), and penicillin-streptomycin (Biological Industries, 03-031-1B). The LNC cultures under the multiple experimental conditions were maintained in flat-bottom plates, in duplicates, in a humidified atmosphere of 5% carbon dioxide at 37°C. The mNPCs were obtained using the method described in Fainstein and Ben-Hur (35) for isolation and growth of mNPCs. The mNPCs were kept in culture with the same media used to culture LNCs. The cells were harvested and analyzed for T-cell amount and proliferation by flow cytometry. Analysis of cells that expressed both Thyl.2 and CD25 determined the percentage of T cells in LNC culture, 24 h after activation with ConA.

BrdU T-cell Proliferation Assay

Co-expression of CD3/BrdU determined the percentage of proliferating T cells in co-cultures with LNC. The LNCs were kept in culture with and without 2.5 µg/ml ConA (Sigma, C5275) for 48 h. The percentage of T cells (Thy1.2$^+$/CD25$^+$) and proliferating T cells (CD3$^+$/BrdU$^+$) of the LNC cultures in the presence of ConA were set as baselines for the T-cell activation—without immunomodulation. The AstroRx® cells were added to LNC culture at ratios of 2:1, 5:1, and 10:1 LNC:AstroRx®, with and without 2.5 µg/ml ConA. Further, the LNCs in 0.5 ml RPMI-1640 were cultured with 0.5 ml conditioned medium with and without 2.5 µg/ml ConA. As a positive control, the mNPCs were added to the LNC culture at a ratio of 2:1 with and without 2.5 µg/ml ConA.

Flow Cytometry

The cells were analyzed by flow cytometry for identity and purity markers using the following antibodies: anti-GLAST (1:20; Miltenibiotec, Germany), anti-CD44 (1:20; BD Pharmingen, CA, USA), anti-CXCR4 (1:20; Biolegend, CA, USA), anti-TRA-1-60 (1:50; Biolegend), anti-EPCAM (1:50; Biolegend), anti-SSEA4 (1:50; Biolegend), anti-GFAP (1:2000; Sigma), anti-Nestin (1:500; BD Pharmingen), and anti-AQP-4 (1:2000; Abcam, UK). The Flow Cytometer FACS Canto II (BD, NJ, USA) was operated with FACSDIVA software (BD). At least 10,000 events were collected per sample. For immune cells identity, the following antibodies were used: FITC Rat Anti-Mouse I-A/I-E Clone 2G9 (RUO) (BD 553623), PerCP-Cy™5.5 Hamster Anti-Mouse CD3e (BD 551163), PerCP-Cy™5.5 Rat Anti-Mouse CD45R/B220 (552771), Mouse CCR3 PE-conjugated Antibody (R&D FAB729P), and APC-anti-mouse CD11 (Biolegend BLG-117310d).

Statistical Analyses

The statistical analyses were performed using GraphPad Prism 7 software (GraphPad Software, San Diego, CA, USA). The p-values were calculated by Mann–Whitney test. The values ≤0.05 were considered significant ($^* p < 0.05$; $^{**} p < 0.01$; and $^{***} p < 0.001$).

DISCUSSION

We are currently evaluating the curative role of AstroRx in patients with ALS. In a Phase I/IIa, open-label, dose-escalating clinical study, we studied the safety, tolerability, and therapeutic effects of AstroRx intrathecal transplantation.

Similarly to ARDS, the levels of circulating chemokines and cytokines in ALS are increased. The patients with a shorter diagnostic delay, which is a marker of more severe rapidly progressing disease (38) display higher levels of the inflammatory chemokine MCP-1/CCL-2. In addition, the increased levels of the inflammatory cytokines IL-17 and IL-6 were detected in the serum of the patients with ALS (39, 40). The increased levels of LPS in patients with ALS suggest systemic inflammation (41).

In preclinical studies, the AstroRx cells demonstrated a neuron-protective phenotype (A2 astrocytes) and secreted neurotrophic factors that were capable to uptake glutamate and regulate oxidative stress (34). Depending on their mode of activation (A1/A0/A2) (23, 25), astrocytes may possibly play an anti-inflammatory (A2) or pro-inflammatory (A1) role.

To test the immunomodulatory effect of AstroRx cells, we chose a rapid and acute inflammation model. LPS lung instillation is one of the most used models for ARDS. This model shares a number of pathological features with COVID-19-related ARDS, such as hypoxemia, neutrophil accumulation, alveolar space thickening, fibrin and tissue pathology, and high levels of inflammatory cytokines (2, 10, 13). The similarities between the LPS-treated rodents and the patients with COVID-19, in terms of lung damage and the inflammatory response, make LPS-induced ARDS a reliable model to evaluate potential COVID-19 therapies.

Administration of cells, mainly MSC has been performed by either local or systemic routes in the different experimental models (42). Local administration via intratracheal or intrathoracic infusion delivers the cells directly to the site of injury, whereas systemic administration *via* intravenous infusion allows wide distribution throughout the body. The cells administered intravenously would encounter the first-class pulmonary effect (43), which might result in the significant retention of cells in the lung, thereby providing advantages for lung tissue repair. The ongoing clinical trials and most experimental studies have used intravenous route for MSC administration (44, 45). Therefore, intravenous infusion of AstroRx cells was selected as a route of administration for testing ARDS.

In the current study, the levels of TNF-alpha, IL-b1, and IL-6 were strongly elevated in LPS-induced animals but could be maintained in steady state in the responder mice of AstroRx and LPS-treated group. The expression of CCL2, a monocyte recruiter, and CXCL1, a neutrophil recruiter, was also increased in the LPS-induced sham animals, and significantly reduced in the AstroRx responder mice. The expression level of IL-6, IL1b, TNFα, and CXCL1 determined if the lung remained in a homeostatic state or became inflamed. The upregulated levels of CXCL1 and TNF were also detected in the peripheral blood. Astrocytes calcium signaling is implicated in regulating inflammation (46–49). Similar to the pathology reported in ALS disease, the levels of pro-inflammatory cytokines, such as TGF-β1, IL-10, IFNγ, and IL-6 are elevated in LPS-induced ARDS animals. Exposure of astrocytes to inflammatory stimuli (e.g., TGF-β1 and IFNγ) demonstrated that inflammatory stimuli can significantly alter the astrocyte calcium signaling elicited by multiple G-protein-coupled receptors (GPCRs) (50). Alterations in the GPCR-evoked astrocyte Ca^{2+} transients may represent mechanisms by which astrocytes regulate inflammation (51) and should be further investigated.

Our current study demonstrated the immunosuppressive capacity of AstroRx cells in the context of lung inflammation and presents AstroRx as an innovative approach for treating ARDS especially in light of the rising unmet need for a treatment for COVID-19-related ARDS.

To make AstroRx cell therapy clinically applicable, further research is needed to elucidate several issues, such as the optimal number of AstroRx cell doses, the time window of AstroRx cell administration, administration routes, and frequency (single vs. multiple-dose regimen). Comprehensive safety investigation on the fate of AstroRx cells was done once the cells were injected intrathecally into the cerebrospinal fluid (34). The safety profile of AstroRx cells upon i.v. injection requires further investigation in the terms of cell survival, homing capacity to different tissues (e.g., lungs, liver, and kidney), cell identity, and reactive state (A1/A2) after cell transplantation.

AUTHOR CONTRIBUTIONS

MR, MI, AR, and JMW conceived and designed the studies. MI, JMW, SGS, TS, and KM performed the experiments, analyzed the data, and interpreted the data. MR, MI, and JMW wrote the manuscript. All authors read and approved the final manuscript.

SUPPLEMENTARY MATERIAL

Supplementary Figure 1 | The percentage analyses of immune cells in bronchoalveolar lavage. Bronchoalveolar lavage (BALF) of mice was analyzed by flow cytometry for lymphocytes and myeloid cells. The results are expressed as mean ± SEM. Mann–Whitney comparison test. $^*p < 0.05$; $^{**}p < 0.01$. Sham ($n = 10$) vs. 200k astrocytes treated mice ($n = 10$): $^*p = 0.0152$ (T cells), sham vs. 500k astrocytes treated mice ($n = 10$): $^*p = 0.0206$ (T cells), sham vs. 500k astrocytes treated mice: $^*p = 0.0274$ (neutrophils and eosinophils).

Supplementary Figure 2 | Immune cell distribution in the lungs resembles naïve, healthy mice. The BALF of mice was analyzed by flow cytometry for the percentage of lymphocytes and myeloid cells divided into responder and non-responders mice. The results are expressed as mean ± SEM. Mann–Whitney comparison test. $^*p < 0.05$; $^{**}p < 0.01$; Naïve vs. sham: $^{**}p = 0.0040$ (T cells, neutrophils, and macrophages), $^{**}p = 0.0028$ (B cells). 500k responders vs. non-responders: $^*p = 0.\ 0286$ (all cell types).

Supplementary Figure 3 | CXCL1 and TNFa levels in the peripheral blood of AstroRx-cell treated mice mirror the situation in the lungs. CXCL1 and TNFa levels in the blood serum were quantified by ELISA. $n = 10$ mice for each experimental group [sham and both groups of human astrocytes (AstroRx) treated mice] and $n = 4$ for naïve mice, results are expressed as mean ± SEM. Mann–Whitney comparison test. $^*p < 0.05$; $^{**}p < 0.01$; $^{***}p < 0.001$.

Supplementary Figure 4 | The CXCL1 and TNFa levels in the peripheral blood of AstroRx-cell treated mice mirror the situation in the lungs. The CXCL1 and TNFa levels divided by responder and non-responder mice in the blood serum were quantified by ELISA. The results are expressed as mean ± SEM. Mann–Whitney comparison test. $^*p < 0.05$.

REFERENCES

Sweeney MD, Zhao Z, Montagne A, Nelson AR, Zlokovic BV. Blood-Brain barrier: from physiology to disease and back. *Physiol Rev.* (2019) 99:21–78. doi: 10.1152/physrev.00050.2017

Lin SH, Zhao YS, Zhou DX, Zhou FC, Xu F. Coronavirus disease 2019 (COVID-19): cytokine storms, hyper-inflammatory phenotypes, and acute respiratory distress syndrome. *Genes Dis.* (2020) 7:520–7. doi: 10.1016/j.gendis.2020.06.009

Jiang F, Deng L, Zhang L, Cai Y, Cheung CW, Xia Z. Review of the clinical characteristics of Coronavirus disease 2019 (COVID-19). *J Gen Intern Med.* (2020) 35:1545–9. doi: 10.1007/s11606-020-05762-w

Zhou F, Yu T, Du R, Fan G, Liu Y, Liu Z, et al. Clinical course and risk factors for mortality of adult inpatients with COVID-19 in Wuhan, China: a retrospective cohort study. *Lancet.* (2020) 395:1054–62. doi: 10.1016/S0140-6736(20)30566-3

Carver C, Jones N. Cardiac injury, ARDS and COVID-19 meta-analysis validity - Correspondence in response to Santoso et al. *Am J Emerg Med.* (2020) 42:252. doi: 10.1016/j.ajem.2020.06.028

Lian J, Jin X, Hao S, Cai H, Zhang S, Zheng L, et al. Analysis of epidemiological and clinical features in older patients with Coronavirus disease 2019 (COVID- 19) outside Wuhan. *Clin Infect Dis.* (2020) 71:740–7. doi: 10.1093/cid/ ciaa242

Rocco PR, Dos Santos C, Pelosi P. Lung parenchyma remodeling in acute respiratory distress syndrome. *Minerva Anestesiol.* (2009) 75:730–40. doi: 10.1590/S0102-35862003000400013

Thille AW, Esteban A, Fernandez-Segoviano P, Rodriguez JM, Aramburu JA, Vargas-Errazuriz P, et al. Chronology of histological lesions in acute respiratory distress syndrome with diffuse alveolar damage: a prospective cohort study of clinical autopsies. *Lancet Respir Med.* (2013) 1:395–401. doi: 10.1016/S2213-2600(13)70053-5

Meduri GU, Eltorky MA. Understanding ARDS-associated fibroproliferation. *Intensive Care Med.* (2015) 41:517–20. doi: 10.1007/s00134-014-3613-0

Akbari H, Tabrizi R, Lankarani KB, Aria H, Vakili S, Asadian F, et al. The role of cytokine profile and lymphocyte subsets in the severity of coronavirus disease 2019 (COVID-19): a systematic review and meta-analysis. *Life Sci.* (2020) 258:118167. doi: 10.1016/j.lfs.2020.118167

Uckun FM. Reducing the fatality rate of COVID-19 by applying clinical insights from immuno-oncology and lung transplantation. *Front Pharmacol.* (2020) 11:796. doi: 10.3389/fphar.2020.00796

Kempuraj D, Selvakumar GP, Ahmed ME, Raikwar SP, Thangavel R, Khan A, et al. COVID-19, mast cells, cytokine storm, psychological stress, and neuroinflammation. *Neuroscientist.* (2020) 26:402–414. doi: 10.1177/1073858420941476

Pelaia C, Tinello C, Vatrella A, De Sarro G, Pelaia G. Lung under attack by COVID-19-induced cytokine storm: pathogenic mechanisms and therapeutic implications. *Ther Adv Respir Dis.* (2020) 14:1753466620933508. doi: 10.1177/1753466620933508

Chen H, Guo J, Wang C, Luo F, Yu X, Zhang W, et al. Clinical characteristics and intrauterine vertical transmission potential of COVID-19 infection in nine pregnant women: a retrospective review of medical records. *Lancet.* (2020) 395:809–15. doi: 10.1016/S0140-6736(20)30360-3

Kandel N, Chungong S, Omaar A, Xing J. Health security capacities in the context of COVID-19 outbreak: an analysis of international health regulations annual report data from 182 countries. *Lancet.* (2020) 395:1047– 53. doi: 10.1016/S0140-6736(20)30553-5

Ferrando C, Suarez-Sipmann F, Mellado-Artigas R, Hernandez M, Gea A, Arruti E, et al. Clinical features, ventilatory management, and outcome of ARDS caused by COVID-19 are similar to other causes of ARDS. *Intensive Care Med.* (2020) 46:2200–11. doi: 10.1007/s00134-020-06251-8

Lopes-Pacheco M, Robba C, Rocco PRM, Pelosi P. Current understanding of the therapeutic benefits of mesenchymal stem cells in acute respiratory distress syndrome. *Cell Biol Toxicol.* (2020) 36:83–102. doi: 10.1007/s10565-019-09493-5

Yen BL, Yen ML, Wang LT, Liu KJ, Sytwu HK. Current status of mesenchymal stem cell therapy for immune/inflammatory lung disorders: gleaning insights for possible use in COVID-19. *Stem Cells Transl Med.* (2020) 9:1163–73. doi: 10.1002/sctm.20-0186

Zhang H, Cui Y, Zhou Z, Ding Y, Nie H. Alveolar type 2 epithelial cells as potential therapeutics for acute lung injury/acute respiratory distress syndrome. *Curr Pharm Des.* (2019) 25:4877–82. doi: 10.2174/1381612825666191204092456

Zhou Y, Li P, Goodwin AJ, Cook JA, Halushka PV, Chang E, et al. Exosomes from endothelial progenitor cells improve outcomes of the lipopolysaccharide-induced acute lung injury. *Crit Care.* (2019) 23:44. doi: 10.1186/s13054-019-2339-3

Allen NJ. Astrocyte regulation of synaptic behavior. *Annu Rev Cell Dev Biol.* (2014) 30:439–63. doi: 10.1146/annurev-cellbio-100913-013053

Allen NJ, Eroglu C. Cell biology of astrocyte-synapse interactions. *Neuron.* (2017) 96:697–708. doi: 10.1016/j.neuron.2017.09.056

Izrael M, Slutsky SG, Revel M. Rising stars: astrocytes as a therapeutic target for ALS disease. *Front Neurosci.* (2020) 14:824. doi: 10.3389/fnins.2020.00824

Fasciani I, Pluta P, Gonzalez-Nieto D, Martinez-Montero P, Molano J, Paino CL, et al. Directional coupling of oligodendrocyte connexin-47 and astrocyte connexin-43 gap junctions. *Glia.* (2018) 66:2340–52. doi: 10.1002/glia.23471

Liddelow SA, Guttenplan KA, Clarke LE, Bennett FC, Bohlen CJ, Schirmer L, et al. Neurotoxic reactive astrocytes are induced by activated microglia. *Nature.* (2017) 541:481–7. doi: 10.1038/nature21029

Liddelow SA, Barres BA. Reactive astrocytes: production, function, therapeutic potential. *Immunity.* (2017) 46:957–67. doi: 10.1016/j.immuni.2017.06.006

Farina C, Aloisi F, Meinl E. Astrocytes are active players in cerebral innate immunity. *Trends Immunol.* (2007) 28:138–45. doi: 10.1016/j.it.2007.01.005

Pekny M, Pekna M, Messing A, Steinhauser C, Lee JM, Parpura V, et al. Astrocytes: a central element in neurological diseases. *Acta Neuropathol.* (2016) 131:323–45. doi: 10.1007/s00401-015-1513-1

Sofroniew MV. Astrogliosis. *Cold Spring Harb Perspect Biol.* (2014) 7:a020420. doi: 10.1101/cshperspect.a020420

Sofroniew MV. Multiple roles for astrocytes as effectors of cytokines and inflammatory mediators. *Neuroscientist.* (2014) 20:160–72. doi: 10.1177/1073858413504466

Owens T, Bechmann I, Engelhardt B. Perivascular spaces and the two steps to neuroinflammation. *J Neuropathol Exp Neurol.* (2008) 67:1113–21. doi: 10.1097/NEN.0b013e31818f9ca8

Wilson EH, Weninger W, Hunter CA. Trafficking of immune cells in the central nervous system. *J Clin Invest.* (2010) 120:1368–79. doi: 10.1172/JCI41911

Thonhoff JR, Simpson EP, Appel SH. Neuroinflammatory mechanisms in amyotrophic lateral sclerosis pathogenesis. *Curr Opin Neurol.* (2018) 31:635– 9. doi: 10.1097/WCO.0000000000000599

Izrael M, Slutsky SG, Admoni T, Cohen L, Granit A, Hasson A, et al. Safety and efficacy of human embryonic stem cell-derived astrocytes following intrathecal transplantation in SOD1(G93A) and NSG animal models. *Stem Cell Res Ther.* (2018) 9:152. doi: 10.1186/s13287-018-0890-5

Einstein O, Fainstein N, Vaknin I, Mizrachi-Kol R, Reihartz E, Grigoriadis N, et al. Neural precursors attenuate autoimmune encephalomyelitis by peripheral immunosuppression. *Ann Neurol.* (2007) 61:209–18. doi: 10.1002/ana.21033

Matute-Bello G, Frevert CW, Martin TR. Animal models of acute lung injury. *Am J Physiol Lung Cell Mol Physiol.* (2008) 295:L379–99. doi: 10.1152/ajplung.00010.2008

Matute-Bello G, Downey G, Moore BB, Groshong SD, Matthay MA, Slutsky AS, et al. An official American thoracic society workshop report: features and measurements of experimental acute lung injury in animals. *Am J Respir Cell Mol Biol.* (2011) 44:725–38. doi: 10.1165/rcmb.2009-0210ST

Kuhle J, Lindberg RL, Regeniter A, Mehling M, Steck AJ, Kappos L, et al. Increased levels of inflammatory chemokines in amyotrophic lateral sclerosis. *Eur J Neurol.* (2009) 16:771–4. doi: 10.1111/j.1468-1331.2009.02 560.x

Fiala M, Chattopadhay M, La Cava A, Tse E, Liu G, Lourenco E, et al. IL-17A is increased in the serum and in spinal cord CD8 and mast cells of ALS patients. *J Neuroinflamm.* (2010) 7:76. doi: 10.1186/1742-2094-7-76

Moreau C, Devos D, Brunaud-Danel V, Defebvre L, Perez T, Destee A, et al. Elevated IL-6 and TNF-alpha levels in patients with ALS: inflammation or hypoxia? *Neurology.* (2005) 65:1958–60. doi: 10.1212/01.wnl.0000188907.97339.76

Zhang R, Miller RG, Gascon R, Champion S, Katz J, Lancero M, et al. Circulating endotoxin and systemic immune activation in sporadic amyotrophic lateral sclerosis (sALS). *J Neuroimmunol.* (2009) 206:121–4. doi: 10.1016/j.jneuroim.2008.09.017

Han J, Liu Y, Liu H, Li Y. Genetically modified mesenchymal stem cell therapy for acute respiratory distress syndrome. *Stem Cell Res Ther.* (2019) 10:386. doi: 10.1186/s13287-019-1518-0

Fischer UM, Harting MT, Jimenez F, Monzon-Posadas WO, Xue H, Savitz SI, et al. Pulmonary passage is a major obstacle for intravenous stem cell delivery: the pulmonary first-pass effect. *Stem Cells Dev.* (2009) 18:683–92. doi: 10.1089/scd.2008.0253

Matthay MA, Calfee CS, Zhuo H, Thompson BT, Wilson JG, Levitt JE, et al. Treatment with allogeneic mesenchymal stromal cells for moderate to severe acute respiratory distress syndrome (START study): a randomised phase 2a safety trial. *Lancet Respir Med.* (2019) 7:154–62. doi: 10.1016/S2213-2600(18)30418-1

Wilson JG, Liu KD, Zhuo H, Caballero L, McMillan M, Fang X, et al. Mesenchymal stem (stromal) cells for treatment of ARDS: a phase 1 clinical trial. *Lancet Respir Med.* (2015) 3:24–32. doi: 10.1016/S2213-2600(14)7 0291-7

Tukhovskaya EA, Turovsky EA, Turovskaya MV, Levin SG, Murashev AN, Zinchenko VP, et al. Anti-inflammatory cytokine interleukin-10 increases resistance to brain ischemia through modulation of ischemia- induced intracellular Ca(2)(+) response. *Neurosci Lett.* (2014) 571:55–60. doi: 10.1016/j.neulet.2014.04.046

Duffy S, MacVicar BA. Adrenergic calcium signaling in astrocyte networks within the hippocampal slice. *J Neurosci.* (1995) 15:5535–50. doi: 10.1523/JNEUROSCI.15-08-05535.1995

Delbro D, Westerlund A, Bjorklund U, Hansson E. In inflammatory reactive astrocytes co-cultured with brain endothelial cells nicotine- evoked Ca(2+) transients are attenuated due to interleukin-1beta release and rearrangement of actin filaments. *Neuroscience.* (2009) 159:770–9. doi: 10.1016/j.neuroscience.2009.01.005

Thrane AS, Rappold PM, Fujita T, Torres A, Bekar LK, Takano T, et al. Critical role of aquaporin-4 (AQP4) in astrocytic Ca2+ signaling events elicited by cerebral edema. *Proc Natl Acad Sci USA.* (2011) 108:846–51. doi: 10.1073/pnas.1015217108

Hamby ME, Coppola G, Ao Y, Geschwind DH, Khakh BS, Sofroniew MV. Inflammatory mediators alter the astrocyte transcriptome and calcium signaling elicited by multiple G-protein-coupled receptors. *J Neurosci.* (2012) 32:14489–510. doi: 10.1523/JNEUROSCI.1256-12.2012

Ortinski PI, Dong J, Mungenast A, Yue C, Takano H, Watson DJ, et al. Selective induction of astrocytic gliosis generates deficits in neuronal inhibition. *Nat Neurosci.* (2010) 13:584–91. doi: 10.1038/nn.2535

9

Mechanical Ventilation in Pediatric and Neonatal Patients

Michaela Kollisch-Singule[1], Harry Ramcharran[1], Joshua Satalin[1], Sarah Blair[1], Louis A. Gatto[1], Penny L. Andrews[2], Nader M. Habashi[2], Gary F. Nieman[1] and Adel Bougatef[3]*

[1] Department of Surgery, SUNY Upstate Medical University, Syracuse, NY, United States, [2] Department of Trauma Critical Care Medicine, R Adams Cowley Shock Trauma Center, University of Maryland School of Medicine, Baltimore, MD, United States, [3] Independent Researcher, San Antonio, TX, United States

***Correspondence:**
Joshua Satalin
SatalinJ@upstate.edu

Pediatric acute respiratory distress syndrome (PARDS) remains a significant cause of morbidity and mortality, with mortality rates as high as 50% in children with severe PARDS. Despite this, pediatric lung injury and mechanical ventilation has been poorly studied, with the majority of investigations being observational or retrospective and with only a few randomized controlled trials to guide intensivists. The most recent and universally accepted guidelines for pediatric lung injury are based on consensus opinion rather than objective data. Therefore, most neonatal and pediatric mechanical ventilation practices have been arbitrarily adapted from adult protocols, neglecting the differences in lung pathophysiology, response to injury, and co-morbidities among the three groups. Low tidal volume ventilation has been generally accepted for pediatric patients, even in the absence of supporting evidence. No target tidal volume range has consistently been associated with outcomes, and compliance with delivering specific tidal volume ranges has been poor. Similarly, optimal PEEP has not been well-studied, with a general acceptance of higher levels of F_iO_2 and less aggressive PEEP titration as compared with adults. Other modes of ventilation including airway pressure release ventilation and high frequency ventilation have not been studied in a systematic fashion and there is too little evidence to recommend supporting or refraining from their use. There have been no consistent outcomes among studies in determining optimal modes or methods of setting them. In this review, the studies performed to date on mechanical ventilation strategies in neonatal and pediatric populations will be analyzed. There may not be a single optimal mechanical ventilation approach, where the best method may simply be one that allows for a personalized approach with settings adapted to the individual patient and disease pathophysiology. The challenges and barriers to conducting well-powered and robust multi-institutional studies will also be addressed, as well as reconsidering outcome measures and study design.

Keywords: PARDS, lung injury, neonatal and pediatric mechanical ventilation, high frequency percussive oscillation, high frequency oscillatory ventilation, airway pressure release ventilation

INTRODUCTION

Pediatric acute respiratory distress syndrome (PARDS) remains a significant cause of morbidity and mortality, with mortality rates as high as 50% in children with severe PARDS (Schouten et al., 2016). Despite this, pediatric lung injury and mechanical ventilation has been poorly studied, with the majority of investigations being observational or retrospective and with only a few randomized controlled trials (RCTs) (Kneyber et al., 2017). The most recent and universally accepted guidelines for pediatric lung injury are based on consensus opinion rather than objective data (Pediatric Acute Lung Injury Consensus Conference Group, 2015). Therefore, most neonatal and pediatric mechanical ventilation practices have been arbitrarily adapted from adult protocols, neglecting the differences in lung pathophysiology, response to injury, and co-morbidities among the groups.

Neonates, in particular, have a complex set of diseases that require mechanical ventilation but have no adult mimic, such as prematurity, congenital diaphragmatic hernia, meconium aspiration syndrome, persistent pulmonary hypertension, and congenital heart disease (Langham et al., 2003). As a reflection of this unique lung pathophysiology, there are a greater number of pulmonary-related ECMO runs in neonates as compared with adults and pediatric patients (Ecmo, 2021). Babies can be born as early as in the canalicular stages of lung development, where the bronchioles are still not fully developed (Iliodromiti et al., 2013). Applying adult ventilation strategies to neonatal lungs that have yet to form alveoli or cells to produce surfactant is erroneous. Even in children, more similar to adults in terms of their lung disease and co-morbidities, the process of alveolarization is thought to continue even up to 8 years of age (Weibel and Gomez, 1962) and possibly even through adolescence (Narayanan et al., 2012). Additionally, the chest walls of infants are more compliant than the chest walls of adults, with stiffening occurring through the first 2 years of age, at which time the lung and chest wall compliance are nearly equal, as they are in adults (Papastamelos et al., 1995). Thus the pleural pressure and response to mechanical ventilation would be expected to be different in infants (Gattinoni et al., 1998; Kollisch-Singule et al., 2015).

One of the challenges to investigating mechanical ventilation in the pediatric population is that mortality is frequently used as a therapeutic endpoint, but the majority of deaths in pediatric patients on mechanical ventilation are due to neurologic causes rather than refractory hypoxemia (Dowell et al., 2018). Up to 44% of children with no previous respiratory co-morbidities have long-term outcomes of pulmonary dysfunction after a pediatric intensive care unit (ICU) stay for acute respiratory failure including persistent need for adjunct therapies such as oxygen supplementation, bronchodilators, and corticosteroids, or persistent asthma or recurrent pneumonia (Keim et al., 2020). These secondary markers of lung injury may therefore make for a useful alternative marker mortality (Keim et al., 2018).

Further challenges associated with pediatric mechanical ventilation trials includes the lower incidence and mortality as compared with adult patients, shorter duration of mechanical ventilation, and diverse population with an estimated need for 60 participating centers to achieve an adequately powered study (Santschi et al., 2010). This has resulted in a lower number of and less recruited RCTs in children with one of the largest recruited studies having only 153 children (Willson et al., 2005).

Mechanical ventilation modes are grouped similarly as in adults: "conventional" ventilation (CV, including both volume- and pressure- regulated modes), airway pressure release ventilation (APRV), and high frequency ventilation (HFV) which can be subdivided into high frequency oscillatory ventilation (HFOV), high frequency jet ventilation (HFJV), and high frequency percussive ventilation (HFPV). CV is the most commonly used ventilation mode in pediatric patients (Pediatric Acute Lung Injury Consensus Conference Group, 2015; Koopman et al., 2019), with the remaining modes often being used as a rescue for refractory hypoxemia. This is in part because many of the non-CV modes (APRV, HFOV, and HFJV) are able to achieve a higher mean airway pressure without increasing peak airway pressures, and all have unique methods of achieving ventilation. There are few well-powered, recent RCTs in both conventional and non-conventional modes: HFOV (Arnold et al., 1994; Samransamruajkit et al., 2016; Snoek et al., 2016), HFJV (Carlo et al., 1990; Keszler et al., 1991; Keszler, 1997), and APRV (Lalgudi Ganesan et al., 2018). Studies that evaluate non-CV as a rescue mode may be providing an unfair evaluation, as many patients have often been on conventional mechanical ventilation for more than 24 h and have refractory hypoxemia. These studies must therefore be interpreted with caution as they are not necessarily comparing one mode vs. another but whether a non-CV mode can rescue a patient from CV. Although matched cohorts and regression can reduce this bias, they may not fully account for it. There can be no recommendations made for a "best mechanical ventilation" strategy, but it is important to understand the benefits and limitations of the ventilation modes available for clinical use. Thus, the focus of this review is to analyze the studies performed to date on mechanical ventilation strategies in neonatal and pediatric populations.

DEFINING LUNG INJURY

Because of the challenges with conducting well-powered pediatric mechanical ventilation trials, the Pediatric Acute Lung Injury Consensus Conference (PALICC) was held over 2 years with 27 experts voting on 151 recommendations in nine different topics varying from definition of lung injury to treatment and adjunctive therapies (Pediatric Acute Lung Injury Consensus Conference Group, 2015). Although the central premise of developing consensus guidelines is laudable, one must be cautious when using these consensus guidelines and applying them to the individual patient. Of the experts, 22 (81%) were located in the United States and Canada with the remaining five from Spain, Netherlands, England, Switzerland, and Australia, with certain experts hailing from the same institution, suggesting some degree of in-group bias (Pediatric Acute Lung Injury Consensus Conference Group, 2015).

Diagnosing PARDS according to standard criteria (Force et al., 2012) with strict reliance on the P_aO_2/F_iO_2 ratio or oxygenation index (OI) is more challenging as children are less likely to have routine arterial blood gases performed. In order to study and compare outcomes in pediatric and neonatal patients, the PALIC Conference determined a definition for PARDS using non-invasive oxygenation criteria. They proposed using an S_pO_2/F_iO_2 ratio or oxygen saturation index (OSI) when P_aO_2 ratio is not available (Pediatric Acute Lung Injury Consensus Conference Group, 2015), as these have been validated in pediatrics (Khemani et al., 2009b). Broadening this inclusion criteria may also help capture children who would otherwise have been excluded due to lack of invasive oxygenation criteria from blood gases (Santschi et al., 2010), also leading to an under-recognition of lung injury (Khemani and Newth, 2010). Embracing non-invasive oxygenation criteria can increase patient eligibility by an estimated 25% (Khemani et al., 2009b). Using this more inclusive definition, the follow-up observational PARDIE study revealed that the PALICC definition of severe PARDS was associated with higher mortality (32.7%) but mortality rates were similar between mild (12.4%) and moderate (10.3%) PARDS (Khemani et al., 2019).

In a meta-analysis of observational and randomized controlled trials investigating PARDS, the overall pooled mortality was determined to be 24% with a marked reduction in mortality over two decades from 40% mortality to an 18% mortality (**Figure 1**; Wong et al., 2019). This improvement in survival is likely due to an increased recognition of milder forms of PARDS, improvement in mechanical ventilators and strategies, and also suggests that children overall fare better than adults, likely due to a decrease in co-morbidities. It is important to consider the results of this meta-analysis (Wong et al., 2019) when comparing studies because trials spanning several years may not accurately reflect differences between ventilator modes but rather with patient inclusion, and advancement in ventilator practices and adjunctive therapies.

CONVENTIONAL MECHANICAL VENTILATION

Conventional ventilation is generally the application of a tidal volume or set inspiratory pressure to a baseline positive-end expiratory pressure (PEEP) with an inspiratory time set shorter than the expiratory time (**Figure 2A**). The majority of pediatric patients (75.2%) are placed on CV with 26.6% of those patients ventilated with a volume control mode and the remainder ventilated with a pressure control or regulated mode (Santschi et al., 2010). There is marked variability in the management of pediatric patients placed on conventional ventilation (Santschi et al., 2010), suggesting the term "conventional" may be a misnomer as there is not yet a convention in terms of mode (pressure- vs. volume-), tidal volume, or PEEP strategy.

Low tidal volume ventilation has become standard-of-care after the ARDSnet trial in adults demonstrated that 6 mL/kg significantly reduced mortality as compared with 12 mL/kg (ARDSnet, 2000). For lack of a similar comparison trial, low tidal volume ventilation has been mostly adopted into the mechanical ventilation strategy of pediatric patients (Pediatric Acute Lung Injury Consensus Conference Group, 2015; Koopman et al., 2019). In neonates, there are similarly no trials supporting one tidal volume goal over another, but tidal volume targets of 5–6 mL/kg are generally well-accepted (Keszler et al., 2009; Patel et al., 2009).

Although translating the practice of low tidal volume ventilation to pediatric patients has been advocated (Hanson and Flori, 2006; Dellinger et al., 2008), and is generally the standard to which other ventilator modes are compared, there are no large well-powered studies on it (Santschi et al., 2010; Koopman et al., 2019). One observational study demonstrated that higher tidal volumes were affiliated with decreased mortality (Erickson et al., 2007) and neonates were less susceptible to lung injury and inflammation with supraphysiologic tidal volumes (Copland et al., 2004; Kornecki et al., 2005; Smith et al., 2010). In a meta-analysis of eight randomized clinical trials and observational studies, there was no association between tidal volumes (7, 8, 10, 12 mL/kg) and mortality both in patients with and without ARDS (de Jager et al., 2014).

Tidal volumes in children tend to average around 8 mL/kg [8.0 mL/kg (Erickson et al., 2007), 8.1 mL/kg (Albuali et al., 2007), and 8.3 mL/kg (Santschi et al., 2010) but with marked variability (with a range from < 4 to > 15 mL/kg], highlighting the absence of a consensus (Santschi et al., 2010). Even PEEP guidelines have not been standardized (Villar, 2005) with more than half of pediatric patients being placed on PEEP < 5 cm H_2O with a range of 0–15 cm H_2O (Santschi et al., 2010). Pediatric intensivists are also more likely to adopt a low PEEP-high F_iO_2 strategy as compared with adults (Khemani et al., 2009a; Koopman et al., 2019). This is particularly relevant because exposure to high F_iO_2 concentrations leads to increased alveolar surface tension, in part due to increased surfactant frangibility (Smallwood, 2017). In addition to an unintended consequence of decreased pulmonary compliance and potential exacerbation of an underlying lung injury, higher F_iO_2 concentrations have been associated with bronchopulmonary dysplasia and longer supplemental oxygen requirements in neonates (No Authors List, 2000; Askie et al., 2003). Caution is deserved when comparing another ventilator mode with "conventional" ventilation since the comparisons will be between one (and possibly two) modes that do not have standardized methods of setting ventilator parameters and a wide variability in practice.

AIRWAY PRESSURE RELEASE VENTILATION

Airway Pressure Release Ventilation (APRV) is a pressure-regulated, time-dependent mode where the upper pressure (P_{High}) is sustained for a prolonged time (T_{High}), creating a continuous positive airway pressure (CPAP) phase to allow for alveolar stabilization and recruitment. The CPAP Phase is interrupted with a lower pressure (P_{Low}) for a brief [millisecond] period of time (T_{Low}) creating a Release Phase to allow for ventilation (**Figure 2B**; Habashi, 2005). A primary advantage to APRV is that it can achieve higher mean airway pressure, promoting recruitment and oxygenation, while limiting peak inspiratory pressures (Anderson and Speicher, 2006). It also

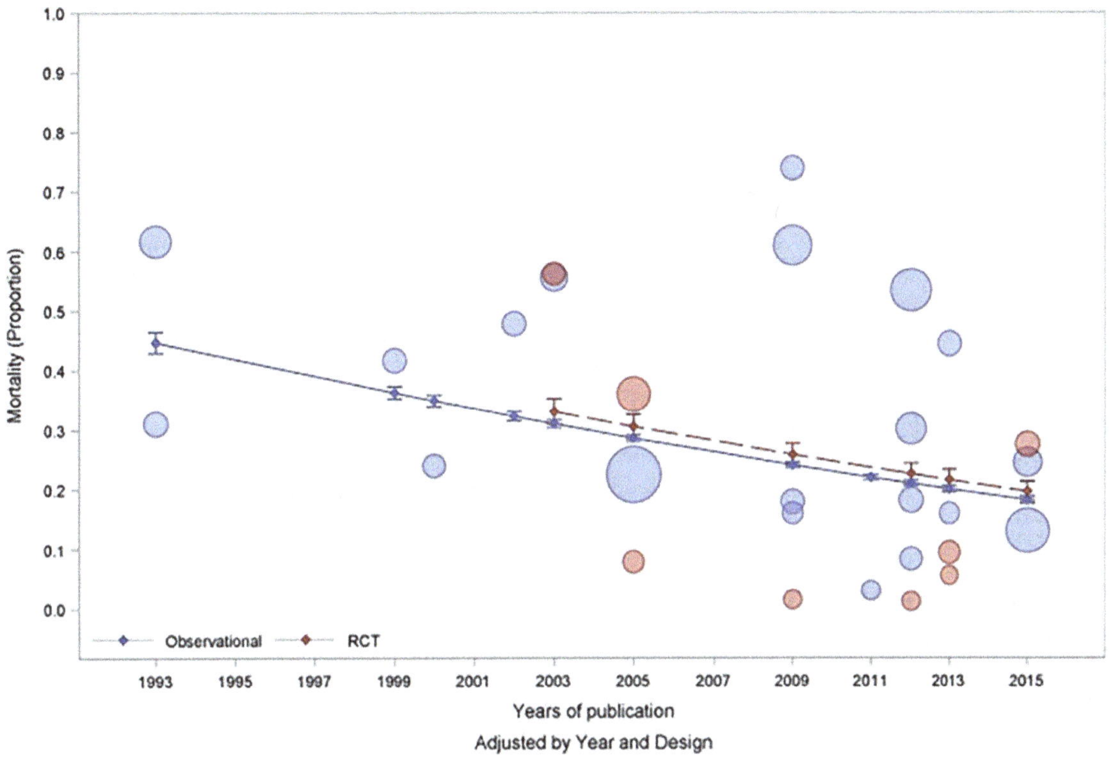

FIGURE 1 | Published with permission from Wong et al. (2019) Bubble plot demonstrating mortality rates associated with pediatric acute respiratory distress syndrome by year of study and study design (observational—blue and RCT—red). The size of the bubbles are proportional to the total number of patients recruited into the individual study.

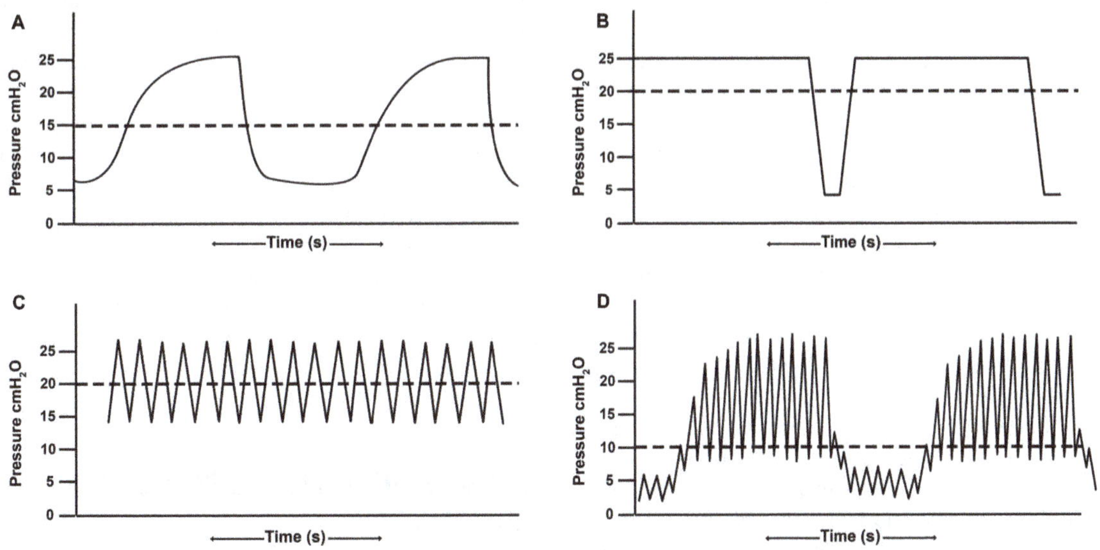

FIGURE 2 | Demonstrative waveforms of **(A)** conventional ventilation **(B)** airway pressure release ventilation, **(C)** high frequency oscillatory ventilation, and **(D)** high-frequency percussive ventilation. Airway pressure release ventilation and high frequency oscillatory ventilation maintain alveolar recruitment by achieving a higher mean airway pressure (horizontal dashed line) as compared with conventional ventilation without raising peak inspiratory pressures.

allows for spontaneous breathing (Krishnan and Morrison, 2007), thereby increasing patient comfort and limiting need for neuromuscular blockade (Frawley and Habashi, 2004; Krishnan and Morrison, 2007). Spontaneous breathing additionally allows for distribution of gas to the dependent regions of the lung, promoting further alveolar recruitment

(Habashi, 2005). Although there is a wide variability in APRV settings, as with any mode (Jain et al., 2016), the most frequently cited is the Time-Controlled Adaptive Ventilation ($TCAV^{TM}$) method which precisely sets the time at expiration (T_{Low}) based on the expiratory flow curve to optimize ventilation while limiting alveolar derecruitment (Frawley and Habashi, 2004; Habashi, 2005; Jain et al., 2016; Nieman et al., 2020).

Although APRV has been an available ventilator mode since 1987 (Stock et al., 1987), it is not widely used in pediatric or neonatal populations (Krishnan and Morrison, 2007). APRV is largely considered a rescue ventilator mode (Gupta et al., 2013) and the incidence of use in pediatric patients in the literature is just 1.6% as compared with 11.3% in adults (Gupta et al., 2013). This lack of clinical experience suggests that patient management can be quite variable from one intensivist to another (Anderson and Speicher, 2006). The sparse APRV studies must therefore be interpreted with caution with close attention to the method by which the mode was set.

PEDIATRIC AIRWAY PRESSURE RELEASE VENTILATION

In pediatric patients, APRV is set similar to adult patients with a P_{High} set at the plateau pressure achieved in the CV mode or at the mean airway pressure on HFOV plus 2–4 cm H_2O (Habashi, 2005). Pediatric patients naturally have a higher respiratory rate and minute ventilation as compared with adults and therefore the T_{High} is often set shorter. As compared with adults with healthy lungs (where the T_{High} is set at 4–6 s), pediatric patients with healthy lungs will have the T_{High} set at 3–5 s. In pediatric patients with injured, derecruited lungs, the T_{High} may be set at a shorter duration of 1–3 s to allow for bulk ventilation. Generally, the longest possible T_{High} is selected that maintains adequate CO_2 clearance (Frawley and Habashi, 2004; Habashi, 2005). The T_{Low} is adjusted as in adults to terminate the expiratory flow at 75% of the peak expiratory flow (Habashi, 2005).

In a prospective, randomized, crossover clinical trial of 15 pediatric patients with mild to moderate lung disease, APRV was found to have similar oxygenation, ventilation, hemodynamics, and patient comfort as compared with SIMV but with a lower peak inspiratory and plateau pressures. The shortcoming of this study was the absence of reported ventilator settings for either group (Schultz et al., 2001). One of the cited concerns for APRV is whether there are hemodynamic consequences given the higher mean airway pressure. In a small case series of pediatric patients, transition to APRV was associated with no alteration of hemodynamics and no need for neuromuscular blockade, while improving oxygenation (Krishnan and Morrison, 2007). Similarly, in patients with refractory hypoxemia transitioned from CV, APRV reduced neuromuscular blockade requirements as compared with HFOV, however, the HFOV group was represented by a younger cohort with a higher OI (Yehya et al., 2014a).

The only published RCT applying APRV to pediatric patients was performed by Lalgudi Ganesan et al. (2018) This was a single-center study conducted over a 2.5-year period but was terminated after 50% enrollment (52 children) due to higher mortality in the APRV arm. This study must be interpreted thoughtfully because it does not necessarily suggest that the APRV mode is harmful but rather that the method of setting it may have been. The authors adjusted the P_{High} to maintain a release tidal volume of 6–7 mL/kg ideal body weight (Lalgudi Ganesan et al., 2018). In doing so, the patients were placed on an open lung technique designed to recruit the lung and number of alveoli available to accommodate a larger tidal volume, but restricted the tidal volumes (Frawley and Habashi, 2004). By comparison, the $TCAV^{TM}$ method does not restrict tidal volumes as the lung opens. Rather, larger tidal volumes are viewed as evidence of increasing lung recruitment and improved compliance (Kollisch-Singule et al., 2014).

NEONATAL AIRWAY PRESSURE RELEASE VENTILATION

In neonatal patients transitioning to APRV, the P_{High} is similarly set at the plateau pressure achieved in the CV mode or at the mean airway pressure on HFOV plus 0–2 cm H_2O. Neonates have a further decrease in their set T_{High} to 1–2 s with the T_{Low} adjusted to terminate the expiratory flow at 75% of the peak expiratory flow (Habashi, 2005). No large studies of APRV have been performed in neonates to date. Gupta et al. (2013) reported a case series of 5 infants ranging in gestational age from 24 to 28 weeks and found that the infants tolerated APRV well with no adverse events.

In a neonatal lamb model with oleic acid induced lung injury, APRV demonstrated improved oxygenation and ventilation as compared with CPAP. APRV and CV had similar ventilation and oxygenation but APRV achieved this with a lower peak airway pressure and with no hemodynamic instability (Martin et al., 1991). In a 24-h model of respiratory distress syndrome, piglets were birthed at the equivalent of a 28-week human gestation. APRV set and adjusted by the $TCAV^{TM}$ method led to increased lung recruitment, improved ventilation, and decreased oxygen requirements without altering hemodynamics (Arrindell et al., 2015). In a subsequent 48-h porcine model of respiratory distress syndrome where piglets were birthed at the equivalent of a 25-week human gestation, APRV set according to the $TCAV^{TM}$ method led to a significant increase in lung compliance with a trend toward improved oxygenation with lower oxygen requirements (Kollisch-Singule et al., 2017).

HIGH-FREQUENCY OSCILLATORY VENTILATION

High frequency oscillatory ventilation operates using a push-pull application of pressure to the airway opening by either piston/diaphragm or microprocessor gas controllers. Fresh gas is supplied within the ventilator circuit as a bias flow, and mean airway pressure is adjusted according to the relationship between fresh gas inflow and any positive or negative pressure placed on the gas outflow from the bias flow circuit. The clinician has the ability to set the oscillatory frequency, pressure amplitude (Δ), oscillator displacement (volume), inspiratory/expiratory ratio, and bias flow. The mean airway pressure or continuous distending pressure (CDP) is generally set at higher value to improve alveolar recruitment and oxygenation (**Figure 2C**). Carbon dioxide elimination is correlated with the coefficient of gas transport (DCO_2), which is the product of frequency (f) and tidal volume-squared ($f * Vt^2$). Thus, a high DCO_2 leads to an improvement in ventilation, as modified by frequency and especially the tidal volume. Increases in frequency can, however, lead to decreases in DCO_2 by secondarily decreasing tidal volume unless the pressure amplitude is simultaneously increased (Sanchez Luna et al., 2013).

High frequency oscillatory ventilation is the most commonly used HFV mode with 16.4% of patients receiving HFOV in a cross-sectional observational study, but with the majority of patients placed on CV (Santschi et al., 2010). This is higher than the 2.9% reported by Arnold et al. (2000) 10 years earlier, which could reflect institutional bias or an increased acceptance of the mode. Intensivists are more apt to start HFOV on infants as an early therapy as compared with their pediatric counterparts, but it is still generally considered a rescue therapy in pediatric populations (Ben Jaballah et al., 2006). Patients are on CV between 2.2 to 11.4 days before being switched to HFOV and with an OI ranging from 27.1 to 36.7 (Arnold et al., 2000). HFOV is also the most studied of the HFV modes, but indications, timing, and strategy of HFOV remain poorly defined (Kneyber et al., 2012). Also, there was a significant difference in performance among earlier generation high-frequency oscillators such that similar settings may have generated opposing results, especially in terms of gas exchange, barotrauma, and intraventricular hemorrhage/periventricular leukomalacia (Jouvet et al., 1997). This is likely contributing to disparate results across earlier studies, particularly when applied to patients who have been transitioned from CV due to refractory hypoxemia. Technological advances have markedly improved the high-frequency oscillators that are available for clinical use such that individual ventilator differences may be less critical. However, even newer generation oscillators have substantive differences ranging from volume delivery and frequency range to required ancillary equipment and available features (Pillow, 2015). Performance among high-frequency oscillators therefore also varies, with discrepancies identified between the set and delivered ΔP in certain machines and disparate tidal volume delivery generation, especially at higher frequencies (Pillow et al., 2001; Tingay et al., 2015). It is therefore important for clinicians to recognize these nuances and understand the high-frequency oscillator that is being applied to the patient in order to improve performance (Pillow, 2015).

PEDIATRIC HIGH FREQUENCY OSCILLATORY VENTILATION

In a RCT of 70 patients, Arnold et al. (1994) demonstrated that HFOV led to an improvement in oxygenation with an increased mean airway pressure but decreased peak airway pressures, however, the study was underpowered to detect significant differences (Arnold et al., 1994). In that study, up to 66% of patients in the CV group crossed over to the HFOV group but only 38% of patients in the HFOV group crossed over to the CV group with the patients not analyzed in the initially randomized group (Arnold et al., 1994). In a smaller RCT, HFOV combined with recruitment maneuvers led to superior oxygenation as compared with CV without a marked change in hemodynamics (Samransamruajkit et al., 2016).

HFOV has been associated with both a shorter (Wong et al., 2020) and longer (Gupta et al., 2014; Curley et al., 2015) intensive care unit length of stay, which may partly be explained by the timing of HFOV application and disease severity. One retrospective study found a shorter duration ICU stay but increased mortality, suggesting that HFOV does not improve outcomes in patients with fatal lung injury, but patients with recoverable lung disease may benefit from improved oxygenation and a decrease in lung injury (Yehya et al., 2014a,b; Wong et al., 2020). In a larger retrospective review of over 9,000 patients from 98 hospitals, the use of HFOV was associated with longer duration of ventilation and ICU length of stay, as well as a higher mortality (Gupta et al., 2014). These results might be explained by the study design in which patients were matched according to propensity score matching rather than pulmonary disease type or ventilator parameters (Gupta et al., 2014). In the patients who were placed on HFOV and survived, earlier application of HFOV (within 24 h) was associated with a shorter ventilation course and length of stay as compared with patients in whom HFOV was applied later (Gupta et al., 2014).

In contrast, the results of a secondary analysis of the Randomized Evaluation of Sedation Titration for Respiratory Failure (RESTORE) trial (Curley et al., 2015) found that earlier application of HFOV was correlated with a greater length of mechanical ventilation as compared with later application of HFOV and conventional mechanical ventilation, however, there was no association with mortality (Bateman et al., 2016). The combination of these results is confusing and the discrepancies may suggest that different methods of setting HFOV were used among patients and between studies. It is important to recognize that the HFOV settings that are applied initially or early will be different from those applied later. The goal for both is to achieve a homogeneously aerated lung, but the acutely injured lung must be nudged open slowly, particularly if it has been subject to a prolonged time on non-open-lung strategies (Froese and Kinsella, 2005).

Optimal settings of HFOV have not been thoroughly illuminated (Kneyber et al., 2012). Most protocols do not involve recruitment maneuvers (Kneyber et al., 2012) and set frequency somewhat arbitrarily based on patient age and weight in the range of 5–8 Hz (Froese and Kinsella, 2005; Kneyber et al., 2012; de Jager et al., 2019), where frequency should rather be optimized to minimize the pressure cost of ventilation to reduce lung injury (Venegas and Fredberg, 1994). As an example of the challenges of standardizing HFOV, the power or amplitude is adjusted according to the chest wiggle factor, or the level to which the chest wiggles on HFOV (Meyers et al., 2019). This is hardly precise and difficult to standardize across intensivists, and especially so among institutions. Animal models have been designed to assist in determining optimal means of setting HFOV. In a saline lavage injury in lambs, stepwise escalation in mean airway pressure modified lung volume and optimized lung recruitment (Pellicano et al., 2009). The ideal method of setting HFOV would be with a mean airway pressure sufficient to stabilize alveoli but as low as reasonable possible, with the smallest superimposed oscillations to minimize alveolar strain (Kneyber and Markhorst, 2016).

NEONATAL HIGH FREQUENCY OSCILLATORY VENTILATION

One of the earliest randomized studies in 1989 comparing CV vs. HFOV was the HiFi study (Group, 1989) in preterm infants (750–2,000 g), in which HFOV did not reduce mortality or BPD rates (Group, 1989; No Authors List, 1990a). They found an increased rate of intraventricular hemorrhage (IVH) and periventricular leukomalacia (PVL) (Group, 1989). In a follow-up study at 16–24 months post-term age, respiratory status was similar between the two groups but neurodevelopmental outcome were worse in the HFOV group with a correlation between cognitive defects and hydrocephalus with IVH (No Authors List, 1990b).

Although HFOV is often used as a rescue therapy with success, it has not yet become a primary mode to use early on ventilated patients. To study this, in 1996, the multicenter Provo trial reported that early application of HFOV to premature newborns born less than 35 weeks gestation with moderate to severe respiratory distress resulted in decreased lung injury, improved oxygenation, and even a lower incidence of necrotizing enterocolitis (Gerstmann et al., 1996). A follow-up study published 5 years later determined that there was no difference in childhood neurodevelopmental outcomes, however, the CV group had some markers of obstructive lung pathology with a decrease in peak expiratory flow but an increase in residual volume (Gerstmann et al., 2001). This study was especially important to illustrate that reducing pulmonary morbidity in neonates can decrease subsequent pulmonary dysfunction into childhood (Gerstmann et al., 2001).

To summarize, in three longer-term observational studies evaluating the neurodevelopmental outcomes of preterm infants with respiratory distress syndrome, one demonstrated worse neurodevelopmental outcome in the HFOV group (No Authors List, 1990b), one showed similar neurodevelopmental outcome in the HFOV group but improved respiratory function (Gerstmann et al., 2001), and another demonstrated similar neurodevelopmental and respiratory outcomes (Marlow et al., 2006). These changes can be attributed to improvement in adjunctive strategies, comfort level with HFOV, and improvement in methods of setting HFOV. For instance, surfactant therapy was not a routine treatment during the HiFi study (Courtney et al., 2002). There was also a higher cross-over rate from HFOV to conventional ventilation which could be interpreted as less comfort with the ventilator given that the methods reported that the oscillator was selected after bench testing available machines (Group, 1989). The oscillator chosen (Senko Medical Instrument Manufacturing, Tokyo, Japan) only has the ability to deliver an I:E ratio of 1:1 leading to higher CDP, and contributing to a higher incidence of barotrauma, and IVH (Bryan and Froese, 1991). The HiFi study also used a low volume HFOV strategy, which is now thought to be sub-optimal for infants (Bryan and Froese, 1991). Nevertheless, with conflicting results from these three RCTs, it is not surprising that there is a lack of consensus on ventilating neonatal patients.

In a later multicenter clinical trial, Courtney et al. (2002) randomized very low birth weight infants (601–1,200 g) to HFOV or synchronized intermittent mandatory ventilation and revealed that infants were more likely to be extubated early with HFOV and with a decreased rate of supplemental oxygen requirements by 36 weeks postmenstrual age. This study did not reveal a difference in IVH or PVL (Courtney et al., 2002). In a separate randomized comparison of pre-term infants born < 30 weeks of age, HFOV led to decreased surfactant requirements but no improvement in pulmonary outcomes (Moriette et al., 2001).

Other studies have revealed that HFOV is successful in preventing ECMO (Erdeve et al., 2019) and with similar (Snoek et al., 2016) or decreased (Erdeve et al., 2019) mortality rates. It has been affiliated with a lower (Courtney et al., 2002) and similar (Snoek et al., 2016) incidence of chronic lung disease and similar rates of death and IVH (Clark et al., 1994). A Cochrane review of elective HFOV RCTs spanning as early as the HiFi trial determined that the 28-and 30-day mortality between HFOV and CV was similar. They also found an increase in pulmonary air leaks in the HFOV group, a decrease in severe retinopathy of prematurity, and a decrease, albeit inconsistent, in chronic lung disease (Cools et al., 2015).

To further illustrate the importance of fully understanding studies, a meta-analysis of 17 randomized trials comparing HFV to CV determined that changes in outcomes between HFV and CV are more likely due to the method by which the mode was set as compared with the mode itself (Thome et al., 2005). Adjunctive therapies in pediatric and neonatal ICU patients have been rapidly progressing, including surfactant therapy and nitric oxide application. Studies must therefore also be taken in context with the year they were performed (Courtney et al., 2002). Recognizing that with the arsenal of critical care techniques available, the limits of what can be done has also expanded, where studies were previously reporting infants born < 35 weeks of age and weighing < 1.751 kg in 1992 (Clark et al., 1994) to infants weighing as little as 601 g in 2002 (Courtney et al., 2002).

HIGH-FREQUENCY PERCUSSIVE VENTILATION

High-frequency percussive ventilation (HFPV) is delivered by a pneumatically powered, flow-regulated, time-cycled, pressure-controlled ventilator. HFPV delivers a small tidal volume (or sub-tidal volume) at a high frequency, in combination with a low frequency bulk distribution of gas similar to that of a pressure limited CV breath (**Figure 2D**). The most unique feature of HFPV is the breathing circuit and the patient airway interface. It uses a sliding venturi, operating simultaneously as inhalation and exhalation valves. It is permanently open to ambient, through which sub-tidal breaths are delivered into the lungs. By venturi effect, flow volume delivery is always inversely proportional to the

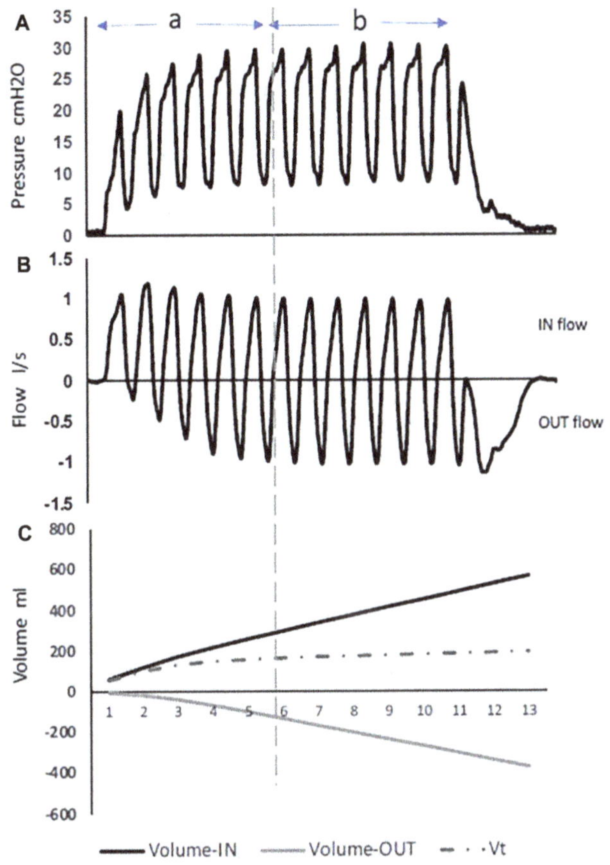

FIGURE 3 | Pressure, flow, and volumes during HFPV inspiratory interval, using a lung model. During phase **(A)** full flow acceleration with an increase in volume-in delivery, while phase **(B)** is characterized with more volume-out. **(C)** The difference between volume-in and volume-out is the tidal volume. Note the tidal volume value remains stable during the whole plateau equilibrium.

pressure reached at the level of the airway. The high frequency flow interrupter generator of the ventilator allows the sliding venturi to be regulated in such a manner that there is a stepwise increase in airway pressure during inspiration to the scheduled peak inspiratory pressure (**Figure 3**; Bougatef et al., 2007).

Two phases describe the inspiration period during HFPV. The first is an initial phase characterized by an inspiratory flow acceleration with a progressive increase in airway pressure. As the inspiratory interval progresses, an expiratory flow component develops. The second phase is where the pressure and flow reach an oscillating plateau equilibrium at the scheduled peak inspiratory pressure, and where the flow signal is characterized by an equilibrium between the inspiratory flow and the expiratory flow components (**Figure 3**). While the second phase is user-controlled (pressure, amplitude, time), the initial phase is dependent on the patient's thoraco-pulmonary mechanics. Unlike the other high-frequency modes (HFOV, HFJV), HFPV does not rely on establishing a higher mean airway pressure to maintain alveolar recruitment. Instead, HFPV maintains gas distribution by synergizing with the time constants of the lung compartments, maintaining open alveoli while preventing overinflation (Lucangelo et al., 2010).

During inspiration, the flow is interrupted between two consecutive pulses, resulting in a pressure drop to a value that depends on the thoraco-pulmonary mechanics. The gradual stacking of the successive pulsed volumes results in a progressive increase in lung volume. Like flow and pressure, sub-tidal volume deliveries during the inspiratory interval follows two phases. At the beginning of inspiration, pulsed volume-in are larger in size, while the exhaled volumes (volume-out) are small. As the inspiratory interval progress, pulsed volume-in decreases and volume-out increases in size to reach an equilibrium characterizing the second phase (**Figure 3**).

After each volume-in, the pulsed flow is interrupted, allowing the exhalation port to vent the proximal airway to ambient, and a volume-out is exhaled by the patient. This represents an important beneficial mechanism of HFPV in the improvement of gas exchange. The tidal volume is calculated by the difference between the cumulative volume-in and the cumulative volume-out (**Figure 3**).

PEDIATRIC HIGH-FREQUENCY PERCUSSIVE VENTILATION

In a retrospective observational study of 31 patients who failed conventional ventilation, application of HFPV led to improved oxygenation and ventilation while decreasing the peak inspiratory pressure from 38 to 26 cm H_2O (Rizkalla et al., 2014). HFPV has found particular application to patients with acute burn injury and respiratory failure, likely because it has been effective in clearing secretions due to percussive bursts (Allan et al., 2010). Three RCTs (Carman et al., 2002; Mlcak et al., 2002; Reper et al., 2002) and one case-controlled series (Cortiella et al., 1999) cumulatively demonstrated improved oxygenation (Cortiella et al., 1999; Carman et al., 2002; Reper et al., 2002) a decrease in peak inspiratory pressures (Cortiella et al., 1999; Carman et al., 2002), and decreased rates of pneumonia (Cortiella et al., 1999; Mlcak et al., 2002) in mechanically ventilated pediatric patients with burns and/or inhalation injury ventilated with HFPV as compared with CV.

NEONATAL HIGH-FREQUENCY PERCUSSIVE VENTILATION

High-frequency percussive ventilation is less well-reported in neonatal studies, often being lumped together with other HFV modes. Only small case series exist in neonates ventilated with HFPV (Pfenninger and Gerber, 1987; Pfenninger and Minder, 1988; Paviotti et al., 2014), but have demonstrated improvements in oxygenation without increasing airway pressures (Pfenninger and Gerber, 1987; Paviotti et al., 2014), and improved static compliance (Pfenninger and Minder, 1988). Nasal high-frequency percussive ventilation has recently been popularized (De La Roque et al., 2011; Moresco et al., 2020; Renesme et al., 2020) and compared with nasal continuous positive airway pressure, demonstrated non-inferiority (Renesme et al., 2013), possible benefit, and that it is well-tolerated (De La Roque et al., 2011). In a piglet model of meconium aspiration syndrome, HFPV and CV were associated with lower mean airway pressures and OI as compared with HFOV, but there was no apparent difference in histologic lung injury (Renesme et al., 2013).

High-Frequency Jet Ventilation

High frequency jet ventilation is seldom used in adults and most often reported in neonates, particularly in preterm infants (Miller et al., 2021a). With HFJV, a high velocity gas jet is delivered *via* an adapter or jet injector inserted into the endotracheal tube. Similar to HFOV, it delivers small tidal volumes at a rapid rate of up to 660 cycles/min with an inspiratory time set as short as 0.02 s (Smith et al., 1993; Miller et al., 2021a). Unlike HFOV, HFJV is set on top of a conventional ventilation mode which regulates the mean airway pressure (Miller et al., 2021a). Additionally, exhalation is passive and dependent on the rate and inspiratory to expiratory ratio, but allows for marked CO_2 elimination (Miller et al., 2021a). The jet pulses and continuous air stream are also hypothesized to improve mucous clearance (Miller et al., 2021a). Like the other HFV modes, HFJV is largely used as a rescue mode when CV has failed (Smith et al., 1993).

PEDIATRIC HIGH FREQUENCY JET VENTILATION

No RCTs exist in the pediatric population and the majority of studies are case series (Miller et al., 2021a), but it has been deemed safe for use as evident in a case series of eleven pediatric patients with respiratory syncytial virus (Valentine et al., 2016). In a physiologic comparison of HFJV vs. CV, HFJV was found to generate a higher intrinsic PEEP leading to an increase in end-expiratory lung volume and improved oxygenation, while also achieving a higher minute ventilation (Berner et al., 1993). In support of this, a retrospective review of 35 pediatric critical care patients (including neonates) transitioned from CV to HFJV were found to have a decrease in acidosis and oxygen requirements (Miller et al., 2021b). HFJV has also been shown to resolve clinically relevant pulmonary barotrauma and air leaks caused by CV at lower mean airway pressures (Smith et al., 1993).

NEONATAL HIGH FREQUENCY JET VENTILATION

In two neonatal RCTs, HFJV was found to improve ventilation at lower peak airway pressures (Keszler et al., 1991; Keszler, 1997). Cross-over was allowed in one of the trials, and 84% of patients who crossed over from CV to HFJV responded well to HFJV, whereas only 9% of those who crossed over from HFJV to CV were successful (Keszler et al., 1991). The incidence of chronic lung disease was similar between CV and HFJV in that study (Keszler et al., 1991), whereas in the other RCT of preterm infants <36 weeks, HFJV was found to reduce the incidence of BPD as well as the need for future supplemental oxygenation (Keszler, 1997). Two different methods of setting HFJV were used in that study: a low airway pressure (Low P_{aw}) strategy and an optimal volume (OV) strategy. In a subgroup analysis, the HFJV-OV strategy was found to have an improvement in oxygenation whereas the HFJV-Low P_{aw} had an increase in ventilation (Keszler, 1997). Other observational studies comparing HFJV with CV have revealed similar oxygenation, ventilation, and hospital days (Wiswell et al., 1996) and no difference in mortality, bronchopulmonary dysplasia, or cross-overs (Carlo et al., 1990), but similar rates of air leaks has been consistent across studies (Carlo et al., 1990; Keszler et al., 1991; Keszler, 1997).

Neurologic outcomes with HFJV have been conflicting. In one of the RCTs, the HFJV-OV strategy was affiliated with a decreased incidence in IVH and PVL as compared with the CV and HFJV-Low P_{aw} groups (Keszler, 1997), whereas the other found no difference (Keszler et al., 1991). In another study of 73 premature infants born less than 33 weeks, HFJV had a higher incidence of PVL or poor neurologic outcome (Wiswell et al., 1996). In another study of 42 infants with severe respiratory distress syndrome there was no difference in IVH incidence between HFJV and CV (Carlo et al., 1990).

Other special considerations that have been studied with HFJV include congenital heart disease, congenital diaphragmatic hernias, and persistent pulmonary hypertension. HFJV in infants with congenital heart disease were found to have decreased acidosis and improved ventilation but no significant difference in oxygenation (Miller et al., 2021c). HFJV has demonstrated improved ventilation in infants with congenital diaphragmatic hernias (Zhang et al., 2013) and a trend toward improved survival as compared with CV (Kuluz et al., 2010). HFJV has been compared against HFOV in infants with persistent pulmonary hypertension (Coates, 2008), but no randomized controlled trials exist (Ethawi et al., 2016). In infants with persistent pulmonary hypertension, HFJV and HFOV led to similar outcomes once adjusted for differences in comparison groups (Coates, 2008). Other special considerations for neonates include meconium aspiration syndrome and pneumonia, in which HFJV may benefit from being combined with surfactant (Davis et al., 1992; Calkovska et al., 2005).

DISCUSSION

Although the results of this review are seemingly bleak, with no consistent outcomes among studies or determination of optimal modes or methods of setting them, a few conclusions may be drawn. The first is that caution must be taken when interpreting studies and comparing modes against one other, particularly when a protocol for setting a mode has not been established, and when comparing studies spanning large periods of time. The second is that there may not be a single optimal mechanical ventilation approach. The best method may simply be one that the intensivist is comfortable with and one that allows for an adaptive approach so the settings are personalized to the individual patient and disease pathophysiology (Gattinoni et al., 2016). Finally, when considering study design, not only does the number of enrolled centers and patients need to be considered, but also patient phenotype. A well-designed multi-center study would ideally also have a centralized method of providing continuous oversight of ventilator settings and waveforms of patients across participating institutions to standardize ventilator adjustments and maximize internal validity.

There has been a call for an increased number and quality of RCTs in pediatric and neonatal mechanical ventilation trials. With the lower incidence of lung injury in pediatric and neonatal patients, it is well-accepted that a properly powered study would require involvement of several institutions over a few year period, not only creating difficulty maintaining inter-institutional protocols and compliance but also over an extended period of time (Khemani and Newth, 2010). Future pediatric mechanical ventilation studies must be carefully designed, not only to ensure adequate power, but also with appropriate age stratification and inclusion/exclusion criteria. Even a perfectly controlled multi-institutional RCT can prompt the question of whether the average of a population with varying clinical characteristics and disease phenotypes can be applied to the individual patient (Goligher et al., 2015). The most prominent example of this is in patients with extrapulmonary vs. pulmonary lung injury. These two quite distinct phenotypes are both lumped together under the umbrella of ARDS yet patients with one vs. the other will respond disparately to ventilator setting adjustments (Kollisch-Singule et al., 2018). Not only should patients be partitioned into pediatric and neonatal categories, but also specific age groups to account for changes in chest wall stiffness and alveolarization. Patients should also be analyzed according to lung injury phenotype in pediatric patients (pulmonary vs. extrapulmonary) and disease type in neonates (persistent pulmonary hypertension, respiratory distress syndrome, congenital heart disease, meconium aspiration syndrome) and whether or not they are on ECMO.

One of the great challenges with RCTs is that a clinician may be expected to set and adjust a mechanical ventilator mode that they are not accustomed to. All clinicians are hostage to their experience, both in training and with previous patients. It is unrealistic to expect improved outcomes in a mode that a clinician is uncomfortable with, particularly if the methods are not well-protocolized. The "best" mechanical ventilation mode is not only dependent on the patient and disease pathophysiology, but also on the experience of the individual making the ventilator adjustments. Therefore, to make an RCT successful requires teaching modules, clinician humility, and consideration toward making ventilator adjustments in a coordinated team fashion.

CONCLUSION

In summary, there are a variety of mechanical ventilation modes available for neonatal and pediatric use, each with benefits and drawbacks but with no definitive indications or protocols for use. In part, this is due to the lack of definitive evidence from trials, however, Froese (Froese and Kinsella, 2005) well-articulated that "*a premature trial can kill a good technique (almost).*" More trials may not provide the answers we are searching for and may provide more conflicting data, particularly without thoughtful study design. There may never be one universalized mechanical ventilation protocol that can be safely and effectively applied to all pediatric and neonatal patients, but it is important to be open to additional strategies and understand the fundamentals of each so they may be titrated to the individual patient. We will likely find that the best mechanical ventilation strategy is that which is personalized and adaptive to the patient.

AUTHOR CONTRIBUTIONS

MK-S: manuscript drafting. GN, PA, JS, HR, SB, LG, NH, and AB: critical revisions. All authors contributed to the article and approved the submitted version.

REFERENCES

Albuali, W. H., Singh, R. N., Fraser, D. D., Seabrook, J. A., Kavanagh, B. P., Parshuram, C. S., et al. (2007). Have changes in ventilation practice improved outcome in children with acute lung injury? *Pediatr. Crit. Care Med.* 8, 324–330. doi: 10.1097/01.PCC.0000269390.48450.AF

Allan, P. F., Osborn, E. C., Chung, K. K., and Wanek, S. M. (2010). High-frequency percussive ventilation revisited. *J. Burn Care Res.* 31, 510–520. doi: 10.1097/BCR.0b013e3181e4d605

Anderson, M., and Speicher, R. (2006). Airway Pressure Release Ventilation in Pediatrics. *U.S. Respir. Dis.* 66–67.

ARDSnet (2000). Ventilation with lower tidal volumes as compared with traditional tidal volumes for acute lung injury and the acute respiratory distress syndrome. The Acute Respiratory Distress Syndrome Network. *N. Engl. J. Med.* 342, 1301–1308.

Arnold, J. H., Anas, N. G., Luckett, P., Cheifetz, I. M., Reyes, G., Newth, C. J., et al. (2000). High-frequency oscillatory ventilation in pediatric respiratory failure: a multicenter experience. *Crit. Care Med.* 28, 3913–3919.

Arnold, J. H., Hanson, J. H., Toro-Figuero, L. O., Gutierrez, J., Berens, R. J., and Anglin, D. L. (1994). Prospective, randomized comparison of high-frequency oscillatory ventilation and conventional mechanical ventilation in pediatric respiratory failure. *Crit. Care Med.* 22, 1530–1539.

Arrindell, E. L. Jr., Krishnan, R., van der, M., Merwe, F. C., Howard, S. C., Zhang, J., et al. (2015). Lung volume recruitment in a preterm pig model of lung immaturity. *Am. J. Physiol. Lung Cell. Mol. Physiol.* 309, L1088–L1092. doi: 10.1152/ajplung.00292.2015

Askie, L. M., Henderson-Smart, D. J., Irwig, L., and Simpson, J. M. (2003). Oxygen-saturation targets and outcomes in extremely preterm infants. *N. Engl. J. Med.* 349, 959–967.

Bateman, S. T., Borasino, S., Asaro, L. A., Cheifetz, I. M., Diane, S., and Wypij, D. (2016). Early High-Frequency Oscillatory Ventilation in Pediatric Acute Respiratory Failure. A Propensity Score Analysis. *Am. J. Respir. Crit. Care Med.* 193, 495–503. doi: 10.1164/rccm.201507-1381OC

Ben Jaballah, N., Khaldi, A., Mnif, K., Bouziri, A., Belhadj, S., Hamdi, A., et al. (2006). High-frequency oscillatory ventilation in pediatric patients with acute respiratory failure. *Pediatr. Crit. Care Med.* 7, 362–367.

Berner, M. E., Cauderay, M., and Suter, P. M. (1993). Assessment of lung volume and alveolar pressure during combined high-frequency jet ventilation in a child with adult respiratory distress syndrome. *Intensive Care Med.* 19, 411–414. doi: 10.1007/BF01724882

Bougatef, A., Casteels, A., Cools, F., De Wolf, D., and Foubert, L. (2007). High Frequency Percussive Ventilation: principle and Fifteen Years of experience in preterm infants with respiratory distress syndrome. *J. Respir. Care Appl. Technol.* 2, 39–50.

Bryan, A. C., and Froese, A. B. (1991). Reflections on the HIFI trial. *Pediatrics* 87, 565–567.

Calkovska, A., Sevecova-Mokra, D., Javorka, K., Petraskova, M., and Adamicova, K. (2005). Exogenous surfactant administration by asymmetric high-frequency jet ventilation in experimental respiratory distress syndrome. *Croat. Med. J.* 46, 209–217.

Carlo, W. A., Siner, B., Chatburn, R. L., Robertson, S., and Martin, R. J. (1990). Early randomized intervention with high-frequency jet ventilation in respiratory distress syndrome. *J. Pediatr.* 117, 765–770. doi: 10.1016/s0022-3476(05)83341-4

Carman, B., Cahill, T., Warden, G., and McCall, J. (2002). A prospective, randomized comparison of the Volume Diffusive Respirator vs conventional ventilation for ventilation of burned children. 2001 ABA paper. *J. Burn Care Rehabil.* 23, 444–448. doi: 10.1097/00004630-200211000-00011

Clark, R. H., Yoder, B. A., and Sell, M. S. (1994). Prospective, randomized comparison of high-frequency oscillation and conventional ventilation in candidates for extracorporeal membrane oxygenation. *J. Pediatr.* 124, 447–454. doi: 10.1016/s0022-3476(94)70374-4

Coates, E. W. (2008). M.E. Klinepeter, and T.M. O'Shea, Neonatal pulmonary hypertension treated with inhaled nitric oxide and high-frequency ventilation. *J. Perinatol.* 28, 675–679. doi: 10.1038/jp.2008.76

Cools, F., Offringa, M., and Askie, L. M. (2015). Elective high frequency oscillatory ventilation versus conventional ventilation for acute pulmonary dysfunction in preterm infants. *Cochrane Database Syst. Rev.* 19:CD000104.

Copland, I. B., Martinez, F., Kavanagh, B. P., Engelberts, D., McKerlie, C., Belik, J., et al. (2004). High tidal volume ventilation causes different inflammatory responses in newborn versus adult lung. *Am. J. Respir. Crit. Care Med.* 169, 739–748. doi: 10.1164/rccm.200310-1417OC

Cortiella, J., Mlcak, R., and Herndon, D. (1999). High frequency percussive ventilation in pediatric patients with inhalation injury. *J. Burn Care Rehabil.* 20, 232–235. doi: 10.1097/00004630-199905000-00014

Courtney, S. E., Durand, D. J., Asselin, J. M., Hudak, M. L., Aschner, J. L., Shoemaker, C. T., et al. (2002). ., High-frequency oscillatory ventilation versus conventional mechanical ventilation for very-low-birth-weight infants. *N. Engl. J. Med.* 347, 643–652. doi: 10.1056/NEJMoa012750

Curley, M. A., Wypij, D., Watson, R. S., Grant, M. J., Asaro, L. A., and Cheifetz, I. M. (2015). Protocolized sedation vs usual care in pediatric patients mechanically ventilated for acute respiratory failure: a randomized clinical trial. *JAMA* 313, 379–389. doi: 10.1001/jama.2014.18399

Davis, J. M., Richter, S. E., Kendig, J. W., and Notter, R. H. (1992). High-frequency jet ventilation and surfactant treatment of newborns with severe respiratory failure. *Pediatr. Pulmonol.* 13, 108–112. doi: 10.1002/ppul.1950130209

de Jager, P., Burgerhof, J. G., van Heerde, M., Albers, M. J., Markhorst, D. G., and Kneyber, M. C. (2014). Tidal volume and mortality in mechanically ventilated children: a systematic review and meta-analysis of observational studies*. *Crit. Care Med.* 42, 2461–2472. doi: 10.1097/CCM.0000000000000546

de Jager, P., Kamp, T., Dijkstra, S. K., Burgerhof, J. G. M., Markhorst, D. G., and Curley, M. A. Q. (2019). Feasibility of an alternative, physiologic, individualized open-lung approach to high-frequency oscillatory ventilation in children. *Ann. Intensive Care* 9:9.

De La Roque, E. D., Bertrand, C., Tandonnet, O., Rebola, M., Roquand, E., Renesme, L., et al. (2011). Nasal high frequency percussive ventilation versus nasal continuous positive airway pressure in transient tachypnea of the newborn: a pilot randomized controlled trial (NCT00556738). *Pediatr. Pulmonol.* 46, 218–223. doi: 10.1002/ppul.21354

Dellinger, R. P., Levy, M. M., Carlet, J. M., Bion, J., Parker, M. M., Jaeschke, R., et al. (2008). Surviving Sepsis Campaign: international guidelines for management of severe sepsis and septic shock: 2008. *Crit. Care Med.* 36, 296–327.

Dowell, J. C., Parvathaneni, K., Thomas, N. J., Khemani, R. G., and Yehya, N. (2018). Epidemiology of Cause of Death in Pediatric Acute Respiratory Distress Syndrome. *Crit. Care Med.* 46, 1811–1819. doi: 10.1097/CCM.0000000000003371

Ecmo. (2021). *ECLS Registry Report - Overall Outcomes.* United States: Extracorporeal Life Support Organization.

Erdeve, O., Okulu, E., Tunc, G., Celik, Y., Kayacan, U., Cetinkaya, M., et al. (2019). An observational, prospective, multicenter study on rescue high-frequency oscillatory ventilation in neonates failing with conventional ventilation. *PLoS One* 14:e0217768. doi: 10.1371/journal.pone.0217768

Erickson, S., Schibler, A., Numa, A., Nuthall, G., Yung, M., Pascoe, E., et al. (2007). Acute lung injury in pediatric intensive care in Australia and New Zealand: a prospective, multicenter, observational study. *Pediatr. Crit. Care Med.* 8, 317–323. doi: 10.1097/01.PCC.0000269408.64179.FF

Ethawi, Y. H., Mehrem, A. A., Minski, J., Ruth, C. A., and Davis, P. G. (2016). High frequency jet ventilation versus high frequency oscillatory ventilation for pulmonary dysfunction in preterm infants. *Cochrane Database Syst .Rev.* 2016:CD010548. doi: 10.1002/14651858.CD010548.pub2

Force, A. D. T., Ranieri, V. M., Rubenfeld, G. D., Thompson, B. T., Ferguson, N. D., Caldwell, E., et al. (2012). Acute respiratory distress syndrome: the Berlin Definition. *JAMA* 307, 2526–2533. doi: 10.1001/jama.2012.5669

Frawley, P. M., and Habashi, N. M. (2004). Airway pressure release ventilation and pediatrics: theory and practice. *Crit. Care Nurs. Clin. North Am.* 16, 337–348. doi: 10.1016/j.ccell.2004.04.003

Froese, A. B., and Kinsella, J. P. (2005). High-frequency oscillatory ventilation: lessons from the neonatal/pediatric experience. *Crit. Care Med.* 33, S115–S121. doi: 10.1097/01.ccm.0000155923.97849.6d

Gattinoni, L., Pelosi, P., Suter, P. M., Pedoto, A., Vercesi, P., and Lissoni, A. (1998). Acute respiratory distress syndrome caused by pulmonary and extrapulmonary disease. Different syndromes? *Am. J. Respir. Crit. Care Med.* 158, 3–11. doi: 10.1164/ajrccm.158.1.9708031

Gattinoni, L., Tonetti, T., and Quintel, M. (2016). Improved survival in critically ill patients: are large RCTs more useful than personalized medicine? We are not sure. *Intensive Care Med.* 42, 1781–1783. doi: 10.1007/s00134-016-4471-8

Gerstmann, D. R., Minton, S. D., Stoddard, R. A., Meredith, K. S., Monaco, F., Bertrand, J. M., et al. (1996). The Provo multicenter early high-frequency oscillatory ventilation trial: improved pulmonary and clinical outcome in respiratory distress syndrome. *Pediatrics* 98, 1044–1057.

Gerstmann, D. R., Wood, K., Miller, A., Steffen, M., Ogden, B., Stoddard, R. A., et al. (2001). Childhood outcome after early high-frequency oscillatory ventilation for neonatal respiratory distress syndrome. *Pediatrics* 108, 617–623. doi: 10.1542/peds.108.3.617

Goligher, E. C., Kavanagh, B. P., Rubenfeld, G. D., and Ferguson, N. D. (2015). Physiologic Responsiveness Should Guide Entry into Randomized Controlled Trials. *Am. J. Respir. Crit. Care Med.* 192, 1416–1419. doi: 10.1164/rccm.201410-1832CP

Group, H. S. (1989). High-frequency oscillatory ventilation compared with conventional mechanical ventilation in the treatment of respiratory failure in preterm infants. *N. Engl. J. Med.* 320, 88–93.

Gupta, P., Green, J. W., Tang, X., Gall, C. M., Gossett, J. M., Rice, T. B., et al. (2014). Comparison of high-frequency oscillatory ventilation and conventional mechanical ventilation in pediatric respiratory failure. *JAMA Pediatr.* 168, 243–249.

Gupta, S., Joshi, V., Joshi, P., Monkman, S., Vaillancourt, K., and Choong, K. (2013). Airway pressure release ventilation: a neonatal case series and review of current practice. *Can. Respir. J.* 20, e86–e91. doi: 10.1155/2013/734729

Habashi, N. M. (2005). Other approaches to open-lung ventilation: airway pressure release ventilation. *Crit. Care Med.* 33, S228–S240. doi: 10.1097/01.ccm.0000155920.11893.37

Hanson, J. H., and Flori, H. (2006). Application of the acute respiratory distress syndrome network low-tidal volume strategy to pediatric acute lung injury. *Respir. Care Clin. N. Am.* 12, 349–357. doi: 10.1016/j.rcc.2006.05.003

Iliodromiti, Z., Zygouris, D., Sifakis, S., Pappa, K. I., Tsikouras, P., Salakos, N., et al. (2013). Acute lung injury in preterm fetuses and neonates: mechanisms and molecular pathways. *J. Matern. Fetal Neonatal. Med.* 26, 1696–1704. doi: 10.3109/14767058.2013.798284

Jain, S. V., Kollisch-Singule, M., Sadowitz, B., Dombert, L., Satalin, J., Andrews, P., et al. (2016). The 30-year evolution of airway pressure release ventilation (APRV). *Intensive Care Med. Exp.* 4:11. doi: 10.1186/s40635-016-0085-2

Jouvet, P., Hubert, P., Isabey, D., Pinquier, D., Dahan, E., Cloup, M., et al. (1997). Assessment of high-frequency neonatal ventilator performances. *Intensive Care Med.* 23, 208–213. doi: 10.1007/s001340050318

Keim, G., Watson, R. S., Thomas, N. J., and Yehya, N. (2018). New Morbidity and Discharge Disposition of Pediatric Acute Respiratory Distress Syndrome Survivors. *Crit Care Med.* 46, 1731–1738. doi: 10.1097/CCM.0000000000003341

Keim, G., Yehya, N., Spear, D., Hall, M. W., Loftis, L. L., Alten, J. A., et al. (2020). Development of Persistent Respiratory Morbidity in Previously Healthy

Children After Acute Respiratory Failure. *Crit Care Med.* 48, 1120–1128. doi: 10.1097/CCM.0000000000004380

Keszler, M. (1997). H.D. Modanlou, D.S. Brudno, F.I. Clark, R.S. Cohen, R.M. Ryan, et al., Multicenter controlled clinical trial of high-frequency jet ventilation in preterm infants with uncomplicated respiratory distress syndrome. *Pediatrics* 100, 593–599. doi: 10.1542/peds.100.4.593

Keszler, M., Donn, S. M., Bucciarelli, R. L., Alverson, D. C., Hart, M., and Lunyong, V. (1991). Multicenter controlled trial comparing high-frequency jet ventilation and conventional mechanical ventilation in newborn infants with pulmonary interstitial emphysema. *J. Pediatr.* 119, 85–93. doi: 10.1016/s0022-3476(05)81046-7

Keszler, M., Nassabeh-Montazami, S., and Abubakar, K. (2009). Evolution of tidal volume requirement during the first 3 weeks of life in infants <800 g ventilated with Volume Guarantee. *Arch. Dis. Child Fetal Neonatal. Ed.* 94, F279–F282. doi: 10.1136/adc.2008.147157

Khemani, R. G., and Newth, C. J. (2010). The design of future pediatric mechanical ventilation trials for acute lung injury. *Am. J. Respir. Crit. Care Med.* 182, 1465–1474. doi: 10.1164/rccm.201004-0606CI

Khemani, R. G., Markovitz, B. P., and Curley, M. A. Q. (2009a). Characteristics of children intubated and mechanically ventilated in 16 PICUs. *Chest* 136, 765–771. doi: 10.1378/chest.09-0207

Khemani, R. G., Patel, N. R., Bart, R. D. III, and Newth, C. J. L. (2009b). Comparison of the pulse oximetric saturation/fraction of inspired oxygen ratio and the PaO2/fraction of inspired oxygen ratio in children. *Chest* 135, 662–668. doi: 10.1378/chest.08-2239

Khemani, R. G., Smith, L., Lopez-Fernandez, Y. M., Kwok, J., Morzov, R., Klein, M. J., et al. (2019). Paediatric acute respiratory distress syndrome incidence and epidemiology (PARDIE): an international, observational study. *Lancet Respir. Med.* 7, 115–128. doi: 10.1016/S2213-2600(18)30344-8

Kneyber, M. C. J., de Luca, D., Calderini, E., Jarreau, P. H., Javouhey, E., Lopez-Herce, J., et al. (2017). Recommendations for mechanical ventilation of critically ill children from the Paediatric Mechanical Ventilation Consensus Conference (PEMVECC). *Intensive Care Med.* 43, 1764–1780. doi: 10.1007/s00134-017-4920-z

Kneyber, M. C., and Markhorst, D. G. (2016). Do We Really Know How to Use High-Frequency Oscillatory Ventilation in Critically Ill Children? *Am. J. Respir. Crit. Care Med.* 193, 1067–1068.

Kneyber, M. C., van Heerde, M., and Markhorst, D. G. (2012). Reflections on pediatric high-frequency oscillatory ventilation from a physiologic perspective. *Respir. Care* 57, 1496–1504. doi: 10.4187/respcare.01571

Kollisch-Singule, M. C., Jain, S. V., Andrews, P. L., Satalin, J., Gatto, L. A., Villar, J., et al. (2018). Looking beyond macroventilatory parameters and rethinking ventilator-induced lung injury. *J. Appl. Physiol.* 124, 1214–1218.

Kollisch-Singule, M., Emr, B., Jain, S. V., Andrews, P., Satalin, J., Liu, J., et al. (2015). The effects of airway pressure release ventilation on respiratory mechanics in extrapulmonary lung injury. *Intensive Care Med. Exp.* 3:35. doi: 10.1186/s40635-015-0071-0

Kollisch-Singule, M., Emr, B., Smith, B., Roy, S., Jain, S., Satalin, J., et al. (2014). Mechanical breath profile of airway pressure release ventilation: the effect on alveolar recruitment and microstrain in acute lung injury. *JAMA Surg.* 149, 1138–1145. doi: 10.1001/jamasurg.2014.1829

Kollisch-Singule, M., Jain, S. V., Satalin, J., Andrews, P., Searles, Q., Liu, Z., et al. (2017). Limiting ventilator-associated lung injury in a preterm porcine neonatal model. *J. Pediatr. Surg.* 52, 50–55. doi: 10.1016/j.jpedsurg.2016.10.020

Koopman, A. A., de Jager, P., Blokpoel, R. G. T., and Kneyber, M. C. J. (2019). Ventilator-induced lung injury in children: a reality? *Ann. Transl. Med.* 7:506. doi: 10.21037/atm.2019.09.13

Kornecki, A., Tsuchida, S., Ondiveeran, H. K., Engelberts, D., Frndova, H., Tanswell, A. K., et al. (2005). Lung development and susceptibility to ventilator-induced lung injury. *Am. J. Respir. Crit. Care Med.* 171, 743–752. doi: 10.1164/rccm.200408-1053OC

Krishnan, J., and Morrison, W. (2007). Airway pressure release ventilation: a pediatric case series. *Pediatr. Pulmonol.* 42, 83–88.

Kuluz, M. A., Smith, P. B., Mears, S. P., Benjamin, J. R., Tracy, E. T., Williford, W. L., et al. (2010). Preliminary observations of the use of high-frequency jet ventilation as rescue therapy in infants with congenital diaphragmatic hernia. *J. Pediatr. Surg.* 45, 698–702. doi: 10.1016/j.jpedsurg.2009.07.025

Lalgudi Ganesan, S., Jayashree, M., Singhi, S. C., and Bansal, A. (2018). Airway Pressure Release Ventilation in Pediatric Acute Respiratory Distress Syndrome: a Randomized Controlled Trial. *Am. J. Respir. Crit. Care Med.* 198, 1199–1207. doi: 10.1164/rccm.201705-0989OC

Langham, M. R. Jr., Kays, D. W., Beierle, E. A., Chen, M. K., Stringfellow, K., and Talbert, J. L. (2003). Expanded application of extracorporeal membrane oxygenation in a pediatric surgery practice. *Ann. Surg.* 237, 766–772. doi: 10.1097/01.SLA.0000067740.05989.45

Lucangelo, U., Accardo, A., Bernardi, A., Ferluga, M., Borelli, M., Antonaglia, V., et al. (2010). Gas distribution in a two-compartment model ventilated in high-frequency percussive and pressure-controlled modes. *Intensive Care Med.* 36, 2125–2131. doi: 10.1007/s00134-010-1993-3

Marlow, N., Greenough, A., Peacock, J. L., Marston, L., Limb, E. S., Johnson, A. H., et al. (2006). Randomised trial of high frequency oscillatory ventilation or conventional ventilation in babies of gestational age 28 weeks or less: respiratory and neurological outcomes at 2 years. *Arch. Dis. Child Fetal. Neonatal. Ed.* 91, F320–F326. doi: 10.1136/adc.2005.079632

Martin, L. D., Wetzel, R. C., and Bilenki, A. L. (1991). Airway pressure release ventilation in a neonatal lamb model of acute lung injury. *Crit. Care Med.* 19, 373–378. doi: 10.1097/00003246-199103000-00016

Meyers, M., Rodrigues, N., and Ari, A. (2019). High-frequency oscillatory ventilation: a narrative review. *Can. J. Respir. Ther.* 55, 40–46. doi: 10.29390/cjrt-2019-004

Miller, A. G., Bartle, R. M., and Rehder, K. J. (2021a). High-Frequency Jet Ventilation in Neonatal and Pediatric Subjects: a Narrative Review. *Respir. Care* 66, 845–856. doi: 10.4187/respcare.08691

Miller, A. G., Haynes, K. E., Gates, R. M., Kumar, K. R., Cheifetz, I. M., and Rotta, A. T. (2021b). High-Frequency Jet Ventilation in Pediatric Acute Respiratory Failure. *Respir. Care* 66, 191–198. doi: 10.4187/respcare.08241

Miller, A. G., Scott, B. L., Gates, R. M., Haynes, K. E., Domowicz, D.A. L., and Rotta, A. T. (2021c). High-Frequency Jet Ventilation in Infants With Congenital Heart Disease. *Respir. Care* 66, 1684–1690. doi: 10.4187/respcare.09186

Mlcak, R. P., Suman, O. E., Sanford, A. P., and Herndon, D. N. (2002). Comparison of high frequency percussive ventilation and conventional. *J. Burns Surg. Wound Care* 1, 1–6.

Moresco, L., Romantsik, O., Calevo, M. G., and Bruschettini, M. (2020). Non-invasive respiratory support for the management of transient tachypnea of the newborn. *Cochrane Database Syst. Rev.* 4:CD013231. doi: 10.1002/14651858.CD013231.pub2

Moriette, G., Paris-Llado, J., Walti, H., Escande, B., Magny, J. F., Cambonie, G., et al. (2001). Prospective randomized multicenter comparison of high-frequency oscillatory ventilation and conventional ventilation in preterm infants of less than 30 weeks with respiratory distress syndrome. *Pediatrics* 107, 363–372. doi: 10.1542/peds.107.2.363

Narayanan, M., Owers-Bradley, J., Beardsmore, C. S., Mada, M., Ball, I., Garipov, R., et al. (2012). Alveolarization continues during childhood and adolescence: new evidence from helium-3 magnetic resonance. *Am. J. Respir. Crit. Care Me.d* 185, 186–191. doi: 10.1164/rccm.201107-1348OC

Nieman, G. F., Gatto, L. A., Andrews, P., Satalin, J., Camporota, L., Daxon, B., et al. (2020). Prevention and treatment of acute lung injury with time-controlled adaptive ventilation: physiologically informed modification of airway pressure release ventilation. *Ann. Intensive Care* 10:3. doi: 10.1186/s13613-019-0619-3

No Authors List. (1990a). High-frequency oscillatory ventilation compared with conventional mechanical ventilation in the treatment of respiratory failure in preterm infants: assessment of pulmonary function at 9 months of corrected age. HiFi Study Group. *J. Pediatr.* 116, 933–941. doi: 10.1016/s0022-3476(05)80657-2

No Authors List. (1990b). High-frequency oscillatory ventilation compared with conventional intermittent mechanical ventilation in the treatment of respiratory failure in preterm infants: neurodevelopmental status at 16 to 24 months of postterm age. The HIFI Study Group. *J. Pediatr.* 117, 939–946. doi: 10.1016/s0022-3476(05)80142-8

No Authors List. (2000). Supplemental Therapeutic Oxygen for Prethreshold Retinopathy Of Prematurity (STOP-ROP), a randomized, controlled trial. Irimary outcomes. *Pediatrics* 105, 295–310.

Papastamelos, C., Panitch, H. B., England, S. E., and Allen, J. L. (1995). Developmental changes in chest wall compliance in infancy and early childhood. *J. Appl. Physiol.* 78, 179–184. doi: 10.1152/jappl.1995.78.1.179

Patel, D. S., Sharma, A., Prendergast, M., Rafferty, G. F., and Greenough, A. (2009). Work of breathing and different levels of volume-targeted ventilation. *Pediatrics* 123, e679–e684. doi: 10.1542/peds.2008-2635

Paviotti, G., Bua, J., Cunto, A. De, Travan, L., and Demarini, S. (2014). High-frequency percussive ventilation as rescue treatment in severe hypoxemic respiratory failure in term neonates. *J. Crit. Care* 29, 662–663. doi: 10.1016/j.jcrc.2014.02.018

Pediatric Acute Lung Injury Consensus Conference Group. (2015). Pediatric acute respiratory distress syndrome: consensus recommendations from the Pediatric Acute Lung Injury Consensus Conference. *Pediatr. Crit. Care Med.* 16, 428–439.

Pellicano, A., Tingay, D. G., Mills, J. F., Fasulakis, S., Morley, C. J., and Dargaville, P. A. (2009). Comparison of four methods of lung volume recruitment during high frequency oscillatory ventilation. *Intensive Care Med.* 35, 1990–1998. doi: 10.1007/s00134-009-1628-8

Pfenninger, J., and Gerber, A. C. (1987). High-frequency ventilation (HFV) in hyaline membrane disease–a preliminary report. *Intensive Care Med.* 13, 71–75. doi: 10.1007/BF00263563

Pfenninger, J., and Minder, C. (1988). Pressure-volume curves, static compliances and gas exchange in hyaline membrane disease during conventional mechanical and high-frequency ventilation. *Intensive Care Med.* 14, 364–372. doi: 10.1007/BF00262890

Pillow, J. J. (2015). Oscillatory Ventilator Performance: what Does It Mean? *Neonatology* 108, 229–232. doi: 10.1159/000438693

Pillow, J. J., Wilkinson, M. H., Neil, H. L., and Ramsden, C. A. (2001). In vitro performance characteristics of high-frequency oscillatory ventilators. *Am. J. Respir. Crit. Care Med.* 164, 1019–1024.

Renesme, L., de la Roque, E. D., Germain, C., Chevrier, A., Rebola, M., Cramaregeas, S., et al. (2020). Nasal high-frequency percussive ventilation vs nasal continuous positive airway pressure in newborn infants respiratory distress: a cross over clinical trial. *Pediatr. Pulmonol.* 55, 2617–2623. doi: 10.1002/ppul.24935

Renesme, L., Elleau, C., Nolent, P., Fayon, M., Marthan, R., and De La Roque, E. D. (2013). Effect of high-frequency oscillation and percussion versus conventional ventilation in a piglet model of meconium aspiration. *Pediatr. Pulmonol.* 48, 257–264. doi: 10.1002/ppul.22590

Reper, P., Wibaux, O., Laeke, P. V., Vandeenen, D., Duinslaeger, L., and Vanderkelen, A. (2002). High frequency percussive ventilation and conventional ventilation after smoke inhalation: a randomised study. *Burns* 28, 503–508. doi: 10.1016/s0305-4179(02)00051-7

Rizkalla, N. A., Dominick, C. L., Fitzgerald, J. C., Thomas, N. J., and Yehya, N. (2014). High-frequency percussive ventilation improves oxygenation and ventilation in pediatric patients with acute respiratory failure. *J. Crit. Care* 29, e1–e7. doi: 10.1016/j.jcrc.2013.11.009

Samransamruajkit, R., Rassameehirun, C., Pongsanon, K., Huntrakul, S., Deerojanawong, J., Sritippayawan, S., et al. (2016). A comparison of clinical efficacy between high frequency oscillatory ventilation and conventional ventilation with lung volume recruitment in pediatric acute respiratory distress syndrome: a randomized controlled trial. *Indian J. Crit. Care Med.* 20, 72–77. doi: 10.4103/0972-5229.175940

Sanchez Luna, M., Gonzalez, M. S., and Cortijo, F. T. (2013). High-frequency oscillatory ventilation combined with volume guarantee in a neonatal animal model of respiratory distress syndrome. *Crit. Care Res. Pract.* 2013:593915. doi: 10.1155/2013/593915

Santschi, M., Jouvet, P., Leclerc, F., Gauvin, F., Newth, C. J., Carroll, C. L., et al. (2010). Acute lung injury in children: therapeutic practice and feasibility of international clinical trials. *Pediatr. Crit. Care Med.* 11, 681–689. doi: 10.1097/PCC.0b013e3181d904c0

Schouten, L. R., Veltkamp, F., Bos, A. P., van Woensel, J. B., Neto, A. Serpa, Schultz, M. J., et al. (2016). Incidence and Mortality of Acute Respiratory Distress Syndrome in Children: a Systematic Review and Meta-Analysis. *Crit. Care Med.* 44, 819–829. doi: 10.1097/CCM.0000000000001388

Schultz, T. R., Costarino, A. J. A., Durning, S. M., Napoli, L. A., Schears, G., Godinez, R. I., et al. (2001). Airway pressure release ventilation in pediatrics. *Pediatr. Crit. Care Med.* 2, 243–246.

Smallwood, C. D. (2017). P. Boloori-Zadeh, M.R. Silva, and A. Gouldstone, High Oxygen Concentrations Adversely Affect the Performance of Pulmonary Surfactant. *Respir. Care* 62, 1085–1090. doi: 10.4187/respcare.05388

Smith, D. W., Frankel, L. R., Derish, M. T., Moody, R. R., Black, L. E. III, Chipps, B. E., et al. (1993). ., High-frequency jet ventilation in children with the adult respiratory distress syndrome complicated by pulmonary barotrauma. *Pediatr. Pulmonol.* 15, 279–286. doi: 10.1002/ppul.1950150504

Smith, L. S., Gharib, S. A., Frevert, C. W., and Martin, T. R. (2010). Effects of age on the synergistic interactions between lipopolysaccharide and mechanical ventilation in mice. *Am. J. Respir. Cell Mol Biol.* 43, 475–486. doi: 10.1165/rcmb.2009-0039OC

Snoek, K. G., Capolupo, I., van Rosmalen, J., Lde, J. Hout, Vijfhuize, S., Greenough, A., et al. (2016). Conventional Mechanical Ventilation Versus High-frequency Oscillatory Ventilation for Congenital Diaphragmatic Hernia: a Randomized Clinical Trial (The VICI-trial). *Ann. Surg.* 263, 867–874. doi: 10.1097/SLA.0000000000001533

Stock, M. C., Downs, J. B., and Frolicher, D. A. (1987). Airway pressure release ventilation. *Crit. Care Med.* 15, 462–466.

Thome, U. H., Carlo, W. A., and Pohlandt, F. (2005). Ventilation strategies and outcome in randomised trials of high frequency ventilation. *Arch. Dis. Child Fetal. Neonatal. Ed.* 90, F466–F473. doi: 10.1136/adc.2004.068437

Tingay, D. G., John, J., Harcourt, E. R., Black, D., Dargaville, P. A., Mills, J. F., et al. (2015). Are All Oscillators Created Equal? In vitro Performance Characteristics of Eight High-Frequency Oscillatory Ventilators. *Neonatology* 108, 220–228. doi: 10.1159/000431216

Valentine, K. M., Sarnaik, A. A., Sandhu, H. S., and Sarnaik, A. P. (2016). High Frequency Jet Ventilation in Respiratory Failure Secondary to Respiratory Syncytial Virus Infection: a Case Series. *Front. Pediatr.* 4:92. doi: 10.3389/fped.2016.00092

Venegas, J. G., and Fredberg, J. J. (1994). Understanding the pressure cost of ventilation: why does high-frequency ventilation work? *Crit. Care Med.* 22, S49–S57. doi: 10.1097/00003246-199422091-00004

Villar, J. (2005). The use of positive end-expiratory pressure in the management of the acute respiratory distress syndrome. *Minerva Anestesiol.* 71, 265–272.

Weibel, E. R., and Gomez, D. M. (1962). A principle for counting tissue structures on random sections. *J. Appl. Physiol.* 17, 343–348. doi: 10.1152/jappl.1962.17.2.343

Willson, D. F., Thomas, N. J., Markovitz, B. P., Bauman, L. A., DiCarlo, J. V., Pon, S., et al. (2005). Effect of exogenous surfactant (calfactant) in pediatric acute lung injury: a randomized controlled trial. *JAMA* 293, 470–476.

Wiswell, T. E., Graziani, L. J., Kornhauser, M. S., Cullen, J., Merton, D. A., McKee, L., et al. (1996). High-frequency jet ventilation in the early management of respiratory distress syndrome is associated with a greater risk for adverse outcomes. *Pediatrics* 98, 1035–1043.

Wong, J. J., Jit, M., Sultana, R., Mok, Y. H., Yeo, J. G., Koh, J., et al. (2019). Mortality in Pediatric Acute Respiratory Distress Syndrome: a Systematic Review and Meta-Analysis. *J. Intensive Care Med.* 34, 563–571. doi: 10.1177/0885066617705109

Wong, J. J., Liu, S., Dang, H., Anantasit, N., Phan, P. H., Phumeetham, S., et al. (2020). The impact of high frequency oscillatory ventilation on mortality in paediatric acute respiratory distress syndrome. *Crit. Care* 24:31. doi: 10.1186/s13054-020-2741-x

Yehya, N., Topjian, A. A., Lin, R., Berg, R. A., Thomas, N. J., and Friess, S. H. (2014a). High frequency oscillation and airway pressure release ventilation in pediatric respiratory failure. *Pediatr. Pulmonol.* 49, 707–715. doi: 10.1002/ppul.22853

10

Unsuccessful and Successful Clinical Trials in Acute Respiratory Distress Syndrome: Addressing Physiology-Based Gaps

Jesús Villar[1,2,3], Carlos Ferrando[1,4,5], Gerardo Tusman[6], Lorenzo Berra[7,8], Pedro Rodríguez-Suárez[9] and Fernando Suárez-Sipmann[1,10,11]*

[1] CIBER de Enfermedades Respiratorias, Instituto de Salud Carlos III, Madrid, Spain, [2] Multidisciplinary Organ Dysfunction Evaluation Research Network (MODERN), Research Unit, Hospital Universitario Dr. Negrín, Las Palmas de Gran Canaria, Spain, [3] Keenan Research Center at the Li Ka Shing Knowledge Institute, St. Michael's Hospital, Toronto, ON, Canada, [4] Department of Anesthesiology and Critical Care, Hospital Clinic, Barcelona, Spain, [5] Institut d'Investigacions Biomèdiques August Pi i Sunyer (IDIBAPS), Hospital Clinic, Barcelona, Spain, [6] Department of Anesthesiology, Hospital Privado de Comunidad, Mar del Plata, Argentina, [7] Harvard Medical School, Boston, MA, United States, [8] Department of Anesthesia, Critical Care and Pain Medicine, Massachusetts General Hospital, Boston, MA, United States, [9] Department of Thoracic Surgery, Hospital Universitario Dr. Negrín, Las Palmas de Gran Canaria, Spain, [10] Intensive Care Unit, Hospital Universitario La Princesa, Madrid, Spain, [11] Hedenstierna Laboratory, Department of Surgical Sciences, Anesthesiology and Critical Care, Uppsala University Hospital, Uppsala, Sweden

***Correspondence:**
Jesús Villar
jesus.villar54@gmail.com

The acute respiratory distress syndrome (ARDS) is a severe form of acute hypoxemic respiratory failure caused by an insult to the alveolar-capillary membrane, resulting in a marked reduction of aerated alveoli, increased vascular permeability and subsequent interstitial and alveolar pulmonary edema, reduced lung compliance, increase of physiological dead space, and hypoxemia. Most ARDS patients improve their systemic oxygenation, as assessed by the ratio between arterial partial pressure of oxygen and inspired oxygen fraction, with conventional intensive care and the application of moderate-to-high levels of positive end-expiratory pressure. However, in some patients hypoxemia persisted because the lungs are markedly injured, remaining unresponsive to increasing the inspiratory fraction of oxygen and positive end-expiratory pressure. For decades, mechanical ventilation was the only standard support technique to provide acceptable oxygenation and carbon dioxide removal. Mechanical ventilation provides time for the specific therapy to reverse the disease-causing lung injury and for the recovery of the respiratory function. The adverse effects of mechanical ventilation are direct consequences of the changes in pulmonary airway pressures and intrathoracic volume changes induced by the repetitive mechanical cycles in a diseased lung. In this article, we review 14 major successful and unsuccessful randomized controlled trials conducted in patients with ARDS on a series of techniques to improve oxygenation and ventilation published since 2010. Those trials tested the effects of adjunctive therapies (neuromuscular blocking agents, prone positioning), methods for selecting the optimum positive end-expiratory pressure (after recruitment maneuvers, or guided by esophageal pressure), high-frequency oscillatory ventilation, extracorporeal oxygenation, and pharmacologic immune modulators of the pulmonary and systemic inflammatory responses in patients affected by ARDS. We will briefly comment physiology-based gaps of negative trials and highlight the possible needs to address in future clinical trials in ARDS.

Keywords: acute respiratory distress syndrome, clinical trials, neuromuscular blockade, prone ventilation, high-frequency ventilation, positive end-expiratory pressure, extracorporeal oxygenation, anti-inflammatory drugs

BACKGROUND

The acute respiratory distress syndrome (ARDS) is a severe form of acute hypoxemic respiratory failure. Caused by an intense direct (pulmonary) or indirect (systemic) inflammatory insult to the alveolar-capillary membrane, it is characterized by the presence of diffuse, non-cardiogenic, high-permeability, protein-rich pulmonary edema, and hypoxemia unresponsive to the application of high inspiratory concentrations of oxygen (FiO_2) (Villar, 2011). The use of mechanical ventilation (MV) is the standard supportive therapy of patients with ARDS. Since the publication in 2000 of the milestone paper by the ARDS Network (Acute Respiratory Distress Syndrome Network, Brower et al., 2000), the aim of MV is to achieve adequate gas-exchange avoiding damaging the lungs by using physiological tidal volumes (VT) of 4–8 ml/kg predicted body weight (PBW), preventing alveolar collapse with positive end-expiratory pressure (PEEP), limiting end-inspiratory plateau pressure (Pplat) to less than 30 cmH_2O, and limiting FiO_2 to maintain an adequate PaO_2. These essential elements are the main components of the framework for lung-protective MV.

INTRODUCTION

Most ARDS patients improve their oxygenation, as assessed by the ratio between the arterial partial pressure of oxygen (PaO_2) and FiO_2 (PaO_2/FiO_2), disease-specific treatment and the application of adequate levels of PEEP. There is no typical ARDS patient. Over the years, hypoxemia has become an infrequent cause of death in ARDS (Slutsky et al., 2016). Physiologically, we are unaware of data linking a specific PaO_2/FiO_2 to predictable morphological changes in the alveolar-capillary membrane at ARDS onset. Recent evidence has shown an association between severity of lung damage and prediction of outcome when the PaO_2/FiO_2 is evaluated at 24 h under standardized ventilator settings using an enrichment strategy (Villar et al., 2019). We lack a standard definition for refractory or persisting hypoxemia, as a predetermined PaO_2 value under a particular FiO_2 and PEEP for a specific time-period. In this review, we will consider hypoxemia for enrolling patients into clinical trials when the PaO_2/FiO_2 is ≤ 200 mmHg on MV and PEEP ≥ 5 cmH_2O, in agreement with the Berlin criteria for moderate-to-severe ARDS (Ranieri et al., 2012). The purpose of this brief review is to summarize the current knowledge based on a number of major randomized controlled trials (RCTs) performed in ARDS patients on MV evaluating interventions applied during the acute phase and published since 2010, independent of whether they reported benefits or not in the primary or secondary outcomes when testing the experimental intervention. Those RCTs were conducted with the aim to improve oxygenation and mortality while the patient was in the intensive care unit (ICU) or after being discharged from ICU. We will discuss the physiology-based gaps of negative trials and highlight the possible needs to address in future trials design in ARDS.

REVIEW OF RANDOMIZED CONTROLLED TRIALS

Since 2010, 14 major RCTs (Papazian et al., 2010; Gao Smith et al., 2012; Ferguson et al., 2013; Guerin et al., 2013; Young et al., 2013; McAuley et al., 2014; Kacmarek et al., 2016; Working group for the Alveolar Recruitment for Acute Respiratory Distress Syndrome Trial (Art) Investigators et al., 2017; Combes et al., 2018; Beitler et al., 2019; Hodgson et al., 2019; The National Heart, Lung, and Blood Institute Petal Clinical Trials Network, Moss et al., 2019; Ranieri et al., 2020; Villar et al., 2020) have been published in patients with ARDS (**Table 1**). In those trials, patients received invasive MV and tested different adjunctive or rescue therapies for improving oxygenation, or different MV approaches to titrate PEEP, or several anti-inflammatory drugs for attenuating the pulmonary and systemic inflammatory responses.

Muscle Paralysis

There is sufficient evidence showing that MV can initiate or aggravate lung injury, a concept labeled as ventilator-induced lung injury (VILI) (Slutsky and Ranieri, 2013). Many of the consequences of VILI bear a resemblance to those of ARDS. Despite limiting VT and pressures during lung-protective MV, ARDS patients could develop tidal hyperinflation during spontaneous respiratory efforts while mechanically ventilated, especially in the early phases of ARDS. VT set in the ventilator does not always correspond to the exact VT delivered to the patient, due to the contribution of inspiratory muscle efforts to inflation pressure and more importantly in the presence of double triggering, reverse triggering, and other types of patient-ventilator asynchronies, which could develop despite receiving deep analgesia or sedation. Papazian et al. (2010) conducted an RCT, the *ARDS et Curarisation Systematique* (ACURASYS) trial, to examine the hypothesis that removing spontaneous respiratory efforts would improve lung mechanics and oxygenation in patients with persistent hypoxemia. It was known that neuromuscular blockade (NMB) decreases the work of breathing and asynchronies in ARDS (Light et al., 1975).

TABLE 1 | Successful and unsuccessful randomized clinical trials since 2010 in ventilated patients with acute respiratory distress syndrome (ARDS).

References publication year	Trial name	Study period, No. ICUs, Country	Criteria for enrollment	Patients	Intervention	Major findings	Remarks
Papazian et al. (2010)	ACURASYS	2006–2008 (24 months) 20 ICUs, France	MV, $PaO_2/FiO_2 < 150$ with PEEP ≥ 5 for < 48 h	340	Neuromuscular blockers (cisatracurium)	Improved adjusted 90-day mortality and VFDs	Control group was deeply sedated
Gao Smith et al. (2012)	BALTI-2	2006–2010 (40 months) 46 ICUs, UK	MV, within 72 h of ARDS onset (AECC criteria)	326	Salbutamol	Salbutamol worsen outcomes	Concerns for use of non-protective MV
Guerin et al. (2013)	PROSEVA	2008–2011 (41 months) 27 ICUs France, Spain	MV < 36 h, $PaO_2/FiO_2 < 150$ on $FiO_2 \geq 0.6$ confirmed at 12–24 MV	466	Prone positioning for at least 12 h/daily	Decreased 28-day and 90-day mortality	Currently, it is standard of care in severe ARDS
Ferguson et al. (2013)	OSCILLATE	2009–2012 (38 months) 39 ICUs in Canada, United States, Saudi Arabia, Chile, India	MV, $PaO_2/FiO_2 \leq 200$ on $FiO_2 \geq 0.5$ and PEEP ≥ 10	548	High-frequency oscillation ventilation (HFOV)	Increased ICU and hospital mortality	Increasing harm from HFOV at higher PaO_2/FiO_2
Young et al. (2013)	OSCAR	2007–2012 (55 months) 29 ICUs, UK	MV, AECC criteria, $PaO_2/FiO_2 \leq 200$ on PEEP ≥ 5	795	High-frequency oscillation (HFOV)	No change in 30-day mortality	HFOV increased harm at higher PaO_2/FiO_2
McAuley et al. (2014)	HARP-2	2010–2014 (39 months) 40 hospitals in UK and Ireland	MV, < 48 h from ARDS onset, $PaO_2/FiO_2 \leq 300$ (AECC criteria)	540	Simvastatin	No effects on outcomes	Concerns for use of non-protective MV
Kacmarek et al. (2016)	OLA	2007–2013 (59 months) 20 ICUs in Spain, South Korea, Brazil	MV, $PaO_2/FiO_2 \leq 200$ (AECC criteria). At 24 h, $PaO_2/FiO_2 \leq 200$ on $FiO_2 \geq 0.5$ and PEEP ≥ 10	200	Open lung approach (lung recruitment and PEEP titration)	Increased oxygenation and decreased driving pressure. No change in ICU mortality	Prognostic enrichment for enrollment at 12–36 h after ARDS onset
Working group for the Alveolar Recruitment for Acute Respiratory Distress Syndrome Trial (Art) Investigators et al. (2017)	ART	2011–2017 (65 months) 120 ICUs in Brazil, Argentina, Colombia, Italy, Poland, Portugal, Malaysia, Spain, Uruguay	MV, ARDS (AECC criteria) < 72 h, enrollment if $PaO_2/FiO_2 \leq 200$ on PEEP ≥ 10 and $FiO_2 = 1$ for 30 min	1,010	Open lung approach (lung recruitment and PEEP titration)	Increased 28-day and 6-month mortality. Decreased VFDs. Increased risk of barotrauma	Concerns with study design, methodology, data analysis, and differences in health care systems
Combes et al. (2018)	EOLIA	2012–2017 (55 months) 23 ICUs in France, Canada, United States	Very severe ARDS: $PaO_2/FiO_2 < 50$ for > 3 h; or $PaO_2/FiO_2 \leq 80$ for > 6 h; or pH < 7.25 with $PaCO_2 \geq 60$ for > 6 h	249	Extracorporeal membrane oxygenation (ECMO)	No significant benefit in 60-day mortality	Control group included crossover to ECMO in 28% patients
The National Heart, Lung, and Blood Institute Petal Clinical Trials Network, Moss et al. (2019)	ROSE	2016–2018 (28 months) 48 hospitals in United States	MV, $PaO_2/FiO_2 < 150$ with PEEP ≥ 8 for < 48 h	1,006	Neuromuscular blockers (cisatracurium)	No significant benefit in 90-day mortality	Control group with lighter sedation
Beitler et al. (2019)	EPVent-2	2012–2017 (59 months) 14 hospitals in United States	MV, $PaO_2/FiO_2 \leq 200$ within 36 h ARDS onset (Berlin criteria)	200	Esophageal pressure-guided for titrating PEEP	No significant benefit in 28-day mortality and VFDs	Median PEEP levels was similar in both groups over time
Hodgson et al. (2019)	PHARLAP	2012–2017 (59 months) 35 ICUs in Australia, New Zealand, Ireland, Saudi Arabia, UK	MV < 72 h, ARDS or other types of respiratory failure with $PaO_2/FiO_2 \leq 200$ on PEEP ≥ 5	113	Lung recruitment maneuvers with PEEP titration	No benefits in VFDs or ICU/hospital mortality	Small sample size, PEEP titration used SpO_2, and treatment crossovers
Ranieri et al. (2020)	INTEREST	2015–2017 (25 months) 74 ICUs, 8 European countries	MV, $PaO_2/FiO_2 \leq 200$ PEEP ≥ 5 (Berlin criteria) within 24 h	301	Interferon β-1a	No significant benefit in 28-day mortality and VFDs	Higher-than-expected use of corticosteroids
Villar et al. (2020)	DEXA-ARDS	2013–2018 (69 months) 17 ICUs, Spain	MV, $PaO_2/FiO_2 \leq 200$ at ARDS onset; at 24 h, $PaO_2/FiO_2 \leq 200$ on $FiO_2 \geq 0.5$ and PEEP ≥ 10	277	Dexamethasone	Increased VFDs. Decreased 60-day mortality	Prognostic enrichment for enrollment at 24 h of ARDS onset

AECC, American-European Consensus Conference; ICU, intensive care unit; MV, mechanical ventilation; PEEP, positive end-expiratory pressure; SpO_2, oxygen saturation; UK, United Kingdom; VFDs, ventilator-free days.

The ACURASYS trial enrolled 340 ARDS patients with moderate-to-severe ARDS (defined by the investigators as a $PaO_2/FiO_2 < 150$ mmHg on PEEP ≥ 5 cmH_2O during the first 2 days of ARDS diagnosis). Patients were randomized to receive either cisatracurium or placebo for 48 h. Patients in the control arm were deeply sedated. The authors found that in patients assigned to NMB, the adjusted 90-day mortality was lower and ventilator free-days (VFDs) were higher than in those not receiving NMB.

The findings of the ACURASYS remained controversial for almost a decade for two reasons: the Kaplan-Meir survival curves of the two treatment arms separated only after 14 days of randomization, and, most importantly, the 90-day all-cause mortality only reached statistical significance with intensity adjustment (Yegneswaran and Murugan, 2011). Thus, additional validation of this trial was required. A RCT termed "*Reevaluation Of Systemic Early neuromuscular blockade (ROSE) trial*" (The National Heart, Lung, and Blood Institute Petal Clinical Trials Network, Moss et al., 2019) was unable to validate ACURASYS results. The ROSE trial was powered for evaluating the efficacy and safety of NMB in decreasing 90-day mortality. The trial stopped for futility when 1006 ARDS patients were enrolled. Although this trial was not an exact replication of ACURACYS (since both arms of the trial received PEEP ≥ 8 cmH_2O, and the control arm received lighter sedation targets), there were no differences between groups in the rate of barotrauma and in the number of VFDs, and 90-day mortality was virtually identical in the two groups.

What are the implications of these two RCTs? First, according to these results routine use of NMB agents are not recommended in moderate-to-severe ARDS patients. Contrary to expectations, the prevalence of patient-ventilator asynchronies in the form of reverse triggering (it occurs when a breath delivered by the ventilator triggers diaphragm contraction, initiating an assisted breath –the reverse of what occurs during assisted MV) increases with deeper sedation levels (Bourenne et al., 2019). Second, from a pathophysiological point of view, there is a basis to use NMB in any patient with ARDS when after ensuring an adequate ventilation and sedation, the patient has a ventilatory pattern that could promote VILI. Therefore, current data suggest that NMB agents can be used when they are physiologically and clinically indicated (Slutsky and Villar, 2019).

Prone Ventilation

Patho-physiologically and histo-pathologically, ARDS is a heterogeneous inflammatory process produced by a variety of insults with collapsed and consolidated areas mainly in the dependent regions, and more healthy units in the non-dependent regions (Villar, 2011). Thus, recruitability of alveolar spaces in ARDS lungs with PEEP is also heterogeneous, both between patients and within the lungs. Changes in body posture could have marked effects on pulmonary function in patients with acute respiratory failure. As normal practice, the critically ill patient is cared for in supine. The usual reduction in function residual capacity (FRC) when adopting the supine position is increased in ARDS ventilated patients, resulting in ventilation-perfusion mismatching and a fall in the PaO_2. Five mechanisms have been proposed to explain the improved oxygenation during prone positioning: (i) increased FRC, (ii) changes in regional diaphragm motion, (iii) improved ventilation-perfusion matching due to a redistribution of regional ventilation to dorsal regions of the lung, (iv) improved clearance of secretions, and (v) removal of the weight of the heart from the lung (Lamm et al., 1994).

Prone ventilation is considered an adjunctive intervention to the ventilatory management of ARDS patients with refractory hypoxemia. Prone ventilation can be performed safely if ICU teams are adequately trained. After several studies reported conflicting results about the efficacy of prone ventilation in persistent hypoxemia, a large RCT, the "*Proning Severe ARDS patients" (PROSEVA)* trial (Guerin et al., 2013), reported survival benefit in moderate-to-severe ARDS. In that trial, 466 patients with persistent ARDS (as defined by a $PaO_2/FiO_2 < 150$ mmHg with $FiO_2 \geq 0.6$ and PEEP ≥ 5 cmH_2O) were randomly assigned to prone position for at least 16 h or to supine position. Patients in both groups were mechanically ventilated following the low PEEP-FiO_2 table from the ARDSnet trial (Acute Respiratory Distress Syndrome Network, Brower et al., 2000). All-cause mortality at 28 days was 33% in the supine group and 16% in the prone group, a highly significant difference that persisted 90 days after randomization.

Proponents of prone ventilation advise that the approach of the PROSEVA trial was a modification of a technique that finally became right at a time when patients were mechanically ventilated with low VT (Beitler et al., 2014). However, although prone positioning improves oxygenation in ARDS patients and could help in recruiting lung regions, there is controversy over its use in clinical practice (Villar et al., 2014). The large treatment effect seems too good to be true: a 28-day mortality of 16% is the lowest, ever reported in a trial, or in any observational study on ARDS. Furthermore, patients assigned to the supine group were mechanically ventilated during the first 72 h with low levels of PEEP (9 ± 3 cmH_2O). Therefore, as with NMB, an additional RCT is required to confirm these findings. Such a trial should guarantee that the control group will receive a higher PEEP approach.

High Frequency Oscillatory Ventilation

Knowledge on the mechanisms and importance of VILI has advanced over the years. Theoretically, from the perspective of lung-protective ventilation, high frequency oscillatory ventilation (HFOV) would be an ideal mode of ventilation for ARDS patients (Ferguson et al., 2007). By definition, it accomplishes adequate gas-exchange by providing very small VT that are typically 1–3 ml/kg, often less than the anatomic dead space, at frequencies from 3 to 15 cycles per second at a constant mean airway pressure. Since HFOV incorporates fewer and simpler controls that are not interrelated, it is an easier technique than conventional MV. However, there is a lack of evidence showing that HFOV is less harmful that using MV with low VT, moderate-to-high PEEP, and limitation of Pplat.

A critical examination of two RCTs comparing HFOV with lung-protective MV published in 2013 (enrolling 1343 ARDS patients) demonstrated no benefits of HFOV. In the OSCILLATE (*OSCILLation for Acute respiratory distress syndrome Treated*

Early) trial (Ferguson et al., 2013), the investigators stopped the trial after 548 of the 1,200 planned patients were randomized. Patients were eligible for inclusion if they had a $PaO_2/FiO_2 \leq 200$ mmHg on $FiO_2 \geq 0.5$. However, only patients with a $PaO_2/FiO_2 \leq 200$ after 30 min of assessment on a VT of 6 ml/kg PBW, PEEP ≥ 10 and FiO_2 of 0.6 were randomized. Patients in the HFOV group received HFOV after lung recruitment with an "open lung approach" (OLA) consisting in the application of a recruitment maneuver (RM) of 40 cmH_2O of pressure for 40 s for a median of 3 days. However, almost 15% of patients in the control group received HFOV as a rescue therapy. The absolute hospital mortality was 12% higher in the HFOV group (relative risk of death 1.33, $p = 0.005$). The relatively high mortality in the HFOV group could be explained by the higher prevalence of hemodynamic compromise (hypotension) after the initiation of HFOV, contributing to extrapulmonary organ dysfunction, and by increased use of sedative agents. In the OSCAR (*OSCillation in ARDS*) trial (Young et al., 2013), the study design was more pragmatic. The authors randomized 795 patients with a $PaO_2/FiO_2 \leq 200$ on PEEP ≥ 5 cmH_2O. Patients in the HFOV arm were ventilated by increasing mean airway pressure and FiO_2. The control group was treated according to local practice in participating ICUs, applying the low PEEP-FiO_2 table from the ARDSnet trial (Acute Respiratory Distress Syndrome Network, Brower et al., 2000). There were no differences in 30-day mortality between the groups.

What are the implications of these two trials? In a recent meta-analysis of 1,552 ARDS patients from four RCTs (Meade et al., 2017), including those from OSCILLATE and OSCAR trials, the investigators reported a significant interaction between PaO_2/FiO_2 at randomization and the effects of HFOV, revealing increased harm from HFOV at higher PaO_2/FiO_2. Although HFOV still have a place as a rescue therapy, especially in centers without access or experience in extracorporeal oxygenation, this meta-analysis strongly question its future use in ARDS (Vincent, 2017).

Recruitment Maneuvers and Transpulmonary Pressure

Therapeutic variation in the distribution of inspired gas for attenuating VILI is the foundation of both prone ventilation and RMs. With the use of computed tomography (CT), it was discovered that radiographically some lung regions in ARDS look relatively normal but other areas are partially collapsed and do not participate in gas-exchange. RMs are applied to reopen collapsed alveolar units and to attenuate the injurious effects of repetitive opening and closing of alveoli. In general, ARDS is a heterogeneous injury in three lung compartments (Nieman et al., 2020): (i) normal alveoli that are inflated at end of expiration –and is referred to as the "baby lung" (Gattinoni and Pesenti, 2005); (ii) alveoli that are collapsed and/or fluid filled; (iii) and alveoli that are in between normal and unstable, and that open and collapse with every breath. Of note, the "baby lung" concept led to the understanding of potential interaction between MV settings and outcome, and to the frequent use of CT as a standard tool for a more precise ventilatory management in ARDS patients. As a result, lung-protective MV is constrained by ventilating this heterogeneous lung to avoid VILI, by protecting the baby lung without overdistending the compliant lung, and by stabilizing the lung using PEEP. Compliance is a property that describes lung distensibility and is calculated as the change in lung volume divided by the change in pressure. Lung compliance of the respiratory system is calculated as the VT divided by the transpulmonary pressure, the pressure across the lung (or alveolar pressure minus pleural pressure) (Kacmarek et al., 2021). Atelectatic areas of the lungs can be expanded by a brief application of high transpulmonary pressure, followed by a PEEP level that maintains open the new re-aerated region (Suárez-Sipmann et al., 2007). PEEP prevents lung collapse at end expiration. Although there are three commonly used RMs (sighs, sustained inflations, and extended sighs) (Guerin et al., 2011), none of these three maneuvers are currently recommended. In fact, none of the above trials used those maneuvers, but favored the use of incremental PEEP steps maintaining a constant driving pressure (Pplat minus PEEP) in a pressure-controlled mode until the recruitment pressures are reached.

There is controversy about the outcome benefits of RMs in patients with ARDS. In a pilot RCT in 200 patients with persistent ARDS (Kacmarek et al., 2016) comparing the ARDSnet protocol (Acute Respiratory Distress Syndrome Network, Brower et al., 2000) with an OLA approach involving RMs and a decremental PEEP trial for identifying the level of PEEP associated with maximum dynamic compliance, OLA improved oxygenation and lung mechanics without harmful effects on all-cause mortality at 60 days, VFDs, or barotrauma. In a large RCT (Working group for the Alveolar Recruitment for Acute Respiratory Distress Syndrome Trial (Art) Investigators et al., 2017), the *Alveolar Recruitment for acute respiratory distress syndrome Trial (ART)* conducted at 120 ICUs in 9 countries (mostly from Brazil) and involving 1010 patients with moderate to severe ARDS, RMs and PEEP titration according to best respiratory system compliance did not show reduced 28-day mortality when compared to patients treated with lower levels of PEEP. By contrary, patients in the RMs group had higher 6-month mortality, lower VFDs, and increased risk of barotrauma. After the publication of the negative results of the ART trial, the *Permissive Hypercapnia, Alveolar Recruitment, and Low Airway Pressure (PHARLAP)* trial (Hodgson et al., 2019) evaluating the effects of an OLA strategy with RMs vs. lung-protective MV was stopped very early when only 113 patients with moderate-to-severe ARDS were randomized (of a planned 340 patients). This small sample size trial (57 patients in the RM group vs. 56 in the control group) had no power to identify differences in VFDs, risk of barotrauma, or 180-day mortality.

Although the findings of the ART trial do not support the routine application of RMs, major concerns about study design, methodology, data analyses, and important differences with health care systems in participating countries, provided solid reasons to distrust the results of the trial and their generalizability to other settings (Villar et al., 2017). Patho-physiologically, there is a rationale for using RM and PEEP titration in ARDS since the ART results are in conflict with previous physiological and clinical data. There is a need for another RCT designed and implemented more appropriately to examine that the principle that "never give the lungs a chance to collapse" (Villar et al., 2017) is associated with better clinical benefits, although all-cause fatality rate might not be reduced further.

A newer technique for titrating PEEP is optimizing the transpulmonary pressure at end of expiration (PEEP minus pleural pressure) (Talmor et al., 2008). Pleural pressure is estimated *via* esophageal manometry employing the measurement of esophageal pressure at the end of expiration, as a surrogate estimate of pleural pressure. It differs among patients with hypoxemic acute respiratory failure, suggesting that lung and chest wall mechanics contribute to respiratory system mechanics, as measured by the mechanical ventilator (Kacmarek et al., 2021). In general, the transpulmonary end-expiratory pressure is equal to zero: the more negative the transpulmonary pressure, the greater the collapse caused by a reduction in lung compliance. A negative transpulmonary pressure reflects that the forces trying to collapse the lung are stronger than the forces maintaining the lung open. This process may reverse if the end-expiratory transpulmonary pressure becomes zero or positive (Fumagalli et al., 2017). That is the main rationale for applying PEEP. PEEP increases the alveolar pressure. When alveolar pressure is equal to or exceeds pleural pressure, the resulting transpulmonary pressure is positive. This mechanism reduces lung collapse if the lung is opened before applying PEEP. That is why performing a RM and setting the appropriate level of PEEP by a decremental titration, augments FRC, decreases atelectasis, improves oxygenation, and increases compliance when compared with the same incremental PEEP level without recruitment (Pirrone et al., 2016).

A multicenter trial (EPVent-2) (Beitler et al., 2019) to validate preliminary results of a previous pilot study on esophageal pressure-guided ventilation (Talmor et al., 2008) was conducted in 200 patients with moderate-to-severe ARDS and examined whether PEEP titration guided by esophageal pressure is more effective than PEEP using a modified PEEP-FiO_2 table adopted from the OSCILLATE trial (Ferguson et al., 2013) using higher PEEP values. The primary outcome was a composite score including mortality and VFDs, calculated in a way that death was a worse outcome than fewer days free of MV. However, values for esophageal end-expiratory pressure, PEEP, Pplat, driving pressure, and PaO_2/FiO_2 were similar between both groups within the first 7 days. Although patients allocated to esophageal pressure-guided PEEP received fewer rescue therapies, the primary endpoint was not different between groups. Although for the investigators these findings did not support the use of PEEP titration using esophageal manometry, there are several reasons that could explain a lack of benefits of this trial (Suarez-Sipmann et al., 2019). First, in the multicenter EPVent-2 trial, participating centers had a wide range of expertise in implementing this novel method, as contrary to the high expertise of investigators in the previous EPVent trial. Second, the study design was not a true validation of the tested hypothesis in the EPVent since the EPVent-2 incorporated the PEEP-FiO_2 table using much higher PEEP levels, and oxygenation was not the primary outcome. This led to similar mean values of PEEP and transpulmonary pressures in both groups, suggesting that, on average, both groups were ventilated similarly! Third, the trial was underpowered: the calculation of the trial sample size was based on an overestimated 22% absolute difference in 28-day mortality. Fourth, a major critique relates to the PEEP titration method. Linking the transpulmonary pressure to the oxygenation level by a non-physiological PEEP-FiO_2 table was an erroneous decision to assess the effects of PEEP in the esophageal manometry group. Changes in oxygenation could not parallel changes in lung mechanics. For example, in the control group patients requiring $FiO_2 \geq 0.5$ could be ventilated with PEEP > 16 cmH_2O, a level that exceeds by far what is considered usual care. On the other hand, there is no guarantee that esophageal pressure recordings were checked for quality control in most participating centers. Fifth, it is plausible that the trial was biased in favor of the control group since both groups were monitored with an esophageal catheter.

A recent *post-hoc* reanalysis of the EPVent-2 trial by the same authors (Sarge et al., 2021) showed that the effect of PEEP strategy on mortality depended on pre-intervention severity of multiorgan dysfunction. Esophageal manometry-guided PEEP was associated with lower mortality among patients with less severe multiorgan dysfunction. Intriguingly, the higher end-inspiratory transpulmonary pressure, a marker of tidal overdistension, was independently correlated with risk of circulatory shock. Future clinical trials should be designed to consider baseline both, esophageal pressure at the end of expiration (to minimize the development of atelectasis) and esophageal pressure at the end of inspiration (to minimize the development of overdistension).

Extracorporeal Membrane Oxygenation

Oxygenation using extracorporeal life support was initially used in patients with severe acute respiratory failure in whom it was impossible to provide adequate gas-exchange by MV (Egan et al., 1988). MV is dependent on the presence of functional lung units for gas diffusion. However, when the number of functional alveoli is markedly reduced, MV is unable to sustain gas-exchange. In those cases, replacing the alveolar gas-exchange by extracorporeal membrane oxygenation (ECMO) can substantially reduce VT, respiratory rate, and FiO_2, and the risk of developing VILI. Most adult ECMO for respiratory support are performed with a veno-venous technique (Munshi et al., 2019). To deliver gas-exchange during ECMO, part of the cardiac output goes through the extracorporeal circuit *via* the femoral, saphenous, or jugular veins. CO_2 is removed by the ECMO circuit while MV is applied at low respiratory rates, high levels of PEEP, and Pplat below 30 cmH_2O by applying very low VTs.

Today, ECMO equipment are simpler, cheaper, and safer. Despite advances in extracorporeal life support and worldwide clinical use of ECMO, the results of a recent RCT in ARDS patients (Combes et al., 2018) has led to a diminished enthusiasm for using it in severe ARDS. Referred to as the EOLIA (*ECMO to rescue Lung Injury in severe ARDS*) trial, this international RCT examined the effects of early use of ECMO in patients with very severe ARDS (**Table 1**). Patients assigned to the control group received MV, and the use of NMB agents, prone positioning, RMs, inhaled nitric oxide, or prostacyclin were strongly encouraged for oxygenation objectives by protocol. Patients assigned to ECMO underwent percutaneous veno-venous cannulation. The data safety monitoring board of the study decided to stop the trial after 75% of the planned patient population had been enrolled because the lower boundary of the predefined stopping rule for futility (defined as < 20% absolute risk reduction in mortality at 60 days) was achieved. The planned sample size was 331 patients, but the trial was terminated when 249 patients were randomized. In retrospect, a 20% absolute risk reduction is an unreasonable very large effect size when calculating sample size. Had the trial been designed with less strict stopping rules and continued to full enrollment, EOLIA may would have reached statistical significance. A major flaw of the trial was that 28% of patients allocated to the control arm (lung protective MV) crossed over to receive ECMO after randomization. This high crossover rate makes it extremely problematic to draw definitive conclusions about the benefits of ECMO in ARDS patients with very severe hypoxemia. Furthermore, the crossover of patients randomized to ECMO in participating ECMO centers could be seen as a weakness since ECMO is not available in most cities of modern countries for treating very severe hypoxemic ARDS.

Despite the results of the EOLIA trial, many clinicians still believe that there is a role for ECMO in severe ARDS patients with single organ failure and potentially reversible pulmonary dysfunction when MV and other adjunctive therapies have failed. Ideally, a comparison among patients who crossed over to ECMO with patients with similar severity randomized to the ECMO group would be an appropriate task to do. However, no such subsets of patients were identified in the ECMO group after a careful systematic review of the EOLIA trial (Munshi et al., 2019).

Pharmacologic Modulators of the Pulmonary and Systemic Inflammatory Responses

Anti-inflammatory drugs have been tested as prophylaxis and/or treatment of ARDS. In 2019, a systematic review provided no conclusive evidence that any pharmacologic intervention could reduce mortality in ARDS patients (Santacruz et al., 2019).

In the last decade in the United Kingdom (UK), two large RCTs (7,11) evaluated pharmacologic therapies to improve outcome in ARDS patients. The BALTI-2 (*beta-2 agonist lung injury trial*) (7) investigated the effects of increasing alveolar water clearance using intravenous salbutamol. This was a multicenter, placebo-controlled, randomized trial at 46 ICUs between 2006 and 2010, where patients within 72 h of ARDS onset, as defined by the American-European Consensus Conference (AECC) criteria (Bernard et al., 1994), were allocated to receive either salbutamol or placebo for 7 days. The primary outcome was death at 28 days of randomization. The trial reported harm in the treatment group and was stopped after the second interim analysis. A total of 324 patients (161 in the salbutamol group vs. 163 in the placebo group) were analyzed. Treatment with salbutamol significantly increased 28-day mortality, and was poorly tolerated. The HARP-2 (*Hydroxymethylglutaryl-CoA reductase inhibition with simvastatin in Acute lung injury to Reduce Pulmonary dysfunction-2*) (11) study tested the use of the anti-inflammatory effects of simvastatin in ARDS. This was a multicenter, double-blind, randomized trial at 40 ICUs from UK and Ireland between 2010 and 2014, where 540 patients within 48 h of ARDS onset, as defined by AECC criteria, were randomized. The primary outcome was the number of VFDs, and secondary outcomes included mortality at 28 days. Treatment with simvastatin was safe, but it did not improve clinical outcomes.

Although the pharmacological mechanisms underlying the increased mortality in patients receiving salbutamol and the no effects of simvastatin are unclear, there are serious concerns about the approach for ventilating ARDS patients in both trials. Despite that leading investigators of both trials recommended the use of lung-protective MV, an audit (Poole et al., 2017) examining the ventilation practice in BALTI-2 and HARP-2 trials found that compliance with the ARDSnet guidelines for VT was very poor across all time points. There was no feedback to participating centers for the MV management in these studies. Baseline data was only available in 49% of patients in the BALTI-2 trial and PEEP levels were not recorded in both trials. This audit analysis revealed that considerably less than half of patients in BALTI-2 and HARP-2 trials received lung protective MV. Given the importance of low VT ventilation in improving outcomes ARDS, the results of those two pharmacologic trials need to be re-examined.

The key pathophysiological event underlying ARDS is injury to both the lung capillary endothelium and the alveolar epithelium with increased pulmonary vascular leakage. It turns out that adenosine has anti-inflammatory properties and reduces endothelial permeability. The enzyme termed cluster of differentiation 73 (CD73) is expressed on endothelial and epithelial cells, and regulates adenosine production by converting extracellular adenosine to active adenosine (Thompson et al., 2004). Since interferon (IFN) β-1a upregulates CD73, preventing vascular leakage, a pilot nonrandomized study reported that treatment with recombinant human IFN-β was associated with a reduction of 28-day mortality in patients with ARDS (Bellingan et al., 2014). In the INTEREST trial (*Efficacy and Safety of Interferon beta-1a in patients with ARDS*), a multicenter, randomized, double-blind, parallel-group in 8 countries, 301 patients with moderate or severe ARDS were randomized to treatment with 10 μg of IFN-1a once daily for 6 days or to placebo (Ranieri et al., 2020). The primary outcome was a composite score combining number of VFDs and number of deaths at 28 days. A total of 296 patients completed the trial, which did not lead to fewer deaths and VFDs when compared to the placebo group. Apart from the lack of efficacy, the trial has two important limitations: (i) the study was underpowered since no enrichment approach was considered to enroll patients; (ii) more than one third of patients received steroids, which inhibit the effects of IFN-β-1a signaling, raising the possibility that the treatment with IFN- β-1a in combination with corticosteroids could increase mortality in ARDS.

Since the first clinical description of ARDS, there has been a great interest in the role of corticosteroids for attenuating the underlying inflammatory state of ARDS because of their potent anti-inflammatory and antifibrotic effects on multiple signaling pathways (Rhen and Cidlowski, 2005). Several doses and types of corticosteroids have been evaluated in the context of ARDS with inconclusive results (Annane et al., 2017). Nevertheless, it is plausible that corticosteroids may benefit ARDS in the early stages of the disease process, a situation that was not evaluated in most RCTs. In addition, dexamethasone was never evaluated in a randomized controlled fashion in ARDS patients, despite its potent anti-inflammatory and weak mineralocorticoid effects. Dexamethasone is 20–30 times more potent than the naturally occurring hormone cortisol and 4–5 times more potent than prednisolone (Rhen and Cidlowski, 2005). In addition, dexamethasone has long-lasting pharmacological effects, allowing for a regime of one dose per day (Meijvis et al., 2011). The beneficial effects of dexamethasone in ARDS were unknown until recently. The DEXA-ARDS (*Dexamethasone in ARDS*) trial, was a multicenter, RCT performed in 277 patients with established moderate-to-severe ARDS (defined by a $PaO_2/FiO_2 \leq 200$ assessed with a PEEP ≥ 10 cmH_2O and $FiO_2 \geq 0.5$ at 24 h after diagnosis of ARDS) (Villar et al., 2020). Patients were randomized to receive treatment with dexamethasone (20 mg once daily from days 1 to 5, which was reduced to 10 mg from days 6 to 10) or continued routine intensive care (control group). The primary outcome was VFDs, and the secondary outcome was mortality at 60 days after randomization. Treatment with dexamethasone markedly increased the number of VFDs and decreased the risk of 60-day mortality by an absolute 15%. These findings paved the road of using steroids to improve survival among critically ill patients with coronavirus disease 19 (COVID-19) (WHO Rapid Evidence Appraisal for Covid-19 Therapies (React) Working Group et al., 2020).

FUTURE TRIAL DESIGN: PERSONALIZED MECHANICAL VENTILATION

The history of interventional clinical trials for ARDS is fraught with many failures and only a few successes in the last decade. Since there is no typical ARDS patient (Villar, 2011), the risk of developing ARDS depends on the underlying disease process but also augments with the number of predisposing factors. Ideally, therapies in ARDS should be personalized to the specific predisposing clinical condition or mechanism of organ injury at any given point in time, rather than being provided uniformly to all patients. The most critical factor in managing ARDS patients is the initiation of lung-protective ventilation instantaneously after endotracheal intubation. However, the development of therapeutic strategies for ARDS is complicated because ARDS is not a disease but a very heterogeneous syndrome (Juschten et al., 2021). The optimal ventilation strategy for ARDS still remains to be refined. For example, the physiological meaning of the end-expiratory transpulmonary pressure could be very useful in managing patients with increased chest wall stiffness or to set optimal PEEP during ventilation and weaning in morbidly obese patients (Kacmarek et al., 2021).

Current lung-protective MV strategies have not significantly decreased ARDS-associated all-cause mortality since the ARDSnet trial (Acute Respiratory Distress Syndrome Network, Brower et al., 2000), possibly because those strategies are reserved to ventilating heterogeneous atelectatic and stable lungs in severe ARDS (Nieman et al., 2020). Furthermore, in most RCTs, an unselected, mixed population of ARDS have been studied, missing the opportunity to test whether the experimental MV approach or adjunctive/pharmacological therapy is beneficial in patients having a single etiology or after assessing their "true" degree of hypoxemia under standardized ventilatory settings prior to randomization (Villar et al., 2007). It is highly plausible that in a substantial proportion of patients in recent RCTs in ARDS, the severity of lung injury was modest. Current definition for ARDS (Ranieri et al., 2012) did not require any specific FiO_2, and only a minimum PEEP level of 5 mH_2O to calculate the PaO_2/FiO_2 for stratifying patients as mild, moderate or severe ARDS. Any change in PEEP or FiO_2 can result in a modification of lung imaging and PaO_2/FiO_2 ratio. Therefore, depending on the applied MV approach, patients may or may not meet criteria for the diagnosis of ARDS. For example, a septic patient with a PaO_2 of 69 mmHg on a FiO_2 of 0.35 and 5 cmH_2O of PEEP satisfies the criteria for moderate ARDS, but there is no need to enroll this type of patients in a trial testing the effects of high PEEP levels and RMs. In addition, systemic inflammation seen in ARDS patients is not specific for ARDS, especially in patients with sepsis, and MV -although it could be considered a curative therapeutic approach in critically ill patients- it is not the cure for sepsis!

Medicine cannot always be provided by a protocol (Florio et al., 2020). Hopefully, it is plausible that in the near future, we will have mechanisms to identify classes or subclasses of ARDS patients that might respond to targeted therapy, including MV, adjunctive therapies, or pharmacological approaches (Sevransky et al., 2021). Research breakthroughs are not enough. To date, attempts to personalize or stratify the care of ARDS patients enrolled in clinical trials using physiologic measures have not been successful, except in the case of the DEXA-ARDS trial where the authors used an enrichment strategy under standardized ventilatory settings to identify patients for enrollment (Villar et al., 2020). If patients enrolled in a trial have a low risk of the condition to prevent, the trial –irrespective of sample size- will not validate the value of the intervention under study (Villar et al., 2005). MV for patients with ARDS would be personalized based on etiology, lung physiology and morphology, and clinical and biological classes or subclasses because explicit numerical values might not apply to individual patients

(Villar et al., 2019; Pelosi et al., 2021). Optimization of patient selection is central to the likelihood of success in future trial design for ARDS (Villar et al., 2020; Pelosi et al., 2021). Both prognostic and predictive enrichment strategies can improve the signal-to-noise ratio, allowing smaller sample sizes and increased effects sizes (Villar et al., 2019; Ware et al., 2020).

AUTHOR CONTRIBUTIONS

JV drafted the first version of the manuscript. JV, CF, GT, and FS-S contributed to the initial concept and design of this review. JV, CF, GT, LB, PR-S, and FS-S critically revised the manuscript. JV, CF, and PR-S obtained funding for the study. All authors read and approved the final manuscript.

REFERENCES

Acute Respiratory Distress Syndrome Network, Brower, R. G., Matthay, M. A., Morris, A., Schoenfeld, D., Thompson, B. T., et al. (2000). Ventilation with lower tidal volumes as compared with traditional tidal volumes for acute lung injury and the acute respiratory distress syndrome. *N. Engl. J. Med.* 342, 1301–1308. doi: 10.1056/nejm200005043421801

Annane, D., Pastores, S. M., Rochwerg, B., Arlt, W., Balk, R. A., Beishuizen, A., et al. (2017). Guidelines for the diagnosis and management of critical illness-related corticosteroids insufficiency (CIRCI) in critically ill patients (Part I): society of critical care medicine (SCCM) and european society of intensive care medicine (ESICM) 2017. *Crit. Care Med.* 45, 2078–2088.

Beitler, J. R., Sarge, T., Banner-Goodspeed, V. M., Gong, M. N., Cook, D., Novack, V., et al. (2019). Effect of titrating positive end-expiratory pressure (PEEP) with an esophageal pressure-guided strategy vs an empirical high PEEP-FiO2 strategy on death and days free from mechanical ventilation among patients with acute respiratory distress syndrome. A randomized clinical trial. *JAMA* 32, 846–857. doi: 10.1001/jama.2019.0555

Beitler, J. R., Shaefi, S., Montesi, S. B., Devlin, A., Loring, S. H., Talmor, D., et al. (2014). Prone positioning reduces mortality from acute respiratory distress syndrome in the low tidal volume era: a meta-analysis. *Intensive Care Med.* 40, 332–341. doi: 10.1007/s00134-013-3194-3

Bellingan, G., Maksimow, M., Howell, D. C., Stotz, M., Beale, R., Beatty, M., et al. (2014). The effect of intravenous interferon-beta-1a (FP-1201) on lung CD73 expression and on acute respiratory distress syndrome mortality: an open-label study. *Lancet Respir. Med.* 2, 98–107. doi: 10.1016/s2213-2600(13)70259-5

Bernard, G. R., Artigas, A., Brigham, K. L., Carlet, J., Falke, K., Hudson, L., et al. (1994). The american-european consensus conference on ARDS. Definitions, mechanisms, relevant outcomes, and clinical trial coordination. *Am. J. Respir. Crit. Care Med.* 149, 818–824. doi: 10.1164/ajrccm.149.3.7509706

Bourenne, J., Guervilly, C., Mechati, M., Hraiech, S., Fraisse, M., and Bisbal, M. (2019). Variability of reverse triggering in deeply sedated ARDS patients. *Intensive Care Med.* 45, 725–726. doi: 10.1007/s00134-018-5500-6

Combes, A., Hajage, D., Capellier, G., Demoule, A., Lavoué, S., Guervilly, C., et al. (2018). Extracorporeal membrane oxygenation for severe acute respiratory distress syndrome. *N. Engl. J. Med.* 378, 1965–1975.

Egan, T. M., Duffin, J., Glynn, M. F., Todd, T. R., DeMajo, W., Murphy, E., et al. (1988). Ten-year experience with extracorporeal membrane oxygenation for severe respiratory failure. *Chest* 94, 681–687.

Ferguson, N. D., Cook, D. J., Guyatt, G. H., Mehta, S., Hand, L., Austin, P., et al. (2013). For the OSCILLATE trail investigators and the canadian critical care trails group: high-frequency oscillation in early acute respiratory distress syndrome. *N. Engl. J. Med.* 368, 795–805. doi: 10.1056/NEJMoa1215554

Ferguson, N. D., Villar, J., and Slutsky, A. S. (2007). Understanding high-frequency oscillation: lessons from the animal kingdom. *Intensive Care Med.* 33, 1316–1318. doi: 10.1007/s00134-007-0706-z

Florio, G., Ferrari, M., Bittner, E. A., De Santis Santiago, R., Pirrone, M., Fumagalli, J., et al. (2020). Investigators of the lung rescue team. A lung rescue team improves survival in obesity with acute respiratory distress syndrome. *Crit. Care* 24:4. doi: 10.1186/s13054-019-2709-x

Fumagalli, J., Berra, L., Zhang, C., Pirrone, M., De Santis Santiago, R. R., Gomes, S., et al. (2017). Transpulmonary pressure describes lung morphology during decremental positive end-expiratory pressure trials in obesity. *Crit. Care Med.* 45, 1374–1381. doi: 10.1097/CCM.0000000000002460

Gao Smith, F., Perkins, G. D., Gates, S., Young, D., McAuley, D. F., Tunnicliffe, W., et al. (2012). Effects of intravenous β-2 agonist treatment on clinical outcomes in acute respiratory distress syndrome (BALTI-2): a multicentre, randomised controlled trial. *Lancet* 379, 229–235.

Gattinoni, L., and Pesenti, A. (2005). The concept of "baby lung". *Intensive Care Med.* 31, 776–784. doi: 10.1007/s00134-005-2627-z

Guerin, C., Debord, S., Leray, V., Delannoy, B., Bayle, F., Bourdinet, G., et al. (2011). Efficacy and safety of recruitment maneuvers in acute respiratory distress syndrome. *Ann. Intensive Care* 1:9.

Guerin, C., Reignier, J., Richard, J. C., Beuret, P., Gacouin, A., Boulain, T., et al. (2013). The PROSEVA Study Group: prone positioning in severe acute respiratory distress syndrome. *N. Engl. J. Med.* 368, 2159–2168.

Hodgson, C. L., Cooper, D. J., Arabi, Y., King, V., Barsten, A., Bihari, S., et al. (2019). Maximal recruitment open lung ventilation in acute respiratiory distress syndrome (PHARLAP). A phase II, multicenter randomized controlled clinical trial. *Am. J. Respir. Crit. Care Med.* 200, 1363–1372.

Juschten, J., Tuinman, P. R., Guo, T., Juffermans, N. P., Schultz, M. J., Loer, S. A., et al. (2021). Between-trial heterogeneity in ARDS research. *Intensive Care Med.* 47, 422–434. doi: 10.1007/s00134-021-06370-w

Kacmarek, R. M., Villar, J., Sulemanji, D., Montiel, R., Ferrando, C., Blanco, J., et al. (2016). Open lung approach for the acute respiratory distress syndrome: a pilot, randomized controlled trial. *Crit. Care Med.* 44, 32–42.

Kacmarek, R. M., Wanderley, H. V., Villar, J., and Berra, L. (2021). Weaning patients with obesity from ventilatory support. *Curr. Opin. Crit. Care* 27, 311–319. doi: 10.1097/mcc.0000000000000823

Lamm, W. J., Graham, M. M., and Albert, R. K. (1994). Mechanisms by which the prone position improves oxygenation in acute lung injury. *Am. J. Respir. Crit. Care Med.* 150, 184–193. doi: 10.1164/ajrccm.150.1.8025748

Light, R. W., Bengfort, J. L., and George, R. B. (1975). The adult respiratory distress syndrome and pancuronium bromide. *Anesth. Analg.* 54, 219–223.

McAuley, D. F., Laffey, J. G., O'Kane, C. M., Perkins, G. D., Mullan, B., Trinder, J., et al. (2014). Simvastatin in the acute respiratory distress syndrome. *N .Engl. J. Med.* 371, 1695–1703.

Meade, M. O., Young, D., Hanna, S., Zhou, Q., Bachman, T. E., Bollen, C., et al. (2017). Severity of hypoxemia and effect of high-frequency oscillatory ventilation in acute respiratory distress syndrome. *Am. J. Respir. Crit. Care Med.* 196, 727–733.

Meijvis, S. C., Hardeman, H., Remmelts, H. H., Heijligenberg, R., Rijkers, G. T., van Velzen-Blad, H., et al. (2011). Dexamethasone and length of hospital stay in patients with community-acquired pneumonia: a randomized, double blind, placebo-controlled trial. *Lancet* 377, 2023–2030. doi: 10.1016/s0140-6736(11)60607-7

Munshi, L., Walkey, A., Goligher, E., Pham, T., Uleryk, E. M., and Fan, E. (2019). Venovenous extracorporeal membrane oxygenation for acute respiratory distress syndrome: a systematic review and meta-analysis. *Lancet Respir. Med.* 7, 163–172. doi: 10.1016/s2213-2600(18)30452-1

Nieman, G. F., Al-Khalisy, H., Kollisch-Singule, M., Satalin, J., Blair, S., Trikha, G., et al. (2020). A physiologically informed strategy to effectively open, stabilize, and protect the acute injured lung. *Front. Physiol.* 11:227. doi: 10.3389/fphys.2020.00227

Papazian, L., Forel, J. M., Gacouin, A., Penot-Ragon, C., Perrin, G., Loundou, A., et al. (2010). For the ACURASYS study investigators: neuromuscular blockers in early acute respiratory distress syndrome. *N. Engl. J. Med.* 363, 1107–1116. doi: 10.1056/NEJMoa1005372

Pelosi, P., Ball, L., Barbas, C. S. V., Bellomo, R., Burns, K. E. A., Einav, S., et al. (2021). Personalized mechanical ventilation in acute respiratory distress syndrome. *Crit. Care* 25:250.

Pirrone, M., Fisher, D., Chipman, D., Imber, D. A. E., Corona, J., Mietto, C., et al. (2016). Recruitment maneuvers and positive end-expiratory pressure titration in morbidly obese ICU patients. *Crit. Care Med.* 44, 300–307. doi: 10.1097/ccm.0000000000001387

Poole, J., MacDowell, C., Lall, R., Perkins, G., McAuley, D., Gao, F., et al. (2017). Individual patient data analysis of tidal volumes used in three large randomized control trials involving patients with acute respiratory distress syndrome. *Brit. J. Anesth.* 118, 570–575. doi: 10.1093/bja/aew465

Ranieri, V. M., Pettilä, V., Karvonen, M. K., Jalkanen, J., Nightingale, P., Brealey, D., et al. (2020). Effects of intravenous interferon β-1a on death and days free from mechanical ventilation among patients with moderate to severe acute respiratory distress syndrome. *JAMA* 323, 725–733. doi: 10.1186/s13063-017-2234-7

Ranieri, V. M., Rubenfeld, G. D., Thompson, B. T., Ferguson, N. D., Caldwell, E., Fan, E., et al. (2012). ARDS definition TASK force: acute respiratory distress syndrome: the berlin definition. *JAMA* 307, 2526–2533.

Rhen, T., and Cidlowski, J. A. (2005). Anti-inflammatory action of glucocorticoids - new mechanisms for old drugs. *N. Engl. J. Med.* 353, 1711–1723. doi: 10.1056/nejmra050541

Santacruz, C. A., Pereira, A. J., Celis, E., and Vincent, J. L. (2019). Which multicenter randomized controlled trials in critical care medicine have shown reduced mortality? A systematic review. *Crit. Care Med.* 47, 1680–1691. doi: 10.1097/ccm.0000000000004000

Sarge, T., Baedorf-Kassis, E., Banner-Goodspeed, V., Novack, V., Loring, S. H., Gong, M. N., et al. (2021). Effect of esophageal pressure-guided positive end-expiratory pressure on survival from acute respiratory distress syndrome: a risk-based and mechanistic reanalysis of the EPVent-2 trial. *Am. J. Respir. Crti. Care Med.* doi: 10.1164/rccm.202009-3539OC [Online ahead of print].

Sevransky, J. E., Agarwal, A., Jabaley, C. S., and Rochwerg, B. (2021). Standardized care is better that individualized care for the majority for critically ill patients. *Crit. Care Med.* 49, 151–155. doi: 10.1097/ccm.0000000000004676

Slutsky, A. S., and Ranieri, V. M. (2013). Ventilator-induced lung injury. *N. Engl. J. Med.* 369, 2126–2136.

Slutsky, A. S., and Villar, J. (2019). Early paralytic agents for ARDS? Yes, no, and sometimes. *N. Engl. J. Med.* 380, 2061–2063. doi: 10.1056/NEJMe1905627

Slutsky, A. S., Villar, J., and Pesenti, A. (2016). Happy 50th birthday ARDS! *Intensive Care Med.* 42, 637–639. doi: 10.1007/s00134-016-4284-9

Suárez-Sipmann, F., Bohm, S. H., Tusman, G., Pesch, T., Thamm, O., Reissmann, H., et al. (2007). Use of dynamic compliance for open lung positive end-expiratiry pressure titration in an experimental study. *Crit. Care Med.* 35, 214–221. doi: 10.1097/01.CCM.0000251131.40301.E2

Suarez-Sipmann, F., Ferrando, C., and Villar, J. (2019). PEEP titration guided by transpulmonary pressure: lessons from a negative trial. *J. Thorac. Dis.* 11(Suppl15), S1957–S1962. doi: 10.21037/jtd.2019.08.03

Talmor, D., Sarge, T., Malhotra, A., O'Donnell, C. R., Ritz, R., Lisbon, A., et al. (2008). Mechanical ventilation guided by esophageal pressure in acute lung injury. *N. Engl. J. Med.* 359, 2095–2104.

The National Heart, Lung, and Blood Institute Petal Clinical Trials Network, Moss, M., Huang, D. T., Brower, R. G., Ferguson, N. D., Ginde, A. A., et al. (2019). Early neuromuscular blockade in the acute respiratory distress syndrome. *N. Engl. J. Med.* 380, 1997–2008.

Thompson, L. F., Eltzschig, H. K., Ibla, J. C., Van De Wiele, C. J., Resta, R., Morote-Garcia, J. C., et al. (2004). Crucial role for ecto-5′-nucleotidase (CD73) in vascular leakage during hypoxia. *J. Exp. Med.* 200, 1395–1405. doi: 10.1084/jem.20040915

Villar, J. (2011). What is the acute respiratory distress syndrome? *Respir. Care* 56, 1539–1545.

Villar, J., Ambrós, A., Mosteiro, F., Martínez, D., Fernández, L., Ferrando, C., et al. (2019). A prognostic enrichment strategy for selection of patients with acute respiratory distress syndrome in clinical trials. *Crit. Care Med.* 47, 377–385.

Villar, J., Ferrando, C., Martínez, D., Ambrós, A., Muñoz, T., Soler, J. A., et al. (2020). Dexamethasone treatment for the acute respiratory distress syndrome: a multicentre, randomised controlled trial. *Lancet Respir. Med.* 8, 267–276.

Villar, J., Kacmarek, R. M., and Guerin, C. (2014). Clinical trials in patients with the acute respiratory distress syndrome: burn after reading. *Intensive Care Med.* 40, 900–902. doi: 10.1007/s00134-014-3288-6

Villar, J., Pérez-Méndez, L., Aguirre-Jaime, A., and Kacmarek, R. M. (2005). Why are physicians so skeptical about positive randomized controlled clinical trials in critical care medicine? *Intensive Care Med.* 31, 196–204.

Villar, J., Pérez-Méndez, L., López, J., Belda, J., Blanco, J., Saralegui, I., et al. (2007). An early PEEP/FiO2 trail identifies different degrees of lung injury in patients with acute respiratory distress syndrome. *Am. J. Respir. Crit. Care Med.* 176, 795–804. doi: 10.1164/rccm.200610-1534OC

Villar, J., Suárez-Sipmann, F., and Kacmarek, R. M. (2017). Should the ART trial change our practice? *J. Thorac. Dis.* 9, 4871–4877. doi: 10.21037/jtd.2017.11.01

Vincent, J. L. (2017). High-frequency oscillation in acute respiratory distress syndrome. The end of the story? *Am. J. Respir. Crit. Care Med.* 196, 670–671. doi: 10.1164/rccm.201703-0475ED

Ware, L. B., Matthay, M. A., and Mebazaa, A. (2020). Designing and ARDS trial for 2020 and beyond: focus on enrichment strategies. *Intensive Care Med.* 46, 2153–2156. doi: 10.1007/s00134-020-06232-x

WHO Rapid Evidence Appraisal for Covid-19 Therapies (React) Working Group, Sterne, J. A. C., Murthy, S., Diaz, J. V., Slutsky, A. S., Villar, J., et al. (2020). Association between administration of systemic corticosteroids and mortality among critically Ill patients with COVID-19: a meta-analysis. *JAMA* 324, 1330–1341.

Working group for the Alveolar Recruitment for Acute Respiratory Distress Syndrome Trial (Art) Investigators, Cavalcanti, A. B., Suzumura, ÉA., Laranjeira, L. N., Paisani, D. M., Damiani, L. P., et al. (2017). Effect of lung recruitment and titrated positive end-expiratory pressure (PEEP) vs. low PEEP on mortality in patients with the acute respiratory distress syndrome. A randomized clinical trial. JAMA 318, 1335–1345. doi: 10.1001/jama.2017.14171

Yegneswaran, B., and Murugan, R. (2011). Neuromuscular blockers and ARDS: thou shall not breathe, move, or die! *Crit. Care* 15:311. doi: 10.1186/cc10470

Young, D., Lamb, S. E., Shah, S., MacKenzie, I., Tunnicliffe, W., Lall, R., et al. (2013). For the OSCAR study group: high-frequency oscillation for acute respiratory distress syndrome. *N. Engl. J. Med.* 368, 806–813. doi: 10.1056/NEJMoa1215716

11

Assessment of Alveolar Macrophage Dysfunction using an *in vitro* Model of Acute Respiratory Distress Syndrome

Rahul Y. Mahida[1], Aaron Scott[1], Dhruv Parekh[1], Sebastian T. Lugg[1], Kylie B. R. Belchamber[1], Rowan S. Hardy[2], Michael A. Matthay[3], Babu Naidu[1] and David R. Thickett[1]*

[1] Birmingham Acute Care Research Group, Institute of Inflammation and Ageing, University of Birmingham, Birmingham, United Kingdom, [2] Institute of Metabolism and Systems Research, University of Birmingham, Birmingham, United Kingdom, [3] Departments of Medicine and of Anaesthesia, Cardiovascular Research Institute, University of California, San Francisco, San Francisco, CA, United States

***Correspondence:**
Rahul Y. Mahida
r.mahida@bham.ac.uk

Background: Impaired alveolar macrophage (AM) efferocytosis may contribute to acute respiratory distress syndrome (ARDS) pathogenesis; however, studies are limited by the difficulty in obtaining primary AMs from patients with ARDS. Our objective was to determine whether an *in vitro* model of ARDS can recapitulate the same AM functional defect observed *in vivo* and be used to further investigate pathophysiological mechanisms.

Methods: AMs were isolated from the lung tissue of patients undergoing lobectomy and then treated with pooled bronchoalveolar lavage (BAL) fluid previously collected from patients with ARDS. AM phenotype and effector functions (efferocytosis and phagocytosis) were assessed by flow cytometry. Rac1 gene expression was assessed using quantitative real-time PCR.

Results: ARDS BAL treatment of AMs decreased efferocytosis ($p = 0.0006$) and Rac1 gene expression ($p = 0.016$); however, bacterial phagocytosis was preserved. Expression of AM efferocytosis receptors MerTK ($p = 0.015$) and CD206 ($p = 0.006$) increased, whereas expression of the antiefferocytosis receptor SIRPα decreased following ARDS BAL treatment ($p = 0.036$). Rho-associated kinase (ROCK) inhibition partially restored AM efferocytosis in an *in vitro* model of ARDS ($p = 0.009$).

Conclusions: Treatment of lung resection tissue AMs with ARDS BAL fluid induces impairment in efferocytosis similar to that observed in patients with ARDS. However, AM phagocytosis is preserved following ARDS BAL treatment. This specific impairment in AM efferocytosis can be partially restored by inhibition of ROCK. This *in vitro* model of ARDS is a useful tool to investigate the mechanisms by which the inflammatory alveolar microenvironment of ARDS induces AM dysfunction.

Keywords: ARDS (acute respiratory disease syndrome), alveolar macrophage (AM), efferocytosis, BAL (bronchoalveolar lavage), Rac1, Rho-associated kinase (ROCK) inhibitor

INTRODUCTION

Acute respiratory distress syndrome (ARDS) is an inflammatory pulmonary disorder, which results in hypoxemic respiratory failure. ARDS may develop in response to various insults, with sepsis being the underlying etiology in > 75% of cases (1). Since December 2019, the emergence of severe acute respiratory syndrome coronavirus-2 (SARS-CoV-2) and the ensuing pandemic has vastly increased the incidence of ARDS; initial studies showed that 41.8% of adult patients admitted with SARS-CoV-2 pneumonia developed ARDS (2, 3). Notwithstanding advances in supportive care and ventilation strategies, mortality for moderate to severe ARDS remains at 40–46%, and ARDS-specific treatment options are limited (1). Pharmacological therapies such as dexamethasone and tocilizumab have only been shown to be efficacious in SARS-CoV-2 ARDS (4, 5). We now understand more about how ARDS develops: It requires damage to the alveolar epithelium and endothelium (6), leading to reduced alveolar fluid clearance (7), increased permeability, exaggerated inflammation, and neutrophilic alveolar edema (8). However, the role of alveolar macrophages (AMs) in ARDS pathogenesis is not fully understood.

We have previously shown that AM efferocytosis is impaired in patients with sepsis-related ARDS, compared to a control group of ventilated sepsis patients without ARDS (9). Impaired AM efferocytosis is associated with increased alveolar neutrophil apoptosis and worse clinical outcomes (increased duration of mechanical ventilation and mortality), indicating this defect in efferocytosis plays a key role in the pathogenesis of ARDS (9). Further studies are required to investigate the pathophysiological role of AM dysfunction in ARDS; however, the difficulty in obtaining relevant cells from these patients is a major barrier to undertaking this work. Safety concerns preclude bronchoscopy in many patients with ARDS due to their ventilation status (9). For those patients in whom bronchoscopy can be performed, the bronchoalveolar lavage (BAL) fluid is highly neutrophilic, resulting in a relatively low AM yield, which is often insufficient to undertake all necessary experiments in every patient (9). This significantly limits the effectiveness of ARDS-related AM research.

Owing to these difficulties with isolating AMs from patients with ARDS, we sought to develop an *in vitro* model of ARDS. A previous study has shown that the treatment of monocyte-derived macrophages (MDMs) with ARDS patient BAL impairs macrophage efferocytosis (10). However, AMs are distinct from MDMs in terms of origin, function, and phenotype. Resident AMs develop from yolk sac progenitors at the embryonic stage (11) and can self-renew throughout life (12, 13), independently from monocytes and hematopoietic stem cells. AMs are crucial for maintaining alveolar immune homeostasis; exposure to the external environment requires AMs to finely balance inflammatory responses to infection against resolving functions to prevent immune-mediated tissue damage (14). The intrinsic protolerogenic characteristic of AMs has likely evolved to prevent excessive inflammation in the face of continuous low-level stimulation from a diverse range of foreign particles (15). Therefore, while previous studies utilizing MDMs are useful, they do not constitute the most representative model of ARDS and, therefore, would not be as appropriate to inform a mechanistic investigation. We postulated that by using AMs from lung resection tissue and treating with pooled ARDS patient BAL, we could develop a more accurate model of the AM defect in ARDS. Since ARDS patient BAL contains high concentrations of proinflammatory cytokines, we hypothesized that following treatment AMs will be driven away from a proresolving phenotype and toward a proinflammatory phenotype, which is associated with reduced efferocytosis capacity (16, 17).

Alveolar macrophage expression of the Mer tyrosine kinase (MerTK) receptor may be critical for efferocytosis (16, 18). MerTK signaling *via* phosphatidylinositol 3′-OH kinase (PI3K) results in activation of Rac1, which causes cytoskeletal rearrangement and engulfment of the apoptotic cell (19, 20). AM surface receptors, namely, CD206 and CD163, are also thought to mediate efferocytosis (14). AMs also express signal regulatory protein-α (SIRPα) on their surface, which binds surfactant proteins or CD47 on healthy cells (21). SIRPα signaling activates Rho-associated kinase (ROCK), and phosphatase and tensin homolog (PTEN), which oppose PI3K signaling, resulting in Rac1 inhibition and suppression of efferocytosis (22). The status of these important efferocytosis-related receptors in ARDS AMs remains unknown.

We hypothesized that treatment of lung resection tissue AMs with pooled ARDS patient BAL will recapitulate the defect in efferocytosis we observed *in vivo* and allow us to determine the mechanism by which this defect occurs. Our study had the following aims:

(1) To determine whether treatment of lung resection tissue AMs with ARDS patient BAL can replicate the impaired efferocytosis observed in patients with ARDS.

(2) To determine whether treatment of lung resection tissue AMs with ARDS patient BAL decreases AM expression of MerTK and increases expression of SIRPα.

(3) To determine whether inhibition of ROCK-PTEN signaling can increase AM efferocytosis in this *in vitro* model of ARDS.

MATERIALS AND METHODS

Ethical Approval

Ethical approval was obtained to recruit ventilated sepsis patients with and without ARDS (REC 16/WA/0169) and for the use of lung tissue samples from patients undergoing routine thoracic surgery (REC 17/WM/0272). For patients who lacked capacity, permission to enroll was sought from a personal legal representative following the UK Mental Capacity Act (2005). For patients with capacity, written informed consent was obtained from the patient.

Patient Recruitment

Invasively ventilated adult patients with ARDS and sepsis were recruited from the intensive care unit of the Queen Elizabeth Hospital, Birmingham, UK, from December 2016 to February 2019, and BAL was collected as previously described (9).

Demographic and physiological details of the patients can also be found in this prior publication. BAL fluid was rendered acellular by centrifuging at 500 g for 5 min. Acellular supernatant BAL was then pooled and stored at −80°C before use in this study.

Adult patients who underwent lung lobectomy as part of their clinical treatment plan for malignancy at Birmingham Heartlands Hospital from September 2017 to July 2019 were also recruited. Recruited patients were never-smokers or long-term ex-smokers (quit > 5 years), with normal spirometry and without airways disease. No patient received chemotherapy before surgery. Following lobectomy, lung tissue resection samples surplus to histopathological requirements were collected.

Alveolar Macrophage Isolation

Macroscopically normal lung tissue samples were perfused with 0.15 M saline *via* pressure bag by inserting a needle (21-gauge) in bronchioles. When saturated, the tissue was gently massaged to facilitate emptying lavage fluid from the tissue, ready for the next instillation. This process was repeated until the lavage fluid contained $<1 \times 10^4$ cells/ml (23).

Cells were pelleted from the lavage fluid by centrifugation at 500 g for 5 min. Mononuclear cells were then separated by gradient centrifugation using Lymphoprep (StemCell Technologies, Vancouver, BC, Canada), according to the instructions of the manufacturer. Mononuclear cells were then cultured in RPMI-1640 media supplemented with 10% fetal calf serum (FCS), 100 U/ml penicillin, 100 µg/ml streptomycin, and 2 mM L-glutamine (Sigma-Aldrich, Darmstadt, Germany) at 37°C and 5% CO_2 for 24 h to allow adherence. After 24-h culture, the wells were washed and media changed, thereby removing non-adherent mononuclear cells (24, 25). AMs were assessed for purity by cytospin (23); AM purity was consistently >95% across all samples.

Alveolar Macrophage Efferocytosis Assay

The efferocytosis assay was modified from published protocols (26–29). Neutrophils were isolated from the blood of healthy volunteers using Percoll density centrifugation (30) as previously described by our group (31). Neutrophil purity was >96% as assessed by cytospin and viability >97% as assessed by trypan blue exclusion. Neutrophils were suspended in a 5 µM solution of CellTracker™ Deep Red fluorescent dye (ThermoFisher, Waltham, MA, USA) in 10% FCS/RPMI at 4×10^6/ml, then incubated for 30 min at 37°C. Stained neutrophils were centrifuged at 1,500 g for 5 min then resuspended at 2×10^6/ml in serum-free RPMI and incubated at 37°C and 5% CO_2 for 24 h to allow apoptosis. Flow cytometric assessment of neutrophil apoptosis was performed using a fluorescein isothiocyanate (FITC)-conjugated Annexin V and 7-aminoactinomycin D (7-AAD) apoptosis detection kit (BioLegend, San Diego, CA, USA): mean neutrophil apoptosis of 93% with necrosis of <2% was observed.

Alveolar macrophages were cultured at 2.5×10^5/well in 24-well plates. As a negative control, 5 µg/ml Cytochalasin D (CytoD, Sigma-Aldrich, Darmstadt, Germany) was added for 30 min to inhibit actin filament polymerization required for efferocytosis. Stained apoptotic neutrophils (ANs) were added to AMs at a 4:1 ratio before incubation for 2 h at 37°C. The optimal assay duration of 2 h had previously been determined by time-course experiments. Media was removed and wells washed two times with ice-cold phosphate-buffered saline (PBS) to remove non-adherent/engulfed neutrophils. Cells were harvested using a 5-min TrypLE™ express (ThermoFisher, Waltham, MA, USA) incubation at 37°C, before acquisition using an Accuri C6 flow cytometer and software (BD Biosciences, Franklin Lakes, NJ, USA). AMs and ANs alone were used to set gates for their respective populations on forward and side-scatter plots. ANs alone were used to set a positive gate on the allophycocyanin (APC) plot, which was subsequently used to identify AMs which had engulfed ANs. Minimum 5,000 events gated as AMs were counted for each experimental condition and the percentage of APC^+ AMs calculated. CytoD-treated AMs (negative control) determined the background fluorescence present due to ANs adhering to the surface of AMs but not being engulfed. This background fluorescence was subtracted from the percentage of APC^+ AMs in other experimental conditions to give a corrected net efferocytosis index representative of neutrophil engulfment (**Supplementary Figure 1**). Steps were taken to avoid bias, including drawing gates based on single-cell populations (ANs and AMs) before assessing efferocytosis.

Alveolar Macrophage Phagocytosis Assay

Alveolar macrophage phagocytosis assays were performed using pHrodo™ red *Escherichia coli* and *Staphylococcus aureus* BioParticle® conjugates (ThermoFisher, Waltham, MA, USA) in a 96-well plate according to the instruction of the manufacturer and as previously described (23). The pHrodo™ beads were prepared according to the instructions of the manufacturer at a final concentration of 1 mg/ml. AMs were seeded at 50,000 cells per well in black well, clear bottomed 96-well plates, and cultured overnight. For negative control wells, 5 µg/ml CytoD (Sigma-Aldrich, Darmstadt, Germany) was added for 30 min. A total of 50 µl of pHrodo bead suspension was added per well and incubated for 6 h at 37°C. After 6 h, cells were washed three times with PBS before adding 100 µl fresh PBS. Fluorescence was measured using a microplate reader (Synergy 2, Bio-Tek, Winooski, VT, USA) set at the excitation/emission spectra of pHrodo™ red dye: 560/585 nm. The negative control (cytochalasin D treated) AMs were used to determine the background fluorescence present due to stained pHrodo™ red BioParticles® adhering to the outside of macrophages but not being engulfed. This background fluorescence value was subtracted from fluorescence values of other experimental conditions, to give the corrected net fluorescence value the representative of phagocytosis. Phagocytosis results were expressed as fold change in relative fluorescence unit from untreated AMs.

Use of Alveolar Macrophages in an *in vitro* Model of ARDS

Bronchoalveolar lavage from 14 recruited patients with sepsis-related ARDS was rendered acellular by centrifugation and then pooled. The acellular pooled BAL was mixed in a 1:1 ratio with 10% FCS/RPMI. To elicit functional changes associated with ARDS, AMs were treated with this 50% ARDS BAL mixture. AMs were also treated with a 1:1 mixture of

0.9% saline and 10% FCS/RPMI, as vehicle control (VC). Other treatments given in conjunction with 50% ARDS BAL or saline included 200 nM Y-27632 dihydrochloride (Rho-associated protein kinase inhibitor, Apexbio, Houston, TX, USA), 2 μM SF1670 (phosphatase and tensin homolog inhibitor, Selleckchem, Houston, TX, USA), and dimethyl sulfoxide (VC for Y-27632 and SF1670, Sigma-Aldrich, Darmstadt, Germany) at a 1:50,000 dilution. ROCK and PTEN inhibitor treatment doses were determined by dose response on untreated AM efferocytosis (**Supplementary Figure 2**). Other treatments not combined with 50% ARDS BAL or saline included 50 ng/ml interferon-γ (IFN-γ, Peprotech, UK), 1 μg/ml ultrapure lipopolysaccharide (LPS, Invitrogen, Waltham, MA, USA), 40 ng/ml interleukin-4 (IL-4, Peprotech, UK), and 40 ng/ml IL-13, (Peprotech, UK). Previous studies have shown that macrophage treatment with IFN-γ and LPS can induce a proinflammatory phenotype, whereas IL-4 and IL-13 treatment can induce a proresolving phenotype (17). Cytokine concentrations were based on published methods (32). The 1 μg/ml dose of LPS was based on the lowest dose required to elicit tumor necrosis factor-α (TNFα) production from AMs (**Supplementary Figure 3**). Efferocytosis, phagocytosis, apoptosis/viability, and RNA extraction for gene expression were performed 24 h after treatment with 50% ARDS BAL. Phenotyping was performed 48 h after treatment. AM apoptosis and viability were assessed using a flow cytometric apoptosis detection kit (BioLegend, San Diego, CA, USA).

Flow Cytometric Assessment of AM Surface Markers

Alveolar macrophages were labeled with the following antihuman antibodies or their isotype controls: CD206-APC, CD80-PE, CD163-FITC, Mer-APC, and SIRPα-FITC (see **Supplementary Table 1**). Surface marker expression was assessed by an Accuri C6 flow cytometer and software (BD Biosciences, Franklin Lakes, NJ, USA). AM population was gated on forward and side-scatter plot. The median fluorescence intensity (MFI) in relevant channels from isotype control AMs was subtracted from the MFIs of stained AMs, to give the net MFI for each antibody fluorophore. Results presented as fold change-corrected MFI, as a measure of change in cell surface expression, compared to VC (50% saline).

Assessment of AM Gene Expression

RNA was isolated from AMs using Nucleospin RNA kits (Machery-Nagel, Düren, Germany) as per the instructions of the manufacturer. RNA quantity was assessed with the NanoDrop 2000 UV-Vis Spectrophotometer (ThermoFisher, Waltham, MA, USA). One-Step Quantifast Probe RT-PCR Kits (Qiagen, Hilden, Germany) were used to assess gene expression with a CFX384 Touch Real-Time PCR Detection System (BioRad, Hercules, CA, USA). Taqman® gene expression assays (ThermoFisher, Waltham, MA, USA) were purchased for 18S on VIC-MGB (ref 4318839) and RAC1 on FAM-MGB (Hs01025984_m1). PCR conditions were used as per the recommendation of the manufacturer. Triplicate data were analyzed using CFX Maestro software (BioRad, Hercules, CA, USA). Relative quantification of target gene mRNA was calculated relative to expression of 18s endogenous control gene.

TABLE 1 | Characterization of pooled ARDS patient BAL.

Characterization of pooled ARDS patient BAL	
IL-6	453 pg/ml
IL-8	4,268 pg/ml
IL-1β	98 pg/ml
IL-1ra	3,023 pg/ml
IL-10	6 pg/ml
TNF-α	3 pg/ml
VEGF	209 pg/ml
MCP-1	1,045 pg/ml
IFN-γ	0 pg/ml
LPS	57 pg/ml
Total protein	2.89 mg/ml

IFN-γ, interferon-γ; IL, interleukin; TNF-α, tumor necrosis factor-α; MCP-1, macrophage chemoattractant protein-1; LPS, lipopolysaccharide; VEGF, vascular endothelial growth factor.

Bronchoalveolar Lavage Cytokine and Protein Quantification

Inflammatory cytokine (IL-6, IL-8, TNF-α, IL-1β, macrophage chemoattractant protein-1, IL-10, IL-1ra, and vascular endothelial growth factor) content of pooled patient BAL fluid was measured by a commercially available custom Magnetic Luminex® Performance Assay (R&D Systems, UK) as per the instructions of the manufacturer. Protein concentration in pooled patient BAL fluid was measured using the Pierce™ BCA (Bicinchoninic Acid) Protein Assay Kit (ThermoFisher Scientific, Waltham, MA, USA) as per the instructions of the manufacturer.

Statistical Analysis

Data were analyzed using Prism 8 software (GraphPad, San Diego, CA, USA). Parametric data are shown as mean and SD. Non-parametric data are shown as the median and interquartile range (IQR). Differences between continuously distributed data were assessed using Welch's t-tests for parametric data or Mann–Whitney tests for non-parametric data. Differences between non-parametric paired data were assessed using Wilcoxon matched-pairs signed-rank test. Differences between three or more unpaired parametric data sets were assessed using ANOVA followed by Dunn's multiple comparison tests. Differences between three or more paired parametric data sets assessed using the repeated measures ANOVA followed by Tukey's multiple comparison tests. Two-tailed p-values of ≤ 0.05 were considered significant.

RESULTS

Patient Characteristics

Samples of BAL from the first 14 patients with sepsis-related ARDS recruited to a previous study (9) were pooled and used to treat AMs isolated from lung resections. This pooled ARDS patient BAL was characterized with regards to inflammatory cytokine and LPS content (**Table 1**). AMs were isolated from the lung tissue of 16 patients who underwent lobectomy (mean yield of 9 million AMs per patient). The mean age of lobectomy

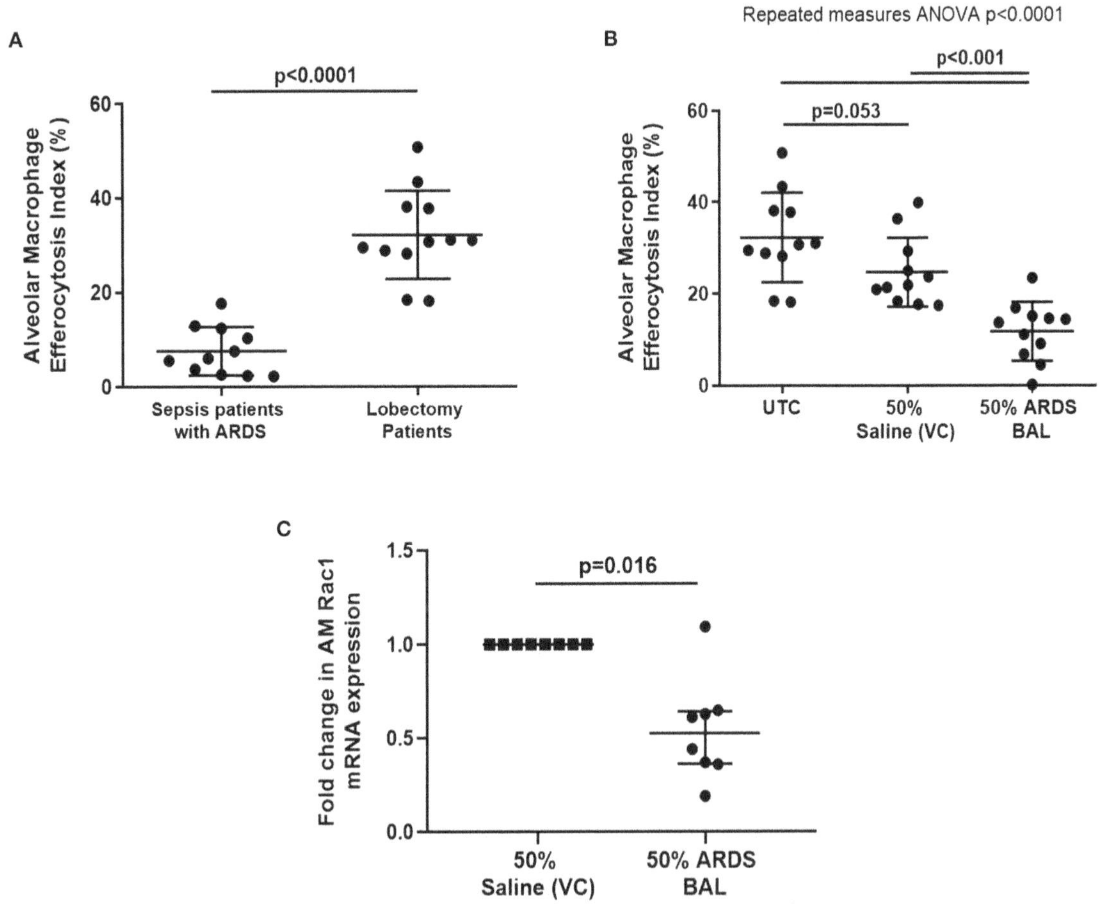

FIGURE 1 | Effect of pooled ARDS BAL treatment on lobectomy patient alveolar macrophage efferocytosis. **(A)** Alveolar macrophages (AMs) from sepsis patients with ARDS have significantly reduced efferocytosis index compared to AMs from lobectomy patients (means 7.6 vs. 32.2%, $p < 0.0001$). Statistical analysis by Welch's *t*-test, $n = 11$–12. **(B)** UTC, Untreated control (cultured in RPMI + 10% FBS); VC, vehicle control (50% saline). Effect of ARDS BAL treatment on lobectomy patient AM efferocytosis. Treatment with 50% ARDS BAL significantly reduced lobectomy patient AM efferocytosis compared to VC treatment (mean of differences 13.0%, $p = 0.0006$) and UTC (mean of differences 20.6%, $p = 0.0009$). Treatment of AMs with VC did not affect efferocytosis compared to UTC (mean of differences 7.6%, $p = 0.053$). Statistical analysis by the repeated measures ANOVA and Tukey's multiple comparisons tests, $n = 11$ for all groups. **(C)** Effect of ARDS BAL treatment on Rac1 gene transcription in lobectomy patient AMs. Data are shown as fold change in AM Rac1 mRNA expression from 50% saline treatment. Statistical analysis by the Wilcoxon matched-pairs signed-rank test, $n = 8$. VC, vehicle control (50% saline). Treatment with 50% ARDS BAL significantly reduced Rac1 mRNA expression in lobectomy patient AMs, compared to VC treatment (median of differences 0.48, $p = 0.016$). Error bars are shown as mean and SD. ARDS, acute respiratory distress syndrome; BAL, bronchoalveolar lavage; FBS, fetal bovine serum.

patients was 70 years (SD = 6.9 years). The male:female split for lobectomy patients was 9:7.

ARDS BAL Treatment of Alveolar Macrophages Impairs Efferocytosis and Preserves Bacterial Phagocytosis

Alveolar macrophage efferocytosis was impaired in sepsis patients with ARDS compared to lobectomy patients (**Figure 1A**, mean 7.6% [SD = 5.1] vs. 32.2% [SD = 9.4], $p < 0.0001$). We established an *in vitro* model of ARDS, by treating lung resection tissue AMs with pooled ARDS BAL to induce AM dysfunction. ARDS BAL or saline VC treatment did not affect AM apoptosis or viability compared to standard culture (**Supplementary Figure 4**). Treatment of AMs with ARDS BAL reduced efferocytosis compared to VC treatment (**Figure 1B**, mean 11.7% [SD = 6.4] vs. 24.7% [SD = 7.6], $p = 0.0006$). Treatment of AMs with ARDS BAL reduced Rac1 mRNA expression compared to VC treatment (**Figure 1C**, median of differences 0.48, $p = 0.016$), which supports our finding that ARDS BAL inhibits AM efferocytosis.

Treatment of AMs with VC reduced phagocytosis of both *S. aureus* and *E. coli* pHrodo® bioparticles compared to untreated controls (**Figures 2A,B**, $p = 0.031$). Treatment of AMs with ARDS BAL increased phagocytosis of *S. aureus* pHrodo® bioparticles compared to VC treatment (**Figure 2A**, median of differences 0.32, $p = 0.031$). There was no difference in AM phagocytosis of *E. coli* pHrodo® bioparticles following ARDS BAL treatment compared to VC treatment (**Figure 3B**, $p =$

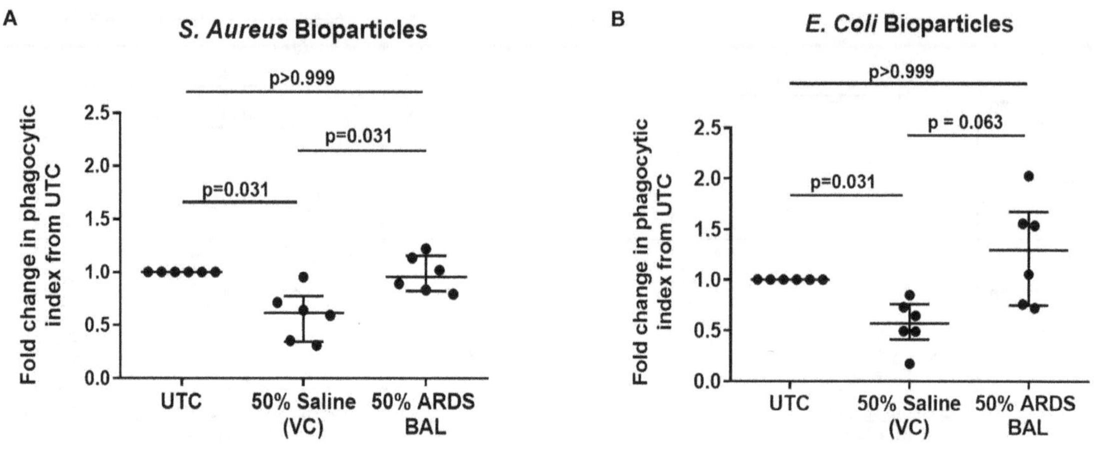

FIGURE 2 | Effect of pooled ARDS BAL treatment on lobectomy patient alveolar macrophage phagocytosis. Alveolar macrophage (AM) phagocytic index in lobectomy AMs treated with 50% ARDS BAL. Data corrected to fold change in the phagocytic index from untreated control (UTC—cultured in RPMI + 10% FBS). Statistical analysis by Wilcoxon matched-pairs signed-rank test, $n = 6$ for all groups. VC, vehicle control (50% saline). VC values are non-identical in graphs C and D. Data are shown as median and interquartile range. ARDS BAL or saline VC-treated AMs receive half the volume of culture media and FCS compared to UTC AMs. **(A)** Treatment of AMs with 50% saline VC reduced phagocytosis of *S. aureus* bioparticles (median of differences −0.38, $p = 0.031$). Treatment with 50% ARDS BAL caused a significant increase in AM phagocytosis of *S. aureus* bioparticles compared to VC (median of differences 0.32, $p = 0.031$). **(B)** Treatment of AMs with 50% saline VC reduced phagocytosis of *E. coli* bioparticles (median of differences −0.43, $p = 0.031$). No significant difference in AM phagocytosis of *E. coli* bioparticles was observed following treatment with 50% ARDS BAL compared to VC (median of differences 0.59, $p = 0.063$). ARDS, acute respiratory distress syndrome; BAL, bronchoalveolar lavage; UTC, untreated control; FCS, fetal calf serum.

0.063). Thus, ARDS BAL treatment had divergent effects on AM efferocytosis and phagocytosis.

ARDS BAL Treatment of Alveolar Macrophages Alters Surface-Receptor Expression

Since ARDS BAL treatment of AMs had divergent effects on efferocytosis and phagocytosis, we used this *in vitro* model to investigate the association between AM phenotype and function. Treatment of AMs with ARDS BAL increased expression of CD206 (**Figure 3A**, mean fold change 0.39, $p = 0.006$) and MerTK (**Figure 3B**, mean fold change 0.3, $p = 0.028$) compared to VC treatment. Treatment of AMs with ARDS BAL decreased SIRPα expression compared to VC treatment (**Figure 3C**, mean fold change −0.26, $p = 0.006$). Treatment of AMs with ARDS BAL did not change the expression of CD163 or CD80 compared to VC treatment (**Figures 3D,E**, $p > 0.05$ for both). These changes in AM surface-receptor expression were incongruent with the observed defect in AM efferocytosis following ARDS BAL treatment.

Treatment of AMs with proinflammatory mediators IFN-γ and LPS also impaired efferocytosis (**Figure 4A**, mean difference 16.5%, $p = 0.008$). However, in contrast to ARDS BAL, proinflammatory mediator treatment decreased expression of both MerTK (**Figure 4B**, mean fold change −0.58, $p = 0.015$) and CD163 (**Figure 4C**, mean fold change −0.58, mean fold change −0.55, $p = 0.005$) while increasing expression of SIRPα (**Figure 4D**, mean fold change 2.48, $p = 0.036$). Proinflammatory mediator treatment had no significant effect on the expression of AM surface markers CD206 or CD80 (**Figures 4E,F**). Treatment with proresolving mediators IL-4 and IL-13 did not affect AM efferocytosis; however, their effect on AM surface-receptor expression was also assessed: expression of MerTK, CD163, and SIRPα was decreased while expression of CD206 was increased (**Figures 4A–E**). These findings indicate that the effect of ARDS BAL treatment on AMs cannot solely be explained by changes in surface-receptor expression.

Rho-Associated Kinase Inhibition Partially Restores Alveolar Macrophage Efferocytosis in an *in vitro* Model of ARDS

Since this model effectively replicated *in vitro* the efferocytosis defect in ARDS AMs evident *in vivo*, we next used this model to explore the mechanism driving this defect. Rac1 intracellular signaling pathways are summarized in **Figure 5**. From this pathway, we identified ROCK and PTEN as potential targets to modify activity. The addition of ROCK-inhibitor to ARDS BAL treatment increased AM efferocytosis compared to treatment with ARDS BAL plus VC (**Figure 6A**, mean fold change 0.17, $p = 0.009$). The addition of PTEN inhibitor to ARDS BAL treatment did not affect efferocytosis compared to treatment with ARDS BAL plus VC (**Figure 6B**). ROCK inhibition did not affect AM phagocytosis of *E. coli* or *S. aureus* bioparticles (**Supplementary Figure 5**). ROCK inhibition also did not affect AM surface marker expression of CD206, CD163, CD80, SIRPα, and MerTK (**Supplementary Figure 6**).

DISCUSSION

Herein, we have established a phenotypically and functionally accurate *in vitro* model through which we can model the effects of ARDS on AM function. In this model, ARDS BAL

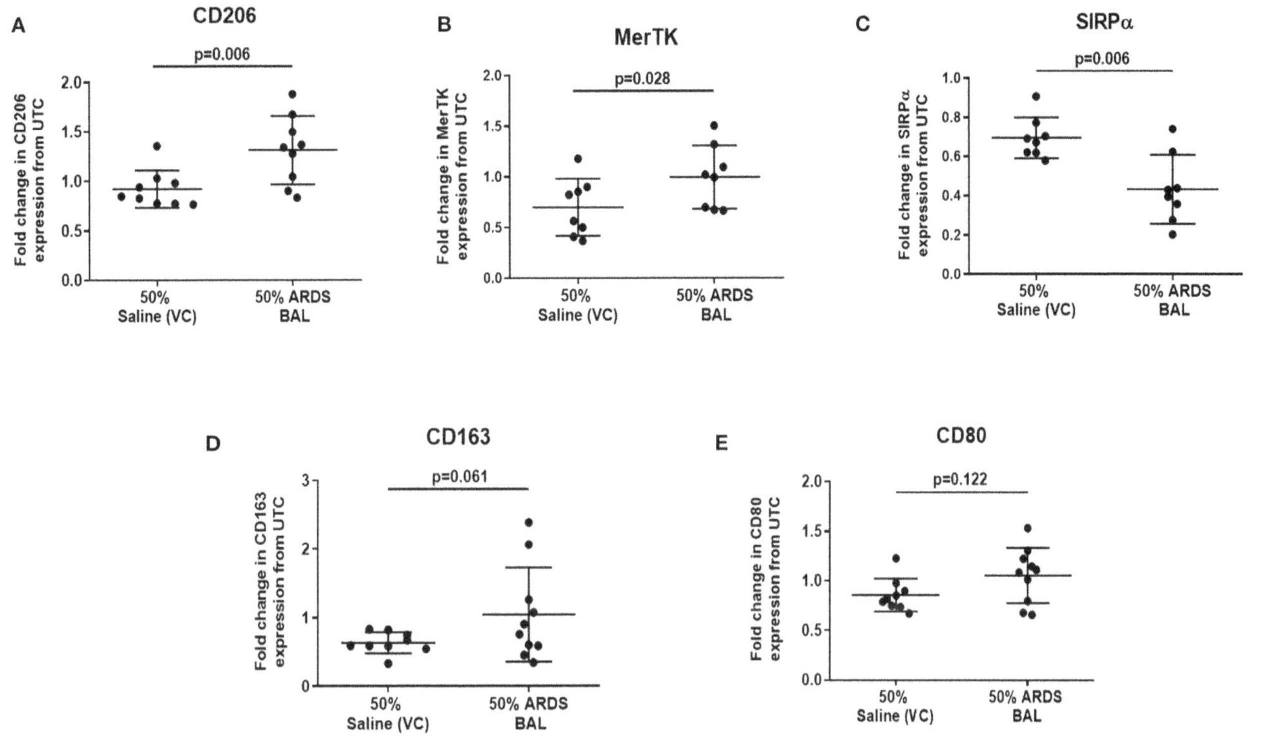

FIGURE 3 | Effect of ARDS BAL treatment on lobectomy patient alveolar macrophage surface-receptor expression. UTC, untreated control (RPMI + 10% FBS); VC, vehicle control (50% saline). Statistical analysis by paired *t*-test, $n \geq 8$ for all groups. **(A)** Treatment with 50% ARDS BAL significantly increased CD206 expression on AMs compared to VC treatment (mean of differences 0.39, $p = 0.006$), **(B)** 50% ARDS BAL treatment significantly increased MerTK expression on AMs compared to VC treatment (mean of differences 0.30, $p = 0.028$), **(C)** 50% ARDS BAL treatment significantly decreased SIRPα expression on AMs compared to VC treatment (mean of differences −0.26, $p = 0.006$), **(D)** 50% ARDS BAL treatment increased CD163 expression on AMs compared to VC treatment; AM, alveolar macrophage; however, this difference did not reach statistical significance (mean of differences 0.44, $p = 0.061$), and **(E)** 50% ARDS BAL treatment did not significantly change CD80 expression on AMs compared to VC treatment (mean of differences 0.19, $p = 0.122$). ARDS, acute respiratory distress syndrome; BAL, bronchoalveolar lavage; FCS, fetal calf serum; MerTK, Mer receptor tyrosine kinase; SIRPα, signal regulatory protein alpha; AMs, alveolar macrophage.

treatment of lung resection tissue AMs induced an impairment in efferocytosis observed in ARDS patients, but preserved AM bacterial phagocytosis. Thus, the inflammatory contents of ARDS BAL do not induce a global impairment in AM function but rather a specific impairment in efferocytosis. The impairment in AM efferocytosis caused by ARDS BAL treatment is not mediated by changes in surface-receptor expression. ROCK inhibition partially restores AM efferocytosis in an *in vitro* model of ARDS. Modulation of the ROCK-PI3K-Rac1 intracellular signaling pathway may offer a therapeutic strategy to upregulate AM efferocytosis in ARDS.

In early ARDS, proinflammatory monocytes migrate to the alveoli and then differentiate into "recruited" AMs (33). A direct correlation was observed between alveolar monocyte influx, the severity of the respiratory failure, and mortality in ARDS (33). Murine models showed that following the initiation of lung injury, the majority of inflammatory cytokines (namely, tumor necrosis factor-alpha, IL-6, and IL-1β) were released by recruited AMs (34). Our study assessed total AM efferocytosis, and did not distinguish between resident and recruited AMs. Therefore, we initially postulated that the decreased AM efferocytosis in ARDS may be due to the polarization of AMs to a proinflammatory phenotype, which is associated with reduced efferocytosis (17). The concentrations of inflammatory cytokines within our pooled ARDS BAL are in keeping with those reported in previous studies (35, 36). We then undertook experiments using the *in vitro* model of ARDS to investigate the association between AM phenotype and function.

Intriguingly, ARDS BAL treatment of AMs increased expression of efferocytosis receptors (CD206 and MerTK) and decreased expression of the antiefferocytosis receptor SIRPα. These phenotypic changes were incongruent with the functional defect in AM efferocytosis induced by ARDS BAL. In comparison, treatment with proinflammatory mediators (IFN-γ and LPS) also decreased AM efferocytosis, but induced SIRPα expression and decreased MerTK expression. Although both ARDS BAL and proinflammatory mediator treatments impaired AM efferocytosis, they had opposite effects on efferocytosis receptor expression. A similar association was observed in cigarette smokers, between decreased AM efferocytosis (37), increased MerTK expression (38), and increased transcription

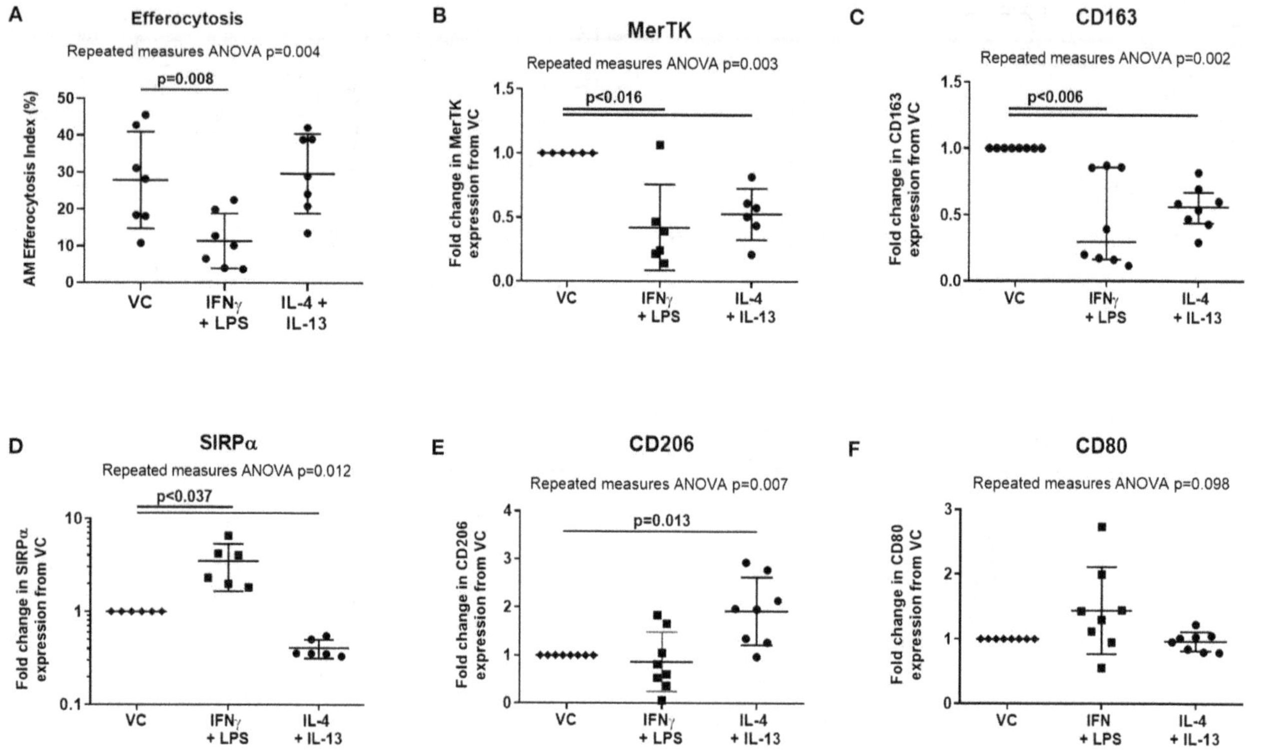

FIGURE 4 | Effect of pro- and anti-inflammatory mediators on alveolar macrophage efferocytosis and surface-receptor expression. VC, vehicle control (distilled water added at 1:500 to RPMI + 10% FBS). IL-4 + IL-13, interleukins 4 and 13 used at 40 ng/ml each; IFN-γ, 50 ng/ml interferon-γ; LPS, 1 μg/ml lipopolysaccharide. **(A)** Data are shown as mean and SD, $n = 7$ for all groups. Cytokine treatment significantly affected alveolar macrophage (AM) efferocytosis (repeated measures ANOVA $p = 0.004$). IFN-γ and LPS treatment significantly reduced AM efferocytosis compared to VC (Dunnett's multiple comparisons test mean difference 16.5%, $p = 0.008$). IL-4 and IL-13 had no significant effect on AM efferocytosis compared to VC (Dunnett's multiple comparisons test mean difference −1.8%, $p = 0.897$). **(B–F)** Statistical analysis by the repeated measures ANOVA with Dunnett's multiple comparison test, $n = 6$–8. Linear *y*-axis was used for all graphs, except SIRPα **(D)** for which a log scale *y*-axis was used. **(B)** Cytokine treatments significantly affected AM surface expression of MerTK (repeated measures ANOVA $p = 0.003$). Compared to treatment with VC, AM surface expression of MerTK was significantly decreased following treatment with IFN-γ + LPS (mean of differences −0.58, $p = 0.015$), and IL-4 + IL-13 (mean of differences −0.47, $p = 0.004$). **(C)** Cytokine treatments significantly affected AM surface expression of CD163 (repeated measures ANOVA $p = 0.002$). Compared to treatment with VC, AM surface expression of CD163 was significantly decreased following treatment with IFN-γ + LPS (mean of differences −0.55, $p = 0.005$), and IL-4 + IL-13 (mean of differences −0.45, $p = 0.002$). **(D)** Cytokine treatments significantly affected AM surface expression of SIRPα (repeated measures ANOVA $p = 0.012$). Compared to treatment with VC, AM surface expression of SIRPα was significantly increased following treatment with IFN-γ + LPS (median of differences 2.48, $p = 0.036$). Compared to treatment with VC, AM surface expression of SIRPα was significantly decreased following treatment with IL-4 + IL-13 (median of differences −0.59, $p < 0.0001$). **(E)** Cytokine treatments significantly affected AM surface expression of CD206 (repeated measures ANOVA $p = 0.007$). Compared to treatment with VC, AM surface expression of CD206 was significantly increased following treatment with IL-4 + IL-13 (mean of differences 0.92, $p = 0.013$). There were no significant changes in CD206 expression following treatment with IFN-γ + LPS (mean of differences −0.13, $p = 0.777$). **(F)** Cytokine treatments did not significantly affect AM surface expression of CD80 (repeated measures ANOVA $p = 0.098$). MerTK, Mer tyrosine kinase receptor; SIRPα, signal regulatory protein-α.

of genes associated with a proresolving phenotype (39). Patients with chronic obstructive pulmonary disease (COPD) also have impaired AM efferocytosis (40) with overexpression of efferocytosis receptors CD206 and CD163 (41). Our data, therefore, suggest that the AM efferocytosis defect induced by ARDS BAL treatment is not mediated by surface-receptor changes.

Strategies to upregulate AM efferocytosis may reduce secondary necrosis of alveolar neutrophils, thereby attenuating inflammation in ARDS. Since *in vitro* ARDS BAL treatment downregulated AM Rac1 gene expression, we sought to upregulate Rac1 expression and restore efferocytosis by inhibiting ROCK and PTEN. The addition of ROCK inhibitor to ARDS BAL treatment partially restored AM efferocytosis function and did not affect bacterial phagocytosis. However, the addition of PTEN inhibitor had no significant effect; this may be because the role of PTEN is less important in antagonizing the PI3K pathway. ROCK inhibitors have been shown to increase efferocytosis in MDMs and AMs from patients with COPD (42). Further studies to investigate the role of the ROCK-PTEN-Rac1 pathway in ARDS AM dysfunction are required. Measurements of Rac1 and PI3K proteins expression in our model, with and without ROCK inhibition, are required to support the hypothesis that Rac1 inhibition is partially responsible for

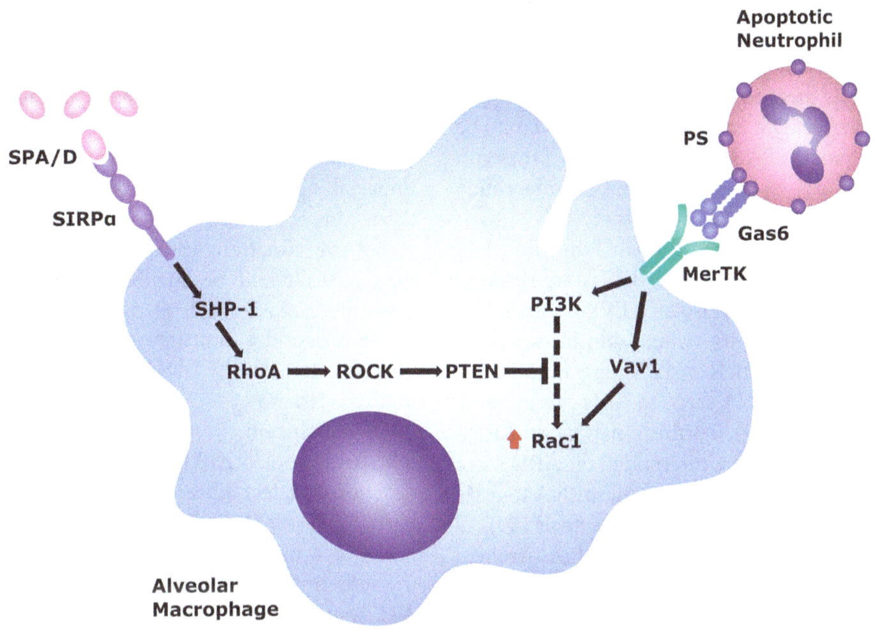

FIGURE 5 | Rac1 intracellular signaling pathways in alveolar macrophages. Alveolar macrophage efferocytosis is regulated by surface receptors MerTK and SIRPα. Gas6 binds to PS on the surface of apoptotic cells. Activation of MerTK by the PS opsonin Gas6 can trigger signaling cascades *via* PI3K and Vav1, which both upregulate Rac1. Activation of Rac1 results in cytoskeletal rearrangement and efferocytosis of the apoptotic cell. Activation of SIRPα by SP-A (or SP-D) triggers a signaling cascade along the SHP1/RhoA/ROCK/PTEN pathway, which inhibits PI3K signaling, and ultimately downregulates Rac1, thereby inhibiting efferocytosis. Gas6, growth arrest specific-6; MerTK, Mer tyrosine kinase receptor; PI3K, phosphatidylinositol 3′-OH kinase; PS, phosphatidylserine; PTEN, phosphatase and tensin homolog; ROCK, Rho-associated kinase; SHP-1, Src homology region 2 domain-containing phosphatase-1; SIRPα, signal regulatory protein-α; SPA/D, surfactant protein A/D.

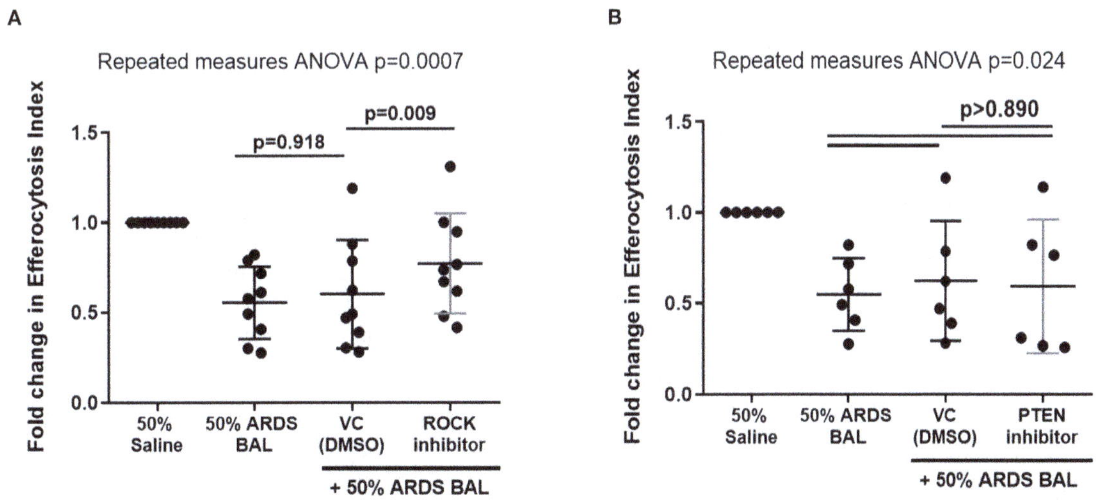

FIGURE 6 | Effect of ROCK and PTEN inhibitors on restoring alveolar macrophage efferocytosis following ARDS BAL treatment. Data are shown as fold change in AM efferocytosis index from 50% saline treatment. ROCK, Rho-associated protein kinase; PTEN, phosphatase and tensin homolog; VC, vehicle control [dimethyl sulfoxide (DMSO) at 1:50,000 dilution]. ROCK inhibitor = 200 nM Y-27632 dihydrochloride. PTEN inhibitor = 2 μM SF1670. Statistical analysis by repeated measures ANOVA with Tukey's multiple comparison test. **(A)** The addition of VC to ARDS BAL mixture had no significant effect on AM efferocytosis (mean of differences 0.05, $p = 0.918$, $n = 9$) compared to ARDS BAL alone. Addition of ROCK inhibitor to ARDS BAL treatment significantly increased efferocytosis compared to treatment with VC + ARDS BAL (mean of differences 0.17, $p = 0.009$, $n = 9$) **(B)** Addition of PTEN inhibitor to 50% ARDS BAL treatment had no significant effect on efferocytosis compared to treatment with VC + ARDS BAL (mean of differences 0.03, $p = 0.924$, $n = 6$).

impaired AM efferocytosis in ARDS. ROCK inhibition promotes PI3K signaling, which has multiple effects on a cellular function beyond upregulation of Rac1, namely, proliferation, chemotaxis, and migration (43). ROCK inhibition would have many off-target effects, thereby limiting its therapeutic potential as a strategy to upregulate AM function in ARDS. Existing medications could be tested using the *in vitro* model of ARDS, to determine if they can restore AM efferocytosis, e.g., N-acetylcysteine (44), macrolide antibiotics (45), statins (46), and glucocorticoids (47).

Studies utilizing an *ex-vivo* perfused human lung model of ARDS have shown that extracellular vesicles (EVs) are released following lung injury with *E. coli*; these isolated EVs subsequently mediated inflammatory lung injury when administered to uninjured lungs (48). Murine models of LPS lung injury have shown that EV transfer of microRNA cargo to AMs can increase inflammatory cytokine release (49). Further analysis of ARDS BAL and studies utilizing our *in vitro* model of ARDS are required to determine whether EV transfer of microRNA to AMs may affect intracellular pathways regulating efferocytosis (50).

Our study had some limitations. Due to logistical constraints, efferocytosis assays were undertaken with heterologous neutrophils, as opposed to autologous neutrophils, which would have more accurately reflected the environment *in vivo*. Although unaffected lung tissue was processed, we cannot rule out contamination with tumor-associated macrophages which are characterized by an immunosuppressive phenotype and may exhibit increased efferocytosis (51), which could account for some of the divergent effects observed. Expression of intracellular signaling mediators (e.g., Rac1) was only measured at the mRNA level. To draw definitive conclusions regarding the mechanism of impaired efferocytosis in ARDS, data on the protein expression of these mediators will be required. Ideally, the use of healthy human BAL would be a more appropriate VC instead of saline in this model; however, healthy BAL is a highly limited resource.

Another limitation to our study is that when assessing AM expression of TAM receptors (key mediators of macrophage efferocytosis), only MerTK was investigated (52). We had predominantly focused on MerTK, as this efferocytosis receptor was best characterized in the context of ARDS within the literature (18, 53–55). However, we omitted to investigate other important TAM receptors: Axl and Tyro3 (52). Impairment of the Axl signaling pathway has been associated with decreased AM efferocytosis in asthma (56). We report a contradictory increase in MerTK expression associated with decreased efferocytosis in AMs treated with ARDS BAL; however, this may, in part, be explained if the expression of TAM receptors Axl and/or Tyro3 were decreased. Further studies will be required to investigate this.

Studies have previously shown that the microenvironment can influence AM metabolism, inflammatory response, and gene expression (57, 58). *In vitro* culture of AMs can alter efferocytosis receptor expression profiles (56), therefore undertaking efferocytosis assays directly *in situ* on lung tissue may provide a more accurate representation of *in vivo* AM function (59). For future studies, precision-cut lung slices could be incubated with ARDS BAL before the assessment of efferocytosis directly on lung tissue (60); terminal deoxynucleotidyl transferase dUTP nick end labeling could be used to identify ANs in a double immunofluorescence method (59).

In conclusion, *in vitro* treatment of lung resection tissue AMs with pooled ARDS patient BAL can recapitulate the same functional defect observed *in vivo*. This dysfunction can be partially restored by ROCK inhibition. The *in vitro* model of ARDS is a useful tool to investigate the mechanisms by which the inflammatory alveolar microenvironment of ARDS induces AM dysfunction.

AUTHOR CONTRIBUTIONS

RM, AS, MM, and DT contributed to the study conception and design. RM, AS, DP, and SL contributed to data acquisition. RM, AS, and DT drafted the manuscript. All the authors contributed to the data analysis and interpretation, critically revised the manuscript for intellectual content, and approved the final version before submission.

ACKNOWLEDGMENTS

We would thank the nurses and thoracic surgeons of the Thoracic Research Team, University Hospitals Birmingham NHS Foundation Trust, for their help consenting patients undergoing thoracic surgery. We also thank Dr. Gerald Langman and Dr. Andrew Robinson, Department of Cellular Pathology, University Hospitals Birmingham NHS Foundation Trust, for their help in obtaining lung tissue samples from patients undergoing lobectomy. We thank Dr. Hui Li for her assistance in processing human lung tissue samples.

REFERENCES

Bellani G, Laffey JG, Pham T, Fan E, Brochard L, Esteban A, et al. Epidemiology, patterns of care, and mortality for patients with acute respiratory distress syndrome in intensive care units in 50 countries. *JAMA.* (2016) 315:788–800. doi: 10.1001/jama.2016.0291

Grasselli G, Tonetti T, Protti A, Langer T, Girardis M, Bellani G, et al. Pathophysiology of COVID-19-associated acute respiratory distress syndrome: a multicentre prospective observational study. *Lancet Respir Med.* (2020) 8:1201–1208. doi: 10.1016/S2213-2600(20)30370-2

Yang X, Yu Y, Xu J, Shu H, Xia J, Liu H, et al. Clinical course and outcomes of critically ill patients with SARS-CoV-2 pneumonia in Wuhan, China: a single-centered, retrospective, observational study. *Lancet Respir Med.* (2020) 8:475–81. doi: 10.1016/S2213-2600(20)30079-5

RECOVERY Collaborative Group. Tocilizumab in patients admitted to hospital with COVID-19 (RECOVERY): a randomised, controlled, open-label, platform trial. *Lancet.* (2021) 397:1637– 45. doi: 10.1016/S0140-6736(21)00676-0

Horby P, Lim WS, Emberson JR, Mafham M, Bell JL, Linsell L, et al. Dexamethasone in hospitalized patients with Covid-19. *N Engl J Med.* (2021) 384:693–704. doi: 10.1056/NEJMoa2021436

Bachofen M, Weibel ER. Alterations of the gas exchange apparatus in adult respiratory insufficiency associated with septicemia. *Am Rev Respir Dis.* (1977) 116:589–615. doi: 10.1164/arrd.1977.116.4.589

Ware LB, Matthay MA. Alveolar fluid clearance is impaired in the majority of

1patients with acute lung injury and the acute respiratory distress syndrome. *Am J Respir Crit Care Med.* (2001) 163:1376– 83. doi: 10.1164/ajrccm.163.6.2004035

Zemans RL, Colgan SP, Downey GP. Transepithelial migration of neutrophils: mechanisms and implications for acute lung injury. *Am J Respir Cell Mol Biol.* (2009) 40:519–35. doi: 10.1165/rcmb.2008-0348TR

Mahida RY, Scott A, Parekh D, Lugg ST, Hardy RS, Lavery GG, et al. Acute Respiratory Distress Syndrome is associated with impaired alveolar macrophage efferocytosis. *Euro Respir J.* (2021) 58:2100829. doi: 10.1183/13993003.00829-2021

Gregoire M, Uhel F, Lesouhaitier M, Gacouin A, Guirriec M, Mourcin F, et al. Impaired efferocytosis and neutrophil extracellular trap clearance by macrophages in ARDS. *Euro Respir J.* (2018) 52:1702590. doi: 10.1183/13993003.02590-2017

Gomez Perdiguero E, Klapproth K, Schulz C, Busch K, Azzoni E, Crozet L, et al. Tissue-resident macrophages originate from yolk-sac-derived erythro- myeloid progenitors. *Nature.* (2015) 518:547–51. doi: 10.1038/nature13989

Hashimoto D, Chow A, Noizat C, Teo P, Beasley MB, Leboeuf M, et al. Tissue-resident macrophages self-maintain locally throughout adult life with minimal contribution from circulating monocytes. *Immunity.* (2013) 38:792– 804. doi: 10.1016/j.immuni.2013.04.004

Yona S, Kim KW, Wolf Y, Mildner A, Varol D, Breker M, et al. Fate mapping reveals origins and dynamics of monocytes and tissue macrophages under homeostasis. *Immunity.* (2013) 38:79–91. doi: 10.1016/j.immuni.2012.12.001

Hussell T, Bell TJ. Alveolar macrophages: plasticity in a tissue-specific context. *Nat Rev Immunol.* (2014) 14:81–93. doi: 10.1038/nri3600

Thepen T, Van Rooijen N, Kraal G. Alveolar macrophage elimination in vivo is associated with an increase in pulmonary immune response in mice. *J Exp Med.* (1989) 170:499–509. doi: 10.1084/jem.170.2.499

Zizzo G, Hilliard BA, Monestier M, Cohen PL. Efficient clearance of early apoptotic cells by human macrophages requires M2c polarization and MerTK induction. *J Immunol.* (2012) 189:3508–20. doi: 10.4049/jimmunol. 1200662

Mosser DM, Edwards JP. Exploring the full spectrum of macrophage activation. *Nat Rev Immunol.* (2008) 8:958–69. doi: 10.1038/ nri2448

Lee YJ, Lee SH, Youn YS, Choi JY, Song KS, Cho MS, et al. Preventing cleavage of Mer promotes efferocytosis and suppresses acute lung injury in bleomycin treated mice. *Toxicol Appl Pharmacol.* (2012) 263:61– 72. doi: 10.1016/j.taap.2012.05.024

Wu Y, Tibrewal N, Birge RB. Phosphatidylserine recognition by phagocytes: a view to a kill. *Trends Cell Biol.* (2006) 16:189–97. doi: 10.1016/j.tcb.2006.02.003

van der Meer JH, van der Poll T, van't Veer C. TAM receptors, Gas6, and protein S: roles in inflammation and hemostasis. *Blood.* (2014) 123:2460– 9. doi: 10.1182/blood-2013-09-528752

Janssen WJ, McPhillips KA, Dickinson MG, Linderman DJ, Morimoto K, Xiao YQ, et al. Surfactant proteins A and D suppress alveolar macrophage phagocytosis via interaction with SIRP alpha. *Am J Respir Crit Care Med.* (2008) 178:158–67. doi: 10.1164/rccm.200711-1661OC

Meili R, Sasaki AT, Firtel RA. Rho rocks PTEN. *Nat Cell Biol.* (2005) 7:334– 5. doi: 10.1038/ncb0405-334

Scott A, Lugg ST, Aldridge K, Lewis KE, Bowden A, Mahida RY, et al. Pro-inflammatory effects of e-cigarette vapour condensate on human alveolar macrophages. *Thorax.* (2018) 73:1161–9. doi: 10.1136/thoraxjnl-2018-211663

O'Kane CM, McKeown SW, Perkins GD, Bassford CR, Gao F, Thickett DR, et al. Salbutamol up-regulates matrix metalloproteinase-9 in the alveolar space in the acute respiratory distress syndrome. *Crit Care Med.* (2009) 37:2242–9. doi: 10.1097/CCM.0b013e3181a5506c

Davies JQ, Gordon S. Isolation and culture of human macrophages. *Methods Mol Biol.* (2005) 290:105–16. doi: 10.1385/1-59259-838-2:105

Michlewska S, Dransfield I, Megson IL, Rossi AG. Macrophage phagocytosis of apoptotic neutrophils is critically regulated by the opposing actions of pro-inflammatory and anti-inflammatory agents: key role for TNF-alpha. *FASEB J.* (2009) 23:844–54. doi: 10.1096/fj.08-121228

Wootton DG, Diggle PJ, Court J, Eneje O, Keogan L, Macfarlane L, et al. Recovery from pneumonia requires efferocytosis which is impaired in smokers and those with low body mass index and enhanced by statins. *Thorax.* (2016) 71:1052–4. doi: 10.1136/thoraxjnl-2016-208505

Zizzo G, Cohen PL. IL-17 stimulates differentiation of human anti- inflammatory macrophages and phagocytosis of apoptotic neutrophils in response to IL-10 and glucocorticoids. *J Immunol.* (2013) 190:5237– 46. doi: 10.4049/jimmunol.1203017

Serban KA, Petrusca DN, Mikosz A, Poirier C, Lockett AD, Saint L, et al. Alpha-1 antitrypsin supplementation improves alveolar macrophages efferocytosis and phagocytosis following cigarette smoke exposure. *PLoS ONE.* (2017) 12:e0176073. doi: 10.1371/journal.pone.0176073

Jepsen LV, Skottun T. A rapid one-step method for the isolation of human granulocytes from whole blood. *Scand J Clin Lab Investig.* (1982) 42:235– 8. doi: 10.3109/00365518209168079

Sapey E, Patel JM, Greenwood H, Walton GM, Grudzinska F, Parekh D, et al. Simvastatin improves neutrophil function and clinical outcomes in pneumonia: a pilot randomised controlled trial. *Am J Respir Crit Care Med.* (2019) 200:1282–93. doi: 10.1164/rccm.201812-2328OC

Bonecchi R, Sozzani S, Stine JT, Luini W, D'Amico G, Allavena P, et al. Divergent effects of interleukin-4 and interferon-gamma on macrophage-derived chemokine production: an amplification circuit of polarized T helper 2 responses. *Blood.* (1998) 92:2668– 71. doi: 10.1182/blood.V92.8.2668.420k39_2668_2671

Rosseau S, Hammerl P, Maus U, Walmrath HD, Schutte H, Grimminger F, et al. Phenotypic characterization of alveolar monocyte recruitment in acute respiratory distress syndrome. *Am J Physiol Lung Cell Mol Physiol.* (2000) 279:L25–35. doi: 10.1152/ajplung.2000.279.1.L25

Mould KJ, Barthel L, Mohning MP, Thomas SM, McCubbrey AL, Danhorn T, et al. Cell origin dictates programming of resident versus recruited macrophages during acute lung injury. *Am J Respir Cell Mol Biol.* (2017) 57:294–306. doi: 10.1165/rcmb.2017-0061OC

Heijnen NFL, Hagens LA, Smit MR, Schultz MJ, van der Poll T, Schnabel RM, et al. Biological subphenotypes of acute respiratory distress syndrome may not reflect differences in alveolar inflammation. *Physiol Rep.* (2021) 9:e14693. doi: 10.14814/phy2.14693

Park WY, Goodman RB, Steinberg KP, Ruzinski JT, Radella F, 2nd, Park DR, et al. Cytokine balance in the lungs of patients with acute respiratory distress syndrome. *Am J Respir Crit Care Med.* (2001) 164(10 Pt 1):1896– 903. doi: 10.1164/ajrccm.164.10.2104013

Hodge S, Hodge G, Ahern J, Jersmann H, Holmes M, Reynolds PN. Smoking alters alveolar macrophage recognition and phagocytic ability: implications in chronic obstructive pulmonary disease. *Am J Respir Cell Mol Biol.* (2007) 37:748–55. doi: 10.1165/rcmb.2007-0025OC

Kazeros A, Harvey BG, Carolan BJ, Vanni H, Krause A, Crystal RG. Overexpression of apoptotic cell removal receptor MERTK in alveolar macrophages of cigarette smokers. *Am J Respir Cell Mol Biol.* (2008) 39:747– 57. doi: 10.1165/rcmb.2007-0306OC

Shaykhiev R, Krause A, Salit J, Strulovici-Barel Y, Harvey BG, O'Connor TP, et al. Smoking-dependent reprogramming of alveolar macrophage polarization: implication for pathogenesis of chronic obstructive pulmonary disease. *J Immunol.* (2009) 183:2867–83. doi: 10.4049/jimmunol.0900473

Hodge S, Hodge G, Scicchitano R, Reynolds PN, Holmes M. Alveolar macrophages from subjects with chronic obstructive pulmonary disease are deficient in their ability to phagocytose apoptotic airway epithelial cells. *Immunol cell Biol.* (2003) 81:289–96. doi: 10.1046/j.1440-1711.2003.t01-1-01170.x

Kaku Y, Imaoka H, Morimatsu Y, Komohara Y, Ohnishi K, Oda H, et al. Overexpression of CD163, CD204 and CD206 on alveolar macrophages in the lungs of patients with severe chronic obstructive pulmonary disease. *PLoS ONE.* (2014) 9:e87400. doi: 10.1371/journal.pone.0087400

Bewley MA, Belchamber KB, Chana KK, Budd RC, Donaldson G, Wedzicha JA, et al. Differential effects of p38, MAPK, PI3K or Rho kinase inhibitors on bacterial phagocytosis and efferocytosis by macrophages in COPD. *PLoS ONE.* (2016) 11:e0163139. doi: 10.1371/journal.pone.0163139

Vanhaesebroeck B, Stephens L, Hawkins P. PI3K signalling: the path to discovery and understanding. *Nat Rev Mol Cell Biol.* (2012) 13:195. doi: 10.1038/nrm3290

Moon C, Lee YJ, Park HJ, Chong YH, Kang JL. N-acetylcysteine inhibits RhoA and promotes apoptotic cell clearance during intense lung inflammation. *Am J Respir Crit Care Med.* (2010) 181:374–87. doi: 10.1164/rccm.200907-1061OC

Hodge S, Hodge G, Jersmann H, Matthews G, Ahern J, Holmes M, et al. Azithromycin improves macrophage phagocytic function and expression of mannose receptor in chronic obstructive pulmonary disease. *Am J Respir Crit Care Med.* (2008) 178:139–48. doi: 10.1164/rccm.200711-1666OC

Morimoto K, Janssen WJ, Fessler MB, McPhillips KA, Borges VM, Bowler RP, et al. Lovastatin enhances clearance of apoptotic cells (efferocytosis) with implications for chronic obstructive pulmonary disease. *J Immunol.* (2006) 176:7657–65. doi: 10.4049/jimmunol.176.12.7657

McColl A, Bournazos S, Franz S, Perretti M, Morgan BP, Haslett C, et al. Glucocorticoids induce protein S-dependent phagocytosis of apoptotic neutrophils by human macrophages. *J Immunol.* (2009) 183:2167– 75. doi: 10.4049/jimmunol.0803503

Liu A, Park JH, Zhang X, Sugita S, Naito Y, Lee JH, et al. Therapeutic effects of hyaluronic acid in bacterial pneumonia in *ex vivo* perfused human lungs. *Am J Respir Crit Care Med.* (2019) 200:1234–45. doi: 10.1164/rccm.201812-2296OC

Shikano S, Gon Y, Maruoka S, Shimizu T, Kozu Y, Iida Y, et al. Increased extracellular vesicle miRNA-466 family in the bronchoalveolar lavage fluid as a precipitating factor of ARDS. *BMC Pulmonary Med.* (2019) 19:110. doi: 10.1186/s12890-019-0876-9

Mahida RY, Matsumoto S, Matthay MA. Extracellular vesicles: a new frontier for research in acute respiratory distress syndrome. *Am J Respir Cell Mol Biol.* (2020) 63:15–24. doi: 10.1165/rcmb.2019-0447TR

Zhou J, Tang Z, Gao S, Li C, Feng Y, Zhou X. Tumor-associated macrophages: recent insights and therapies. *Front Oncol.* (2020) 10:188. doi: 10.3389/fonc.2020.00188

Lemke G, Rothlin CV. Immunobiology of the TAM receptors. *Nat Rev Immunol.* (2008) 8:327–36. doi: 10.1038/nri2303

Choi JY, Park HJ, Lee YJ, Byun J, Youn YS, Choi JH, et al. Upregulation of Mer receptor tyrosine kinase signaling attenuated lipopolysaccharide- induced lung inflammation. *J Pharmacol Exp Ther.* (2013) 344:447– 58. doi: 10.1124/jpet.112.199778

Lee YJ, Han JY, Byun J, Park HJ, Park EM, Chong YH, et al. Inhibiting Mer receptor tyrosine kinase suppresses STAT1, SOCS1/3, and NF-κB activation and enhances inflammatory responses in lipopolysaccharide-induced acute lung injury. *J Leukocyte Biol.* (2012) 91:921–32. doi: 10.1189/jlb.0611289

Mohning MP, Thomas SM, Barthel L, Mould KJ, McCubbrey AL, Frasch SC, et al. Phagocytosis of microparticles by alveolar macrophages during acute lung injury requires MerTK. *Am J Physiol Lung Cell Mol Physiol.* (2018) 314:L69–82. doi: 10.1152/ajplung.00058.2017

Grabiec AM, Denny N, Doherty JA, Happonen KE, Hankinson J, Connolly E, et al. Diminished airway macrophage expression of the Axl receptor tyrosine kinase is associated with defective efferocytosis in asthma. *J Allergy Clin Immunol.* (2017) 140:1144–6.e4. doi: 10.1016/j.jaci.2017.03.024

Svedberg FR, Brown SL, Krauss MZ, Campbell L, Sharpe C, Clausen M, et al. The lung environment controls alveolar macrophage metabolism and responsiveness in type 2 inflammation. *Nat Immunol.* (2019) 20:571– 80. doi: 10.1038/s41590-019-0352-y

Lavin Y, Winter D, Blecher-Gonen R, David E, Keren-Shaul H, Merad M, et al. Tissue-resident macrophage enhancer landscapes are shaped by the local microenvironment. *Cell.* (2014) 159:1312–26. doi: 10.1016/j.cell.2014.11.018

Proto JD, Doran AC, Gusarova G, Yurdagul A, Jr., Sozen E, et al. Regulatory T Cells Promote Macrophage Efferocytosis during Inflammation Resolution. *Immunity.* (2018) 49:666–77.e6. doi: 10.1016/j.immuni.2018.07.015

Dutra Silva J, Su Y, Calfee CS, Delucchi KL, Weiss D, McAuley DF, et al. Mesenchymal stromal cell extracellular vesicles rescue mitochondrial dysfunction and improve barrier integrity in clinically relevant models of ARDS. *Euro Respir J.* (2021) 58:2002978. doi: 10.1183/13993003.02978-2020

12

Gene Therapy for Acute Respiratory Distress Syndrome

Jing Liu[1,2] *and David A. Dean*[1,2*]

[1] Department of Pediatrics, University of Rochester, Rochester, NY, United States, [2] Department of Pharmacology and Physiology, University of Rochester, Rochester, NY, United States

***Correspondence:**
David A. Dean
David_dean@urmc.rochester.edu

Acute respiratory distress syndrome (ARDS) is a devastating clinical syndrome that leads to acute respiratory failure and accounts for over 70,000 deaths per year in the United States alone, even prior to the COVID-19 pandemic. While its molecular details have been teased apart and its pathophysiology largely established over the past 30 years, relatively few pharmacological advances in treatment have been made based on this knowledge. Indeed, mortality remains very close to what it was 30 years ago. As an alternative to traditional pharmacological approaches, gene therapy offers a highly controlled and targeted strategy to treat the disease at the molecular level. Although there is no single gene or combination of genes responsible for ARDS, there are a number of genes that can be targeted for upregulation or downregulation that could alleviate many of the symptoms and address the underlying mechanisms of this syndrome. This review will focus on the pathophysiology of ARDS and how gene therapy has been used for prevention and treatment. Strategies for gene delivery to the lung, such as barriers encountered during gene transfer, specific classes of genes that have been targeted, and the outcomes of these approaches on ARDS pathogenesis and resolution will be discussed.

Keywords: viral vectors, non-viral vectors, sepsis, acute lung injury, electroporation, alveolar fluid clearance, barrier function

INTRODUCTION

Acute respiratory distress syndrome (ARDS) is a devastating clinical syndrome that leads to acute respiratory failure (Ware, 2006; Thompson et al., 2017; Matthay et al., 2019). ARDS can be directly caused by bacterial or viral infection of or chemical damage to the lung, or indirect due to injuries outside the lung or systemic inflammatory response, such as non-pulmonary sepsis, blood transfusions, and non-pulmonary injury (Pelosi et al., 2003; Rezoagli et al., 2017). In all cases, bacterial or viral infection is most commonly seen clinically. Most recently, the global pandemic of the coronavirus disease-2019 (COVID-19) has caused a high number of severe ARDS cases in the United States and around the world. As of October 24, 2021, there have been more than 45 million COVID 19 cases and more than 733,000 deaths in the United States (CDC, 2021). From multiple studies, approximately 33% of hospitalized COVID-19 patients develop ARDS, and there is a ~70% mortality rate for COVID-19 patient-associated ARDS (Hasan et al., 2020; Tzotzos et al., 2020). The incidence of ARDS among non-survivors of COVID-19 is even higher, up to 90%, indicating that ARDS accounts for the majority of COVID-19 deaths (Tzotzos et al., 2020). Although the molecular mechanisms regarding the pathogenesis and progress of ARDS have been studied for decades, the development of effective treatments has lagged, and clinical management strategies still rely on supportive care, broad activity pharmacological treatment, ventilation, prone positioning, and other supportive strategies (Matthay et al., 2020). This review will focus on the pathophysiological features of ARDS and summarize the state of gene therapy treatments for ARDS.

CELLULAR AND MOLECULAR MECHANISMS OF ACUTE RESPIRATORY DISTRESS SYNDROME

The key features of ARDS are pulmonary edema of noncardiogenic origin and pathologic diffuse alveolar damage (DAD; Thompson et al., 2017; Matthay et al., 2019), which is primarily caused by alveolar capillary barrier dysfunction and the resulting flooding of alveoli and lung interstitial space with protein-rich fluid (Matthay et al., 2019). The clinical hallmarks of ARDS include refractory hypoxemia due to insufficient gas exchange, fluffy bilateral infiltrates on X-ray radiographs, decreased lung compliance due to alveolar collapse and edema, and increased physiological dead space fraction due to lung microvascular destruction (Lewis and Jobe, 1993; Ware and Matthay, 2000; Nuckton et al., 2002; Matthay and Zemans, 2011). Although ARDS is defined by its pulmonary versus extrapulmonary origin, lung mechanical dysfunction is etiologically independent (Menezes et al., 2005). The observed edema and inflammation in both direct and indirect injured lungs indicate several significant events, namely, alveolar capillary barrier dysfunction, impaired alveolar fluid resolution, and uncontrolled neutrophil activation, sequestration, and their metabolite-mediated inflammatory responses (Ware and Matthay, 2001; Ware, 2006; Matthay and Zemans, 2011; Herrero et al., 2018). Perhaps the best illustration of these mechanisms remains the classic figure of the healthy and injured alveoli introduced by Lorraine Ware and Michael Matthay in 2000, although a relatively recent update incorporates several features now realized to be central to ARDS pathogenesis (**Figure 1**; Ware and Matthay, 2000). Understanding the mechanisms behind these events would provide insights to identify therapeutic targets for ARDS gene therapy.

Alveolar-Capillary Barrier Dysfunction

One early event during the exudative phase that defines ARDS is the accumulation of pulmonary edema, the major factor causing hypoxemia (**Box 1**; Bhattacharya and Matthay, 2013; Matthay et al., 2019). In the normal lung, fluid homeostasis is maintained by microvascular filtration, which provides the fluid source, and lymphatic clearance, which drains the filtrate flow away (Bhattacharya and Matthay, 2013). Vascular endothelial permeability is the determining factor for microvascular filtration (Staub, 1978; Mehta and Malik, 2006). It shows selectivity to sieve large protein molecules (e.g., albumin) in the plasma (Siflinger-Birnboim et al., 1987; Mehta and Malik, 2006; Sukriti et al., 2014), creating high osmotic pressure to encounter the pro-filtration force (hydrostatic pressure) and promote water retention in the circulation (Bhattacharya and Matthay, 2013). Besides the lymphatic system, the filtrate also flows into alveoli forming a protective liquid layer with surfactant (Lindert et al., 2007). Alveolar fluid balance is mainly determined by epithelial integrity, which provides a tight barrier preventing fluid influx and alveolar fluid clearance (AFC), which drives water out of the alveolar space based on the Na^+ osmotic gradient (Matthay et al., 2002; Johnson et al., 2006; Bhattacharya and Matthay, 2013; Herrero et al., 2018). The importance of the alveolar-capillary barrier and AFC can be reflected from the cardiogenic lung edema, which shows much less protein content (Sprung et al., 1981; Ware et al., 2010), and could be quickly resolved because of the relatively intact alveolar epithelial and capillary endothelial integrity and fluid clearance capacity (Matthay, 2014; Hamacher et al., 2018). However, in ARDS, accumulated pulmonary edema results from the loss of the alveolar-capillary barrier, hyperpermeability, and impaired AFC, allowing the influx of fluid and large amounts of proteins to accumulate in the interstitial and alveolar spaces (Ware and Matthay, 2000, 2001; Matthay et al., 2012; Matthay, 2014). In patients with ARDS, various endothelial injury markers, e.g., von Willebrand factor (VWF; Ware et al., 2004), can be detected in blood and epithelial apoptotic markers, e.g., cytokeratin-18 (Lee et al., 2008; Galani et al., 2010), and can be measured in bronchoalveolar lavage (BAL) fluid. Clinically, the decreased AFC capacity is associated with prolonged acute respiratory failure and higher mortality rate (Ware and Matthay, 2001); and the degree of injury to the alveolar epithelium appears to be a determinant of the severity of ARDS (Matthay et al., 2005; Yanagi et al., 2015). Multiple mechanisms are involved in alveolar-capillary barrier and AFC dysfunction, such as cell death, loss of cell-cell adhesion molecules and ion transporter activities, and activation of neutrophils and their products. Apoptosis induces alveolar epithelial cell death, and many studies show that apoptosis is the main route of cell death detectable immediately following lung injury (Albertine et al., 2002; Martin et al., 2003; Tang et al., 2008; Perl et al., 2010; Herrero et al., 2013; Jagrosse et al., 2019). In addition, cellular necrosis is also seen in patients with ARDS (Tomashefski, 2000; Cardinal-Fernández et al., 2017). Many studies have shown that Fas/Fas ligand (FasL) extrinsic pathway-mediated apoptosis contributes to ARDS (Herrero et al., 2013). The Fas/FasL system is significantly upregulated in the pulmonary edema fluid of patients with ARDS and is associated with increased mortality (Matute-Bello et al., 1999; Albertine et al., 2002). In animal models of ARDS, there is increased expression of Fas in epithelial cells and FasL in BAL (Fine et al., 1997; Hamann et al., 1998; Perl et al., 2007). A study using chimeric mice expressing Fas receptor exclusively on non-myeloid cells, including lung epithelial cells, demonstrated that lung injury is primarily via the activation of the pro-apoptotic pathway in alveolar epithelial cellsand is associated with increased alveolar permeability and edema formation (Matute-Bello et al., 2005a). Besides the Fas/FasL-mediated extrinsic apoptotic pathway, Bcl-2-mediated intrinsic apoptosis is also involved, which might be relevant to the mitochondrial dysfunction seen in this disease (Tang et al., 2008). During ARDS, cell death is greatly due to multiple cellular dysfunctions: elevated CO_2 levels and oxidative imbalance lead to mitochondrial DNA damage and cell toxicity (Herold et al., 2013), ventilator-induced

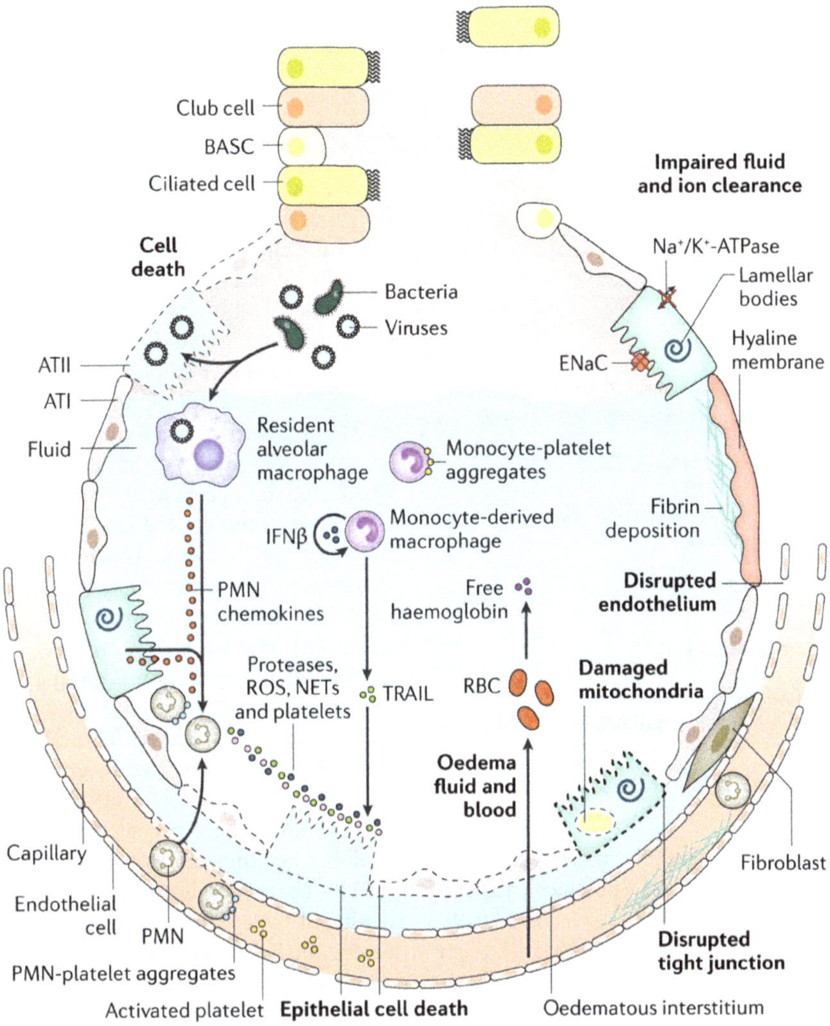

FIGURE 1 | Injured alveolus in the acute phase of lung injury and acute respiratory distress syndrome. A variety of insults (such as acid, viruses, ventilator-associated lung injury, hyperoxia, and bacteria) can injure the epithelium, either directly or by inducing inflammation, which in turn injures the epithelium. Direct injury is inevitably exacerbated by a secondary wave of inflammatory injury. Activation of toll-like receptors (not shown) on alveolar type II (ATII) cells and resident macrophages induces the secretion of chemokines, which recruit circulating immune cells into the airspaces. As neutrophils migrate across the epithelium, they release toxic mediators, such as proteases, reactive oxygen species (ROS), and neutrophil extracellular traps (NETs), which have an important role in host defense but cause endothelial and epithelial injury. Monocytes also migrate into the lungs and can cause an injury, such as epithelial cell apoptosis *via* IFNβ-dependent release of tumor necrosis factor (TNF)-related apoptosis-inducing ligand (TRAIL), which activates death receptors. Activated platelets form aggregates with polymorphonuclear (PMN) leukocytes, which are involved in NET formation, and monocyte–platelet aggregates. Red blood cells (RBCs) release cell-free hemoglobin, which exacerbates injury *via* oxidant-dependent mechanisms. Angiopoietin 2 inhibits TIE2-stabilization of vascular endothelial cadherin (VE-cadherin); vascular endothelial growth factor and other permeability-promoting agonists also destabilize VE-cadherin *via* dissociation from p120-catenin, resulting in its internalization and enhanced paracellular permeability. Additionally, loss of cell–cell adhesion in the setting of actomyosin contraction results in the formation of occasional gaps between endothelial cells. Epithelial injury also includes wounding of the plasma membrane, which can be induced by bacterial pore-forming toxins or mechanical stretch, and mitochondrial dysfunction. Together, these effects result in endothelial and epithelial permeability, which further facilitates the transmigration of leukocytes and leads to the influx of edematous fluid and RBCs. Airspace filling with edematous fluid causes hypoxemia, resulting in the need for mechanical ventilation. Vascular injury and alveolar edema contribute to the decreased ability to excrete CO_2 (hypercapnia), accounting for the elevated pulmonary dead space in acute respiratory distress syndrome. In turn, hypoxemia and hypercapnia impair vectorial sodium transport, reducing alveolar edema clearance. ATI, alveolar type I cell; BASC, bronchioalveolar stem cell; ENaC, epithelial sodium channel. Reproduced with permission (Ware and Matthay, 2000).

mechanical stress (Syrkina et al., 2008), hypoxia (Tang et al., 2008), NO formation by iNOS (Rudkowski et al., 2004), and LPS-activated apoptotic signaling (Zeng et al., 2018). Since gene therapy requires living cells as targets in order for any gene expression to take place, the level of apoptotic or necrotic cells can have a profound effect on any such treatment. Thus, in order for gene therapy to be effective, the level of cell death needs to be relatively low or the treatment must be administered prior to significant cell loss.

The alveolar capillary barrier is composed of two physical barriers: a tight alveolar epithelial monolayer of flat ATI cells (95% of alveolar surface area) and cuboidal ATII cells (5%

BOX 1 | Mechanisms for edema formation.

I) **Alveolar-capillary barrier dysfunction**

- **Epithelial and endothelial cell injury markers:** Fas/FasL, RAGE (epithelial) VWF, Angiopoietin 2 (endothelial)
- **Cell death:** apoptosis; necrosis
- **Adhesion junction disruption and downregulation:** Proteolytic degradation: ZO-1; VE-cadherin; E-cadherin Claudin-4,5,18 Phosphorylation and internalization: occludin; VE-cadherin
- **Inducing factors:** oxidative stress; ROS; ventilation; mitochondrial damage NETs; cytokines; LPS; virus

II) **Alveolar fluid clearance dysfunction**

- **Decreased cell membrane abundance of Na, K, ENaC** hypoxia; ROS; IAV; IFNs; TRAIL; coagulation proteases; decreased adrenergic stimulation
- **Decreased mRNA and protein level of Na, k, ENaC, CFTR** hypoxia; IL-lb; TGFbl; TNFa; oxidant; INFr
- **Decreased transepithelial ion transport activities** loss of epithelial polarity reduced channel open probability

III) **PMN activation and inflammation mediators**

- **Increased PMN recruitment**
- **NETosis induced lung barrier disruption** DNA; histone; MPO; NE
- **extracellular matrix modeling** increased MM P-2,9
- **Increased cytokine level in plasma and BAL fluid** IL-lb, TNFa, IL-6 and IL-8

of alveolar surface area), and a relatively more permeable microvascular endothelial cell monolayer (Bhattacharya and Matthay, 2013; Knudsen and Ochs, 2018; Katz et al., 2019). A study measuring (Matthay and Zimmerman, 2005) I-labeled albumin flux in blood, surrounding interstitium, and alveolar space in sheep lungs indicates that more than 92% of resistance to albumin flux across the alveolar capillary barrier lies in the epithelial barrier (Gorin and Stewart, 1979). Adhesion molecules holding together neighboring cells in the monolayer are the major structural components regulating the paracellular permeability pathway, the major route for passage of large molecules, such as albumin, across both barriers (Mehta and Malik, 2006; Overgaard et al., 2012; Bhattacharya and Matthay, 2013). Tight junctions (TJs) are located in the most apical side of the alveolar epithelium and largely determine barrier tightness (Overgaard et al., 2012; Gunzel and Yu, 2013). Damage to TJs greatly contributes to epithelial barrier leakage, further increasing edema accumulation without necessary cell death (Hook et al., 2018; Matthay et al., 2019). Claudins, key tight junction proteins, are highly expressed in the alveolar epithelium with the predominant isoforms being claudin-3, 4, and 18 (Overgaard et al., 2012). Knockout (KO) of claudin18 in mice shows significant accumulation of FITC-albumin in the BAL 4 h after intraperitoneal instillation of labeled tracer, indicating increased alveolar epithelial permeability (LaFemina et al., 2014). Morphological disruption of this barrier is further confirmed by ultrastructural analysis of ATI and ATII cells (Bachofen and Weibel, 1977, 1982). In cultured alveolar epithelial cells, silencing of claudin 18 by siRNA shows decreased transepithelial electrical resistance (TEER), a measurement of epithelial tightness *in vitro*, and increased permeability to small size tracer markers (LaFemina et al., 2014; Srinivasan et al., 2015). Similarly, overexpression of claudin 4 increases TEER by nearly 50% (Mitchell et al., 2011); KO of claudin 4 in mice not only increases barrier permeability to solute but also, surprisingly, decreases AFC, which might be relevant to decrease in Na^+, K^+-ATPase activity (Wray et al., 2009; Overgaard et al., 2012). The promotion of AFC by claudin 4 in the alveolar epithelium is also indicated by the property of Cl^--selective paracellular permeability, since claudin4 limits paracellular Na flux but favors transepithelial Cl^- transport for electrical neutrality during Na^+ active transport for fluid clearance (Colegio et al., 2002, 2003). Occludin is another important transmembrane a TJ molecule expresses in both the epithelium and endothelium (Förster, 2008). The internalization and phosphorylation of occludin are associated with lung barrier dysfunction (Hirase et al., 2001; Förster, 2008). TJ proteins are targets of numerous factors during ARDS, namely, excessive ROS (Rao, 2008), pathogens (Lu et al., 2014), e.g., LPS, viruses and bacteria, ventilation (Liu et al., 2014), inflammatory mediators (Al-Sadi et al., 2009), hypoxia (Caraballo et al., 2011), hyperoxia (You et al., 2012), and inhaled particulate matter (PM; Wang et al., 2012).

Endothelial dysfunction is another important contributor to alveolar capillary barrier disruption, leading to uncontrolled extravascular fluid leakage. The microvascular endothelium is the first barrier encountered by fluid and neutrophils infiltrating from vessels into the alveoli. Under normal conditions, the endothelium is more permeable to large macromolecules than the alveolar epithelium. However, upon activation by pathogens, e.g., LPS-containing bacteria, the endothelial barrier properties are altered by a series of events, such as structural damage to the endothelial barrier, significant proinflammatory response, coagulation and micro-thrombosis formation, and vascular tone dysregulation (Vassiliou et al., 2020).

Endothelial hyperpermeability can directly result from structural damage to the endothelial barrier, through both endothelial cell apoptosis and inter-endothelial cell junctional complex disruption. For the former, mitochondrial DNA (mtDNA) damage may initiate endothelial cell death (Ruchko et al., 2005). Mitochondria are a major source of ROS in the endothelium (Ince et al., 2016). Under oxidative stress, mtDNA released from mitochondria, in turn, triggers mitochondrial dysfunction and induces apoptosis through cytochrome c and the intrinsic apoptosis pathway. Circulating mtDNA has been reported as a plasma biomarker for the severity of sepsis or sepsis-related ARDS with higher plasma cell-free mtDNA levels observed in ICU patients who died within 28 days of medical ICU admission, as well as in ICU patients with sepsis or ARDS (Nakahira et al., 2014). Receptor agonism-initiated extrinsic apoptosis also contributes to endothelial cell death. Tumor necrosis factor alpha (TNFα) receptor and Fas are also expressed in endothelial cells, and their activation has been shown to induce caspases 8 and 3 signaling, resulting in apoptosis (Hotchkiss et al., 2002). Recently, more types of cell death programs have been identified in dysfunctional endothelium during sepsis, such as necrosis and pyroptosis (Singla and Machado, 2018). Pyroptosis is of particular interest in sepsis, since it is triggered by proinflammatory signals and is vital for endothelial injury when overactivated (Gao et al., 2018). Knockout of one of key pyroptosis mediators, such as caspase 1 or 11, displays resistance to endotoxic shock in mice and provides increased survival and protection against vascular injury, endothelial hyperpermeability, lung edema, and histological damage (Li et al., 1995; Cheng et al., 2017; Mitra et al., 2018).

The endothelial paracellular pathway is the major filtration route of the microvasculature, and disruption of inter-endothelial junction structures may account for another mechanism of barrier hyperpermeability (Bhattacharya and Matthay, 2013). Inter-endothelial junction molecules include tight junctions, adherens junctions, junctional adhesion molecules (JAMs), and other endothelial specific molecules, such as platelet endothelial cell adhesion molecules (PECAMs; Komarova and Malik, 2010). In contrast to the alveolar epithelium where tight junctions play a major role in the integrity of epithelial barrier function, in the capillary endothelium, tight junctions are secondary, while adherens junctions play a more significant role (Mehta and Malik, 2006; Aird, 2007). Vascular endothelial cadherin (VE-cadherin), a key component of the endothelial adherens junction, primarily maintains the architectural integrity of the endothelial barrier, rendering high permeability to plasma proteins, a key property in establishing protein (e.g., albumin) gradients for fluid balance in the lungs. Claudin-5 is the predominant tight junction molecule expressed in pulmonary endothelial cells (Kaarteenaho-Wiik and Soini, 2009) and has been found to be downregulated in various models of ALI, such as influenza infection (Armstrong et al., 2012). Pathogen-induced VE-cadherin phosphorylation, internalization, and lysosomal degradation are major forms of VE-cadherin disruption (Chan et al., 2020). All of these junctional molecules are also targets of oxidative stress, ROS, IL-1β and other stimuli (Xiong et al., 2020). In addition, some sepsis mediators, e.g., high-mobility group protein B1, have been shown to activate acto-myosin contraction, inducing endothelial cell retraction, which mechanically breaks apart adhesion junctions, leading to hyperpermeability (Wolfson et al., 2011). Such cytoskeletal contraction due to phosphorylation of myosin light chain (MLC) is a common cause of endothelial cell retraction, and signaling pathways involved in the activation of MLC have been extensively studied and shown to be mediated through a number of pathways, most notably RhoA/ROCK (Reutershan et al., 2007). Furthermore, influx of Ca2+ has been shown to increase vascular permeability and allow for migration of neutrophils across the alveolocapillary barrier, as well as overall vascular leakage (Alvarez et al., 2006).

Glycocalyx shedding has been recognized in recent years as another crucial mechanism undermining endothelial barrier integrity, leading to edema formation and sepsis-induced organ failure. The glycocalyx is a thin multicomponent fibrous matrix layer lining the luminal endothelial surface, which includes proteoglycans, glycoproteins, and glycosaminoglycans that protect the vascular endothelium from oxidants, hyperglycemia, cytokines, and bacterial endotoxins (Weinbaum et al., 2007; Ince et al., 2016). However, these toxins, in turn, often induce glycocalyx degradation, and that layer becomes thinner as a result of and during sepsis. Glycocalyx fragments, such as syndecan-1, shed into the blood and have been reported as potential clinical biomarkers for sepsis survival and respiratory failure (Smart et al., 2018). Bacteria, TNF-α, and ROS all induce degradation of the glycocalyx layer, making the endothelial lining more vulnerable to pathogens and leading to barrier disruption and protein-rich extravascular fluid leakage. That the glycocalyx provides such a protective layer to the endothelium is exemplified by the fact that Crocin, a chemical compound, has been shown to prevent LPS-induced ARDS by protecting against glycocalyx degradation (Zhang et al., 2020). Glycocalyx shedding also decreases the sensitivity of endothelial cell responses to sheer stress, leading to unbalanced release of nitric oxide and vascular tone dysregulation (Ince et al., 2016). In addition, glycocalyx shedding may exacerbate endothelial proinflammatory response by promoting neutrophil adhesion to endothelial cells.

Neutrophil activation and transmigration from the circulation into lung tissue are perhaps the most significant events of the proinflammatory response during the early stage of ALI. However, excessive neutrophil activation induces endothelial barrier damage and, ultimately, lung damage. Neutrophil transendothelial migration requires temporal and spatial increases in endothelial paracellular permeability, which is a process found in normal host defense. However, uncontrolled neutrophil transmigration results in the prolonged opening of intercellular junction structures and increased paracellular permeability, which leads to fluid accumulation and edema in the interstitial tissue, and, ultimately, ARDS (Tsushima et al., 2009). Moreover, toxic mediators (e.g., proteases and ROS, etc.) and cytokines released from activated neutrophils also damage endothelial cells, inducing vascular leakage. More details are addressed below in "Neutrophil activation and inflammatory mediators." In addition, endothelial homeostasis is disrupted during sepsis or ARDS, shifting to a pro-coagulant condition with massive production of thrombin, which directly affects the endothelial barrier, leading to hyperpermeability (Bogatcheva et al., 2002).

Alveolar Fluid Clearance Dysfunction

Alveolar fluid clearance, or AFC, is important for maintaining fluid homeostasis in the lungs and is regulated by osmotic pressure (Matthay et al., 2002; Huppert and Matthay, 2017). The active transport of Na^+ ions is the main contributor for the creation of the osmotic gradient: Na^+ is primarily transported through the amiloride-sensitive ENaC, as well as by the nonselective (NCC) or highly selective cation channels (SCC) and cyclic nucleotide-gated (CNG) channels on the apical epithelial surface and then extruded out of the cell by the Na^+, K^+ ATPase on the basolateral surface into the interstitium and the circulation (Matthay, 2014). The Na^+, K^+ ATPase is the primary determining factor for AFC since it is the major active Na^+ transporter expressed in the epithelial basolateral membrane, which continuously pumps Na^+ out of the alveoli by utilizing ATP (Mutlu and Sznajder, 2005). Instillation of ouabain, a cardiac aminoglycoside inhibitor of the Na^+, K^+ ATPase, into animal and *ex vivo* human lungs decreases AFC by more than 50% (Matthay et al., 2002). Conversely, adenovirus- or electroporation-mediated overexpression of the

Na^+, K^+ ATPase increased AFC by ~100% in rat lungs (Machado-Aranda et al., 2005).

During lung injury, fluid clearance is impaired, ultimately resulting in hypoxemia (Huppert and Matthay, 2017). Majority of patients with ARDS show severe fluid clearance impairment, whereas 25% of all patients with hydrostatic lung edema have ARDS (Ware and Matthay, 2001). Multiple factors result in AFC impairment during ARDS (Vadasz et al., 2007). Loss of epithelial polarity due to disrupted epithelial TJs decreases AFC (Han et al., 2004; Zemans and Matthay, 2004). Hypoxia induces the downregulation of both ENaC and Na^+, K^+ ATPase at the mRNA level and membrane abundance of the Na^+, K^+ ATPase (Planès et al., 1997; Zhou G. et al., 2008). The Na^+, K^+ ATPase is most vulnerable to hypoxic effects, since it works by consuming ATP. Indeed, ~40% of a cell's total energy is consumed by this transporter to maintain homeostasis, and during injury, reduced oxygenation limits ATP production (Milligan and McBride, 1985). Excessive resulting ROS triggers Na^+, K^+ ATPase endocytosis through α1 subunit phosphorylation (Dada et al., 2003). Pathogens, such as influenza A virus, induce degradation of membrane-localized Na^+, K^+ ATPase in nearby noninfected alveolar epithelial cells by activating pathways in the infected epithelium and resident macrophages that produce cytokines like type I IFN and IFN- related apoptosis-inducing ligand (TRAIL; Peteranderl et al., 2016). Proinflammatory cytokines, such as IL-1β, IL-8, and TGFβ1, are detected at high levels in the edema fluid of patients in the early stage of ARDS (Pugin et al., 1999; Lee et al., 2011). They downregulate the expression and function of ENaC and the Na^+, K^+ ATPase through activation of various pathways in the epithelium, causing decreased AFC (Pugin et al., 1999). Furthermore, mechanical ventilation also negatively affects Na^+ transport activity and AFC (Lecuona et al., 1999), although it is commonly used in the ICU to facilitate breathing and oxygenation. Indeed, in ATII cells isolated from rats after high tidal volume ventilation, the activity of Na^+, K^+ ATPase decreased by 50% compared to the control group (Lecuona et al., 1999).

Besides being critical for AFC, the expression and function of the Na^+, K^+ ATPase are closely involved in the regulation of epithelial barrier integrity (Rajasekaran et al., 2001b; Rajasekaran and Rajasekaran, 2003; Vadasz et al., 2007). Increasing evidence indicates that the role of the Na^+, K^+ ATPase in barrier junction formation is independent of its ion transport activity. For example, (1) the Na^+, K^+ ATPaseβ1 subunit may be necessary for membrane localization of TJs (Rajasekaran et al., 2007); silencing of β1 by siRNA disrupts the continuous staining pattern of ZO-1 and occludin, indicating that β1 might be directly or indirectly associated with TJs (Madan et al., 2007); (2) the Na^+, K^+ ATPase is required for establishing epithelial polarization in MDCK cells and co-expression of the Na^+, K^+ ATPaseβ1 subunit, and E-cadherin recovers the lost polarity and junctions seen in MSV-MDCK cells, a highly invasive cell line (Rajasekaran et al., 2001b); (3) the basolateral localized Na^+, K^+ ATPase also acts as an adhesion molecule, forming a trans-dimer junction structure mediated through the N-glycosylation of β1's extracellular domain (Vagin et al., 2012). The mechanisms by which the Na^+, K^+ ATPase regulates epithelial barrier function has not completely been characterized, but it appears related to stress fiber formation and actin assembly (Rajasekaran and Rajasekaran, 2003). RhoA GTPase, a small GTP-binding protein involved in stress fiber formation (Guasch et al., 1998), has been implicated as a downstream effector of Na^+, K^+ ATPase signaling for TJ assembly and function (Rajasekaran et al., 2001a). We recently identified MRCKα (CDC42-binding protein kinase alpha) by mass spectrometry as an interacting partner of the β1 subunit (Bai et al., 2021). These findings point to the interdependency of alveolar capillary barrier and AFC dysfunction in edema formation during ARDS. MRCKα is a Rho GTPase effector kinase that regulates diverse cell behaviors, such as actomyosin contraction-mediated junction formation (**Figure 2**; Unbekandt and Olson, 2014). Silencing of MRCKα by siRNA abolished the increased TEER seen in cultured AT1 cells following transfection with the β1 subunit, indicating that β1 signals through MRCKα to upregulate tight junction proteins and epithelial barrier function, at least in cells (Bai et al., 2021).

Neutrophil Activation, Inflammatory Mediators, and Coagulation

Recruitment of neutrophils is a hallmark of ARDS and is considered to play a key role in the progression of ARDS. An analysis of BAL fluid cellularity in patients with ARDS or animals in various injury models demonstrates elevated neutrophil infiltration into alveoli. This is correlated with ARDS outcomes and severity, with non-survivors having higher levels of chemotactic IL-8 than survivors of ARDS. Neutrophils are important components of the innate immune system. In response to stimuli, they are activated, recruited, and secrete various antimicrobial molecules, such as ROS, proteases, and cationic peptides, to destroy invading microorganisms. However, under some disease conditions, e.g., ARDS, excessive neutrophil activation and imbalanced inflammatory responses can cause additional tissue damage. NETosis is an important mechanism of neutrophil defense against invading pathogens, in which neutrophils release DNA combined with histones, myeloperoxidase, neutrophil elastase, and extracellular fibers into the extracellular environment to form a network for microorganism trapping (Thiam et al., 2020). This increased extracellular NET production is correlated with ARDS severity and alveolar capillary barrier dysfunction in experimental models. Elastase in NETs degrades alveolar capillary barrier integrity, contributing to edema formation. It proteolytically degrades junctional molecules, such as ZO-1, E-cadherin, and VE-cadherin, to induce intercellular adhesion disruption in cultured epithelial and endothelial monolayers. Histones are the most abundant proteins in NETs, and it has been shown that incubation of endothelial cells or ATII cells with histones induces cell death, suggesting a role in damage to alveolar capillary barrier integrity. Finally, matrix metalloproteinases (MMPs) are produced by a variety of cell types, such as neutrophils, and the levels of MMP-2 and 9 are increased in BAL of patients and are correlated with ARDS severity.

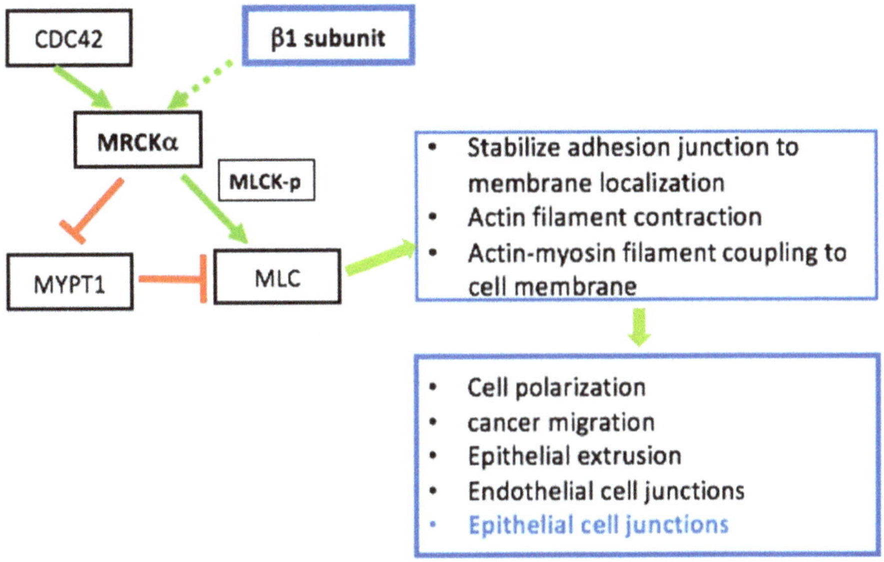

FIGURE 2 | MRCKα signaling pathway is involved in epithelial intercellular junction regulation. MRCKα is activated (solid green arrow) by cdc42, a Rho family of small GTPases. The MRCKα kinase activates myosin light chain (MLC) either by directly phosphorylating/activating (green arrow) myosin light chain kinase (MLCK) or by inactivating (red arrow) myosin phosphatase target subunit 1 (MYPT1), which dephosphorylates/ inactivates (red arrow) MLC. The two consecutive negative activities (red arrows) result in the indirect activation of MLC by reducing MLC dephosphorylation/ inactivation. These events regulate multiple cellular functions such as actin-myosin contraction, which is involved in epithelial junction regulation. In addition, our previous data indicate that overexpression of β1- Na^+, K^+-ATPase increases activation/phosphorylation of MLC (Bai et al., 2021).

Uncontrolled inflammatory response is another hallmark of the early stage of ARDS that contributes to lung barrier disruption and AFC impairment, leading to edema formation (Ware and Matthay, 2000; Matthay and Zimmerman, 2005). Inflammatory response is initiated, amplified, and regulated by a network of various cytokines and other inflammatory molecules (Park et al., 2001). High concentrations of cytokines, such as IL-1β, TNFα, IL-6, and IL-8, are detected in plasma and BAL fluids and are associated with poor clinical outcomes of ARDS, such as mortality rate (Pugin et al., 1996; Parsons et al., 2005; McClintock et al., 2008). In several experimental models, highly expressed TNFα in BAL fluid triggers caspase-8-mediated apoptotic signaling in the epithelium, inducing cell death, and consequently, alveolar epithelial barrier dysfunction (Patel B. V. et al., 2013).

Coagulation is a critical host response to infection. However, it is also involved in ARDS pathogenesis with markedly increased release of soluble tissue factor and microthrombi formation in the pulmonary microvasculature and decreased fibrinolytic activities with diffuse alveolar and interstitial fibrin deposition (Grinnell et al., 1980; Nagy et al., 1995). Some studies have shown that pro-coagulant activities observed during ARDS can increase alveolar capillary barrier permeability (Abraham, 2000; Mosnier et al., 2007). As seen in both patients and experimental animal models, upregulated levels of soluble tissue factor, thrombin, and fibrinolysis inhibitors are present in BAL fluid (Idell et al., 1991; Fuchs-Buder et al., 1996). In cultured epithelial cells, thrombin induces F-actin polymerization and stress fiber formation, which further increases cell contraction, stiffness, and epithelial barrier permeability (Hayashi et al., 2006). Platelets are another important component of the host defense system and may contribute to the neutrophil-dependent lung injury (Rossaint et al., 2018). Activated platelets have been shown to directly interact with neutrophils, facilitating their extravasation and recruitment to the lungs (Zarbock and Ley, 2009; Rossaint et al., 2018). In acid-induced lung injury, platelet-neutrophil interactions in the vascular endothelium could be visualized by electron microscopy within 30 min of injury (Zarbock et al., 2006). These studies showed that platelet depletion significantly reduces neutrophil rolling and adherence to the endothelium, thereby markedly reducing lung edema and increasing mouse survival.

Current Pharmacological Treatments for Acute Respiratory Distress Syndrome

Over the past several decades, considerable research efforts have made ARDS well-understood in terms of pathogenesis, risk factors, genetic predispositions, and various signaling pathways and molecules involved. Although large efforts have been committed to developing pharmacological therapies for ARDS, the results have been discouraging. A review from 2018 summarized that large-scale clinical trials with positive results only account for 5% of the 20 most recent large pharmacological studies on both sepsis and ARDS (Laffey and Kavanagh, 2018). The incidence and overall hospital mortality of ARDS have not changed considerably in the past 10 years (Villar et al., 2016). In the 2016 cross-country study LUNG SAFE, the mortality rate remained at 40% for moderate ARDS and even higher at 46% for severe ARDS (Bellani et al., 2016). In the evolving COVID-19 pandemic, the mortality rate for patients with COVID-19 associated ARDS is even higher, which further highlights the importance of developing novel treatments or therapies for ARDS.

β_2 Adrenergic agonists have been demonstrated to enhance AFC *in vivo* through the activation of the cAMP pathway, which increases transepithelial ion transport by upregulating the activity and membrane abundance of ENaC, Na^+, K^+-ATPases and chloride channels (Bertorello et al., 1999; Matalon and O'Brodovich, 1999; Fang et al., 2002; Mutlu et al., 2004; Mutlu and Sznajder, 2005). While treatment of mice with existing acute lung injury with several different β_2 agonists, such as albuterol and salmeterol, can treat the disease and give positive outcomes in lung function, inflammation, edema clearance, and survival, none of these treatments have been proven effective in patients. Indeed, it has even been suggested to avoid using these drugs in patients with ARDS (Boyle et al., 2013). In several clinical studies, β_2 adrenergic therapy showed no significance in the primary outcome of ventilator-free days and even worsened the outcome of increased mortality, although there was some amelioration in pulmonary fluid accumulation (Perkins et al., 2006; National Heart Lung Blood Institute Acute Respiratory Distress Syndrome (ARDS) Clinical Trials Network et al., 2011; Gao Smith et al., 2012; Matthay et al., 2017; Laffey and Kavanagh, 2018). Several possibilities might account for the failure of β_2 receptor agonist therapy. For example, prolonged β_2 adrenergic agonism by endogenous catecholamines could desensitize β_2 receptors, which would prevent further receptor stimulation with exogenous catecholamines (Berthiaume et al., 2002). In some patients with no response to β adrenergic therapy, the alveolar epithelium might be too injured to benefit from any transporter upregulation (Hamacher et al., 2018). In addition, some circulating factors could limit the action of β-adrenergic agonists (Berthiaume et al., 2002).

Corticosteroids are commonly used for both prevention and treatment of ARDS, given their anti-inflammation properties (Khilnani and Hadda, 2011). Although nearly 20% of patients with ARDS receive systemic steroids, there is no clear-cut efficacy of steroids in attenuating lung injury (Boyle et al., 2013; Bellani et al., 2016). Similarly, non-steroidal anti-inflammatory agents ketoconazole and lisofylline also failed in clinical trials for the early treatment of ARDS (The ARDS Network, 2000; The ARDS Clinical Trials Network, 2002). However, the recent identification of ARDS sub-phenotypes (hypo- vs. hyper-inflammatory phenotypes) may help to specify ARDS cohorts and show promise for anti-inflammation therapy to ARDS. For example, statins have been proposed for use in ARDS because of their anti-inflammatory function beyond lowering cholesterol, and they have shown to significantly improve the 28-day survival of patients compared to placebo in a "hyper-inflammatory" subgroup (Calfee et al., 2018). However, no difference was detected in a "hypo-inflammatory" subgroup in terms of the same outcome. Nitric oxide (NO) is crucial in regulating vascular tone and blood flow. Inhaled NO has also been shown to improve pulmonary gas exchange and oxygenation in animal models of ARDS, but as for most other drugs, in patients, inhaled NO has shown no long-term survival benefits (Putensen et al., 1994; Rossaint et al., 1995; Adhikari et al., 2007).

N-Acetylcysteine (NAC) is a common antioxidant widely used for treating conditions characterized by the generation of free oxygen radicals (Shahin et al., 2009). It has been tested in multiple trials on sepsis and lung-injury related ARDS, as well as COVID-19-induced ARDS. However, the benefit of antioxidant therapy with NAC is not consistent among studies, including early mortality rate, duration of ICU stay, and oxygenation (Adhikari et al., 2004; Shahin et al., 2009; Lu et al., 2019). A recent clinical study using NAC for COVID-19 treatment, a high dose of NAC showed no significant benefit in terms of mortality, ICU admission, or time of invasive mechanical ventilation compared to the placebo group (de Alencar et al., 2020).

Apart from these examples, a number of potential therapies have shown promising results in preclinical studies but have been proven ineffective or even harmful in clinical trials. These include surfactant replacement, neutrophil elastase (NE) inhibitors, aspirin, heparin, and angiotensin-converting enzyme (ACE) inhibitors. The use of ACE inhibitors has been limited in preclinical studies because of their side effects on systemic hypotension (Arndt et al., 2006). However, ACE2, which counteracts the activity of ACE, was demonstrated to have a treatment effect on patients with ARDS in a pilot study (Imai et al., 2005; Khan et al., 2017). In addition, ACE2 is a functional receptor for SARS-CoV-2, the coronavirus that caused the COVID-19 pandemic in 2020, and recombinant ACE2 has entered clinical trials (NCT04335136) for COVID-19 (Bao et al., 2020).

PULMONARY STRUCTURAL BARRIERS FOR GENE DELIVERY

The lung is a highly specialized and delicate organ that has evolved to maximumly expose blood to air for gas exchange (Hsia et al., 2016). Functionally, conducting airways connecting the inner and outer pulmonary environments dominate the airflow during inhalation and exhalation. Thus, easy access to both the airways and vascular network makes the lung attractive for gene delivery (Pouton and Seymour, 2001; Gautam et al., 2002). Genes can be easily administered through intranasal or oral inhalation using nebulizers or by bronchoscopy-mediated intratracheal administration (Gautam et al., 2002; Katz et al., 2019). For small rodents, oropharyngeal aspiration is a straightforward and simple method for gene delivery into the lung (Zhang S. et al., 2013; Bale et al., 2016; Lin et al., 2016). Compared to intravascular injection, airway delivery shows lower DNA and RNA degradation by nuclease activities (Liu et al., 2007; Henning et al., 2010). Normally, the human lung has approximately 480 million alveoli, which compose a large surface area (~140 m; Guggino and Cebotaru, 2017) for any gene delivery and account for more than 99% of total lung internal surface area (Crapo et al., 1983; Ochs et al., 2004). Furthermore, there is a massive pulmonary micro-capillary network surrounding alveoli for gas exchange. The thin alveolar epithelial monolayer (0.1–0.5 μm; Weibel, 1973) and its formed massive lung surface area, together with the high permeability of the alveolar-capillary membrane, provide superior conditions for gene and/or particle deposition and uptake into the lung (Labiris and Dolovich, 2003).

Although the lung is unique and has advantages for gene delivery, low transfection efficiency has hindered the progress of gene therapy for lung diseases because of multiple barriers, such as complex branching of the conducting airways, alveolar-capillary barrier, surfactant, lining fluid and mucus, basement membrane, and host immunological defenses. The conducting airways defend the lungs from exogenous particles and bacterial and viral insults through mucociliary clearance (Nicod, 2005). However, they also trap therapeutic genes and decrease the efficiency of delivery (Duncan et al., 2016; Bustamante-Marin and Ostrowski, 2017). For patients with cystic fibrosis, their airways are progressively filled with thickened mucus that forms a solid barrier hindering viral vector or nonviral liposomal vector penetration into the lungs (Sanders et al., 2009; Schuster et al., 2014). Sufficient delivery of gene materials into the parenchymal session of the lungs is also challenging since it heavily relies on particle deposition (Paranjpe and Müller-Goymann, 2014). The respiratory airway branches multiple times to the distal terminal bronchioles and ends in the alveolar sacs (Patwa and Shah, 2015; Hsia et al., 2016; Sondhi et al., 2017). Once delivered cargos, e.g., plasmids, viral vectors, peptides, and siRNA, reach the alveoli, they face the risk of phagocytosis by resident alveolar macrophages (Patton, 1996; Patton et al., 2004; Katz et al., 2019). Localization of a Cy3-labeled adenoviral vector by fluorescence microscopy shows that adenoviral vectors are rapidly internalized (~1 min) by alveolar macrophages after reaching the alveolar surface (Zsengellér et al., 2000). In a mouse model, within 24 h following administration, 70–90% of adenovirus genomes were cleared, indicating the significance of macrophages in transfection efficiency (Worgall et al., 1997). Surfactant proteins, SP-A and SP-D, can interact with gene delivery agents containing carbohydrate domains, decreasing their transfection efficiency (Vadolas et al., 2002). In addition, the thin alveolar epithelial monolayer provides a large surface area for particle deposition (Labiris and Dolovich, 2003); meanwhile, the tightness formed by junction molecules between cells increases difficulties for gene transfer to subepithelial cells (Patton and Byron, 2007; Murgia et al., 2014).

In addition, the pathological conditions of several diseases would complicate those barrier mechanisms, and metabolic products could also be potential barriers hindering gene delivery (Weiss, 2002). For example, sputum from patients with CF could slow down the adeno-associated virus (AAV) vector diffusion rate by >1,000 fold compared to water (Schuster et al., 2014), and some patients' sputum also contains adenovirus-specific antibodies that neutralize the Ad vectors for further inhibition (Perricone et al., 2000). During acute lung injury and ARDS, pulmonary edema influx, which results from the loss of the alveolar epithelium and alveolar capillary barrier dysfunction, collapsed alveoli, excessive mucus secretion, and the proinflammatory environment make it hard to transduce the injured lung (Zhang et al., 1998; Weiss, 2002; Matthay et al., 2019).

GENE DELIVERY SYSTEMS

Because both the cell membrane and nucleic acids are highly negatively charged and, thus, repel each other, delivering exogenous genetic materials into cells requires either a carrier or vector to mask the nucleic acid's charge or a physical method to circumvent the membrane. Vectors usually refer to virus particles, and carriers typically imply nonviral chemical agents. Ideally, the vector/carrier should show high transduction efficiency with a sufficient number of cells transduced, cell or tissue specificity, enough stability to protect the transgene from extracellular and intracellular degradation, and, perhaps most importantly, minimal immune and inflammatory responses (Mehier-Humbert and Guy, 2005; Katz et al., 2013, 2019). Gene delivery vectors can be classified into two broad categories: viral vectors and nonviral physical or chemical methods (Nishikawa and Huang, 2001; Nayerossadat et al., 2012; Ginn et al., 2018). In either case, high-quality, clinical-grade vectors (viral or nonviral) could be used for any clinical trial. Currently, a number of biotechnology and pharmaceutical companies are focusing on the development of virus- and nonvirus-based systems for gene therapy with the goal of providing single-dose medications available for use in the ICU or even in the outpatient setting (depending on the indication). Thus, like the mRNA-based Covid19 vaccine, any nucleic acid-based gene therapy approach would be available from hospital pharmacies for direct use in patients.

Viral Vectors

Viral vectors are widely used for gene therapy because of their high transduction efficiency and oftentimes long duration of transgene expression (Bouard et al., 2009). For use as a gene transfer vector, the viral genome is modified to limit viral replication by removing critical viral genes, for example, Gag, Pol, and Env genes in retroviruses, and replacing them with the desired transgene for the target protein (Verma and Weitzman, 2005). Both RNA and DNA viruses have been employed extensively for lung gene delivery (Driskell and Engelhardt, 2003; Sondhi et al., 2017). In the case of RNA viruses, the retrovirus was first used in *ex vivo* lung gene therapy for α1AT deficiency (Garver et al., 1987). Because the RNA genome requires conversion into double-stranded DNA, which then can integrate into the host chromosomal genome (Chiu and Davies, 2004; Yi et al., 2011; Sondhi et al., 2017), it was seen as an ideal vector for long-term durable expression. However, retroviruses are only able to transduce proliferating cells (Hu and Pathak, 2000; Schambach and Morgan, 2016) and have been of limited use for *in vivo* lung gene delivery, since most of the cells in the lungs are not dividing at any given time (Driskell and Engelhardt, 2003; Sondhi et al., 2017). Compared to retroviruses, lentiviral vectors are able to infect nondividing cells (Naldini et al., 1996)and have been proven to be more useful for lung gene delivery (Driskell and Engelhardt, 2003; Patel M. et al., 2013; Marquez Loza et al., 2019). Two types of lentivirus, human immunodeficiency virus (HIV; Goldman et al., 1997) and feline immunodeficiency virus (FIV; Wang et al., 1999), have been shown to infect the airway epithelium for cystic fibrosis gene therapy. However, their application is hindered by the lack of suitable receptors expressed on the epithelial apical surface for viral approach (Walters et al., 1999). In the face of this disadvantage, envelope glycoprotein-pseudotyped lentiviruses were developed to widen their host range (James et al., 2005). For example, pseudotyped lentiviral vectors from filoviruses (Kobinger et al., 2001; Sinn et al., 2017a), baculovirus (Sinn et al., 2012, 2017b), Ebolavirus (Kobinger et al., 2001), influenza virus (Patel M. et al., 2013), and Sendai virus (Mitomo et al., 2010; Griesenbach et al., 2012) all confer access to receptors on the apical side of airway epithelial cells, allowing gene transfer to these cells. In contrast, vesicular stomatitis virus (VSV) glycoprotein-pseudotyped vectors predominantly enter from the epithelial basolateral surface (Goldman et al., 1997; Johnson et al., 2000; Kremer et al., 2007), which limits their direct translation into clinical use. Since RNA viruses integrate the transgene into the host genome in a random fashion, there exists the possibility of oncogene activation or induced mutagenesis for these vectors (Anson, 2004; Bushman, 2007; Milone and O'Doherty, 2018). So far, most application of lentivirus to the lung has focused on chronic diseases, e.g., cystic fibrosis, rather than ARDS, and it is being used for RNA interference-mediated gene knockdown (Tiscornia et al., 2003; Copreni et al., 2004). One study using lentivirus delivered shRNA to silence CD36, which is required for latent TGF-β1 activation, and showed antifibrotic effects after injury to the lung in a silicosis model (Wang et al., 2009). However, since short-term gene expression is more desirable for acute indications like ARDS, such integrating vectors are not appropriate.

The most studied and widely used DNA viral vectors include replication-deficient adenovirus (Ad) and adeno-associated virus (AAV) derived vectors (Crystal, 2014; Katz et al., 2019). Ad contains a large, double-stranded linear DNA genome (~36 kb), whereas AAV contains a single-stranded DNA genome that is relatively small (~4.7 kb) (Verma and Weitzman, 2005). Since the Ad genome can be transcribed and replicated episomally (Samulski and Muzyczka, 2014; Sondhi et al., 2017), without necessary integration into the host genome, Ad vectors can confer moderate duration expression and show high transduction efficiency in non-dividing cells of the airway (Crystal, 2014). Unfortunately, Ad vectors are highly immunogenic and induce strong host inflammatory and immune responses specifically against products of these viral genes (Schiedner et al., 1998; Ahi et al., 2011; Lundstrom, 2018), which hinder repetitive administration of the vector and limit gene expression to 2–3 weeks (Crystal, 2014). Several generations of Ad vectors have been developed in order to minimize the host inflammatory and immune responses (Capasso et al., 2014). Compared to the first and second generations of Ad vectors with partial viral genome deletion (Verma and Weitzman, 2005; Capasso et al., 2014), the third generation, called "gutted/helper dependent" Ad vector (Kochanek et al., 2001; Capasso et al., 2014), has had the whole viral coding region deleted to minimize viral antigen expression (Alba et al., 2005; Verma and Weitzman, 2005). Although these advanced Ad vectors enable *in vivo* gene delivery by maximally reducing initial inflammatory responses to administration (Koehler et al., 2006), their capsid proteins can still induce cytotoxic T-cell destruction of the infected cells by antigen presentation and induce antibody production, again preventing subsequent vector administration (Alba et al., 2005; Katz et al., 2019). Of note, a common drawback to *in vivo* viral delivery is immune responses that might confront animals or patients with preexisting lung injuries to a higher risk of inflammatory toxicities (Lin and Dean, 2011). For example, adenovirus transfected rat lungs with high efficiency and uniform distribution of marker genes; however, all end point measurements, such as AFC, were taken 7 days after animal recovery because of viral infection-induced inflammatory responses (Factor et al., 1998). In comparison, electroporation is an effective method to deliver plasmid DNA to living animal lungs with no extra damage and high-level gene expression (Somiari et al., 2000; Dean et al., 2003).

Compared to Ad vectors, AAV vectors show less immunogenicity but have high transduction efficiency, persistent transgene expression, and broad host range (Mingozzi and High, 2013; Samulski and Muzyczka, 2014). Several serotypes of AAV vectors, for example, 2, 5, 6, and 9, have been shown to effectively transduce the airway and alveolar epithelium, and have allowed limited re-administration in experimental animals (Limberis et al., 2009; Li et al., 2011). In a rat model of ARDS, delivery of aerosolized AAV serotypes 2 and 6 to rat lung showed high transduction efficiency of transgene expression, which significantly prevented subsequent LPS-induced lung injury in a protection model (MacLoughlin et al., 2015). AAV-mediated gene therapy for CF has even moved into phase I/II clinical trials (Guggino and Cebotaru, 2017). However, the application of AAV for clinical trials is still limited because of its small packaging capacity, difficulty producing large quantities, issues with re-dosing, and various immune responses in different organs (Mingozzi and High, 2011; Sondhi et al., 2017; Wang et al., 2019).

Nonviral Gene Delivery: Chemical Vectors

Although viral vectors remain the major delivery method for gene therapy, accounting for approximately two-thirds of total vectors used in clinical trials in 2017 (Ginn et al., 2018), nonviral vectors have been increasingly used in clinical trials since 2004 (~23%) (Ginn et al., 2018). Compared to viral vectors, nonviral vectors possess some inherent advantages for gene delivery (Nayerossadat et al., 2012; Yin et al., 2014; Ginn et al., 2018; Patil et al., 2019): (1) much larger transgene packaging capacity; (2) much better safety profile; (3) ability to carry and deliver DNA or RNA by chemical carriers; (4) ability for repeat administration; (5) low immunogenicity due to lack of antigen presentation to adaptive immune system; and (6) ease of synthesis and production in large quantities. Indeed, DNA- and RNA-based vectors (plasmids, minicircles, mRNA, and siRNA) are simple and relatively inexpensive to produce on a large scale, especially when compared to their viral counterparts. Although nonviral gene transfer has been widely performed in research in laboratories, its applications in clinical trials have been hindered by several obstacles, such as lower transfection efficiency, lack of specific cell targeting, and lack of stability compared to viral vectors (Glover et al., 2005; Ramamoorth and Narvekar, 2015; Ginn et al., 2018). For example, naked plasmid DNA delivered systemically is degraded quickly, and its half-life is estimated to be only 10 min following intravenous (IV) injection in mice (Kawabata et al., 1995). Thus, various physical and chemical methods have been developed to enhance gene transfection efficiency *in vivo* (Nayerossadat et al., 2012). Cationic lipid- (lipoplexes) and cationic polymer- (polyplexes) based vectors are the most commonly used chemical transfection reagents and are extensively used in gene transfer to the lungs (Davis and Cooper, 2007; Aneja et al., 2009; Jones et al., 2013). Both types of delivery agent interact electrostatically with the negatively charged DNA, forming a net positively charged lipoplex- or polyplex-DNA complex for further interaction with the cell membrane (Zuidam and Barenholz, 1998; Zhu and Mahato, 2010; Jones et al., 2013). Consistent with fundamental purposes of using vectors for gene delivery, namely to overcome multiple extracellular and intracellular barriers and facilitate therapeutic nucleic acids reaching target cells or tissues, chemical vectors are designed to increase the stability and transfection efficiency of DNA complexes and decrease their biodegradability (Zhu and Mahato, 2010). Following intravenous administration, DNA complexes face multiple barriers, such as endonuclease degradation, traversing the vascular wall, intercellular junctions, the cytoplasmic membrane of target cells, and avoiding entrapment in endosomal vesicles (Song et al., 1997; Pack et al., 2005; Hill et al., 2016). Thus, it is important to investigate vector structure-activity relationships and their optimization for lung gene delivery.

Cationic lipids are diverse in structure, but there are three basic structural components, a cationic head group, a hydrophobic tail, and a linker connecting both the head and tail groups (Zhu and Mahato, 2010; Jones et al., 2013). The positively charged hydrophilic head group is the major domain that interacts with negatively charged DNA molecules, leading to plasmid condensation, enhanced cellular uptake, and endosomal escape (Miller et al., 1998; Tseng et al., 2009; Zhu and Mahato, 2010). The hydrophobic tail group is usually composed of saturated or monounsaturated fatty acid chains (aliphatic chains) with various lengths (Niculescu-Duvaz et al., 2003; Kou et al., 2011). It is widely accepted that gene transfection efficiency is inversely correlated with chain length, which means the shorter the chain length (e.g., C14), the higher the transfection efficiency. This is presumably due to increased lipoplex stability (Felgner et al., 1994; Adir et al., 2008; Jones et al., 2013). Cholesterol is a commonly used alternative for the hydrophobic tail domain and shows enhanced fusion with the host cell membrane (Mahato et al., 1997; Jones et al., 2013; Monteiro et al., 2014). The linker that connects the cationic head to the hydrophobic tail domain can greatly impact the stability and biodegradability of the lipoplex (Mahato et al., 1999). Ether bonds, such as those in DOTMA, are indicated to render good gene delivery efficiency because of their stable and nondegradable properties, but their cytotoxicity is higher than that of other linker chemicals, such as esters and amides (Singhal and Huang, 1994; Freedland et al., 1996; Zhu and Mahato, 2010; Jones et al., 2013). Cleavable linkers are also used as an alternative. Additionally, the cationic nature of the head group can be another source of cytotoxicity, since it can interact non-specifically with negatively charged serum proteins (albumin, lipoproteins, and IgG), resulting in charge neutralization, reduced cellular uptake, hemolysis, and decreased transfection efficiency (Escriou et al., 1998; Zelphati et al., 1998; Lv et al., 2006; Jones et al., 2013). It has been shown that intravenous injection of DNA lipoplexes actually induces embolization in the lungs because of large complex size (>5 μm) by interaction with blood components, leading to failure to pass through capillaries (Litzinger et al., 1996; Nishikawa and Huang, 2001).

Cationic polymers also form complexes with DNA through electrostatic interactions and coat the complex with a net positive charge (Nishikawa and Huang, 2001; Eliyahu et al., 2005). Polyethylenimine (PEI) is one of the most commonly used synthetic polymers with a highly positive charge (Eliyahu et al., 2005; Jin L. et al., 2014). The different amine groups in PEI's structure affect the polyplex's endosomal escape after uptake by displaying buffering capacities over a wide range of pH (Zhu and Mahato, 2010). It has been proposed that different types of amines work as a "proton sponge", which can be protonated to different levels as the endosomal environment acidifies, leading to ultimate endosomal breakup and release of their contents (i.e., DNA) (Boussif et al., 1995; Eliyahu et al., 2005; Pack et al., 2005; Jin L. et al., 2014). Compared to linear PEI, which contains almost all secondary amines in its backbone, branched PEI contains primary, secondary, and tertiary amino groups (Fischer et al., 1999; Zhu and Mahato, 2010), which confers PEI with larger buffering capacity (Boussif et al., 1995), leading to early endosomal escape of plasmids, and offers protection of the DNA from lysosomal degradation (Zhu and Mahato, 2010). In PEI, the nitrogen to DNA phosphate (N/P) ratio, one indicator of the properties of DNA polyplex, along with complex size, net surface charge, and stability, is associated with transfection efficiency (Nimesh et al., 2007; Vu et al., 2012; Gary et al., 2013). With an N/P ratio < 1, the PEI /DNA complex is characterized by incomplete DNA condensation, whereas when the ratio > 3, the free PEI is thought to enhance endosomal escape, contributing to DNA intracellular release (Mislick and Baldeschwieler, 1996; Boeckle et al., 2004; Perevyazko et al., 2012; Jin L. et al., 2014). The molecular weight of PEI is another determinant of transfection efficiency (Jones et al., 2013; Jin L. et al., 2014).

Physical Methods for Gene Delivery

Gene transfer of naked or plasmid DNA by physical means is an attractive delivery system for gene therapy because it is simple and has low cytotoxicity (Gao et al., 2007). Physical delivery approaches are popular in clinical trials, accounting for 14% in 2004, 18% in 2007, 18.3% in 2012, and 16.6% in 2017, of total gene therapy clinical trials (Edelstein et al., 2004, 2007; Ginn et al., 2013, 2018). Physical methods to introduce exogenous genes into cells have been explored both *in vitro* and *in vivo* (Dean et al., 2003; Gehl, 2003; Matsuda and Cepko, 2004; Dean, 2005). Basically, a physical force, produced by mechanical force, electrical pulses, ultrasound, laser irradiation, or magnetic fields, is employed to transiently disrupt the cell membrane and create small pores, so that DNA can diffuse into cells (Schneckenburger et al., 2002; Gehl, 2003; Mehier-Humbert and Guy, 2005; Li et al., 2008; Liu et al., 2012; Nayerossadat et al., 2012). Although naked DNA can be directly injected into local tissues, e.g., skeletal muscles or liver, and into the systemic circulation *via* tail vein, this "simplest" delivery method shows low transfection efficiency due to rapid *in vivo* degradation by nucleases and clearance by tissue-resident macrophage (e.g., Kupffer cells in the liver), limited extravasation from the circulation, and high interindividual variability (Kawabata et al., 1995; Mahato et al., 1995; Mir et al., 1999; Heller et al., 2000; Zhang et al., 2012; Yin et al., 2014). Plasmid DNA incubated in isolated rat plasma can degrade quickly with a half-life of 1.2 min for the supercoiled form, 21 min for the open circular plasmid DNA, and 11 min for the linear form (Houk et al., 1999). Cytoplasmic nucleases are another barrier impeding the efficient expression of plasmid DNA (Lechardeur et al., 1999; Bai et al., 2017). In contrast to direct injection of naked DNA into tissues, the "gene gun" or gene-mediated particle bombardment takes advantage of the high velocity of a particle carrier (e.g., gold beads) to deliver DNA into target tissues, such as skin, liver, and muscle (Wolff et al., 1992; Nishikawa and Huang, 2001). This method demonstrates increased transfection efficiency, for example, for epidermal tissues with 10–20% transfection of cells in the bombarded area, but is still limited in clinical trials because of concerns of poor penetration (<0.5 mm depth) into organs (Yang et al., 1990; Williams et al., 1991; Zelenin et al., 1997). The major application of gene gun in human trials is for DNA vaccination or suicide gene therapy to treat cancers (Trimble et al., 2003; Fuller et al., 2006). To date, this approach has not been used successfully in the lungs.

Electroporation, or EP, has been widely used in clinical settings to treat cancer (electrochemotherapy) and deliver drugs or vaccines to target cells. It was first used for DNA transfection of cultured mouse lyoma cells in 1982 (Neumann et al., 1982). It is a fast and reproducible approach, and requires a relatively low dose of DNA (Dean et al., 2003). In principle, when the transmembrane potential applied by the external electric field exceeds the cell resting potential, EP transiently disrupts the cell membrane and forms hydrophilic pores so that various molecules surrounding cell surface, such as DNA, RNA, oligonucleotides, ions, drugs and antibodies, can pass into the cells (Weaver and Chizmadzhev, 1996; Somiari et al., 2000). This delivery approach is not limited to small DNAs like AAV or other viruses. Indeed, delivery of plasmids with large loading capacity (e.g., 100 kb) and co-transfection of several plasmids to cells can be achieved through EP (Magin-Lachmann et al., 2004). For *in vivo* applications, DNA is delivered to the tissue, usually by injection, and then the electric field is applied with penetrating needles or surface electrodes. Several advantages are highlighted for EP in gene transfer *in vivo*. First, EP shows high transfection efficiency with relatively little interindividual variability and increases tissue transgene expression by 100–1,000 folds compared to direct injection of naked DNA. For example, EP of plasmid-encoding IL-5 into mouse tibialis muscle produced 20 ng/ml of IL-5, while direct delivery of plasmids without EP generated only 0.2 ng/ml of IL-5 in the blood (Aihara and Miyazaki, 1998; Mir et al., 1999; Wells, 2004). One critical step for gene transfer by EP is that EP should be applied immediately after DNA administration (Gao et al., 2007). For one thing, the short time interval between these two procedures would minimize DNA degradation by extracellular nucleases (Gao et al., 2007). For another, several studies indicate that there is almost no gene transfection, comparable to direct injection of plasmids, if naked DNA is injected into tissue (e.g., skeletal muscle) after EP application, suggesting that DNA must be present while the electric pulse is being applied (Mir et al., 1999; Satkauskas et al., 2002). Second, EP can be used to deliver genes locally to tissues, rather than by systemic delivery, which avoids the unnecessary exposure of other tissues to electric fields and also reduces the DNA dose needed (Mir et al., 1991; Gilbert et al., 1997; Gehl, 2003; Mir, 2014). Any solid tissue, for example, skin, liver, skeletal muscle, lung, kidney, cornea, and retina, prone to exposure to electric fields could be subject to EP-mediated gene delivery (Mir et al., 1999; Blair-Parks et al., 2002; Dean, 2003; Dean et al., 2003; Franquesa et al., 2005; Jaichandran et al., 2006; Zhou and Dean, 2007; Matsuda and Cepko, 2008; Medi and Singh, 2008). The electrodes delineate the area for gene transfer, which increases gene targeting specificity (Gehl, 2003). Third, EP can be applied to all cell types and cells in the dividing and non-dividing stages, since the mechanism of transfection does not depend on the uptake function of cells, but rather the transiently formed pores on the plasma membrane and the electrophoretic force during EP (Wells, 2004; Hirao et al., 2008; Escobar-Chávez et al., 2009). Additionally, EP does not induce any immune response, which is a significant safety concern in viral vector delivery system. However, a recent report indicated that a small transient increase in neutrophils could be detected in the lungs of mice within the first hour of electroporation, but that this returned to normal within 24 h; whether this has any lasting effects is unknown at this point, but, given that EP has been used by multiple groups to treat ARDS in mouse and pig models, suggests that this is not of a great concern (Eliseeva et al., 2021). Some inflammatory responses can be potentially provoked by any unmethylated CpG motifs in plasmids, but this can be reduced by plasmid modification (Krieg et al., 1995; Nishikawa and Huang, 2001).

Electroporation has been developed to deliver plasmid DNA into the lungs to treat diseases (Dean et al., 2003; Hasson et al., 2005; Jones et al., 2005). Traditionally, solid tissues (e.g., skeletal muscle, heart, and liver) have been directly injected with plasmids, and then the electric field is applied for *in vivo* gene delivery (Dean, 2005). However, lungs are not completely amenable to this approach (Dean, 2003; Young et al., 2014). For one thing, plasmid solution usually needs to be injected through some syringe or needle into solid tissues (Wolff et al., 1990), whereas the structure of the lungs is not appropriate for direct injection. For another, the electrodes designed for solid tissues, such as penetrating electrodes and caliper plate electrodes (Somiari et al., 2000), are not suitable for lungs. The lung is a delicate organ, which directly contacts the external environment through the airway and has a large epithelial surface area for gas exchange (Katz et al., 2019). This easy access *via* the airways makes the lung amenable to plasmid delivery through intratracheal administration (Zhou R. et al., 2008). Our laboratory and others have developed protocols for DNA delivery into the lungs (i.e., aspiration or inhalation) followed by EP, which show high transfection efficiency (Dean et al., 2003; Jones et al., 2005; Machado-Aranda et al., 2005; Gazdhar et al., 2006). Specifically, a plasmid solution containing 140 mM NaCl is administered to the lungs by aspiration in anesthetized mice, and then a pair of pre-gelled pediatric pacemaker surface electrodes is placed on either side of the chest under the armpits to deliver electric pulses that would travel through multiple tissue layers, e.g., skin, fat, and muscle, to reach the lungs (Dean, 2003). The parameters for optimal field strength have been determined to be 200 V/cm, using eight continuous 10 ms square wave pulses with 1 s interval (Dean et al., 2003). These parameters are also optimal in rats for lung delivery (Machado-Aranda et al., 2005). For larger animals such as 50-kg pigs, the DNA is delivered to anesthetized animals by bronchoscope to the desired lobe(s), and surface electrodes (in this case defibrillation pads) are used to deliver a train of eight pulses of ~150 V/cm but with a shorter duration (~100 to 150 μs each) (Dean et al., 2011; Emr et al., 2015). The distribution of transgene expression in the lungs has been evaluated by transferring reporter genes such as lacZ and GFP (Dean et al., 1999, 2003; Dean, 2003; Gottfried et al., 2016; Lin et al., 2016). Histological, immunohistochemical, and immunofluorescent analyses of mouse lung sections indicate that most cells receive and express transgenes throughout the lungs and in all cell types, such as the airway epithelium, alveolar epithelium (both ATI and ATII cells), endothelial cells, smooth muscle cells (both airway and vascular), and fibroblasts (Dean et al., 2003). Although plasmids could be administered intravenously to target the lungs, DNA nucleases are much higher in the serum than in the airway, and the injected DNA would be quickly degraded in the blood, resulting in low transfection efficiency (Song et al., 1997; Barron et al., 1999).

Choice of Gene Therapy Approach

Apart from their various properties, the choice of which type of gene therapy vector to use depends in great part on the disease being treated and its presentation. For example, in the case of a monogenetic disease such as sickle cell disease or cystic fibrosis, replacement of the defective genomic copy of the gene may be desired. If this is the case, homologous recombination methods such as CRISPR/Cas9 may be used, delivered either virally or by plasmid. Alternatively, the long-term expression of wild type copies of these genes may be sufficient to overcome the phenotype of the disease (e.g., overexpression of fetal hemoglobin in sickle cell patients), in which case using a viral vector that integrates into the genome such as a retrovirus or lentivirus would be desired. However, in the case of ARDS, three main issues should be considered. First, this is an acute disease that requires limited term expression of transferred genes. For example, if treatment involves overexpressing a Na^+ transporter such as ENaC or the Na^+, K^+-ATPase to reduce pulmonary edema, overexpression should be only for a short time so that disease-associated edema is cleared. If the gene was expressed long-term (e.g., by integration of the vector) in healthy individuals after resolution, increased fluid clearance from the lungs could result in mucus-rich, dehydrated lungs. Second, since ARDS is an acute-onset disease, any gene that is transferred to the lungs should be turned on quickly so that it would have maximal time to elicit benefit. In this case, mRNA could be a great choice, since it leads to almost immediate translation of proteins upon entry into the cell. However, the only drawback to mRNA approaches is that they are transient (perhaps too transient in this case), and unstable since mRNA is rapidly degraded by host nucleases. Plasmid DNA can also elicit rapid gene expression following entry into cells and tissues, with significant levels of expression seen in skeletal muscle in mice being detected within minutes of injection (Doh et al., 1997). Finally, in inflammatory diseases such as ARDS, the last thing that is wanted is using a gene delivery system that exacerbates the injury by causing more inflammation. Thus, viral vectors are not the best choice; nonviral vectors, with their greater safety profile, would be a more appropriate choice.

Current Gene Therapy for Acute Respiratory Distress Syndrome

A number of gene-based therapies have been developed over the past few decades for ARDS treatment (**Table 1**). In contrast to hereditary diseases, which require permanent alteration of the defective genome, ARDS is an acute disease of lung dysfunction, so short-lived or transiently altered gene expression is sufficient to treat the disease (Devaney et al., 2011). Gene delivery systems, such as viral vectors and conventional nonviral vectors, and physical delivery approaches have been well- developed to target the lungs for overexpression or silencing and make pulmonary gene transfer clinically possible (Jin L. et al., 2014; Ginn et al., 2018). Unfortunately, ARDS is not caused by a single gene, making gene therapy more difficult. However, a number of obvious target genes exist to promote AFC and edema resolution, repair the alveolar capillary barrier function, and relieve inflammation (**Figure 3**).

Gene Therapy to Improve Alveolar Fluid Clearance

In the setting of lung injury or ARDS, fluid clearance is impaired, and reduction in AFC rate correlates with increased mortality (Ware and Matthay, 2001; Huppert and Matthay, 2017). Thus, enhancing AFC has been considered one of the primary therapeutic goals for gene therapy for ARDS. Fluid clearance is based on the osmotic pressure created by transepithelial ion transport. Thus, similar to the principle of using β_2 agonists to enhance fluid clearance, gene delivery to potentiate AFC is based on the rationale that by introducing genes encoding various ion channels or transporters into the lungs, ion transport activities can be directly or indirectly upregulated. However, underlying the complexity of the disease, many factors need to be considered to develop any ARDS gene therapy. First, are the mechanisms known to stimulate AFC in normal lungs also effective in acutely injured lungs? One possible reason accounting for the failure of β_2 agonist therapy is the desensitization and internalization of β_2 receptors by long-term endogenous catecholamine stimulation, leading to decreased response during disease. Adenovirus-mediated gene transfer of the β_2-adrenergic receptor into healthy rat lungs increased receptor sensitivity to endogenous catecholamines and consequently upregulated Na^+,

TABLE 1 | Gene therapy approaches for acute respiratory distress syndrome (ARDS).

Target gene	Vector	Results	Clinical significance	Lung injury model	References
Gene therapy to enhance AFC					
ATP1 b1	Ad	Basal AFC, 100%	–	Normal rat without injury	Factor et al., 1998
ATP1 a2	Ad	+Na, K-ATPase activity; AFC	–	Normal rat without injury	Ridge et al., 2003
ATP1 b1	Ad	+AFC +Survival	Prevention	Hyperoxia and rat	Factor et al., 1999, 2000
ATP1 b1	Ad	+AFC, 100%	Prevention	Acutely elevated left atrial pressure	Azzam et al., 2002
b2 Adrenergic receptor	Ad	+AFC, 100% +Receptor function	–	Normal rat without injury	Dumasius et al., 2001
ATP1 a1 and ATP1b1	Cationic lipoplex	-W/D ratio +Na pump activity	Prevention	Thiourea, I.P injection, and mouse	Stern et al., 2000
ATP1 b1	Ad	+AFC	Prevention	High tidal volume ventilation and *ex vivo* rat	Adir et al., 2003
ATP1 a2	Ad	+AFC +Na pump activity -Barrier permeability	Prevention	High tidal volume ventilation and *ex vivo* rat	Adir et al., 2008
ATP1 b1	EP	+AFC, 100%	–	Normal rat without injury	Machado-Aranda et al., 2005
ATP1 b1	EP	+AFC, -W/D ratio -Cellularity, -protein in BAL, -barrier permeability	Prevention; treatment	I.t. delivery of LPS and mouse	Mutlu et al., 2007; Lin et al., 2016
ATP1 b1 ENaC-α1	EP	-W/D ratio, +survival, +Compliance, +PaO2/FiO2 ratio	Treatment	PS + I/R in gut, pig	Emr et al., 2015
CFTR	Ad	AFC, 100%	–	Normal rat without injury	Mutlu et al., 2005
Gene therapy to target pulmonary inflammation					
IL-10	Ad	-TNFα, IL-1, MPO in BAL -Inflammation -Histological injury +IL-10 level	Prevention	I.t. delivery of bacteria, pig	Morrison et al., 2000
IL-10	AAV	-Proinflammatory cytokines (IL-1β, TNFα, MIP-1α, and KC) -Histological injury	Prevention	I.t. delivery of bacteria, mouse	Buff et al., 2010
IL-10	Cationic lipoplex	-Lung, liver, and kidney injury (PMNs, MPO, and MDA) -TNFα	Prevention	Cecal ligation and puncture model of sepsis, mouse	Kabay et al., 2007
IL-10	Ad	Dose of adv vector inversely correlates to survival rate	Prevention	I.p. injection of zymosan, mouse	McAuliffe et al., 2006
IL-12	Ad	+Survival +IL-12 level in tissue and BAL	Prevention	I.t. delivery of bacteria, mouse	Greenberger et al., 1996
TGFb1	Cationic lipoplex	-Histologic score of rejection +Oxygenation	Prevention	Acute lung allograft rejection by left rat lung transplantation	Mora et al., 2000
Manganese SOD	Ad	+AFC +Na pump activity	Prevention	Hypoxia and rat	Litvan et al., 2006
CuZn-SOD; catalase	Ad	-Histologic injury score, inflammation +SOD, catalase activity	Prevention	100% oxygen, rat	Danel et al., 1998
Extracellular SOD	AAV	+Oxygen saturation +Lung compliance -PMNs, protein in BAL	Prevention	I.t. delivery of LPS, rat	Hassett et al., 2011
HO-1	Ad	+Survival -PMNs in BAL -Histologic injury	Prevention	Hyperoxia and rat	Otterbein et al., 1999
HO-1	Ad	-Histologic injury -Cytokine (KC, TNFα, and IL-10) in BAL	Prevention	Inhalation of aerolized LPS, mouse	Inoue et al., 2001
HO-1	Ad	-PMNs, KC, and TNFα in BAL -Epithelial cell death	Prevention	I.t. delivery of bacteria, mouse	Tsuburai et al., 2004
HO-1	Ad	+Survival -PMNs, total cell, cytokine in BAL -Histologic injury	Prevention	I.n. delivery of influenza A virus, mouse	Hashiba et al., 2001

(Continued)

TABLE 1 | (Continued)

Target gene	Vector	Results	Clinical significance	Lung injury model	References
HO-1	Cationic polyplex	PMNs, total cell, cytokine in BAL -Histologic injury	Treatment 2 h post	I.t. delivery of LPS, rat, mouse	Kim et al., 2019; Park et al., 2012
Ang-1	Ad	+Survival -Lung barrier permeability	Prevention	Septic shock model by i.p. injection of LPS, mouse	Huang et al., 2008
Ang-1	EP mediated transfection of MSC, *ex vivo*	-Lung barrier permeability (protein, Albumin, and IgM in BAL) -Proinflammatory cytokine, chemokine -Histologic injury	Treatment 30 mins post	I.t. delivery of LPS, mouse	Mei et al., 2007
HSP-70	Ad	-PMN infiltration -Mortality rate -Histologic injury	Prevention	Cecal ligation and double puncture model of sepsis, rat	Weiss et al., 2002
Adiponectin	Cationic polyplex	-TNFα, IL-1β in BAL and tissue -Histologic injury	Prevention	I.t. delivery of LPS, mouse	Piao et al., 2017
PGD synthase	Retroviral infection of fibroblast *ex vivo*	-BAL total cells -Edema +Survival	Prevention	I.t. delivery of bleomycin, mouse	Ando et al., 2003
NF-κB p65	siRNA	-NF-κB, MMP9 -W/D, histology -total cell, IL-6,17 in BAL	Prevention	Cecal ligation and puncture model of sepsis, mouse	Jin L.-Y. et al., 2014
NF-κB	siRNA	-NF-κB, TNFa level -W/D, white blood cell +Rectal temperature	Prevention	I.p. injection of LPS, rat	Li et al., 2016
KC, MIP-1	siRNA	-IL-6, MPO, and MIP-2 KC and PMNs	Prevention	Cecal ligation and puncture after hemorrhage induction, mouse	Lomas-Neira et al., 2005
FER	EP	+Survival, lung compliance, anti-bacterial immune response, and bacterial clearance -Total cells in BAL -Histological injury	Prevention	Lung contusion with secondary bacterial pneumonia, mouse	Dolgachev et al., 2016
FER	EP	+Survival, anti-bacterial immune response (IFN-γ, TNF-α, and KC), bacterial clearance	Prevention Treatment	Bacterial pneumonia and mouse	Dolgachev et al., 2018
Gene delivery to restore alveolar capillary barrier function					
ATP1 b1	EP	+AFC, -W/D ratio -Cellularity, -protein in BAL, -barrier permeability	Treatment	I.t. delivery of LPS, mouse	Lin et al., 2016
ATP1 b1	EP	+AFC, -W/D ratio -Cellularity, protein in BAL	Treatment	I.t. delivery of LPS, mouse	Mutlu et al., 2007
ATP1 b1 and ATP1 a2	EP	+Lung compliance -Lung barrier permeability -Histologic injury	Treatment (immediately after trauma)	Lung contusion by blunt chest injury, mouse	Machado-Aranda et al., 2012
MRCKα	EP	-W/D ratio -Cellularity, -protein in BAL, -barrier permeability	Treatment	I.t. delivery of LPS, mouse	Liu and Dean, 2021
FER	EP	+Survival, lung compliance -Lung permeability -Total cells in BAL -Histological injury	Prevention	Lung contusion with secondary bacterial pneumonia, mouse	Dolgachev et al., 2016
Ang-1	Ad	+Survival -Lung barrier permeability -W/D, MPO	Prevention	Septic shock model by i.p. injection of LPS, mouse	Witzenbichler et al., 2005; Huang et al., 2008

+, increase; –, decrease. ATP1, Na$^+$, K$^+$-ATPase; W/D, wet to dry ratio; CFTR, cystic fibrosis transmembrane conductance regulator; KC, murine chemokine CXCL1; MIP2, murine chemokine CXCL2; MIP-1a, macrophage inflammatory protein-1 alpha; PMN, neutrophil; MPO, myeloperoxidase; MMP9, matrix metallopeptidase 9; MDA, malondialdehyde; SOD, superoxide dismutase; NOS-2, nitric oxide synthase; PGD synthase, prostaglandin D synthase; HSP-70, heat shock protein 70; HO-1, heme oxygenase-1; MRCKa, CDC42-binding protein kinase alpha; AFC, alveolar fluid clearance; BAL, bronchoalveolar lavage fluid; TEER, transepithelial/trans-endothelial electrical resistance; EP, electroporation.

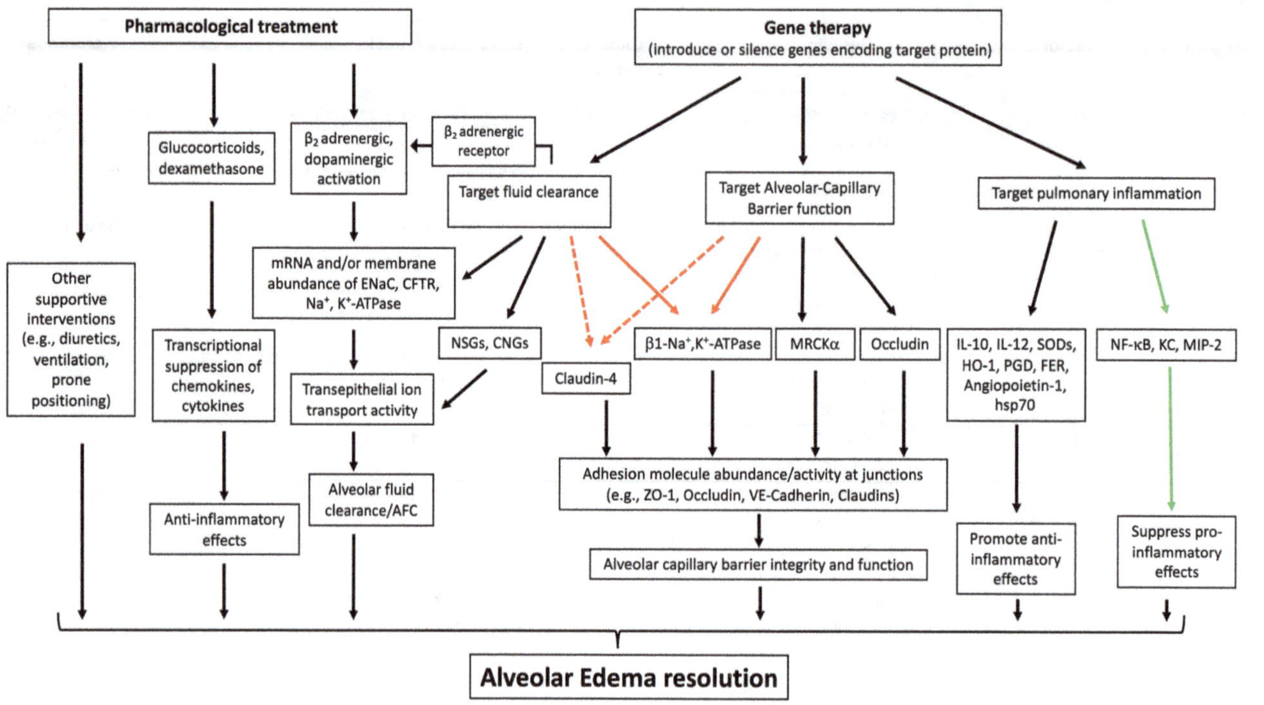

FIGURE 3 | Therapeutic approaches to treat acute lung injury (ALI)/ARDS. Pharmacological interventions primarily focus on enhancing fluid clearance through b2 adrenergic or dopaminergic activation, dampening inflammation with glucocorticoids, and use of supportive strategies, all of which have led to limited therapeutic effects. Gene therapies to overexpress or silence target genes have targeted alveolar fluid clearance, alveolar capillary barrier function, and pulmonary inflammation. The protein targets of gene therapy for ARDS/ALI have been validated in various animal or *ex vivo* organ models, indicating their therapeutic potential. Black solid arrow: increase, upregulate or target downstream effects; green solid arrow: decrease or inhibit target proteins; red solid arrow: has been validated in various animal models to have a dual role in both upregulating fluid clearance and lung barrier function; red dotted arrow: has the potential for dually upregulating fluid clearance and lung barrier integrity. ENaC, epithelial sodium channel; CFTR, cystic fibrosis transmembrane conductance regulator; NSGs, non-selective cation channels; CNGs, cyclic nucleotide-gated channels; MRCKa, CDC42 binding protein kinase alpha; ZO-1, zonula occludens-1; VE-cadherin, vascular endothelial-cadherin; HSP-70, heat shock protein 70; HO-1, heme oxygenase-1; KC, murine chemokine CXCL1; MIP2, murine chemokine CXCL2; PGDsyn, prostaglandin D synthase.

K^+-ATPase activity and ENaC expression in the lungs, leading to improved AFC (Dumasius et al., 2001, 2003). In a hyperoxia-induced injury model, gene transfer of the β_2 receptor protected animal lungs from subsequent injury, showing decreased lung edema and increased survival (Mutlu et al., 2004). However, most studies showing beneficial effects by upregulating β_2 receptors in lung injury have been limited to animal models with gene delivery prior to inducing injury, and such protection studies have limited clinical significance.

Second, what aspects really matter for the upregulation of fluid clearance by delivered genes encoding different ion transporters or channels? The underlying mechanisms of catecholamine-activated Na^+ transport include increased protein synthesis and membrane recruitment of the Na^+, K^+-ATPase and ENaC, as well as increased open probability of the channels (Yue et al., 1995; Minakata et al., 1998; Bertorello et al., 1999; Saldías et al., 1999). Although catecholamine activation significantly increases edema clearance in various animal models and in isolated human lungs (Sakuma et al., 1994; Lecuona et al., 1999; Frank et al., 2000), the experimental design of these studies is not entirely reflective of the pathophysiology of ARDS in which the alveolar-capillary barrier is at least partially disrupted. In all these experimental cases, there is an intact alveolar epithelial barrier, allowing for effective AFC by upregulating Na^+ transport (Mutlu and Sznajder, 2004). This brings up the fact that effective net AFC depends on an intact epithelial barrier that can transport ions across the alveolar epithelium (Huppert and Matthay, 2017). Overexpression of Na^+, K^+-ATPase, ENaC, cystic fibrosis transmembrane conductance regulator (CFTR), or other ion channels through gene delivery directly increases ion transport activity, accelerating fluid clearance. For example, overexpression of the Na^+, K^+-ATPase $\alpha 2$, or $\beta 1$ subunit through adenoviral transfer or electroporation of $\beta 1$ subunit plasmids into healthy rat lungs increased fluid clearance rates by >100 (Factor et al., 1998), 250 (Ridge et al., 2003), and 74% (Machado-Aranda et al., 2005), respectively. Adenoviral delivery of the Na^+, K^+-ATPase into rat lungs before induction of lung injury (e.g., by hypoxic injury or VILI) prevented and even somewhat reversed the decrease in AFC, compared to injury alone (Factor et al., 2000; Adir et al., 2003, 2008). However, in most *in vivo* studies, adenoviral vectors were delivered either to healthy lungs or prior to induction of lung injury by various insults, such as ventilation, acute elevation of lung pressure, or 100% oxygen, demonstrating that gene therapy to enhance AFC could protect against experimental lung injury. These studies could be implied to suggest that gene delivery to an intact alveolar epithelium was required for upregulating transepithelial ion transport and net AFC. In this respect, the β1 subunit of the Na^+, K^+-ATPase has been identified as a unique target for gene delivery to treat acute lung injury, since the Na^+, K^+-ATPase is not only the major driver of AFC but is also closely involved in the regulation of epithelial barrier integrity (Rajasekaran and Rajasekaran, 2003; Vadasz et al., 2007). Our laboratory has focused on β1 subunit gene therapy using different animal models, such as mice (Mutlu et al., 2007), rats (Machado-Aranda et al., 2005), and pigs (Emr et al., 2015), and our previously published data have shown that electroporation-mediated gene delivery of the β1 subunit of the Na^+, K^+-ATPase can rescue endotoxin pre-injured mouse lungs by both increasing AFC and, more importantly, restoring lung barrier function. These studies indicate that lung barrier integrity is important for gene therapy targeted at increasing net AFC (Lin et al., 2016).

Apart from ion channel transporters, some paracellular tight junction molecules, for example, claudin-4, play roles as regulators of ion transport across the epithelium, showing selective permeability to ions (Brune et al., 2015). For one thing, they are required for maximal epithelial barrier function and are upregulated during epithelial repair (Wray et al., 2009). For another, they are not ion transporters but are closely involved in paracellular ion conductance and have an impact on fluid clearance (Rokkam et al., 2011). Because of this, claudin-4 could be a potential target for gene therapy to increase AFC and barrier integrity. Claudin-4 is highly expressed in both ATI and ATII cells (LaFemina et al., 2010), and staining of human lungs shows a positive correlation of claudin-4 with AFC, indicating that higher claudin-4 expression is associated with higher rates of fluid clearance (Rokkam et al., 2011). It is still not clear whether claudin-4 levels are altered from baseline during injury in human lungs, although its expression was increased during early experimental lung injury.

Nonselective cation channels (NSCs), cyclic nucleotide-gated channels (CNGs), and the CFTR Cl channel are also expressed apically and contribute to the creation of the transepithelial osmotic gradient (Mutlu and Sznajder, 2005). In fluid-filled lungs of mice with genetic KO of acid-sensing ion channel 1 (ASIC1), a nonselective cation channel, fluid clearance was reduced by more than 50% compared to wild type, which is comparable to the AFC reduction seen in mice with ENaC inhibition, indicating that ASIC1 could also be a potential target for gene delivery for AFC (Trac et al., 2017). CFTR is important for maintaining alveolar fluid homeostasis and has been identified contributing to lung fluid reabsorption (Fang et al., 2002). Indeed, overexpression of CFTR by adenoviral infection of mouse lungs increases AFC 90% over that seen following infection with empty vector control (Mutlu et al., 2005).

Gene Therapy to Target Pulmonary Inflammation

In the early stage of ARDS, the uncontrolled production of cytokines and chemokines initiate proinflammatory responses, which further exacerbates lung injury. Therefore, gene delivery of target proteins to suppress or dampen proinflammatory effects or enhance anti-inflammatory effects has been studied on various experimental models of ARDS and proven successful *in vivo*. One strategy has been to deliver genes to overexpress anti-inflammatory cytokines, anti-oxidant enzymes, antiproteases, and other protective proteins to attenuate inflammation-associated lung injury during ARDS (Liu and Slutsky, 1997). However, most experiments delivered target genes before inducing injury and primarily demonstrated the protection effect with less clinical significance. IL-10 is an anti-inflammatory cytokine and is produced to suppress proinflammatory responses by inhibiting proinflammatory cytokine release, thus limiting the excessive injury induced by inflammation (Couper et al., 2008). Ad delivered IL-10 into animal lungs prior to bacterial infection significantly prevented histological lung injury, release of proinflammatory TNα in BAL, and overall inflammation (Morrison et al., 2000; Buff et al., 2010). Furthermore, in a systematic sepsis model in mice, lipoplex-delivered IL-10 significantly prevented lung and other organ injury (Kabay et al., 2007). However, it was reported that adenoviral-delivered IL-10 protected lungs with improved outcome only when a relatively low dose of vector was administered and that survival rates actually worsened at higher doses (McAuliffe et al., 2006). This highlights the inherent problems associated with using a proinflammatory viral vector to treat an inflammatory disease. Other cytokine therapeutic targets for gene delivery have included IL-12, which has shown protection from subsequent lethal doses of Klebsiella in a pneumonia model (Greenberger et al., 1996).

Superoxide dismutases (SODs) are a group of metalloenzymes that form the front line of defense against oxidative stress, e.g., ROS, in the body (Landis and Tower, 2005). During ARDS, the overwhelmed inflammatory response leads to excessive ROS, contributing to disease progression (Ware and Matthay, 2000). Overexpression of SOD in transgenic mice has been shown to have a protective effect on lung injury induced by hyperoxia (Ahmed et al., 2003), hypoxia (Litvan et al., 2006), LPS (Bowler et al., 2004), and influenza virus (Suliman et al., 2001). However, the pharmacological administration of SODs for clinical treatment of ARDS has shown limited success due to the enzyme's short half-life in circulation, rapid renal excretion, and inability to penetrate cells to remove ROS, leading to low accumulation within injured lungs (Danel et al., 1998). Adenoviral-mediated gene transfer of SODs prevented hypoxia-induced lung injury, counteracting ROS-induced endocytosis of the Na^+,K^+-ATPase and subsequent decrease in alveolar fluid reabsorption (Litvan et al., 2006). Another study further demonstrated the protection effects of SODs on LPS-induced injury, in terms of physiological oxygen saturation and lung compliance, lung barrier function, and inflammation (Hassett et al., 2011). However, again, all studies have used protection, not treatment protocols, thus calling into question the utility to treat ARDS clinically.

Heme oxygenase-1 (HO-1) is another candidate for gene delivery to fight against excessive oxidative stress during lung injury. It is a critical enzyme for catabolizing heme and shows antioxidant, anti-inflammatory, and anti-apoptotic properties for vascular protection (Araujo et al., 2012). Chemical inhibition or genetic silencing of HO-1 significantly increases proinflammatory cytokine release, immune cell infiltration, and apoptosis, indicating that HO-1 has a protective role in LPS-induced ALI (Wiesel et al., 2000; Gong et al., 2008; Zhang Y. et al., 2013). Ad transfer of HO-1 has been shown to confer protection against hyperoxia, aerosolized endotoxin, and bacteria- or virus-induced lung injury (Otterbein et al., 1999; Hashiba et al., 2001; Inoue et al., 2001; Tsuburai et al., 2004). In a more recent study, the treatment effect of HO-1 nonviral gene delivery was tested, in which HO-1 plasmids were co-delivered *via* a polymeric complex with an anti-inflammatory compound after LPS had been administered intratracheally to induce injury. Thus, gene delivery was carried out in lungs that were already injured. From the results, the histological lung injury and proinflammatory cytokine release were significantly rescued (Kim et al., 2019). Other gene therapeutic targets for anti-inflammatory strategy include angiopoietin-1 (see below), heat shock protein 70, and adiponectin, but while all have shown some promise in limiting inflammation, improving edema resolution, and/or improving survival, all have either carried out protection studies only, or have failed to have an effect when tested in a treatment strategy to decrease damage and disease in lungs with pre-existing injury (Weiss et al., 2002; Huang et al., 2008; Piao et al., 2017).

Prostaglandins (PGs) are a group of lipid compounds that mediate inflammatory responses (Ricciotti and FitzGerald, 2011). They are converted from arachidonic acid through various PG synthases, the rate-limiting enzymes in the cyclooxygenase pathway of arachidonic acid metabolism (DeWitt, 1991). Multiple observations have indicated that PGs, such as PG E2 (PGE_2) and PG D2 (PGD_2), have anti-inflammatory and protective effects on ARDS (Birukova et al., 2007; Scher and Pillinger, 2009; Murata et al., 2013). Thus, gene transfer of PG synthase has been evaluated to upregulate endogenous PGs for treating lung injury. This approach worked in protection studies to reduce bleomycin-induced lung injury, but more importantly, retrovirally introduced PGD2 synthase into murine lungs that were pre-injured by bleomycin remarkedly increased animal survival rate and reduced edema accumulation, leukocyte infiltration, and plasma extravasation (Ando et al., 2003).

Another interesting approach has been to mine high-throughput sequencing analyses to identify potential therapeutic targets for ARDS. A recent genome-wide association study (GWAS) identified the non-receptor cytosolic tyrosine kinase FER as being associated with increased survival in patients with pneumonia and sepsis (Rautanen et al., 2015). In a mouse model of combined lung contusion and pneumonia, the expression of FER was down compared to controls. When FER was overexpressed in the lungs by electroporation-mediated gene transfer, survival of the animals was improved and antibacterial response genes were activated (Dolgachev et al., 2016). In follow-up studies, it was shown that in a Klebsiella pneumonia model in mice, electroporation-mediated delivery of FER plasmids to the lungs of mice previously infected with Klebsiella not only improved survival but also reduced bacterial counts in the lungs. Further experiments suggested that FER gene transfer activates the STAT pathway to enhance innate immunity and accelerate bacterial clearance in the lung (Dolgachev et al., 2018).

Another strategy to fight against the overwhelming inflammation in early ARDS is to suppress the proinflammatory effects by silencing genes that directly regulate the production of proinflammatory cytokines and chemokines or indirectly promote inflammation through RNAi (Lomas-Neira et al., 2008). Intratracheal delivery of siRNA could target the local lungs with high efficiency (Lomas-Neira et al., 2005). NF-κB is an important inflammation inducer that regulates the transcription of a number of downstream proinflammatory cytokines or mediators, such as IL-1b, IL-6, and TNF-α (Jha and Das, 2017). In recent studies, siRNA-mediated local or systematical silencing of NF-κB significantly protected animals against further increased proinflammatory cytokine (TNF-α, IL-6) release, histological and other lung injury scores in animals subsequently injured with LPS compared with injury and scramble control, indicating that NF-κB could be a potential target for developing RNAi gene therapy for ARDS (Jin L.-Y. et al., 2014; Li et al., 2016). A decoy strategy has also been employed to target the NF-κB inflammatory pathway, to block the binding of NF-κB to promoter regions of its targeted genes, resulting in the inhibition of proinflammatory gene transcription. In this approach, multiple copies of oligonucleotides encoding the NF-κB consensus binding site are delivered to cells or tissues to compete for activated NF-κB binding, thereby reducing normal signaling. In a sepsis model of cecal ligation and puncture (CLP), tail-vein injection of synthetic double stranded oligodeoxynucleotides (ODNs) to decoy NF-κB showed protective effects on septic lung injury, such as decreased transcription of sepsis-induced proinflammatory genes (iNOS, COX-2), decreased histological damage in terms of alveolar wall thickening, immune cell infiltration and hemorrhage, decreased vascular permeability, and improved blood gas exchange capacity (Matsuda et al., 2005). Other proteins that have a potential for siRNA therapeutics include neutrophil chemo-attractant Keratinocyte derived-chemokine (KC) and macrophage inflammatory protein-2 (MIP-2), which alleviate neutrophil activation-induced excessive inflammation and injury (Lomas-Neira et al., 2005). Similarly, in a hemorrhage induced sepsis mouse model, intratracheal delivery of siRNA to locally silence chemoattractant cytokines KC and MIP-2 significantly suppressed neutrophil influx into the lungs and decreased tissue or plasma level of IL-6, MIP-2 and MPO, activity (Lomas-Neira et al., 2005).

Gene Delivery to Restore Alveolar Capillary Barrier Function

Alveolar capillary barrier disruption is a primary cause of ARDS leading to the influx of protein-rich fluid into alveoli and accumulation of pulmonary edema. Damage to junctional structures between epithelial cells and/or between endothelial cells, and cell death both result in alveolar capillary barrier dysfunction.

In recent years, gene delivery of target proteins to repair lung barrier function has been investigated. The Na^+, K^+-ATPase has been primarily studied for its function in promoting AFC, although increasing evidence demonstrates that the expression and function of the Na^+, K^+-ATPase are also closely involved in the regulation of epithelial barrier integrity (Rajasekaran et al., 2001b; Rajasekaran and Rajasekaran, 2003; Vadasz et al., 2007). For example, the Na^+, K^+-ATPase β1 subunit has been shown to be necessary for membrane localization of TJs, e.g., ZO-1, occluding. Furthermore, silencing of the β1subunit by siRNA disrupts the continuous staining pattern of ZO-1, indicating that the β1subunit might be directly or indirectly associated with TJ proteins (Madan et al., 2007; Rajasekaran et al., 2007). The Na^+, K^+-ATPase is required for establishing epithelial polarization and co-expression of the Na^+, K^+-ATPase β1 subunit, and E-cadherin has been shown to recover the lost polarity and junctions in MSV-MDCK cells, a highly invasive cell line (Rajasekaran et al., 2001b). In addition, the basolateral membrane-localized Na^+, K^+-ATPase acts as an adhesion molecule, forming a trans-dimer junction structure between cells. This structure appears dependent on the N-glycosylation of the β1 subunit's extracellular domain (Vagin et al., 2012). Because of the dual role of Na^+, K^+-ATPase in enhancing both AFC and epithelial barrier function, this transporter has been targeted for gene delivery to treat ALI in various experimental animal models. Recent data from our laboratory showed that overexpression of the rat or human Na^+, K^+-ATPase β1 subunit upregulated the protein expression and membrane localization of TJ proteins occludin and ZO-1 (Lin et al., 2016; Bai et al., 2021). Furthermore, in cultured monolayers of rat alveolar epithelial ATI cells, overexpression of the β1 subunit increased transmembrane epithelial electrical resistance (TEER) by 30% compared to untransfected cells or those transfected with empty plasmids (Bai et al., 2021). More importantly, electroporation-mediated gene delivery of the rat or the human β1-subunit of the Na^+, K^+-ATPase to the lungs of mice with existing LPS-induced lung injury rescued experimental ALI by upregulating both AFC and TJ protein abundance, and pulmonary barrier function, as demonstrated by decreased lung permeability, total protein, and cellularity in BAL fluid, and improved overall histological injury outcomes (Mutlu et al., 2007; Lin et al., 2016).

Based on these findings, our laboratory pursued two avenues for further treatment: evaluation of the ability of gene transfer of individual tight junction protein genes to protect and treat ARDS in animal models, and identification of the pathway(s) by which the β1-subunit of the Na^+, K^+-ATPase upregulates barrier function. Occludin plays a central role in the formation, maintenance, regulation, and structure of tight junctions. In unpublished studies, when an occludin-expressing plasmid was delivered to the lungs of mice that had been injured 24 h previously with intratracheal LPS, occludin was overexpressed, which resulted in decreased pulmonary edema, improved histology, and reduced inflammation (numbers of infiltrating neutrophils and reduced levels of proinflammatory cytokines), compared to animals that received empty plasmids or no treatment at all (Lin et al., submitted for publication). However, it was not determined whether expression was localized to the alveolar epithelium or the capillary endothelium. Either way, these results suggest that gene therapy to increase levels of tight junction proteins directly may be a viable approach to treat ARDS.

Claudin family TJ proteins are critical components that are required to form apical junction complexes for alveolar epithelial barrier function. The major claudins expressed in ATI and ATII cells include claudins 3 and 4 (Frank, 2012). Although claudins 3 and 4 are highly homologous in a peptide sequence, they have opposite effects on the regulation of alveolar barrier function: overexpression of claudin 4 leads to decreased epithelial permeability and increased TEER, while opposite responses are observed for claudin 3 (Mitchell et al., 2011). In response to various injury-inducing stimuli (e.g., hyperoxia, ventilation, and septic shock), claudin 4 expression has been shown to be downregulated in mice, although an early upregulation of claudin 4 mRNA level was observed at 4 h in a ventilation-induced ALI mouse model (Wray et al., 2009; Cohen et al., 2010; Herrero et al., 2018; Vyas-Read et al., 2018). So far, there is no direct *in vivo* evidence indicating that overexpression of claudin 4 could benefit or protect from injury in living lungs, but claudin 4 could be a potential target for ARDS by gene therapy. Taken with the fact that levels of claudins show a positive correlation with AFC in human lungs, it suggests that this approach may have merit (Rokkam et al., 2011). In addition, claudin 5 is a primary tight junction component expressed in pulmonary endothelial cells (Kaarteenaho-Wiik and Soini, 2009) and has been shown to be downregulated in the lungs during influenza infection and other models of ALI (Armstrong et al., 2012). In several cell culture experiments, the overexpression of claudin 5 significantly protected endothelial cells from LPS-induced decreased permeability to molecules and restored TEER in these cells, indicating a role for claudin 5 in barrier protection and pulmonary leakage (Soma et al., 2004; Armstrong et al., 2012). The therapeutic potential of claudin 5 was further confirmed in a study investigating the beneficial effects of simvastatin on ALI, which concluded that claudin 5 is an important mediator of ALI protection by simvastatin (Chen et al., 2014). These studies indicate that claudin 5 might be a promising target for gene therapy for lung barrier protection.

Claudin-18 is another major tight junction protein expressed specifically in alveolar epithelial cells. So far, there has been no study directly reporting the effects, of claudin-18, by gene delivery, on ALI in an animal model. This is probably due to the complex role of claudin-18 in edema resolution. Claudin-18-knocked out mice did not exhibit apparent respiratory dysfunction and showed unchanged wet-to-dry weight ratios from baseline, although claudin-18 was downregulated at the protein and transcriptional levels during injury (Ohta et al., 2012; Li et al., 2014). However, the claudin-18-knocked out mice showed increased lung permeability to ions and solutes of various sizes, significantly enhanced fluid clearance rates with increased ion transport activities, and altered expression of claudins 3 and 4 (LaFemina et al., 2014; Li et al., 2014). These results suggest that the overexpression of claudin-18 may have actually exacerbated the injury, although because of its ability to regulate other claudins, cytoskeletal organization, b_2 adrenergic signaling, and CFTR activity, it is difficult to say what ultimate effects its overexpression could have.

Fas/FasL apoptosis signaling has been identified as a main form of lung epithelial cell death, leading to alveolar capillary barrier damage. The Fas/FasL system is significantly upregulated in the BAL fluid of ARDS patients (Albertine et al., 2002). Using a FasL analog to compete with FasL for Fas binding improved pneumococcal bacterial clearance from the lungs of mice, indicating that the Fas/FasL axis might have a therapeutic potential (Matute-Bello et al., 2005b). In another study on hemorrhage-induced septic ALI, intratracheal instillation of siRNA 4 h after hemorrhagic shock and sepsis induction to silence local Fas in the lung showed markedly decreased levels of cytokines, such as TNFα, IL-6, and IL-10, and caspase 3 activity, indicating a protective effect by blocking Fas/FasL (Perl et al., 2005). Although this study primarily targeted local alveolar epithelial cells, the Fas receptor is also expressed in vascular endothelial cells, resulting in endothelial apoptosis (Hotchkiss et al., 2002). Thus, targeting Fas expression in the vascular endothelium for ARSD or sepsis endothelial injury might be a possible direction for future study.

Lung microvascular endothelial dysfunction plays an important role in the pathogenesis of ARDS and sepsis, and numerous approaches to modulate endothelial cell activation and decrease vascular leakage have been and are being investigated. For example, the bioactive sphingolipid metabolite sphingosine-1-phosphate (S1P) and its receptor, S1PR, have been reported to have protective effects on the endothelial barrier. S1P-mediated cellular events induce MLC phosphorylation, activation of Rho GTPase, and recruitment and assembly of adhesion junction molecules. Furthermore, genetic variants of the S1P receptor, such as S1PR3, have been shown to be positively associated with risk of ARDS (Natarajan et al., 2013). A recent publication reported that S1P receptor 1 (S1PR1) deletion resulted in increased endothelial permeability, and that S1PR1-expressing endothelial cells are required for barrier repair, suggesting a therapeutic potential of the S1P pathway in endothelial barrier dysfunction (Akhter et al., 2021).

Angiopoietin-1 (Ang-1) is an agonist for the endothelial-specific receptor tyrosine kinase Tie2 and has been shown to protect from microvascular endothelial permeability and plasma leakage both *in vitro* and *in vivo*. The Ang-1-Tie2 axis signals to downstream effector proteins and regulates intercellular junction complexes, like VE-cadherin or other adhesion molecules (e.g., PECAM-1, ICAM-1, VCAM-1, and E-selectin) (Gamble et al., 2000; Parikh, 2017). The anti-inflammatory role of Ang-1 has also been shown to be due to its suppression of neutrophils' adherence to the endothelium during transmigration in ALI (Gamble et al., 2000). In mice with LPS-induced lung injury, Ang-1 expression was decreased in the lungs (Karmpaliotis et al., 2002). In mouse models of endotoxin-induced septic shock, animals pre-treated with adenoviral-mediated delivery of Ang-1 showed more resistance to subsequent injury, demonstrating significantly decreased lung edema, vascular permeability, histological damage, and mortality rate (Witzenbichler et al., 2005; Huang et al., 2008).

Mesenchymal stem cell (MSC)-mediated gene therapy has been reported to have a promising therapeutic potential for treating diseases such as sepsis. There are several advantages in using MSC therapy to treat ALI and sepsis. MSCs can be stably expanded *in vitro* to produce sufficient quantities for use while maintaining an undifferentiated state (Laffey and Matthay, 2017). This means that from another perspective, delivering target genes to manipulate endothelial damage, inflammation, or vascular injury could be more easily achieved through plasmid transfection of MSCs *in vitro*. In recent studies, systemic delivery of MSCs that overexpress an Ang-1 transgene to animals before LPS injury showed protective effects such as decreased lung leakage of plasma protein and decreased neutrophil infiltration (McCarter et al., 2007; Xu et al., 2008). Although these are promising results, there are fewer studies showing that Ang-1 overexpression could benefit the pre-injured lungs in animals. In addition, potential side effects of Ang-1 treatment were also reported (Sullivan et al., 2003; Long et al., 2008). Second, MSCs can easily access and traverse the vascular endothelium and incorporate into injured lungs *via* intravenous infusion, all while maintaining the ability to divide and self-renew. In addition, MSCs have good safety records with minimal immunogenicity, which helps avoid immune responses, a common adverse effect seen during viral vector-mediated gene delivery (Laffey and Matthay, 2017).

Several studies have reported that MSC-mediated gene therapy could repair alveolar capillary barrier disruption by targeting various genes. Ang-1 is the most studied one. Administration of MSCs overexpressing Ang-1 decreased IgM and albumin levels in BAL by more than 50% compared to LPS-induced lung hyperpermeability alone in mice, indicating significant restoration of lung barrier function (Mei et al., 2007). Growth factor genes, e.g., fibroblast growth factor (FGF), keratinocyte growth factor (KGF), and vascular endothelial growth factor (VEGF), also show a therapeutic potential for MSC-mediated gene therapy (Lee et al., 2011). FGF-activated signaling is required for the maintenance of interendothelial adhesion, the inhibition of which results in dissociation of the VE-cadherin/p120-catenin complex and disassembly of adherens and tight junctions, and eventually leads to endothelial barrier disruption and vascular leakage (Murakami et al., 2008). Moreover, FGF signaling is necessary for glycocalyx reconstitution, protecting against glycocalyx shedding during sepsis (Yang et al., 2017). Tail vein injection of MSCs overexpressing FGF2 into mice in an LPS-induced sepsis model significantly decreased the level of total protein and cytokines in BAL, lung edema, and histological lung damage, indicating the treatment potential of MSC-mediated FGF in lung injury (Zhao et al., 2015). KGF signaling is critical for pulmonary epithelial repair and proliferation. In animal lungs injured by intratracheal LPS administration, KGF gene-modified MSCs protected lung permeability, significantly decreased total protein levels in BAL, decreased edema (wet to dry ratio), attenuated inflammation with decreased expression of cytokines (IL-1β and TNF-α) and myeloperoxidase (MPO) activity in BAL fluid, and increased animal survival (Chen et al., 2013). Finally, VEGF is notable as a vascular permeability factor that has been shown to induce endothelial barrier disruption. In addition, paracrine factors secreted by MSCs, such as hepatocyte growth factor (HGF) and VEGF, were also investigated as having protective effects on endothelial barrier integrity in experimental LPS-induced lung injury models (Yang et al., 2015, 2016).

As a second approach to repair barrier function in ARDS, our lab has worked to identify the pathway(s) by which the β1 subunit of the Na^+, K^+-ATPase upregulates barrier function in cells and mouse models. Using a proteomics approach, we recently demonstrated that the novel CDC42-related kinase MRCKα is a specific interacting partner of the Na^+, K^+-ATPase β1-subunit, and that it is responsible for the upregulation of tight junction protein abundance in the membrane and activity seen following β1 overexpression (**Figure 2**; Bai et al., 2021). Interestingly, MRCKα expression appears down in the lungs of patients with ARDS compared to control lungs (Bai et al., 2021). In cultured rat ATI cells, we demonstrated that MRCKα was both necessary for β1's ability to upregulate tight junction expression and TEER in cells using siRNA to knock down MRCKα expression and using specific inhibitors of the kinase (Bai et al., 2021). Furthermore, we also showed that the overexpression of MRCKα itself was sufficient to increase TEER seen in the monolayers. More recently, we have asked whether MRCKα overexpression in the lungs of mice in which lung injury had been previously induced by administration of LPS and have found that the overexpression of MRCKα leads to the same upregulation of tight junction proteins as does the transfer of the β1 subunit of the Na^+, K^+-ATPase, and provides the same degree of treatment of the disease, reducing pulmonary edema, lung permeability, measures of inflammation, and histological health of the lungs (Liu and Dean, 2021). As expected, the overexpression of MRCKα had no effect on the rates of AFC in mice. Taken together, these results suggest that repair of the epithelial and endothelial barrier activities is more important than upregulation of AFC alone.

While mouse models are often the first test of a given gene therapy, or for any therapeutic, approach for utility *in vivo*, they do not always reflect what will actually be of use therapeutically in patients. Indeed, this has been a major problem in developing effective treatments for ARDS in the past. An animal model that accurately duplicates the complex inflammatory and hemodynamic response that occurs in humans over several days during the development of sepsis-induced ARDS is critical to the understanding and treatment of lung injury. It has been shown that the success of clinical trials testing sepsis therapies depends on sound preclinical data using appropriate animal models (Piper et al., 1996). The best model, termed a "good evidence" model, is one in which the results of the study would be similar in a clinical trial (Piper et al., 1996). For example, while studies testing anti-endotoxin HA-1A demonstrated improved survival in a murine model of sepsis (Teng et al., 1985), a phase III clinical trial did not show survival benefit (Ziegler et al., 1991). However, when a clinically relevant "good evidence" large animal model of chronic septic shock was utilized to test the efficacy of HA-1A, the results were very similar to those of the clinical trial (Quezado et al., 1993). Similarly, a provocative article in PNAS several years ago generated great interest and press since it suggested that findings from mouse models alone do not always translate to larger species or humans (Seok et al., 2013).

There is a consensus that chronic, insidious-onset large animal models that mimic the pathogenesis of sepsis-induced ARDS are superior to small animal models as predictors of clinical efficacy (Parker and Watkins, 2001). To this end, Nieman et al. developed a chronic (48 h) two-hit sepsis and gut ischemia/reperfusion porcine model that accurately resembles the pathologic progression from injury to systemic inflammatory response syndrome, to septic shock, and finally to ARDS seen in human patients (Steinberg et al., 2005). Following injury, the animals are maintained and sedated according to the ARDSnet treatment paradigm (Network, 2000), making comparisons to existing human clinical trial data, more relevant and clear. Since sepsis is the leading cause of indirect ARDS, this model is highly germane developing any ARDS treatment (Sigurdsson et al., 2013). This model contains all of the key components of a "good evidence" animal model, such as a randomized, controlled study with supportive therapy (fluids, antibiotics) in a large animal, insidious-onset, chronic model of septic shock and ARDS (Piper et al., 1996). Moreover, the injury induced in this model yields all the features of ALI identified in the ATS consensus report on ALI in animals (Matute-Bello et al., 2011). The data generated from this model, which includes inflammatory mediator response, hemodynamic measures, lung function, and blood chemistry have allowed us to demonstrate that electroporation-mediated gene delivery of ENaC and Na^+, K^+-ATPase subunits 4 h after injury provides effective treatment of lung injury and statistically significant survival benefit in the pig.

Emr et al. (2015) transferred a mixture of two plasmids expressing GFP-tagged rat Na^+, K^+-ATPase β1 subunit and DDK-tagged α1 subunit of ENaC, or a non-coding, empty plasmid as control, to pigs in this two-hit model of lung injury (**Figure 4**). Four h after injury (to mimic when a patient would present in the ER after traumatic injury leading to ALI), a bronchoscope was used to deliver 50 ml of DNA in saline (50 mg endotoxin-free plasmid), each into the left lower and right lobes, within a 2-min period. The bronchoscope was removed, and the animals were electroporated using external defibrillator pads placed on either side of the chest ("external electroporation"). Alternatively, in several experiments, the bronchoscope was left in the lung and used as an internal electrode coupled to one external electrode ("Internal electroporation"). Eight pulses (2,000 V at 150 μs each; ~150 V/cm) were then applied to the animals. The anesthetized animals were maintained on mechanical ventilation and administered vasopressors according to the human ARDSnet and Early Goal Directed Therapy protocols (Network, 2000; Rivers et al., 2001). Initially, the animals were ventilated at 10 cc/kg tidal volume (V_T) with a PEEP of 5 cmH_2O, respiratory rate of 12, FiO_2 30%, and inspiratory to expiratory Ratio 1:2. The animals were transitioned to low V_T (6 cc/kg) when they met ARDSnet clinical criteria of $PaO_2/FiO_2 < 300$ (mild ARDS) the per ARDSnet protocol (Network, 2000). Appropriate adjustments were made to maintain adequate minute volume. PEEP and FiO_2 were adjusted in response to changes in SaO_2 along the "High PEEP, Low FiO_2" scale (Network, 2000). If airway plateau pressure (P_{plat}) rose above 30 cm H_2O, V_T was further reduced by 1 cc/kg increments to 4 cc/kg with appropriate adjustments in respiratory rate to maintain equivalent minute volume per ARDSnet guidelines. The upper limit for respiratory rate was 35 BPM, with titrations made in V_T if respiratory acidosis

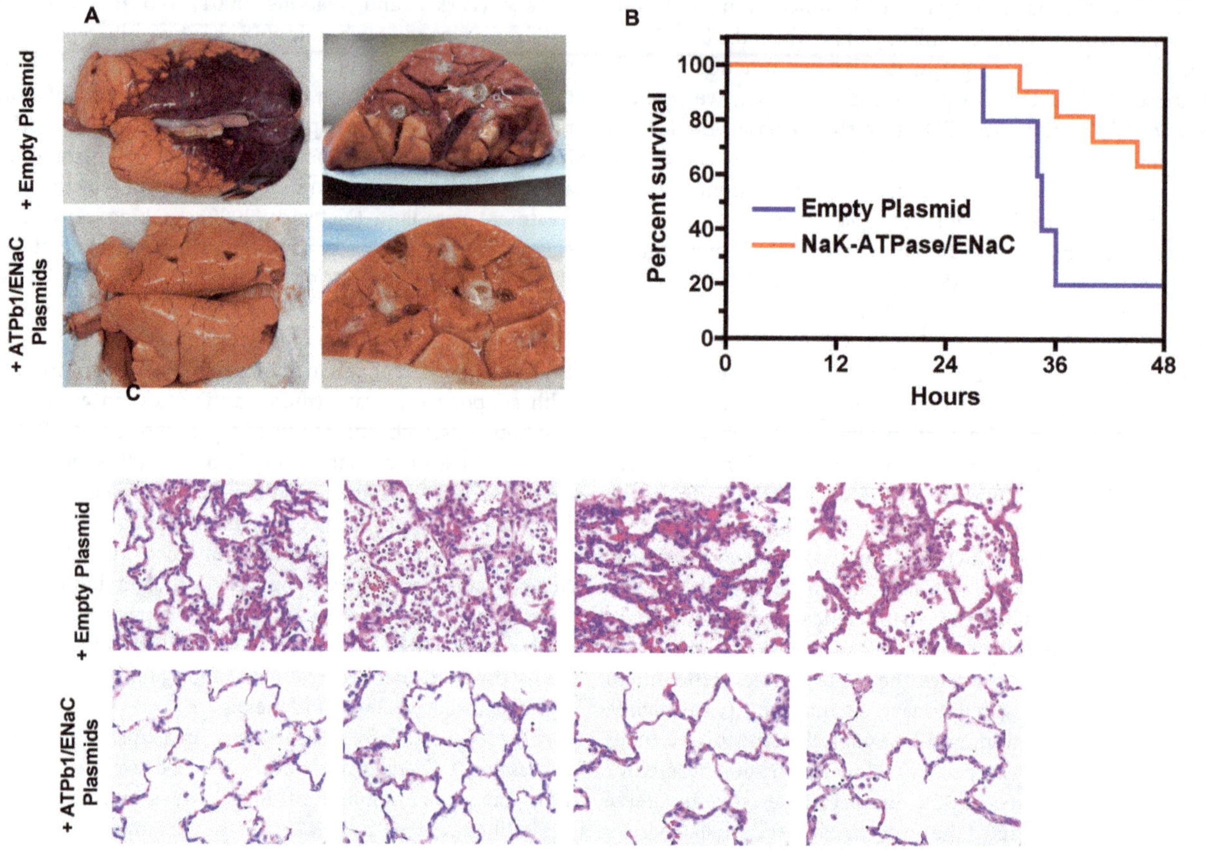

FIGURE 4 | Electroporation-mediated gene transfer of Na^+,K^+-ATPase β1 subunit and α-ENaC plasmids can treat lung injury in a severe septic pig model of ARDS. Lung injury was induced in pigs (40 kg) at $t = 0$ by inducement of a fecal clot into the abdomen and ischemia-reperfusion injury of the superior mesenteric artery for 30 min and 4 h later, either empty plasmids or plasmids expressing α-ENaC and the Na^+, K^+-ATPase β1 subunit (ATP1b1) were delivered to the right and left lower lobes by electroporation. ARDSnet ventilation and vasopressor protocols (Network, 2000) were followed until death or the 48-h pre-set endpoint. **(A)** Gross histology of lungs from both groups of animals. Note the high degree of atelectasis and glossy presence of excess fluid in lungs from animals receiving empty plasmids. **(B)** Histology of lungs shows a much lower degree of injury in animals receiving the plasmid treatment. **(C)** Survival curves show that gene transfer of Na^+, K^+-ATPase β1 and α-ENaC plasmids increases survival (Dean, unpublished).

was detected (pH < 7.15) according to the ARDSnet protocol. Broad-spectrum antibiotics (ampicillin 2 g IV and metronidazole 500 mg IV) were given following abdominal closure and every 12 h until the end of the study. The results seen following electroporation-mediated gene transfer of the Na^+, K^+-ATPase and ENaC genes were remarkable (**Figure 4**).

First, gene transfer of an empty plasmid (pCDNA3) did not change the course of the injury compared to animals with no intervention. In contrast, the transfer of Na^+, K^+-ATPase/α-ENaC plasmids lead to improved lung function, improved kidney function, less injured lungs upon gross and microscopic histological analysis, and greater survival. In terms of lung function, electroporation of the treatment plasmids increased P/F ratios and compliance in the pigs, while the amount of PEEP needed to keep the lungs open was less in these animals, as was plateau pressure. As in mice, gene transfer of Na^+,K^+- ATPase/α-ENaC plasmids increased the abundance of tight junction proteins ZO-1 and occludin in the septic pigs (Emr et al., 2015; Lin et al., 2016). This upregulation may indeed result in improved barrier function and may account in part for the improved outcome. Gene transfer also had an effect on cellular death with 3.5 ± 1.4% (mean ± SD) of alveolar cells staining tunnel positive for apoptosis in empty plasmid-treated pigs compared to 1.9 ± 0.9% in Na^+,K^+-ATPase/α-ENaC pigs ($p < 0.01$). The health of the lungs was evident upon visual inspection of lungs removed from the euthanized animals (Emr et al., 2015). Histologically, the animals receiving either no intervention or empty plasmid showed all the signs of ALI/ARDS, namely, thickened alveolar septa, cell infiltrates, hemorrhage, edema, fibrin deposits, hyaline membranes, and vascular congestion, while animals receiving the Na^+,K^+-ATPase/α-ENaC plasmids presented much more like healthy lungs (**Figure 4**). Quantitative histological analysis revealed statistically significant differences between these groups (Emr et al., 2015). Wet to dry ratios showed significantly drier lungs in the animals receiving the Na^+,K^+-ATPase/α-ENaC plasmids. Finally, survival was also improved. The success of this electroporation-mediated gene therapy in such a stringent model demonstrates the robust nature and promise of this approach for possible use in critically ill patients.

CONCLUSION

Despite the fact that there has been no single gene or combination of genes identified that are responsible for ARDS, a number of genes have been effectively targeted for up- or down-regulation in multiple animal models that have shown varied degrees of alleviation of many of the symptoms and severity of ARDS. While in the past, most focus has been aimed at increasing the expression of ion channels and transporters to aid in alveolar fluid removal, these have not been as successful in treatment studies. More promising strategies are targeted toward dampening inflammatory responses and repairing or strengthening the alveolar-capillary barrier. In both cases, a number of genes have shown promise.

Perhaps the major problem with developing treatments for ARDS at the gene therapy level has been that most studies have relied on prevention approaches as opposed to treatment. In these instances, genes are transferred to healthy lungs before any lung injury is induced. While this allows for maximal gene delivery, since healthy lungs allow for greater distribution of any viral or nonviral gene delivery agent and maximal transcription from delivered transgenes, it is not reflective of how any gene therapy or other treatment would be given clinically (i.e., after development of lung injury). Furthermore, a myriad of studies have clearly shown that mice are not humans, and that ALI and ARDS in mice do not show all of the same pathological hallmarks as the human disease. Larger animals that more closely reflect human pathophysiology are needed to make any advancement toward the clinic. Thus, greater emphasis should be placed on those studies that (1) use experimental designs aimed at treating existing disease and (2) use larger, clinically relevant animal models of ARDS.

Using a number of different animal models and humans, many of the molecular mechanisms that contribute directly and indirectly to the pathogenesis of ARDS have been identified over the past 30 years. Developing strategies to treat this and any disease at the genetic level using gene therapy is perhaps the most direct way to change the pathophysiology and resolve injury, if concerns for safety and appropriate gene expression are kept in balance. While a number of different families or types of targets have been studied (inflammatory, edema clearance, and barrier, etc.), perhaps the major limitation for effective gene therapy remains optimizing gene delivery itself. Gene delivery systems that are nontoxic and non-inflammatory allow for repeat dosing and produce therapeutic levels of gene product, all the while being targeted to desired cell types is needed. Although each different viral vector or nonviral chemical or physical technology may address one or more of these problems, none has yet solved all of them. However, advances are rapid in both the areas of gene delivery and our understanding of the disease itself, so it is highly likely that safe and efficacious treatments for ARDS are within reach.

AUTHOR CONTRIBUTIONS

JL and DD contributed to, wrote, revised the manuscript, and approved the submitted version.

REFERENCES

Abraham, E. (2000). Coagulation abnormalities in acute lung injury and sepsis. *Am. J. Respir. Cell Mol. Biol.* 22, 401–404. doi: 10.1165/ajrcmb.22.4.f184

Adhikari, N., Burns, K. E., and Meade, M. O. (2004). Pharmacologic therapies for adults with acute lung injury and acute respiratory distress syndrome. *Cochrane Database Syst. Rev.* 2004:Cd004477. doi: 10.1002/14651858.CD004477.pub2

Adhikari, N. K., Burns, K. E., Friedrich, J. O., Granton, J. T., Cook, D. J., and Meade, M. O. (2007). Effect of nitric oxide on oxygenation and mortality in acute lung injury: systematic review and meta-analysis. *BMJ* 334:779. doi: 10.1136/bmj.39139.716794.55

Adir, Y., Factor, P., Dumasius, V., Ridge, K. M., and Sznajder, J. I. (2003). Na,K-ATPase gene transfer increases liquid clearance during ventilation-induced lung injury. *Am. J. Respir. Crit. Care Med.* 168, 1445–1448. doi: 10.1164/rccm.200207-702OC

Adir, Y., Welch, L. C., Dumasius, V., Factor, P., Sznajder, J. I., and Ridge, K. M. (2008). Overexpression of the Na-K-ATPase alpha2-subunit improves lung liquid clearance during ventilation-induced lung injury. *Am. J. Physiol. Lung Cell. Mol. Physiol.* 294, L1233–L1237. doi: 10.1152/ajplung.00076.2007

Ahi, Y. S., Bangari, D. S., and Mittal, S. K. (2011). Adenoviral vector immunity: its implications and circumvention strategies. *Curr. Gene Ther.* 11, 307–320. doi: 10.2174/156652311796150372

Ahmed, M. N., Suliman, H. B., Folz, R. J., Nozik-Grayck, E., Golson, M. L., Mason, S. N., et al. (2003). Extracellular superoxide dismutase protects lung development in hyperoxia-exposed newborn mice. *Am. J. Respir. Crit. Med.* 167, 400–405. doi: 10.1164/rccm.200202-108OC

Aihara, H., and Miyazaki, J. (1998). Gene transfer into muscle by electroporation in vivo. *Nat. Biotechnol.* 16, 867–870. doi: 10.1038/nbt0998-867

Aird, W. C. (2007). Phenotypic heterogeneity of the endothelium: II. Representative vascular beds. *Circ. Res.* 100, 174–190. doi: 10.1161/01.RES.0000255690.03436.ae

Akhter, M. Z., Joshi, J. C., Balaji Ragunathrao, V. A., Maienschein-Cline, M., Proia, R. L., Malik, A. B., et al. (2021). Programming to $S1PR1^{+}$ endothelial cells promote restoration of vascular integrity. *Circ. Res.* 129, 221–236. doi: 10.1161/CIRCRESAHA.120.318412

Alba, R., Bosch, A., and Chillon, M. (2005). Gutless adenovirus: last-generation adenovirus for gene therapy. *Gene Ther.* 12, S18–S27. doi: 10.1038/sj.gt.3302612

Albertine, K. H., Soulier, M. F., Wang, Z., Ishizaka, A., Hashimoto, S., Zimmerman, G. A., et al. (2002). Fas and fas ligand are up-regulated in pulmonary edema fluid and lung tissue of patients with acute lung injury and the acute respiratory distress syndrome. *Am. J. Pathol.* 161, 1783–1796. doi: 10.1016/S0002-9440(10)64455-0

Al-Sadi, R., Boivin, M., and Ma, T. (2009). Mechanism of cytokine modulation of epithelial tight junction barrier. *Front. Biosci.* 14:2765–2778. doi: 10.2741/3413

Alvarez, D. F., King, J. A., Weber, D., Addison, E., Liedtke, W., and Townsley, M. I. (2006). Transient receptor potential vanilloid 4-mediated disruption of the alveolar septal barrier: a novel mechanism of acute lung injury. *Circ. Res.* 99, 988–995. doi: 10.1161/01.RES.0000247065.11756.19

Ando, M., Murakami, Y., Kojima, F., Endo, H., Kitasato, H., Hashimoto, A., et al. (2003). Retrovirally introduced prostaglandin D2 synthase suppresses lung injury induced by bleomycin. *Am. J. Respir. Cell Mol. Biol.* 28, 582–591. doi: 10.1165/rcmb.2002-0162OC

Aneja, M. K., Geiger, J. P., Himmel, A., and Rudolph, C. (2009). Targeted gene delivery to the lung. *Expert Opin. Drug Deliv.* 6, 567–583. doi: 10.1517/17425240902927841

Anson, D. S. (2004). The use of retroviral vectors for gene therapy-what are the risks? A review of retroviral pathogenesis and its relevance to retroviral vector-mediated gene delivery. *Genet. Vaccines Ther.* 2:9. doi: 10.1186/1479-0556-2-9

Araujo, J., Zhang, M., and Yin, F. (2012). Heme oxygenase-1, oxidation, inflammation, and atherosclerosis. *Front. Pharmacol.* 3:119. doi: 10.3389/fphar.2012.00119

Armstrong, S. M., Wang, C., Tigdi, J., Si, X., Dumpit, C., Charles, S., et al. (2012). Influenza infects lung microvascular endothelium leading to microvascular leak: role of apoptosis and claudin-5. *PLoS One* 7:e47323. doi: 10.1371/journal.pone.0047323

Arndt, P. G., Young, S. K., Poch, K. R., Nick, J. A., Falk, S., Schrier, R. W., et al. (2006). Systemic inhibition of the angiotensin-converting enzyme limits lipopolysaccharide-induced lung neutrophil recruitment through both bradykinin and angiotensin II-regulated pathways. *J. Immunol.* 177, 7233–7241. doi: 10.4049/jimmunol.177.10.7233

Azzam, Z. S., Dumasius, V., Saldias, F. J., Adir, Y., Sznajder, J. I., and Factor, P. (2002). Na,K-ATPase overexpression improves alveolar fluid clearance in a rat model of elevated left atrial pressure. *Circulation* 105, 497–501. doi: 10.1161/hc0402.102848

Bachofen, M., and Weibel, E. R. (1977). Alterations of the gas exchange apparatus in adult respiratory insufficiency associated with septicemia. *Am. Rev. Respir. Dis.* 116, 589–615. doi: 10.1164/arrd.1977.116.4.589

Bachofen, M., and Weibel, E. R. (1982). Structural alterations of lung parenchyma in the adult respiratory distress syndrome. *Clin. Chest Med.* 3, 35–56. doi: 10.1016/s0272-5231(21)00143-x

Bai, H., Lester, G. M. S., Petishnok, L. C., and Dean, D. A. (2017). Cytoplasmic transport and nuclear import of plasmid DNA. *Biosci. Rep.* 37:BSR20160616. doi: 10.1042/BSR20160616

Bai, H., Zhou, R., Barravecchia, M., Norman, R., Friedman, A., Yu, D., et al. (2021). The Na^+, K^+-ATPase β1 subunit regulates epithelial tight junctions via MRCKα. *JCI Insight* 6:e134881.

Bale, S., Sunkoju, M., Reddy, S. S., Swamy, V., and Godugu, C. (2016). Oropharyngeal aspiration of bleomycin: an alternative experimental model of pulmonary fibrosis developed in Swiss mice. *Indian J. Pharmacol.* 48, 643–648. doi: 10.4103/0253-7613.194859

Bao, L., Deng, W., Huang, B., Gao, H., Liu, J., Ren, L., et al. (2020). The pathogenicity of SARS-CoV-2 in hACE2 transgenic mice. *Nature* 583, 830–833. doi: 10.1038/s41586-020-2312-y

Barron, L. G., Uyechi, L. S., and Szoka, F. C. (1999). Cationic lipids are essential for gene delivery mediated by intravenous administration of lipoplexes. *Gene Ther.* 6, 1179–1183. doi: 10.1038/sj.gt.3300929

Bellani, G., Laffey, J. G., Pham, T., Fan, E., Brochard, L., Esteban, A., et al. (2016). Epidemiology, patterns of care, and mortality for patients with acute respiratory distress syndrome in intensive care units in 50 countries. *JAMA* 315, 788–800. doi: 10.1001/jama.2016.0291

Berthiaume, Y., Folkesson, H. G., and Matthay, M. A. (2002). Invited review: alveolar edema fluid clearance in the injured lung. *J. Appl. Physiol.* 93, 2207–2213. doi: 10.1152/japplphysiol.01201.2001

Bertorello, A. M., Ridge, K. M., Chibalin, A. V., Katz, A. I., and Sznajder, J. I. (1999). Isoproterenol increases Na^+-K^+-ATPase activity by membrane insertion of α-subunits in lung alveolar cells. *Am. J. Physiol. Lung Cell. Mol. Physiol.* 276, L20–L27. doi: 10.1152/ajplung.1999.276.1.L20

Bhattacharya, J., and Matthay, M. A. (2013). Regulation and repair of the alveolar-capillary barrier in acute lung injury. *Annu. Rev. Physiol.* 75, 593–615. doi: 10.1146/annurev-physiol-030212-183756

Birukova, A. A., Zagranichnaya, T., Fu, P., Alekseeva, E., Chen, W., Jacobson, J. R., et al. (2007). Prostaglandins PGE_2 and PGI_2 promote endothelial barrier enhancement via PKA- and Epac1/Rap1-dependent Rac activation. *Exp. Cell Res.* 313, 2504–2520. doi: 10.1016/j.yexcr.2007.03.036

Blair-Parks, K., Weston, B. C., and Dean, D. A. (2002). Gene delivery to the cornea by plasmid injection and electroporation. *J. Gene Med.* 4, 92–100.

Boeckle, S., von Gersdorff, K., van der Piepen, S., Culmsee, C., Wagner, E., and Ogris, M. (2004). Purification of polyethylenimine polyplexes highlights the role of free polycations in gene transfer. *J. Gene Med.* 6, 1102–1111. doi: 10.1002/jgm.598

Bogatcheva, N. V., Garcia, J. G., and Verin, A. D. (2002). Molecular mechanisms of thrombin-induced endothelial cell permeability. *Biochemistry (Mosc.)* 67, 75–84. doi: 10.1023/a:1013904231324

Bouard, D., Alazard-Dany, D., and Cosset, F. L. (2009). Viral vectors: from virology to transgene expression. *Br. J. Pharmacol.* 157, 153–165. doi: 10.1038/bjp.2008.349

Boussif, O., Lezoualc'h, F., Zanta, M. A., Mergny, M. D., Scherman, D., Demeneix, B., et al. (1995). A versatile vector for gene and oligonucleotide transfer into cells in culture and in vivo: polyethylenimine. *Proc. Natl. Acad. Sci. U.S.A.* 92, 7297–7301. doi: 10.1073/pnas.92.16.7297

Bowler, R. P., Nicks, M., Tran, K., Tanner, G., Chang, L.-Y., Young, S. K., et al. (2004). Extracellular superoxide dismutase attenuates lipopolysaccharide-induced neutrophilic inflammation. *Am. J. Respir. Cell Mol. Biol.* 31, 432–439. doi: 10.1165/rcmb.2004-0057OC

Boyle, A. J., Mac Sweeney, R., and McAuley, D. F. (2013). Pharmacological treatments in ARDS; a state-of-the-art update. *BMC Med.* 11:166. doi: 10.1186/1741-7015-11-166

Brune, K., Frank, J. A., Schwingshackl, A., Finigan, J. H., and Sidhaye, V. K. (2015). Pulmonary epithelial barrier function- some new players and mechanisms. *Am. J. Physiol. Lung Cell Mol. Physiol.* 308, L731–L745. doi: 10.1152/ajplung.00309.2014

Buff, S. M., Yu, H., McCall, J. N., Caldwell, S. M., Ferkol, T. W., Flotte, T. R., et al. (2010). IL-10 delivery by AAV5 vector attenuates inflammation in mice with *pseudomonas* pneumonia. *Gene Ther.* 17, 567–576. doi: 10.1038/gt.2010.28

Bushman, F. D. (2007). Retroviral integration and human gene therapy. *J. Clin. Invest.* 117, 2083–2086. doi: 10.1172/jci32949

Bustamante-Marin, X. M., and Ostrowski, L. E. (2017). Cilia and mucociliary clearance. *Cold Spring Harb. Perspect. Biol.* 9:a028241.

Calfee, C. S., Delucchi, K. L., Sinha, P., Matthay, M. A., Hackett, J., Shankar-Hari, M., et al. (2018). Acute respiratory distress syndrome subphenotypes and differential response to simvastatin: secondary analysis of a randomised controlled trial. *Lancet Respir. Med.* 6, 691–698.

Capasso, C., Garofalo, M., Hirvinen, M., and Cerullo, V. (2014). The evolution of adenoviral vectors through genetic and chemical surface modifications. *Viruses* 6, 832–855.

Caraballo, J. C., Yshii, C., Butti, M. L., Westphal, W., Borcherding, J. A., Allamargot, C., et al. (2011). Hypoxia increases transepithelial electrical conductance and reduces occludin at the plasma membrane in alveolar epithelial cells via PKC-ζ and PP2A pathway. *Am. J. physiol. Lung Cell. Mol. Physiol.* 300, L569–L578.

Cardinal-Fernández, P., Lorente, J. A., Ballén-Barragán, A., and Matute-Bello, G. (2017). Acute respiratory distress syndrome and diffuse alveolar damage. new insights on a complex relationship. *Ann. Am. Thorac. Soc.* 14, 844–850. doi: 10.1513/AnnalsATS.201609-728PS

CDC (2021). *Centers for Disease Control and Prevention Coronavirus Disease 2019 (COVID-19) Data Tracker.* Available online at: https://covid.cdc.gov/covid-data-tracker/#cases_casesper100klast7days (accessed October 24, 2021).

Chan, Y. H., Harith, H. H., Israf, D. A., and Tham, C. L. (2020). Differential regulation of LPS-mediated VE-cadherin disruption in human endothelial cells and the underlying signaling pathways: a mini review. *Front. Cell Dev. Biol.* 7:280. doi: 10.3389/fcell.2019.00280

Chen, J., Li, C., Gao, X., Li, C., Liang, Z., Yu, L., et al. (2013). Keratinocyte growth factor gene delivery via mesenchymal stem cells protects against lipopolysaccharide-induced acute lung injury in mice. *PLoS One* 8:e83303. doi: 10.1371/journal.pone.0083303

Chen, W., Sharma, R., Rizzo, A. N., Siegler, J. H., Garcia, J. G., and Jacobson, J. R. (2014). Role of claudin-5 in the attenuation of murine acute lung injury by simvastatin. *Am. J. Respir. Cell Mol. Biol.* 50, 328–336. doi: 10.1165/rcmb.2013-0058OC

Cheng, K. T., Xiong, S., Ye, Z., Hong, Z., Di, A., Tsang, K. M., et al. (2017). Caspase-11-mediated endothelial pyroptosis underlies endotoxemia-induced lung injury. *J. Clin. Invest.* 127, 4124–4135. doi: 10.1172/JCI94495

Chiu, T. K., and Davies, D. R. (2004). Structure and function of HIV-1 integrase. *Curr. Top. Med.Chem.* 4, 965–977. doi: 10.2174/1568026043388547

Cohen, T. S., Gray Lawrence, G., and Margulies, S. S. (2010). Cultured alveolar epithelial cells from septic rats mimic in vivo septic lung. *PLoS One* 5:e11322. doi: 10.1371/journal.pone.0011322

Colegio, O. R., Van Itallie, C., Rahner, C., and Anderson, J. M. (2003). Claudin extracellular domains determine paracellular charge selectivity and resistance but not tight junction fibril architecture. *Am. J. Physiol. Cell Physiol.* 284, C1346–C1354. doi: 10.1152/ajpcell.00547.2002

Colegio, O. R., Van Itallie, C. M., McCrea, H. J., Rahner, C., and Anderson, J. M. (2002). Claudins create charge-selective channels in the paracellular pathway between epithelial cells. *Am. J. Physiol. Cell Physiol.* 283, C142–C147.

Copreni, E., Penzo, M., Carrabino, S., and Conese, M. (2004). Lentivirus-mediated gene transfer to the respiratory epithelium: a promising approach to gene therapy of cystic fibrosis. *Gene Ther.* 11, S67–S75. doi: 10.1038/sj.gt.3302372

Couper, K. N., Blount, D. G., and Riley, E. M. (2008). IL-10: the Master regulator of Immunity to Infection. *J. Immunol.* 180:5771. doi: 10.4049/jimmunol.180.9.5771

Crapo, J. D., Young, S. L., Fram, E. K., Pinkerton, K. E., Barry, B. E., and Crapo, R. O. (1983). Morphometric characteristics of cells in the alveolar region of mammalian lungs. *Am. Rev. Respir. Dis.* 128, S42–S46. doi: 10.1164/arrd.1983.128.2P2.S42

Crystal, R. G. (2014). Adenovirus: the first effective in vivo gene delivery vector. *Hum. Gene Ther.* 25, 3–11. doi: 10.1089/hum.2013.2527

Dada, L. A., Chandel, N. S., Ridge, K. M., Pedemonte, C., Bertorello, A. M., and Sznajder, J. I. (2003). Hypoxia-induced endocytosis of Na,K-ATPase in alveolar epithelial cells is mediated by mitochondrial reactive oxygen species and PKC-zeta. *J. Clin. Invest.* 111, 1057–1064. doi: 10.1172/JCI16826

Danel, C., Erzurum, S. C., Prayssac, P., Eissa, N. T., Crystal, R. G., Hervé, P., et al. (1998). Gene therapy for oxidant injury-related diseases: adenovirus-mediated transfer of superoxide dismutase and catalase cDNAs protects against hyperoxia but not against ischemia-reperfusion lung injury. *Hum. Gene Ther.* 9, 1487–1496. doi: 10.1089/hum.1998.9.10-1487

Davis, P. B., and Cooper, M. J. (2007). Vectors for airway gene delivery. *AAPS J.* 9, E11–E17.

de Alencar, J. C. G., Moreira, C. D. L., Müller, A. D., Chaves, C. E., Fukuhara, M. A., da Silva, E. A., et al. (2020). Double-blind, randomized, placebo-controlled trial with N-acetylcysteine for treatment of severe acute respiratory syndrome caused by Coronavirus disease 2019 (COVID-19). *Clin. Infect. Dis.* 72, e736–e741. doi: 10.1093/cid/ciaa1443

Dean, D. A. (2003). Electroporation of the vasculature and the lung. *DNA Cell Biol* 22, 797–806. doi: 10.1089/104454903322625000

Dean, D. A. (2005). Nonviral gene transfer to skeletal, smooth, and cardiac muscle in living animals. *Am. J. Physiol. Cell Physiol.* 289, C233–C245. doi: 10.1152/ajpcell.00613.2004

Dean, D. A., Barravecchia, M., Danziger, B., and Lin, X. (2011). Use of electroporation for efficacious gene delivery to the lungs. *ECS Trans.* 35, 167–177. doi: 10.1149/1.3571989

Dean, D. A., Dean, B. S., Muller, S., and Smith, L. C. (1999). Sequence requirements for plasmid nuclear entry. *Exp. Cell Res.* 253, 713–722. doi: 10.1006/excr.1999.4716

Dean, D. A., Machado-Aranda, D., Blair-Parks, K., Yeldandi, A. V., and Young, J. L. (2003). Electroporation as a method for high-level nonviral gene transfer to the lung. *Gene Ther.* 10, 1608–1615. doi: 10.1038/sj.gt.3302053

Devaney, J., Contreras, M., and Laffey, J. G. (2011). Clinical review: gene-based therapies for ALI/ARDS: where are we now? *Crit. Care (London, England)* 15, 224–224. doi: 10.1186/cc10216

DeWitt, D. L. (1991). Prostaglandin endoperoxide synthase: regulation of enzyme expression. *Biochim. Biophys. Acta* 1083, 121–134. doi: 10.1016/0005-2760(91)90032-d

Doh, S. G., Vahlsing, H. L., Hartikka, J., Liang, X., and Manthorpe, M. (1997). Spatial-temporal patterns of gene expression in mouse skeletal muscle after injection of lacZ plasmid DNA. *Gene Ther.* 4, 648–663. doi: 10.1038/sj.gt.3300460

Dolgachev, V., Panicker, S., Balijepalli, S., McCandless, L. K., Yin, Y., Swamy, S., et al. (2018). Electroporation-mediated delivery of FER gene enhances innate immune response and improves survival in a murine model of pneumonia. *Gene Ther.* 25, 359–375. doi: 10.1038/s41434-018-0022-y

Dolgachev, V. A., Goldberg, R., Suresh, M. V., Thomas, B., Talarico, N., Hemmila, M. R., et al. (2016). Electroporation-mediated delivery of the FER gene in the resolution of trauma-related fatal pneumonia. *Gene Ther.* 23, 785–796. doi: 10.1038/gt.2016.58

Driskell, R. A., and Engelhardt, J. F. (2003). Current status of gene therapy for inherited lung diseases. *Annu. Rev. Physiol.* 65, 585–612. doi: 10.1146/annurev.physiol.65.092101.142426

Dumasius, V., Jameel, M., Burhop, J., Meng, F. J., Welch, L. C., Mutlu, G. G., et al. (2003). In vivo timing of onset of transgene expression following adenoviral-mediated gene transfer. *Virology* 308, 243–249. doi: 10.1016/s0042-6822(02)00138-1

Dumasius, V., Sznajder, J. I., Azzam, Z. S., Boja, J., Mutlu, G. K. M., Maron, M. B., et al. (2001). β2-Adrenergic receptor overexpression increases alveolar fluid clearance and responsiveness to endogenous catecholamines in rats. *Circ. Res.* 89, 907–914. doi: 10.1161/hh2201.100204

Duncan, G. A., Jung, J., Hanes, J., and Suk, J. S. (2016). The mucus barrier to inhaled gene therapy. *Mol. Ther.* 24, 2043–2053. doi: 10.1038/mt.2016.182

Edelstein, M. L., Abedi, M. R., and Wixon, J. (2007). Gene therapy clinical trials worldwide to 2007–an update. *J. Gene Med.* 9, 833–842. doi: 10.1002/jgm.1100

Edelstein, M. L., Abedi, M. R., Wixon, J., and Edelstein, R. M. (2004). Gene therapy clinical trials worldwide 1989–2004—an overview. *J. Gene Med.* 6, 597–602. doi: 10.1002/jgm.619

Eliseeva, S. I., Knowlden, Z. A., Lester, G. M., Dean, D. A., Georas, S. N., and Chapman, T. J. (2021). Changes in lung immune cell infiltrates after electric field treatment in mice. *Sci. Rep.* 11:1453. doi: 10.1038/s41598-021-81174-y

Eliyahu, H., Barenholz, Y., and Domb, A. J. (2005). Polymers for DNA delivery. *Molecules* 10, 34–64. doi: 10.3390/10010034

Emr, B. M., Roy, S., Kollisch-Singule, M., Gatto, L. A., Barravecchia, M., Lin, X., et al. (2015). Electroporation-mediated gene delivery of Na^+,K^+ -ATPase, and ENaC subunits to the lung attenuates acute respiratory distress syndrome in a two-hit porcine model. *Shock* 43, 16–23. doi: 10.1097/SHK.0000000000000228

Escobar-Chávez, J. J., Bonilla-Martínez, D., Villegas-González, M. A., and Revilla-Vázquez, A. L. (2009). Electroporation as an efficient physical enhancer for skin drug delivery. *J. Clin. Pharmacol.* 49, 1262–1283. doi: 10.1177/0091270009344984

Escriou, V., Ciolina, C., Helbling-Leclerc, A., Wils, P., and Scherman, D. (1998). Cationic lipid-mediated gene transfer: analysis of cellular uptake and nuclear import of plasmid DNA. *Cell Biol. Toxicol.* 14, 95–104. doi: 10.1023/a:1007425803756

Factor, P., Dumasius, V., Saldias, F., Brown, L. A., and Sznajder, J. I. (2000). Adenovirus-mediated transfer of an Na^+/K^+-ATPase beta1 subunit gene improves alveolar fluid clearance and survival in hyperoxic rats. *Hum. Gene Ther.* 11, 2231–2242. doi: 10.1089/104303400750035753

Factor, P., Dumasius, V., Saldias, F., and Sznajder, J. I. (1999). Adenoviral-mediated overexpression of the NA,K-ATPase beta1 subunit gene increases lung edema clearance and improves survival during acute hyperoxic lung injury in rats. *Chest* 116, 24S–25S. doi: 10.1378/chest.116.suppl_1.24s

Factor, P., Saldias, F., Ridge, K., Dumasius, V., Zabner, J., Jaffe, H. A., et al. (1998). Augmentation of lung liquid clearance via adenovirus-mediated transfer of a Na,K-ATPase beta1 subunit gene. *J. Clin. Invest.* 102, 1421–1430. doi: 10.1172/JCI3214

Fang, X., Fukuda, N., Barbry, P., Sartori, C., Verkman, A. S., and Matthay, M. A. (2002). Novel role for CFTR in fluid absorption from the distal airspaces of the lung. *J. Gen. Physiol.* 119, 199–207. doi: 10.1085/jgp.119.2.199

Felgner, J. H., Kumar, R., Sridhar, C. N., Wheeler, C. J., Tsai, Y. J., Border, R., et al. (1994). Enhanced gene delivery and mechanism studies with a novel series of cationic lipid formulations. *J. Biol. Chem.* 269, 2550–2561. doi: 10.1016/s0021-9258(17)41980-6

Fine, A., Anderson, N. L., Rothstein, T. L., Williams, M. C., and Gochuico, B. R. (1997). Fas expression in pulmonary alveolar type II cells. *Am. J. Physiol.* 273, L64–L71. doi: 10.1152/ajplung.1997.273.1.L64

Fischer, D., Bieber, T., Li, Y., Elsasser, H. P., and Kissel, T. (1999). A novel non-viral vector for DNA delivery based on low molecular weight, branched polyethylenimine: effect of molecular weight on transfection efficiency and cytotoxicity. *Pharm. Res.* 16, 1273–1279. doi: 10.1023/a:1014861900478

Förster, C. (2008). Tight junctions and the modulation of barrier function in disease. *Histochem. Cell Biol.* 130, 55–70. doi: 10.1007/s00418-008-0424-9

Frank, J. A. (2012). Claudins and alveolar epithelial barrier function in the lung. *Ann. N. Y. Acad. Sci.* 1257, 175–183. doi: 10.1111/j.1749-6632.2012.06533.x

Frank, J. A., Wang, Y., Osorio, O., and Matthay, M. A. (2000). Beta-adrenergic agonist therapy accelerates the resolution of hydrostatic pulmonary edema in sheep and rats. *J. Appl. Physiol. (1985)* 89, 1255–1265. doi: 10.1152/jappl.2000.89.4.1255

Franquesa, M., Alperovich, G., Herrero-Fresneda, I., Lloberas, N., Bolaños, N., Fillat, C., et al. (2005). Direct electrotransfer of hHGF gene into kidney ameliorates ischemic acute renal failure. *Gene Ther.* 12, 1551–1558. doi: 10.1038/sj.gt.3302569

Freedland, S. J., Malone, R. W., Borchers, H. M., Zadourian, Z., Malone, J. G., Bennett, M. J., et al. (1996). Toxicity of cationic lipid-ribozyme complexes in human prostate tumor cells can mimic ribozyme activity. *Biochem. Mol. Med.* 59, 144–153. doi: 10.1006/bmme.1996.0080

Fuchs-Buder, T., de Moerloose, P., Ricou, B., Reber, G., Vifian, C., Nicod, L., et al. (1996). Time course of procoagulant activity and D dimer in bronchoalveolar fluid of patients at risk for or with acute respiratory distress syndrome. *Am. J Respir. Crit. Care Med.* 153, 163–167. doi: 10.1164/ajrccm.153.1.8542111

Fuller, D. H., Loudon, P., and Schmaljohn, C. (2006). Preclinical and clinical progress of particle-mediated DNA vaccines for infectious diseases. *Methods* 40, 86–97. doi: 10.1016/j.ymeth.2006.05.022

Galani, V., Tatsaki, E., Bai, M., Kitsoulis, P., Lekka, M., Nakos, G., et al. (2010). The role of apoptosis in the pathophysiology of acute respiratory distress syndrome (ARDS): an up-to-date cell-specific review. *Pathol. Res. Pract.* 206, 145–150. doi: 10.1016/j.prp.2009.12.002

Gamble, J. R., Drew, J., Trezise, L., Underwood, A., Parsons, M., Kasminkas, L., et al. (2000). Angiopoietin-1 is an antipermeability and anti-inflammatory agent in vitro and targets cell junctions. *Circ. Res.* 87, 603–607. doi: 10.1161/01.res.87.7.603

Gao, X., Kim, K. S., and Liu, D. (2007). Nonviral gene delivery: what we know and what is next. *AAPS J.* 9, E92–E104. doi: 10.1208/aapsj0901009

Gao, Y.-L., Zhai, J.-H., and Chai, Y.-F. (2018). Recent advances in the molecular mechanisms underlying pyroptosis in sepsis. *Mediators Inflamm.* 2018:5823823. doi: 10.1155/2018/5823823

Gao Smith, F., Perkins, G. D., Gates, S., Young, D., McAuley, D. F., Tunnicliffe, W., et al. (2012). Effect of intravenous β-2 agonist treatment on clinical outcomes in acute respiratory distress syndrome (BALTI-2): a multicentre, randomised controlled trial. *Lancet* 379, 229–235. doi: 10.1016/S0140-6736(11)61623-1

Garver, R. I. Jr., Chytil, A., Courtney, M., and Crystal, R. G. (1987). Clonal gene therapy: transplanted mouse fibroblast clones express human alpha 1-antitrypsin gene in vivo. *Science* 237, 762–764. doi: 10.1126/science.3497452

Gary, D. J., Min, J., Kim, Y., Park, K., and Won, Y. Y. (2013). The effect of N/P ratio on the in vitro and in vivo interaction properties of PEGylated poly[2-(dimethylamino)ethyl methacrylate]-based siRNA complexes. *Macromol. Biosci.* 13, 1059–1071. doi: 10.1002/mabi.201300046

Gautam, A., Waldrep, C. J., and Densmore, C. L. (2002). Delivery systems for pulmonary gene therapy. *Am. J. respir. Med.* 1, 35–46. doi: 10.1007/BF03257161

Gazdhar, A., Bilici, M., Pierog, J., Ayuni, E. L., Gugger, M., Wetterwald, A., et al. (2006). In vivo electroporation and ubiquitin promoter–a protocol for sustained gene expression in the lung. *J. Gene Med.* 8, 910–918. doi: 10.1002/jgm.911

Gehl, J. (2003). Electroporation: theory and methods, perspectives for drug delivery, gene therapy and research. *Acta Physiol. Scand.* 177, 437–447. doi: 10.1046/j.1365-201X.2003.01093.x

Gilbert, R. A., Jaroszeski, M. J., and Heller, R. (1997). Novel electrode designs for electrochemotherapy. *Biochim. Biophys. Acta* 1334, 9–14. doi: 10.1016/s0304-4165(96)00119-5

Ginn, S. L. I, Alexander, E., Edelstein, M. L., Abedi, M. R., and Wixon, J. (2013). Gene therapy clinical trials worldwide to 2012 - an update. *J. Gene Med.* 15, 65–77. doi: 10.1002/jgm.2698

Ginn, S. L., Amaya, A. K. I, Alexander, E., Edelstein, M., and Abedi, M. R. (2018). Gene therapy clinical trials worldwide to 2017: an update. *J. Gene Med.* 20:e3015.

Glover, D. J., Lipps, H. J., and Jans, D. A. (2005). Towards safe, non-viral therapeutic gene expression in humans. *Nat. Rev. Genet.* 6, 299–310. doi: 10.1038/nrg1577

Goldman, M. J., Lee, P. S., Yang, J. S., and Wilson, J. M. (1997). Lentiviral vectors for gene therapy of cystic fibrosis. *Hum. Gene Ther.* 8, 2261–2268. doi: 10.1089/hum.1997.8.18-2261

Gong, Q., Yin, H., Fang, M., Xiang, Y., Yuan, C. L., Zheng, G.-Y., et al. (2008). Heme oxygenase-1 upregulation significantly inhibits TNF-α and Hmgb1 releasing and attenuates lipopolysaccharide-induced acute lung injury in mice. *Int. Immunopharmacol.* 8, 792–798. doi: 10.1016/j.intimp.2008.01.026

Gorin, A. B., and Stewart, P. A. (1979). Differential permeability of endothelial and epithelial barriers to albumin flux. *J. Appl. Physiol. Respir. Environ. Exerc. Physiol.* 47, 1315–1324. doi: 10.1152/jappl.1979.47.6.1315

Gottfried, L., Lin, X., Barravecchia, M., and Dean, D. A. (2016). Identification of an alveolar type I epithelial cell-specific DNA nuclear import sequence for gene delivery. *Gene Ther.* 23, 734–742. doi: 10.1038/gt.2016.52

Greenberger, M. J., Kunkel, S. L., Strieter, R. M., Lukacs, N. W., Bramson, J., Gauldie, J., et al. (1996). IL-12 gene therapy protects mice in lethal *Klebsiella pneumonia. J. Immunol.* 157, 3006–3012.

Griesenbach, U., Inoue, M., Meng, C., Farley, R., Chan, M., Newman, N. K., et al. (2012). Assessment of F/HN-pseudotyped lentivirus as a clinically relevant vector for lung gene therapy. *Am. J. Respir. Crit. Care Med.* 186, 846–856. doi: 10.1164/rccm.201206-1056OC

Grinnell, F., Feld, M., and Minter, D. (1980). Fibroblast adhesion to fibrinogen and fibrin substrata: requirement for cold-insoluble globulin (plasma fibronectin). *Cell* 19, 517–525. doi: 10.1016/0092-8674(80)90526-7

Guasch, R. M., Scambler, P., Jones, G. E., and Ridley, A. J. (1998). RhoE regulates actin cytoskeleton organization and cell migration. *Mol. Cell. Biol.* 18, 4761–4771. doi: 10.1128/MCB.18.8.4761

Guggino, W. B., and Cebotaru, L. (2017). Adeno-associated virus (AAV) gene therapy for cystic fibrosis: current barriers and recent developments. *Expert Opin. Biol. Ther.* 17, 1265–1273. doi: 10.1080/14712598.2017.1347630

Gunzel, D., and Yu, A. S. (2013). Claudins and the modulation of tight junction permeability. *Physiol. Rev.* 93, 525–569. doi: 10.1152/physrev.00019.2012

Hamacher, J., Hadizamani, Y., Borgmann, M., Mohaupt, M., Männel, D. N., Moehrlen, U., et al. (2018). Cytokine–ion channel interactions in pulmonary inflammation. *Frontiers in Immunology* 8:1644. doi: 10.3389/fimmu.2017.01644

Hamann, K. J., Dorscheid, D. R., Ko, F. D., Conforti, A. E., Sperling, A. I., Rabe, K. F., et al. (1998). Expression of Fas (CD95) and FasL (CD95L) in human airway epithelium. *Am. J. Respir. Cell Mol. Biol.* 19, 537–542. doi: 10.1165/ajrcmb.19.4.3100

Han, X., Fink, M. P., Uchiyama, T., Yang, R., and Delude, R. L. (2004). Increased iNOS activity is essential for pulmonary epithelial tight junction dysfunction in endotoxemic mice. *Am. J. Physiol. Lung Cell. Mol. Physiol.* 286, L259–L267. doi: 10.1152/ajplung.00187.2003

Hasan, S. S., Capstick, T., Ahmed, R., Kow, C. S., Mazhar, F., Merchant, H. A., et al. (2020). Mortality in COVID-19 patients with acute respiratory distress syndrome and corticosteroids use: a systematic review and meta-analysis. *Expert Rev. Respir. Med.* 14, 1149–1163. doi: 10.1080/17476348.2020.1804365

Hashiba, T., Suzuki, M., Nagashima, Y., Suzuki, S., Inoue, S., Tsuburai, T., et al. (2001). Adenovirus-mediated transfer of heme oxygenase-1 cDNA attenuates severe lung injury induced by the influenza virus in mice. *Gene Ther.* 8, 1499–1507. doi: 10.1038/sj.gt.3301540

Hassett, P., Curley, G. F., Contreras, M., Masterson, C., Higgins, B. D., O'Brien, T., et al. (2011). Overexpression of pulmonary extracellular superoxide dismutase attenuates endotoxin-induced acute lung injury. *Intensive Care Med.* 37:1680. doi: 10.1007/s00134-011-2309-y

Hasson, E., Slovatizky, Y., Shimoni, Y., Falk, H., Panet, A., and Mitrani, E. (2005). Solid tissues can be manipulated ex vivo and used as vehicles for gene therapy. *J. Gene Med.* 7, 926–935. doi: 10.1002/jgm.740

Hayashi, S., Takeuchi, K., Suzuki, S., Tsunoda, T., Tanaka, C., and Majima, Y. (2006). Effect of thrombin on permeability of human epithelial cell monolayers. *Pharmacology* 76, 46–52. doi: 10.1159/000089718

Heller, L., Jaroszeski, M. J., Coppola, D., Pottinger, C., Gilbert, R., and Heller, R. (2000). Electrically mediated plasmid DNA delivery to hepatocellular carcinomas in vivo. *Gene Ther.* 7, 826–829. doi: 10.1038/sj.gt.3301173

Henning, A., Hein, S., Schneider, M., Bur, M., and Lehr, C. M. (2010). Pulmonary drug delivery: medicines for inhalation. *Handb. Exp. Pharmacol.* 197, 171–192. doi: 10.1007/978-3-642-00477-3_6

Herold, S., Gabrielli, N. M., and Vadasz, I. (2013). Novel concepts of acute lung injury and alveolar-capillary barrier dysfunction. *Am. J. Physiol. Lung Cell. Mol. Physiol.* 305, L665–L681. doi: 10.1152/ajplung.00232.2013

Herrero, R., Sanchez, G., and Lorente, J. A. (2018). New insights into the mechanisms of pulmonary edema in acute lung injury. *Ann. Transl. Med.* 6, 32. doi: 10.21037/atm.2017.12.18

Herrero, R., Tanino, M., Smith, L. S., Kajikawa, O., Wong, V. A., Mongovin, S., et al. (2013). The Fas/FasL pathway impairs the alveolar fluid clearance in mouse lungs. *Am. J. Physiol. Lung Cell. Mol. Physiol.* 305, L377–L388. doi: 10.1152/ajplung.00271.2012

Hill, A. B., Chen, M., Chen, C. K., Pfeifer, B. A., and Jones, C. H. (2016). Overcoming gene-delivery hurdles: physiological considerations for nonviral vectors. *Trends Biotechnol.* 34, 91–105. doi: 10.1016/j.tibtech.2015.11.004

Hirao, L. A., Wu, L., Khan, A. S., Satishchandran, A., Draghia-Akli, R., and Weiner, D. B. (2008). Intradermal/subcutaneous immunization by electroporation improves plasmid vaccine delivery and potency in pigs and rhesus macaques. *Vaccine* 26, 440–448. doi: 10.1016/j.vaccine.2007.10.041

Hirase, T., Kawashima, S., Wong, E. Y., Ueyama, T., Rikitake, Y., Tsukita, S., et al. (2001). Regulation of tight junction permeability and occludin phosphorylation by Rhoa-p160ROCK-dependent and -independent mechanisms. *J. Biol. Chem.* 276, 10423–10431. doi: 10.1074/jbc.M007136200

Hook, J. L., Islam, M. N., Parker, D., Prince, A. S., Bhattacharya, S., and Bhattacharya, J. (2018). Disruption of staphylococcal aggregation protects against lethal lung injury. *J. Clin. Invest.* 128, 1074–1086. doi: 10.1172/JCI95823

Hotchkiss, R. S., Tinsley, K. W., Swanson, P. E., and Karl, I. E. (2002). Endothelial cell apoptosis in sepsis. *Crit. Care Med.* 30, S225–S228.

Houk, B. E., Hochhaus, G., and Hughes, J. A. (1999). Kinetic modeling of plasmid DNA degradation in rat plasma. *AAPS PharmSci* 1:E9. doi: 10.1208/ps010309

Hsia, C. C. W., Hyde, D. M., and Weibel, E. R. (2016). Lung structure and the intrinsic challenges of gas exchange. *Compr. Physiol.* 6, 827–895. doi: 10.1002/cphy.c150028

Hu, W. S., and Pathak, V. K. (2000). Design of retroviral vectors and helper cells for gene therapy. *Pharmacol. Rev.* 52, 493–511.

Huang, Y. Q., Sauthoff, H., Herscovici, P., Pipiya, T., Cheng, J., Heitner, S., et al. (2008). Angiopoietin-1 increases survival and reduces the development of lung edema induced by endotoxin administration in a murine model of acute lung injury. *Crit. Care Med.* 36, 262–267. doi: 10.1097/01.CCM.0000297955.02633.A4

Huppert, L. A., and Matthay, M. A. (2017). Alveolar fluid clearance in pathologically relevant conditions: in vitro and in vivo models of acute respiratory distress syndrome. *Front. Immunol.* 8:371. doi: 10.3389/fimmu.2017.00371

Idell, S., Koenig, K. B., Fair, D. S., Martin, T. R., McLarty, J., and Maunder, R. J. (1991). Serial abnormalities of fibrin turnover in evolving adult respiratory distress syndrome. *Am. J. Physiol.* 261, L240–L248. doi: 10.1152/ajplung.1991.261.4.L240

Imai, Y., Kuba, K., Rao, S., Huan, Y., Guo, F., Guan, B., et al. (2005). Angiotensin-converting enzyme 2 protects from severe acute lung failure. *Nature* 436, 112–116. doi: 10.1038/nature03712

Ince, C., Mayeux, P. R., Nguyen, T., Gomez, H., Kellum, J. A., Ospina-Tascón, G. A., et al. (2016). The endothelium in sepsis. *Shock* 45, 259–270.

Inoue, S., Suzuki, M., Nagashima, Y., Suzuki, S., Hashiba, T., Tsuburai, T., et al. (2001). Transfer of heme oxygenase 1 cDNA by a replication-deficient adenovirus enhances interleukin 10 production from alveolar macrophages that attenuates lipopolysaccharide-induced acute lung injury in mice. *Hum. Gene Ther.* 12, 967–979. doi: 10.1089/104303401750195926

Jagrosse, M. L., Dean, D. A., Rahman, A., and Nilsson, B. L. (2019). RNAi therapeutic strategies for acute respiratory distress syndrome. *Transl. Res.* 214, 30–49. doi: 10.1016/j.trsl.2019.07.011

Jaichandran, S., Yap, S. T., Khoo, A. B., Ho, L. P., Tien, S. L., and Kon, O. L. (2006). In vivo liver electroporation: optimization and demonstration of therapeutic efficacy. *Hum. Gene Ther.* 17, 362–375. doi: 10.1089/hum.2006.17.362

James, C., Xian-Yang, Z., and Jakob, R. (2005). Altering the tropism of lentiviral vectors through pseudotyping. *Curr. Gene Ther.* 5, 387–398. doi: 10.2174/1566523054546224

Jha, P., and Das, H. (2017). KLF2 in Regulation of NF-κB-Mediated Immune Cell Function and Inflammation. *Int. J. Mol. Sci.* 18:2383.

Jin, L., Zeng, X., Liu, M., Deng, Y., and He, N. (2014). Current progress in gene delivery technology based on chemical methods and nano-carriers. *Theranostics* 4, 240–255. doi: 10.7150/thno.6914

Jin, L.-Y., Li, C.-F., Zhu, G.-F., Wu, C.-T., Wang, J., and Yan, S.-F. (2014). Effect of siRNA against NF-κB on sepsis-induced acute lung injury in a mouse model. *Mol. Med. Rep.* 10, 631–637.

Johnson, L., Olsen, J., Naldini, L., and Boucher, R. (2000). Pseudotyped human lentiviral vector-mediated gene transfer to airway epithelia in vivo. *Gene Ther.* 7, 568–574. doi: 10.1038/sj.gt.3301138

Johnson, M. D., Bao, H.-F., Helms, M. N., Chen, X.-J., Tigue, Z., Jain, L., et al. (2006). Functional ion channels in pulmonary alveolar type I cells support a role for type I cells in lung ion transport. *Proc. Natl. Acad. Sci. U.S.A.* 103, 4964–4969. doi: 10.1073/pnas.0600855103

Jones, C. H., Chen, C. K., Ravikrishnan, A., Rane, S., and Pfeifer, B. A. (2013). Overcoming nonviral gene delivery barriers: perspective and future. *Mol. Pharm.* 10, 4082–4098. doi: 10.1021/mp400467x

Jones, M. R., Simms, B. T., Lupa, M. M., Kogan, M. S., and Mizgerd, J. P. (2005). Lung NF-kappaB activation and neutrophil recruitment require IL-1 and TNF receptor signaling during pneumococcal pneumonia. *J. immunol.* 175, 7530–7535. doi: 10.4049/jimmunol.175.11.7530

Kaarteenaho-Wiik, R., and Soini, Y. (2009). Claudin-1,- 2,- 3,- 4,- 5, and- 7 in usual interstitial pneumonia and sarcoidosis. *J. Histochem. Cytochem.* 57, 187–195. doi: 10.1369/jhc.2008.951566

Kabay, B., Kocaefe, C., Baykal, A., Özden, H., Baycu, C., Oner, Z., et al. (2007). Interleukin-10 gene transfer: prevention of multiple organ injury in a murine cecal ligation and puncture model of sepsis. *World J. Surg.* 31, 105–115. doi: 10.1007/s00268-006-0066-9

Karmpaliotis, D., Kosmidou, I., Ingenito, E. P., Hong, K., Malhotra, A., Sunday, M. E., et al. (2002). Angiogenic growth factors in the pathophysiology of a murine model of acute lung injury. *Am. J. Physiol. Lung Cell. Mol. Physiol.ogy* 283, L585–L595. doi: 10.1152/ajplung.00048.2002

Katz, M. G., Fargnoli, A. S., Gubara, S. M., Fish, K., Weber, T., Bridges, C. R., et al. (2019). Targeted gene delivery through the respiratory system: rationale for intratracheal gene transfer. *J. Cardiovasc. Dev. Dis.* 6:8. doi: 10.3390/jcdd6010008

Katz, M. G., Fargnoli, A. S., Williams, R. D., and Bridges, C. R. (2013). Gene therapy delivery systems for enhancing viral and nonviral vectors for cardiac diseases: current concepts and future applications. *Hum. Gene Ther.* 24, 914–927. doi: 10.1089/hum.2013.2517

Kawabata, K., Takakura, Y., and Hashida, M. (1995). The fate of plasmid DNA after intravenous injection in mice: involvement of scavenger receptors in its hepatic uptake. *Pharm. Res.* 12, 825–830. doi: 10.1023/a:1016248701505

Khan, A., Benthin, C., Zeno, B., Albertson, T. E., Boyd, J., Christie, J. D., et al. (2017). A pilot clinical trial of recombinant human angiotensin-converting enzyme 2 in acute respiratory distress syndrome. *Crit. Care* 21:234. doi: 10.1186/s13054-017-1823-x

Khilnani, G. C., and Hadda, V. (2011). Corticosteroids and ARDS: a review of treatment and prevention evidence. *Lung India* 28, 114–119. doi: 10.4103/0970-2113.80324

Kim, G., Piao, C., Oh, J., and Lee, M. (2019). Combined delivery of curcumin and the heme oxygenase-1 gene using cholesterol-conjugated polyamidoamine for anti-inflammatory therapy in acute lung injury. *Phytomedicine* 56, 165–174. doi: 10.1016/j.phymed.2018.09.240

Knudsen, L., and Ochs, M. (2018). The micromechanics of lung alveoli: structure and function of surfactant and tissue components. *Histochem. Cell Biol.* 150, 661–676. doi: 10.1007/s00418-018-1747-9

Kobinger, G. P., Weiner, D. J., Yu, Q.-C., and Wilson, J. M. (2001). Filovirus-pseudotyped lentiviral vector can efficiently and stably transduce airway epithelia in vivo. *Nat. Biotechnol.* 19, 225–230. doi: 10.1038/85664

Kochanek, S., Schiedner, G., and Volpers, C. (2001). High-capacity'gutless' adenoviral vectors. *Curr. Opin. Mol. Ther.* 3, 454–463.

Koehler, D. R., Martin, B., Corey, M., Palmer, D., Ng, P., Tanswell, A. K., et al. (2006). Readministration of helper-dependent adenovirus to mouse lung. *Gene Ther.* 13, 773–780. doi: 10.1038/sj.gt.3302712

Komarova, Y., and Malik, A. B. (2010). Regulation of endothelial permeability via paracellular and transcellular transport pathways. *Annu. Rev. Physiol.* 72, 463–493. doi: 10.1146/annurev-physiol-021909-135833

Kou, Z., Lim, J. Y., Beltramello, M., Quinn, M., Chen, H., Liu, S., et al. (2011). Human antibodies against dengue enhance dengue viral infectivity without suppressing type I interferon secretion in primary human monocytes. *Virology* 410, 240–247. doi: 10.1016/j.virol.2010.11.007

Kremer, K. L., Dunning, K. R., Parsons, D. W., and Anson, D. S. (2007). Gene delivery to airway epithelial cells in vivo: a direct comparison of apical and basolateral transduction strategies using pseudotyped lentivirus vectors. *J. Gene Med.* 9, 362–368. doi: 10.1002/jgm.1025

Krieg, A. M., Yi, A.-K., Matson, S., Waldschmidt, T. J., Bishop, G. A., Teasdale, R., et al. (1995). CpG motifs in bacterial DNA trigger direct B-cell activation. *Nature* 374, 546–549. doi: 10.1038/374546a0

Labiris, N. R., and Dolovich, M. B. (2003). Pulmonary drug delivery. Part I: physiological factors affecting therapeutic effectiveness of aerosolized medications. *Br. J. Clin. Pharmacol.* 56, 588–599. doi: 10.1046/j.1365-2125.2003.01892.x

LaFemina, M. J., Rokkam, D., Chandrasena, A., Pan, J., Bajaj, A., Johnson, M., et al. (2010). Keratinocyte growth factor enhances barrier function without altering claudin expression in primary alveolar epithelial cells. *Am. J. Physiol. Lung Cell. Mol. Physiol.* 299, L724–L734. doi: 10.1152/ajplung.00233.2010

LaFemina, M. J., Sutherland, K. M., Bentley, T., Gonzales, L. W., Allen, L., Chapin, C. J., et al. (2014). Claudin-18 deficiency results in alveolar barrier dysfunction and impaired alveologenesis in mice. *Am. J. Respir. Cell Mol. Biol.* 51, 550–558. doi: 10.1165/rcmb.2013-0456OC

Laffey, J. G., and Kavanagh, B. P. (2018). Negative trials in critical care: why most research is probably wrong. *Lancet Respir. Med.* 6, 659–660. doi: 10.1016/S2213-2600(18)30279-0

Laffey, J. G., and Matthay, M. A. (2017). Fifty years of research in ARDS. Cell-based therapy for acute respiratory distress syndrome. biology and potential therapeutic value. *Am. J. Respir. Crit. Care Med.* 196, 266–273. doi: 10.1164/rccm.201701-0107CP

Landis, G. N., and Tower, J. (2005). Superoxide dismutase evolution and life span regulation. *Mech. Ageing Dev.* 126, 365–379. doi: 10.1016/j.mad.2004.08.012

Lechardeur, D., Sohn, K. J., Haardt, M., Joshi, P. B., Monck, M., Graham, R. W., et al. (1999). Metabolic instability of plasmid DNA in the cytosol: a potential barrier to gene transfer. *Gene Ther.* 6, 482–497. doi: 10.1038/sj.gt.3300867

Lecuona, E., Saldías, F., Comellas, A., Ridge, K., Guerrero, C., and Sznajder, J. I. (1999). Ventilator-associated lung injury decreases lung ability to clear edema in rats. *Am. J. Respir. Crit. Care Med.* 159, 603–609. doi: 10.1164/ajrccm.159.2.9805050

Lee, J. W., Fang, X., Krasnodembskaya, A., Howard, J. P., and Matthay, M. A. (2011). Concise review: mesenchymal stem cells for acute lung injury: role of paracrine soluble factors. *Stem Cells* 29, 913–919. doi: 10.1002/stem.643

Lee, K. S., Choi, Y. H., Kim, Y. S., Baik, S. H., Oh, Y. J., Sheen, S. S., et al. (2008). Evaluation of bronchoalveolar lavage fluid from ARDS patients with regard to apoptosis. *Respir. Med.* 102, 464–469. doi: 10.1016/j.rmed.2007.10.001

Lewis, J. F., and Jobe, A. H. (1993). Surfactant and the adult respiratory distress syndrome. *Am. Rev. Respir. Dis.* 147, 218–233. doi: 10.1164/ajrccm/147.1.218

Li, G., Flodby, P., Luo, J., Kage, H., Sipos, A., Gao, D., et al. (2014). Knockout mice reveal key roles for claudin 18 in alveolar barrier properties and fluid homeostasis. *Am. J. Respir. Cell Mol. Biol.* 51, 210–222. doi: 10.1165/rcmb.2013-0353OC

Li, N., Song, Y., Zhao, W., Han, T., Lin, S., Ramirez, O., et al. (2016). Small interfering RNA targeting NF-κB attenuates lipopolysaccharide-induced acute lung injury in rats. *BMC Physiol.* 16:7. doi: 10.1186/s12899-016-0027-y

Li, P., Allen, H., Banerjee, S., Franklin, S., Herzog, L., Johnston, C., et al. (1995). Mice deficient in IL-1β-converting enzyme are defective in production of mature IL-1β and resistant to endotoxic shock. *Cell* 80, 401–411. doi: 10.1016/0092-8674(95)90490-5

Li, W., Ma, N., Ong, L. L., Kaminski, A., Skrabal, C., Ugurlucan, M., et al. (2008). Enhanced thoracic gene delivery by magnetic nanobead-mediated vector. *J. Gene Med.* 10, 897–909. doi: 10.1002/jgm.1208

Li, W., Zhang, L., Wu, Z., Pickles, R. J., and Samulski, R. J. (2011). AAV-6 mediated efficient transduction of mouse lower airways. *Virology* 417, 327–333. doi: 10.1016/j.virol.2011.06.009

Limberis, M. P., Vandenberghe, L. H., Zhang, L., Pickles, R. J., and Wilson, J. M. (2009). Transduction efficiencies of novel AAV vectors in mouse airway epithelium in vivo and human ciliated airway epithelium in vitro. *Mol. Ther.* 17, 294–301. doi: 10.1038/mt.2008.261

Lin, X., Barravecchia, M., Kothari, P., Young, J. L., and Dean, D. A. (2016). beta1-Na^+,K^+-ATPase gene therapy upregulates tight junctions to rescue lipopolysaccharide-induced acute lung injury. *Gene Ther.* 23, 489–499. doi: 10.1038/gt.2016.19

Lin, X., and Dean, D. A. (2011). Gene therapy for ALI/ARDS. *Crit. Care Clin.* 27, 705–718. doi: 10.1016/j.ccc.2011.04.002

Lindert, J., Perlman, C. E., Parthasarathi, K., and Bhattacharya, J. (2007). Chloride-dependent secretion of alveolar wall liquid determined by optical-sectioning microscopy. *Am. J. Respir. Cell Mol. Biol.* 36, 688–696. doi: 10.1165/rcmb.2006-0347OC

Litvan, J., Briva, A., Wilson, M. S., Budinger, G. R. S., Sznajder, J. I., and Ridge, K. M. (2006). β-adrenergic receptor stimulation and adenoviral overexpression of superoxide dismutase prevent the hypoxia-mediated decrease in Na,K-ATPase and alveolar fluid reabsorption. *J. Biol. Chem.* 281, 19892–19898. doi: 10.1074/jbc.M602064200

Litzinger, D. C., Brown, J. M., Wala, I., Kaufman, S. A., Van, G. Y., Farrell, C. L., et al. (1996). Fate of cationic liposomes and their complex with oligonucleotide in vivo. *Biochim. Biophys. Acta* 1281, 139–149. doi: 10.1016/0005-2736(95)00268-5

Liu, D., Wang, L., Wang, Z., and Cuschieri, A. (2012). Magnetoporation and magnetolysis of cancer cells via carbon nanotubes induced by rotating magnetic fields. *Nano Lett.* 12, 5117–5121. doi: 10.1021/nl301928z

Liu, F., Shollenberger, L., Conwell, C., Yuan, X., and Huang, L. (2007). Mechanism of naked DNA clearance after intravenous injection. *J. Gene Med.* 9, 613–619. doi: 10.1002/jgm.1054

Liu, J., and Dean, D. A. (2021). Gene transfer of MRCKa rescues lipopolysaccharide-induced acute lung injury by restoring alveolar capillary barrier function. *Sci. Rep.* 11:20862. doi: 10.1038/s41598-021-99897-3

Liu, M., Gu, C., and Wang, Y. (2014). Upregulation of the tight junction protein occludin: effects on ventilation-induced lung injury and mechanisms of action. *BMC Pulm. Med.* 14:94. doi: 10.1186/1471-2466-14-94

Liu, M., and Slutsky, A. S. (1997). Anti-inflammatory therapies: application of molecular biology techniques in intensive care medicine. *Intensive Care Med.* 23, 718–731. doi: 10.1007/s001340050400

Lomas-Neira, J., Chung, C. S., and Ayala, A. (2008). RNA interference as a potential therapeutic treatment for inflammation associated lung injury. *Int. J. Clin. Exp. Med.* 1, 154–160.

Lomas-Neira, J. L., Chung, C. S., Wesche, D. E., Perl, M., and Ayala, A. (2005). In vivo gene silencing (with siRNA) of pulmonary expression of MIP-2 versus KC results in divergent effects on hemorrhage-induced, neutrophil-mediated septic acute lung injury. *J. Leukoc. Biol.* 77, 846–853. doi: 10.1189/jlb.1004617

Long, D. A., Price, K. L., Ioffe, E., Gannon, C. M., Gnudi, L., White, K. E., et al. (2008). Angiopoietin-1 therapy enhances fibrosis and inflammation following folic acid-induced acute renal injury. *Kidney Int.* 74, 300–309. doi: 10.1038/ki.2008.179

Lu, R.-Y., Yang, W.-X., and Hu, Y.-J. (2014). The role of epithelial tight junctions involved in pathogen infections. *Mol. Biol. Rep.* 41, 6591–6610. doi: 10.1007/s11033-014-3543-5

Lu, X., Ma, Y., He, J., Li, Y., Zhu, H., and Yu, X. (2019). N-acetylcysteine for adults with acute respiratory distress syndrome: a meta-analysis of randomized controlled trials. *Hong Kong J. Emerg. Med.* 26, 288–298. doi: 10.1177/1024907918794559

Lundstrom, K. (2018). Viral vectors in gene therapy. *Diseases* 6:42.

Lv, H., Zhang, S., Wang, B., Cui, S., and Yan, J. (2006). Toxicity of cationic lipids and cationic polymers in gene delivery. *J. Control Release* 114, 100–109. doi: 10.1016/j.jconrel.2006.04.014

Machado-Aranda, D., Adir, Y., Young, J. L., Briva, A., Budinger, G. R. S., Yeldandi, A., et al. (2005). Gene transfer of the Na^+,K^+-ATPase b1 subunit using electroporation increases lung liquid clearance in rats. *Am. J. Respir. Crit. Care Med.* 171, 204–211. doi: 10.1164/rccm.200403-313OC

Machado-Aranda, D. A., Suresh, M. V., Yu, B., and Raghavendran, K. (2012). Electroporation-mediated in vivo gene delivery of the Na^+/K^+-ATPase pump reduced lung injury in a mouse model of lung contusion. *J. Trauma Acute Care Surg.* 72, 32–39; discussion 39–40. doi: 10.1097/TA.0b013e31823f0606

MacLoughlin, R. J., Higgins, B. D., Devaney, J., O'Toole, D., Laffey, J. G., and O'Brien, T. (2015). Aerosol-mediated delivery of AAV2/6-IκBα attenuates lipopolysaccharide-induced acute lung injury in rats. *Hum. Gene Ther.* 26, 36–46. doi: 10.1089/hum.2014.053

Madan, P., Rose, K., and Watson, A. J. (2007). Na/K-ATPase beta1 subunit expression is required for blastocyst formation and normal assembly of trophectoderm tight junction-associated proteins. *J. Biol. Chem.* 282, 12127–12134. doi: 10.1074/jbc.M700696200

Magin-Lachmann, C., Kotzamanis, G., D'Aiuto, L., Cooke, H., Huxley, C., and Wagner, E. (2004). In vitro and in vivo delivery of intact BAC DNA –

comparison of different methods. *J. Gene Med.* 6, 195–209. doi: 10.1002/jgm.481

Mahato, R. I., Kawabata, K., Takakura, Y., and Hashida, M. (1995). In vivo disposition characteristics of plasmid DNA complexed with cationic liposomes. *J. Drug Target* 3, 149–157. doi: 10.3109/10611869509059214

Mahato, R. I., Rolland, A., and Tomlinson, E. (1997). Cationic lipid-based gene delivery systems: pharmaceutical perspectives. *Pharm. Res.* 14, 853–859. doi: 10.1023/a:1012187414126

Mahato, R. I., Smith, L. C., and Rolland, A. (1999). Pharmaceutical perspectives of nonviral gene therapy. *Adv. Genet.* 41, 95–156. doi: 10.1016/s0065-2660(08)60152-2

Marquez Loza, L. I., Yuen, E. C., and McCray, P. B. Jr. (2019). Lentiviral vectors for the treatment and prevention of cystic fibrosis lung disease. *Genes* 10:218. doi: 10.3390/genes10030218

Martin, T. R., Nakamura, M., and Matute-Bello, G. (2003). The role of apoptosis in acute lung injury. *Crit. Care Med.* 31, S184–S188.

Matalon, S., and O'Brodovich, H. (1999). Sodium channels in alveolar epithelial cells: molecular characterization, biophysical properties, and physiological significance. *Annu. Rev. Physiol.* 61, 627–661. doi: 10.1146/annurev.physiol.61.1.627

Matsuda, N., Hattori, Y., Jesmin, S., and Gando, S. (2005). Nuclear factor-kappaB decoy oligodeoxynucleotides prevent acute lung injury in mice with cecal ligation and puncture-induced sepsis. *Mol. Pharmacol.* 67, 1018–1025. doi: 10.1124/mol.104.005926

Matsuda, T., and Cepko, C. L. (2004). Electroporation and RNA interference in the rodent retina in vivo and in vitro. *Proc. Natl. Acad. Sci. U.S.A.* 101, 16–22. doi: 10.1073/pnas.2235688100

Matsuda, T., and Cepko, C. L. (2008). Analysis of gene function in the retina. *Methods Mol. Biol.* 423, 259–278. doi: 10.1007/978-1-59745-194-9_19

Matthay, M. A. (2014). Resolution of pulmonary edema. Thirty years of progress. *Am. J. Respir. Crit. Care Med.* 189, 1301–1308. doi: 10.1164/rccm.201403-0535OE

Matthay, M. A., Aldrich, J. M., and Gotts, J. E. (2020). Treatment for severe acute respiratory distress syndrome from COVID-19. *Lancet Respir. Med.* 8, 433–434. doi: 10.1016/s2213-2600(20)30127-2

Matthay, M. A., Folkesson, H. G., and Clerici, C. (2002). Lung epithelial fluid transport and the resolution of pulmonary edema. *Physiol. Rev.* 82, 569–600. doi: 10.1152/physrev.00003.2002

Matthay, M. A., McAuley, D. F., and Ware, L. B. (2017). Clinical trials in acute respiratory distress syndrome: challenges and opportunities. *Lancet Respir. Med.* 5, 524–534. doi: 10.1016/S2213-2600(17)30188-1

Matthay, M. A., Robriquet, L., and Fang, X. (2005). Alveolar epithelium. *Proc. Am. Thoracic Soc.* 2, 206–213.

Matthay, M. A., Ware, L. B., and Zimmerman, G. A. (2012). The acute respiratory distress syndrome. *J. Clin. Invest.* 122, 2731–2740.

Matthay, M. A., and Zemans, R. L. (2011). The acute respiratory distress syndrome: pathogenesis and treatment. *Annu. Rev. Pathol.* 6, 147–163.

Matthay, M. A., Zemans, R. L., Zimmerman, G. A., Arabi, Y. M., Beitler, J. R., Mercat, A., et al. (2019). Acute respiratory distress syndrome. *Nat. Rev. Dis. Primers* 5, 18–18.

Matthay, M. A., and Zimmerman, G. A. (2005). Acute lung injury and the acute respiratory distress syndrome: four decades of inquiry into pathogenesis and rational management. *Am. J. Respir. Cell Mol. Biol.* 33, 319–327. doi: 10.1165/rcmb.F305

Matute-Bello, G., Downey, G., Moore, B. B., Groshong, S. D., Matthay, M. A., Slutsky, A. S., et al. (2011). An official American Thoracic Society workshop report: features and measurements of experimental acute lung injury in animals. *Am. J Respir. Cell Mol. Biol.* 44, 725–738. doi: 10.1165/rcmb.2009-0210ST

Matute-Bello, G., Lee, J. S., Liles, W. C., Frevert, C. W., Mongovin, S., Wong, V., et al. (2005a). Fas-mediated acute lung injury requires fas expression on nonmyeloid cells of the lung. *J. Immunol.* 175, 4069–4075. doi: 10.4049/jimmunol.175.6.4069

Matute-Bello, G., Liles, W. C., Frevert, C. W., Dhanireddy, S., Ballman, K., Wong, V., et al. (2005b). Blockade of the Fas/FasL system improves pneumococcal clearance from the lungs without preventing dissemination of bacteria to the spleen. *J. Infect. Dis.* 191, 596–606. doi: 10.1086/427261

Matute-Bello, G., Liles, W. C., Steinberg, K. P., Kiener, P. A., Mongovin, S., Chi, E. Y., et al. (1999). Soluble fas ligand induces epithelial cell apoptosis in humans with acute lung injury (ARDS). *J. Immunol.* 163, 2217–2225.

McAuliffe, P. F., Murday, M. E., Efron, P. A., Scumpia, P. O., Ungaro, R., Abouhamze, A., et al. (2006). Dose-dependent improvements in outcome with adenoviral expression of interleukin-10 in a murine model of multisystem organ failure. *Gene Ther.* 13, 276–282. doi: 10.1038/sj.gt.3302600

McCarter, S. D., Mei, S. H., Lai, P. F., Zhang, Q. W., Parker, C. H., Suen, R. S., et al. (2007). Cell-based angiopoietin-1 gene therapy for acute lung injury. *Am. J. Respir. Crit. Care Med.* 175, 1014–1026.

McClintock, D., Zhuo, H., Wickersham, N., Matthay, M. A., and Ware, L. B. (2008). Biomarkers of inflammation, coagulation and fibrinolysis predict mortality in acute lung injury. *Crit. Care* 12, R41–R41. doi: 10.1186/cc6846

Medi, B. M., and Singh, J. (2008). Delivery of DNA into skin via electroporation. *Methods Mol. Biol.* 423, 225–232. doi: 10.1007/978-1-59745-194-9_16

Mehier-Humbert, S., and Guy, R. H. (2005). Physical methods for gene transfer: improving the kinetics of gene delivery into cells. *Adv. Drug Deliv. Rev.* 57, 733–753. doi: 10.1016/j.addr.2004.12.007

Mehta, D., and Malik, A. B. (2006). Signaling mechanisms regulating endothelial permeability. *Physiol. Rev.* 86, 279–367. doi: 10.1152/physrev.00012.2005

Mei, S. H., McCarter, S. D., Deng, Y., Parker, C. H., Liles, W. C., and Stewart, D. J. (2007). Prevention of LPS-induced acute lung injury in mice by mesenchymal stem cells overexpressing angiopoietin 1. *PLoS Med.* 4:e269. doi: 10.1371/journal.pmed.0040269

Menezes, S. L., Bozza, P. T., Neto, H. C., Laranjeira, A. P., Negri, E. M., Capelozzi, V. L., et al. (2005). Pulmonary and extrapulmonary acute lung injury: inflammatory and ultrastructural analyses. *J. Appl. Physiol. (1985)* 98, 1777–1783. doi: 10.1152/japplphysiol.01182.2004

Miller, C. R., Bondurant, B., McLean, S. D., McGovern, K. A., and O'Brien, D. F. (1998). Liposome-cell interactions in vitro: effect of liposome surface charge on the binding and endocytosis of conventional and sterically stabilized liposomes. *Biochemistry* 37, 12875–12883. doi: 10.1021/bi980096y

Milligan, L. P., and McBride, B. W. (1985). Energy costs of ion pumping by animal tissues. *J. Nutr.* 115, 1374–1382. doi: 10.1093/jn/115.10.1374

Milone, M. C., and O'Doherty, U. (2018). Clinical use of lentiviral vectors. *Leukemia* 32, 1529–1541. doi: 10.1038/s41375-018-0106-0

Minakata, Y., Suzuki, S., Grygorczyk, C., Dagenais, A., and Berthiaume, Y. (1998). Impact of beta-adrenergic agonist on Na^+ channel and Na^+-K^+-ATPase expression in alveolar type II cells. *Am. J. Physiol.* 275, L414–L422. doi: 10.1152/ajplung.1998.275.2.L414

Mingozzi, F., and High, K. A. (2011). Therapeutic in vivo gene transfer for genetic disease using AAV: progress and challenges. *Nat. Rev. Genet.* 12, 341–355. doi: 10.1038/nrg2988

Mingozzi, F., and High, K. A. (2013). Immune responses to AAV vectors: overcoming barriers to successful gene therapy. *Blood* 122, 23–36. doi: 10.1182/blood-2013-01-306647

Mir, L. M. (2014). Electroporation-based gene therapy: recent evolution in the mechanism description and technology developments. *Methods Mol. Biol.* 1121, 3–23. doi: 10.1007/978-1-4614-9632-8_1

Mir, L. M., Belehradek, M., Domenge, C., Orlowski, S., Poddevin, B., Belehradek, J. Jr., et al. (1991). [Electrochemotherapy, a new antitumor treatment: first clinical trial]. *C R Acad. Sci. III* 313, 613–618.

Mir, L. M., Bureau, M. F., Gehl, J., Rangara, R., Rouy, D., Caillaud, J.-M., et al. (1999). High-efficiency gene transfer into skeletal muscle mediated by electric pulses. *Proc. Natl. Acad. Sci. U.S.A.* 96, 4262–4267. doi: 10.1073/pnas.96.8.4262

Mislick, K. A., and Baldeschwieler, J. D. (1996). Evidence for the role of proteoglycans in cation-mediated gene transfer. *Proc. Natl. Acad. Sci. U.S.A.* 93, 12349–12354. doi: 10.1073/pnas.93.22.12349

Mitchell, L. A., Overgaard, C. E., Ward, C., Margulies, S. S., and Koval, M. (2011). Differential effects of claudin-3 and claudin-4 on alveolar epithelial barrier function. *Am. J. Physiol. Lung Cell. Mol. Physiol.* 301, L40–L49. doi: 10.1152/ajplung.00299.2010

Mitomo, K., Griesenbach, U., Inoue, M., Somerton, L., Meng, C., Akiba, E., et al. (2010). Toward gene therapy for cystic fibrosis using a lentivirus pseudotyped with sendai virus envelopes. *Mol. Ther.* 18, 1173–1182. doi: 10.1038/mt.2010.13

Mitra, S., Exline, M., Habyarimana, F., Gavrilin, M. A., Baker, P. J., Masters, S. L., et al. (2018). Microparticulate caspase 1 regulates gasdermin D and pulmonary vascular endothelial cell injury. *Am. J. Respir. Cell Mol. Biol.* 59, 56–64. doi: 10.1165/rcmb.2017-0393OC

Monteiro, N., Martins, A., Reis, R. L., and Neves, N. M. (2014). Liposomes in tissue engineering and regenerative medicine. *J. R. Soc. Interface* 11:20140459.

Mora, B. N., Boasquevisque, C. H. R., Boglione, M., Ritter, J. M., Scheule, R. K., Yew, N. S., et al. (2000). Transforming growth factor-β1 gene transfer ameliorates acute lung allograft rejection. *J. Thorac. Cardiovasc. Surg.* 119, 913–920. doi: 10.1016/s0022-5223(00)70086-9

Morrison, D. F., Foss, D. L., and Murtaugh, M. P. (2000). Interleukin-10 gene therapy-mediated amelioration of bacterial pneumonia. *Infect. Immun.* 68, 4752–4758. doi: 10.1128/IAI.68.8.4752-4758.2000

Mosnier, L. O., Yang, X. V., and Griffin, J. H. (2007). Activated protein C mutant with minimal anticoagulant activity, normal cytoprotective activity, and preservation of thrombin activable fibrinolysis inhibitor-dependent cytoprotective functions. *J. Biol. Chem.* 282, 33022–33033. doi: 10.1074/jbc.M705824200

Murakami, M., Nguyen, L. T., Zhang, Z. W., Moodie, K. L., Carmeliet, P., Stan, R. V., et al. (2008). The FGF system has a key role in regulating vascular integrity. *J. Clin. Invest.* 118, 3355–3366. doi: 10.1172/JCI35298

Murata, T., Aritake, K., Tsubosaka, Y., Maruyama, T., Nakagawa, T., Hori, M., et al. (2013). Anti-inflammatory role of PGD_2 in acute lung inflammation and therapeutic application of its signal enhancement. *Proc. Natl. Acad. Sci. U.S.A.* 110, 5205–5210. doi: 10.1073/pnas.1218091110

Murgia, X., Carvalho, C. D. S., and Lehr, C.-M. (2014). Overcoming the pulmonary barrier: new insights to improve the efficiency of inhaled therapeutics. *Eur. J. Nanomed.* 6:157.

Mutlu, G. M., Adir, Y., Jameel, M., Akhmedov, A. T., Welch, L., Dumasius, V., et al. (2005). Interdependency of beta-adrenergic receptors and CFTR in regulation of alveolar active Na^+ transport. *Circ. Res.* 96, 999–1005. doi: 10.1161/01.RES.0000164554.21993.AC

Mutlu, G. M., Dumasius, V., Burhop, J., McShane, P. J., Meng, F. J., Welch, L., et al. (2004). Upregulation of alveolar epithelial active Na^+ transport is dependent on beta2-adrenergic receptor signaling. *Circ. Res.* 94, 1091–1100. doi: 10.1161/01.RES.0000125623.56442.20

Mutlu, G. M., Machado-Aranda, D., Norton, J. E., Bellmeyer, A., Urich, D., Zhou, R., et al. (2007). Electroporation-mediated gene transfer of the Na^+,K^+ -ATPase rescues endotoxin-induced lung injury. *Am. J. Respir. Crit. Care Med.* 176, 582–590. doi: 10.1164/rccm.200608-1246OC

Mutlu, G. M., and Sznajder, J. I. (2004). β2-agonists for treatment of pulmonary edema: ready for clinical studies?*. *Crit. Care Med.* 32, 1607–1608. doi: 10.1097/01.ccm.0000130825.84691.e2

Mutlu, G. M., and Sznajder, J. I. (2005). Mechanisms of pulmonary edema clearance. *Am. J. Physiol. Lung Cell. Mol. Physiol.* 289, L685–L695.

Nagy, Z., Kolev, K., Csonka, E., Pék, M., and Machovich, R. (1995). Contraction of human brain endothelial cells induced by thrombogenic and fibrinolytic factors. An in vitro cell culture model. *Stroke* 26, 265–270. doi: 10.1161/01.str.26.2.265

Nakahira, K., Kyung, S.-Y., Rogers, A. J., Gazourian, L., Youn, S., Massaro, A. F., et al. (2014). Circulating mitochondrial DNA in patients in the ICU as a marker of mortality: derivation and validation. *PLoS Med.* 10:e1001577. doi: 10.1371/journal.pmed.1001577

Naldini, L., Blomer, U., Gallay, P., Ory, D., Mulligan, R., Gage, F. H. I, et al. (1996). In vivo gene delivery and stable transduction of nondividing cells by a lentiviral vector. *Science* 272, 263–267. doi: 10.1126/science.272.5259.263

Natarajan, V., Dudek, S. M., Jacobson, J. R., Moreno-Vinasco, L., Huang, L. S., Abassi, T., et al. (2013). Sphingosine-1-phosphate, FTY720, and sphingosine-1-phosphate receptors in the pathobiology of acute lung injury. *Am. J. Respir. Cell Mol. Biol.* 49, 6–17. doi: 10.1165/rcmb.2012-0411TR

National Heart, Lung, and Blood Institute Acute Respiratory Distress Syndrome (ARDS) Clinical Trials Network, Matthay, M. A., Brower, R. G., Carson, S., Douglas, I. S., Eisner, M., et al. (2011). Randomized, placebo-controlled clinical trial of an aerosolized β2-agonist for treatment of acute lung injury. *Am. J. Respir. Crit. Care Med.* 184, 561–568. doi: 10.1164/rccm.201012-2090OC

Nayerossadat, N., Maedeh, T., and Ali, P. A. (2012). Viral and nonviral delivery systems for gene delivery. *Adv. Biomed. Res.* 1, 27–27. doi: 10.4103/2277-9175.98152

Network, A. (2000). Ventilation with lower tidal volumes as compared with traditional tidal volumes for acute lung injury and the acute respiratory distress syndrome. *N. Engl. J. Med.* 342, 1301–1308. doi: 10.1056/NEJM200005043421801

Neumann, E., Schaefer-Ridder, M., Wang, Y., and Hofschneider, P. H. (1982). Gene transfer into mouse lyoma cells by electroporation in high electric fields. *EMBO J.* 1, 841–845.

Nicod, L. P. (2005). Lung defences: an overview. *Eur. Respir. Rev.* 14, 45–50. doi: 10.1183/09059180.05.00009501

Niculescu-Duvaz, D., Heyes, J., and Springer, C. J. (2003). Structure-activity relationship in cationic lipid mediated gene transfection. *Curr. Med. Chem.* 10, 1233–1261. doi: 10.2174/0929867033457476

Nimesh, S., Aggarwal, A., Kumar, P., Singh, Y., Gupta, K. C., and Chandra, R. (2007). Influence of acyl chain length on transfection mediated by acylated PEI nanoparticles. *Int. J. Pharm.* 337, 265–274. doi: 10.1016/j.ijpharm.2006.12.032

Nishikawa, M., and Huang, L. (2001). Nonviral vectors in the new millennium: delivery barriers in gene transfer. *Hum. Gene Ther.* 12, 861–870. doi: 10.1089/104303401750195836

Nuckton, T., Alonso, J., Kallet, R., Daniel, B., Pittet, J.-F., Eisner, M., et al. (2002). Pulmonary dead-space fraction as a risk factor for death in the acute respiratory distress syndrome. *N. Engl. J. Med.* 346, 1281–1286. doi: 10.1056/NEJMoa012835

Ochs, M., Nyengaard, J. R., Jung, A., Knudsen, L., Voigt, M., Wahlers, T., et al. (2004). The number of alveoli in the human lung. *Am. J. Respir. Crit. Care Med.* 169, 120–124.

Ohta, H., Chiba, S., Ebina, M., Furuse, M., and Nukiwa, T. (2012). Altered expression of tight junction molecules in alveolar septa in lung injury and fibrosis. *Am. J. Physiol. Lung Cell. Mol. Physiol.* 302, L193–L205. doi: 10.1152/ajplung.00349.2010

Otterbein, L. E., Kolls, J. K., Mantell, L. L., Cook, J. L., Alam, J., and Choi, A. M. (1999). Exogenous administration of heme oxygenase-1 by gene transfer provides protection against hyperoxia-induced lung injury. *J. Clin. Invest.* 103, 1047–1054. doi: 10.1172/JCI5342

Overgaard, C. E., Mitchell, L. A., and Koval, M. (2012). Roles for claudins in alveolar epithelial barrier function. *Ann. N. Y. Acad. Sci.* 1257, 167–174. doi: 10.1111/j.1749-6632.2012.06545.x

Pack, D. W., Hoffman, A. S., Pun, S., and Stayton, P. S. (2005). Design and development of polymers for gene delivery. *Nat. Rev. Drug Discov.* 4, 581–593. doi: 10.1038/nrd1775

Paranjpe, M., and Müller-Goymann, C. C. (2014). Nanoparticle-mediated pulmonary drug delivery: a review. *Int. J. Mol. Sci.* 15, 5852–5873. doi: 10.3390/ijms15045852

Parikh, S. M. (2017). The angiopoietin-Tie2 signaling axis in systemic inflammation. *J. Am. Soc. Nephrol.* 28, 1973–1982.

Park, J. H., Kim, H. A., Park, J. H., and Lee, M. (2012). Amphiphilic peptide carrier for the combined delivery of curcumin and plasmid DNA into the lungs. *Biomaterials* 33, 6542–6550. doi: 10.1016/j.biomaterials.2012.05.046

Park, W. Y., Goodman, R. B., Steinberg, K. P., Ruzinski, J. T., Radella, F. II, Park, D. R., et al. (2001). Cytokine balance in the lungs of patients with acute respiratory distress syndrome. *Am. J. Respir. Crit. Care Med.* 164, 1896–1903. doi: 10.1164/ajrccm.164.10.2104013

Parker, S. J., and Watkins, P. E. (2001). Experimental models of gram-negative sepsis. *Br. J. Surg.* 88, 22–30. doi: 10.1046/j.1365-2168.2001.01632.x

Parsons, P. E., Matthay, M. A., Ware, L. B., and Eisner, M. D. (2005). Elevated plasma levels of soluble TNF receptors are associated with morbidity and mortality in patients with acute lung injury. *Am. J. Physiol. Lung Cell. Mol. Physiol.* 288, L426–L431. doi: 10.1152/ajplung.00302.2004

Patel, B. V., Wilson, M. R., O'Dea, K. P., and Takata, M. (2013). TNF-induced death signaling triggers alveolar epithelial dysfunction in acute lung injury. *J. Immunol.* 190, 4274–4282. doi: 10.4049/jimmunol.1202437

Patel, M., Giddings, A. M., Sechelski, J., and Olsen, J. C. (2013). High efficiency gene transfer to airways of mice using influenza hemagglutinin pseudotyped lentiviral vectors. *J. Gene Med.* 15, 51–62. doi: 10.1002/jgm.2695

Patil, S., Gao, Y.-G., Lin, X., Li, Y., Dang, K., Tian, Y., et al. (2019). The development of functional non-viral vectors for gene delivery. *Int. J. Mol. Sci.* 20:5491. doi: 10.3390/ijms20215491

Patton, J. S. (1996). Mechanisms of macromolecule absorption by the lungs. *Adv. Drug Deliv. Rev.* 19, 3–36.

Patton, J. S., and Byron, P. R. (2007). Inhaling medicines: delivering drugs to the body through the lungs. *Nat. Rev. Drug Discov.* 6, 67–74. doi: 10.1038/nrd2153

Patton, J. S., Fishburn, C. S., and Weers, J. G. (2004). The lungs as a portal of entry for systemic drug delivery. *Proc. Am. Thorac. Soc.* 1, 338–344. doi: 10.1513/pats.200409-049TA

Patwa, A., and Shah, A. (2015). Anatomy and physiology of respiratory system relevant to anaesthesia. *Indian J. Anaesth.* 59, 533–541. doi: 10.4103/0019-5049.165849

Pelosi, P., D'onofrio, D., Chiumello, D., Paolo, S., Chiara, G., Capelozzi, V., et al. (2003). Pulmonary and extrapulmonary acute respiratory distress syndrome are different. *Eur. Respir. J.* 22, 48s–56s.

Perevyazko, I. Y., Bauer, M., Pavlov, G. M., Hoeppener, S., Schubert, S., Fischer, D., et al. (2012). Polyelectrolyte complexes of DNA and linear PEI: formation, composition and properties. *Langmuir* 28, 16167–16176. doi: 10.1021/la303094b

Perkins, G. D., McAuley, D. F., Thickett, D. R., and Gao, F. (2006). The beta-agonist lung injury trial (BALTI): a randomized placebo-controlled clinical trial. *Am. J. Respir. Crit. Care Med.* 173, 281–287. doi: 10.1164/rccm.200508-1302OC

Perl, M., Chung, C.-S., Lomas-Neira, J., Rachel, T.-M., Biffl, W. L., Cioffi, W. G., et al. (2005). Silencing of Fas, but not caspase-8, in lung epithelial cells ameliorates pulmonary apoptosis, inflammation, and neutrophil influx after hemorrhagic shock and sepsis. *Am. J. Pathol.* 167, 1545–1559. doi: 10.1016/S0002-9440(10)61240-0

Perl, M., Chung, C.-S., Perl, U., Lomas-Neira, J., de Paepe, M., Cioffi, W. G., et al. (2007). Fas-induced pulmonary apoptosis and inflammation during indirect acute lung injury. *Am. J. Respir. Crit. Care Med.* 176, 591–601. doi: 10.1164/rccm.200611-1743OC

Perl, M., Chung, C.-S., Perl, U., Thakkar, R., Lomas-Neira, J., and Ayala, A. (2010). Therapeutic accessibility of caspase-mediated cell death as a key pathomechanism in indirect acute lung injury. *Crit. Care Med.* 38, 1179–1186. doi: 10.1097/CCM.0b013e3181d4563f

Perricone, M. A., Rees, D. D., Sacks, C. R., Smith, K. A., Kaplan, J. M., and St George, J. A. (2000). Inhibitory effect of cystic fibrosis sputum on adenovirus-mediated gene transfer in cultured epithelial cells. *Hum. Gene Ther.* 11, 1997–2008. doi: 10.1089/10430340050143426

Peteranderl, C., Morales-Nebreda, L., Selvakumar, B., Lecuona, E., Vadász, I., Morty, R. E., et al. (2016). Macrophage-epithelial paracrine crosstalk inhibits lung edema clearance during influenza infection. *J. Clin. Invest.* 126, 1566–1580. doi: 10.1172/JCI83931

Piao, C., Park, J. H., and Lee, M. (2017). Anti-inflammatory therapeutic effect of adiponectin gene delivery using a polymeric carrier in an acute lung injury model. *Pharm. Res.* 34, 1517–1526. doi: 10.1007/s11095-017-2175-6

Piper, R. D., Cook, D. J., Bone, R. C., and Sibbald, W. J. (1996). Introducing critical appraisal to studies of animal models investigating novel therapies in sepsis. *Crit. Care Med.* 24, 2059–2070. doi: 10.1097/00003246-199612000-00021

Planès, C., Escoubet, B., Blot-Chabaud, M., Friedlander, G., Farman, N., and Clerici, C. (1997). Hypoxia downregulates expression and activity of epithelial sodium channels in rat alveolar epithelial cells. *Am. J. Respir. Cell Mol. Biol.* 17, 508–518. doi: 10.1165/ajrcmb.17.4.2680

Pouton, C. W., and Seymour, L. W. (2001). Key issues in non-viral gene delivery1PII of original article: S0169-409X(98)00048-9. The article was originally published in advanced drug delivery reviews 34 (1998) 3–19.1. *Adv. Drug Deliv. Rev.* 46, 187–203. doi: 10.1016/s0169-409x(98)00048-9

Pugin, J., Ricou, B., Steinberg, K. P., Suter, P. M., and Martin, T. R. (1996). Proinflammatory activity in bronchoalveolar lavage fluids from patients with ARDS, a prominent role for interleukin-1. *Am. J. Respir. Crit. Care Med.* 153, 1850–1856. doi: 10.1164/ajrccm.153.6.8665045

Pugin, J., Verghese, G., Widmer, M.-C., and Matthay, M. A. (1999). The alveolar space is the site of intense inflammatory and profibrotic reactions in the early phase of acute respiratory distress syndrome. *Crit. Care Med.* 27, 304–312. doi: 10.1097/00003246-199902000-00036

Putensen, C., Räsänen, J., and Downs, J. B. (1994). Effect of endogenous and inhaled nitric oxide on the ventilation-perfusion relationships in oleic-acid lung injury. *Am. J. Respir. Crit. Care Med.* 150, 330–336. doi: 10.1164/ajrccm.150.2.8049811

Quezado, Z. M., Natanson, C., Alling, D. W., Banks, S. M., Koev, C. A., Elin, R. J., et al. (1993). A controlled trial of HA-1A in a canine model of gram-negative septic shock. *JAMA* 269, 2221–2227.

Rajasekaran, A. K., and Rajasekaran, S. A. (2003). Role of Na-K-ATPase in the assembly of tight junctions. *Am. J. Physiol. Renal Physiol.* 285, F388–F396. doi: 10.1152/ajprenal.00439.2002

Rajasekaran, S. A., Barwe, S. P., Gopal, J., Ryazantsev, S., Schneeberger, E. E., and Rajasekaran, A. K. (2007). Na-K-ATPase regulates tight junction permeability through occludin phosphorylation in pancreatic epithelial cells. *Am. J. Physiol. Gastrointest. Liver Physiol.* 292, G124–G133. doi: 10.1152/ajpgi.00297.2006

Rajasekaran, S. A., Palmer, L. G., Quan, K., Harper, J. F., Ball, W. J. Jr., Bander, N. H., et al. (2001b). Na,K-ATPase beta-subunit is required for epithelial polarization, suppression of invasion, and cell motility. *Mol. Biol. Cell* 12, 279–295. doi: 10.1091/mbc.12.2.279

Rajasekaran, S. A., Palmer, L. G., Moon, S. Y., Peralta Soler, A., Apodaca, G. L., Harper, J. F., et al. (2001a). Na,K-ATPase activity is required for formation of tight junctions, desmosomes, and induction of polarity in epithelial cells. *Mol. Biol. Cell* 12, 3717–3732. doi: 10.1091/mbc.12.12.3717

Ramamoorth, M., and Narvekar, A. (2015). Non viral vectors in gene therapy- an overview. *J. Clin. Diagn. Res.* 9, GE01–GE6. doi: 10.7860/JCDR/2015/10443.5394

Rao, R. (2008). Oxidative stress-induced disruption of epithelial and endothelial tight junctions. *Front. Biosci.* 13:7210–7226. doi: 10.2741/3223

Rautanen, A., Mills, T. C., Gordon, A. C., Hutton, P., Steffens, M., Nuamah, R., et al. (2015). Genome-wide association study of survival from sepsis due to pneumonia: an observational cohort study. *Lancet Respir. Med.* 3, 53–60. doi: 10.1016/S2213-2600(14)70290-5

Reutershan, J., Stockton, R., Zarbock, A., Sullivan, G. W., Chang, D., Scott, D., et al. (2007). Blocking p21-activated kinase reduces lipopolysaccharide-induced acute lung injury by preventing polymorphonuclear leukocyte infiltration. *Am. J. Respir. Crit. Care Med.* 175, 1027–1035. doi: 10.1164/rccm.200612-1822OC

Rezoagli, E., Fumagalli, R., and Bellani, G. (2017). Definition and epidemiology of acute respiratory distress syndrome. *Ann. Transl. Med.* 5, 282–282.

Ricciotti, E., and FitzGerald, G. A. (2011). Prostaglandins and inflammation. *Arterioscler Thromb. Vasc. Biol.* 31, 986–1000.

Ridge, K. M., Olivera, W. G., Saldias, F., Azzam, Z., Horowitz, S., Rutschman, D. H., et al. (2003). Alveolar type 1 cells express the alpha2 Na,K-ATPase, which contributes to lung liquid clearance. *Circ. Res.* 92, 453–460. doi: 10.1161/01.RES.0000059414.10360.F2

Rivers, E., Nguyen, B., Havstad, S., Ressler, J., Muzzin, A., Knoblich, B., et al. (2001). Early goal-directed therapy in the treatment of severe sepsis and septic shock. *N. Engl. J. Med.* 345, 1368–1377.

Rokkam, D., Lafemina, M. J., Lee, J. W., Matthay, M. A., and Frank, J. A. (2011). Claudin-4 levels are associated with intact alveolar fluid clearance in human lungs. *Am. J. Pathol.* 179, 1081–1087. doi: 10.1016/j.ajpath.2011.05.017

Rossaint, J., Margraf, A., and Zarbock, A. (2018). Role of platelets in leukocyte recruitment and resolution of inflammation. *Front. Immunol.* 9:2712. doi: 10.3389/fimmu.2018.02712

Rossaint, R., Gerlach, H., Schmidt-Ruhnke, H., Pappert, D., Lewandowski, K., Steudel, W., et al. (1995). Efficacy of inhaled nitric oxide in patients with severe ARDS. *Chest* 107, 1107–1115. doi: 10.1378/chest.107.4.1107

Ruchko, M., Gorodnya, O., LeDoux, S. P., Alexeyev, M. F., Al-Mehdi, A.-B., and Gillespie, M. N. (2005). Mitochondrial DNA damage triggers mitochondrial dysfunction and apoptosis in oxidant-challenged lung endothelial cells. *Am. J. Physiol. Lung Cell. Mol. Physiol.* 288, L530–L535. doi: 10.1152/ajplung.00255.2004

Rudkowski, J. C., Barreiro, E., Harfouche, R., Goldberg, P., Kishta, O., D'Orleans-Juste, P., et al. (2004). Roles of iNOS and nNOS in sepsis-induced pulmonary apoptosis. *Am. J. Physiol. Lung Cell. Mol. Physiol.* 286, L793–L800. doi: 10.1152/ajplung.00266.2003

Sakuma, T., Okaniwa, G., Nakada, T., Nishimura, T., Fujimura, S., and Matthay, M. A. (1994). Alveolar fluid clearance in the resected human lung. *Am. J. Respir. Crit. Care Med.* 150, 305–310.

Saldías, F. J., Comellas, A., Ridge, K. M., Lecuona, E., and Sznajder, J. I. (1999). Isoproterenol improves ability of lung to clear edema in rats exposed to hyperoxia. *J. Appl. Physiol. (1985)* 87, 30–35. doi: 10.1152/jappl.1999.87.1.30

Samulski, R. J., and Muzyczka, N. (2014). AAV-mediated gene therapy for research and therapeutic purposes. *Annu. Rev. Virol.* 1, 427–451. doi: 10.1146/annurev-virology-031413-085355

Sanders, N., Rudolph, C., Braeckmans, K., De Smedt, S. C., and Demeester, J. (2009). Extracellular barriers in respiratory gene therapy. *Adv. Drug. Deliv. Rev.* 61, 115–127. doi: 10.1016/j.addr.2008.09.011

Satkauskas, S., Bureau, M. F., Puc, M., Mahfoudi, A., Scherman, D., Miklavcic, D., et al. (2002). Mechanisms of in vivo DNA electrotransfer: respective contributions of cell electropermeabilization and DNA electrophoresis. *Mol. Ther.* 5, 133–140. doi: 10.1006/mthe.2002.0526

Schambach, A., and Morgan, M. (2016). Retroviral vectors for cancer gene therapy. *Recent Results Cancer Res.* 209, 17–35.

Scher, J. U., and Pillinger, M. H. (2009). The anti-inflammatory effects of prostaglandins. *J. Invest. Med.* 57, 703–708. doi: 10.1016/0090-6980(78)90 074-6

Schiedner, G., Morral, N., Parks, R. J., Wu, Y., Koopmans, S. C., Langston, C., et al. (1998). Genomic DNA transfer with a high-capacity adenovirus vector results in improved in vivo gene expression and decreased toxicity. *Nat. Genet.* 18, 180–183. doi: 10.1038/ng0298-180

Schneckenburger, H., Hendinger, A., Sailer, R., Strauss, W. S., and Schmitt, M. (2002). Laser-assisted optoporation of single cells. *J. Biomed. Opt.* 7, 410–416.

Schuster, B. S., Kim, A. J., Kays, J. C., Kanzawa, M. M., Guggino, W. B., Boyle, M. P., et al. (2014). Overcoming the cystic fibrosis sputum barrier to leading adeno-associated virus gene therapy vectors. *Mol. Ther.* 22, 1484–1493. doi: 10.1038/mt.2014.89

Seok, J., Warren, H. S., Cuenca, A. G., Mindrinos, M. N., Baker, H. V., Xu, W., et al. (2013). Genomic responses in mouse models poorly mimic human inflammatory diseases. *Proc. Natl. Acad. Sci. U.S.A.* 110, 3507–3512.

Shahin, A. Y. I, Hassanin, M., Ismail, A. M., Kruessel, J. S., and Hirchenhain, J. (2009). Effect of oral N-acetyl cysteine on recurrent preterm labor following treatment for bacterial vaginosis. *Int. J. Gynaecol. Obstet.* 104, 44–48. doi: 10. 1016/j.ijgo.2008.08.026

Siflinger-Birnboim, A., del Vecchio, P. J., Cooper, J. A., Blumenstock, F. A., Shepard, J. M., and Malik, A. B. (1987). Molecular sieving characteristics of the cultured endothelial monolayer. *J. Cell. Physiol.* 132, 111–117. doi: 10.1002/jcp. 1041320115

Sigurdsson, M. I., Sigvaldason, K., Gunnarsson, T. S., Moller, A., and Sigurdsson, G. H. (2013). Acute respiratory distress syndrome: nationwide changes in incidence, treatment and mortality over 23 years. *Acta Anaesthesiol. Scand.* 57, 37–45. doi: 10.1111/aas.12001

Singhal, A., and Huang, L. (1994). "Gene transfer in mammalian cells using liposomes as carriers," in *Gene Therapeutics: Methods and Applications of Direct Gene Transfer*, ed. J. A. Wolff (Boston, MA: Birkhäuser Boston), 118–142. doi: 10.1007/978-1-4684-6822-9_7

Singla, S., and Machado, R. F. (2018). Death of the endothelium in sepsis: understanding the crime scene. *Am. J. Respir. Cell Mol. Biol.* 59, 3–4. doi: 10.1165/rcmb.2018-0051ED

Sinn, P. L., Coffin, J. E., Ayithan, N., Holt, K. H., and Maury, W. (2017a). Lentiviral vectors pseudotyped with filoviral glycoproteins. *Methods Mol. Biol.* 1628, 65–78. doi: 10.1007/978-1-4939-7116-9_5

Sinn, P. L., Hwang, B. Y., Li, N., Ortiz, J. L. S., Shirazi, E., Parekh, K. R., et al. (2017b). Novel GP64 envelope variants for improved delivery to human airway epithelial cells. *Gene Ther.* 24, 674–679. doi: 10.1038/gt. 2017.78

Sinn, P. L., Cooney, A. L., Oakland, M., Dylla, D. E., Wallen, T. J., Pezzulo, A. A., et al. (2012). Lentiviral vector gene transfer to porcine airways. *Mol. Ther. Nucleic Acids* 1:e56. doi: 10.1038/mtna.2012.47

Smart, L., Bosio, E., Macdonald, S. P. J., Dull, R., Fatovich, D. M., Neil, C., et al. (2018). Glycocalyx biomarker syndecan-1 is a stronger predictor of respiratory failure in patients with sepsis due to pneumonia, compared to endocan. *J. Crit. Care* 47, 93–98. doi: 10.1016/j.jcrc.2018.06.015

Soma, T., Chiba, H., Kato-Mori, Y., Wada, T., Yamashita, T., Kojima, T., et al. (2004). Thr207 of claudin-5 is involved in size-selective loosening of the endothelial barrier by cyclic AMP. *Exp. Cell Res.* 300, 202–212. doi: 10.1016/ j.yexcr.2004.07.012

Somiari, S., Glasspool-Malone, J., Drabick, J. J., Gilbert, R. A., Heller, R., Jaroszeski, M. J., et al. (2000). Theory and in vivo application of electroporative gene delivery. *Mol. Ther.* 2, 178–187. doi: 10.1006/mthe.2000.0124

Sondhi, D., Stiles, K. M., De, B. P., and Crystal, R. G. (2017). Genetic modification of the lung directed toward treatment of human disease. *Hum. Gene Ther.* 28, 3–84. doi: 10.1089/hum.2016.152

Song, Y. K., Liu, F., Chu, S., and Liu, D. (1997). Characterization of cationic liposome-mediated gene transfer in vivo by intravenous administration. *Hum. Gene Ther.* 8, 1585–1594. doi: 10.1089/hum.1997.8.13-1585

Sprung, C. L., Rackow, E. C., Fein, I. A., Jacob, A. I., and Isikoff, S. K. (1981). The spectrum of pulmonary edema: differentiation of cardiogenic, intermediate, and noncardiogenic forms of pulmonary edema. *Am. Rev. Respir. Dis.* 124, 718–722. doi: 10.1164/arrd.1981.124.6.718

Srinivasan, B., Kolli, A. R., Esch, M. B., Abaci, H. E., Shuler, M. L., and Hickman, J. J. (2015). TEER measurement techniques for in vitro barrier model systems. *J. Lab. Autom.* 20, 107–126. doi: 10.1177/2211068214561025

Staub, N. C. (1978). Pulmonary edema due to increased microvascular permeability to fluid and protein. *Circ. Res.* 43, 143–151. doi: 10.1161/01.res.43.2.143

Steinberg, J., Halter, J., Schiller, H., Gatto, L., and Nieman, G. (2005). The development of acute respiratory distress syndrome after gut ischemia/reperfusion injury followed by fecal peritonitis in pigs: a clinically relevant model. *Shock* 23, 129–137. doi: 10.1097/01.shk.0000148053.66645.2e

Stern, M., Ulrich, K., Robinson, C., Copeland, J., Griesenbach, U., Masse, C., et al. (2000). Pretreatment with cationic lipid-mediated transfer of the Na^+K^+-ATPase pump in a mouse model in vivo augments resolution of high permeability pulmonary oedema. *Gene Ther.* 7, 960–966. doi: 10.1038/sj.gt. 3301193

Sukriti, S., Tauseef, M., Yazbeck, P., and Mehta, D. (2014). Mechanisms regulating endothelial permeability. *Pulm. Circ.* 4, 535–551.

Suliman, H. B., Ryan, L. K., Bishop, L., and Folz, R. J. (2001). Prevention of influenza-induced lung injury in mice overexpressing extracellular superoxide dismutase. *Am. J. Physiol. Lung Cell. Mol. Physiol.* 280, L69–L78. doi: 10.1152/ ajplung.2001.280.1.L69

Sullivan, C. C., Du, L., Chu, D., Cho, A. J., Kido, M., Wolf, P. L., et al. (2003). Induction of pulmonary hypertension by an angiopoietin 1/TIE2/serotonin pathway. *Proc. Natl. Acad. Sci. U.S.A.* 100, 12331–12336. doi: 10.1073/pnas. 1933740100

Syrkina, O., Jafari, B., Hales, C. A., and Quinn, D. A. (2008). Oxidant stress mediates inflammation and apoptosis in ventilator-induced lung injury. *Respirology* 13, 333–340. doi: 10.1111/j.1440-1843.2008.01279.x

Tang, P. S., Mura, M., Seth, R., and Liu, M. (2008). Acute lung injury and cell death: how many ways can cells die? *Am. J. Physiol. Lung Cell. Mol. Physiol.* 294, L632–L641. doi: 10.1152/ajplung.00262.2007

Teng, N. N., Kaplan, H. S., Hebert, J. M., Moore, C., Douglas, H., Wunderlich, A., et al. (1985). Protection against gram-negative bacteremia and endotoxemia with human monoclonal IgM antibodies. *Proc. Natl. Acad. Sci. U.S.A.* 82, 1790–1794. doi: 10.1073/pnas.82.6.1790

The ARDS Clinical Trials Network (2002). Randomized, placebo-controlled trial of lisofylline for early treatment of acute lung injury and acute respiratory distress syndrome. *Crit. Care Med.* 30, 1–6. doi: 10.1097/00003246-200201000-00001

The ARDS Network (2000). Ketoconazole for early treatment of acute lung injury and acute respiratory distress syndrome: a randomized controlled trial. The ARDS Network. *JAMA* 283, 1995–2002. doi: 10.1001/jama.283.15.1995

Thiam, H. R., Wong, S. L., Wagner, D. D., and Waterman, C. M. (2020). Cellular mechanisms of NETosis. *Annu. Rev. Cell Dev. Biol.* 36, 191–218. doi: 10.1146/ annurev-cellbio-020520-111016

Thompson, B. T., Chambers, R. C., and Liu, K. D. (2017). Acute respiratory distress syndrome. *N. Engl. J. Med.* 377, 562–572.

Tiscornia, G., Singer, O., Ikawa, M., and Verma, I. M. (2003). A general method for gene knockdown in mice by using lentiviral vectors expressing small interfering RNA. *Proc. Natl. Acad. Sci. U.S.A.* 100, 1844–1848. doi: 10.1073/ pnas.0437912100

Tomashefski, J. F. (2000). Pulmonary pathology of acute respiratory distress syndrome. *Clin. Chest Med.* 21, 435–466.

Trac, P. T., Thai, T. L., Linck, V., Zou, L., Greenlee, M., Yue, Q., et al. (2017). Alveolar nonselective channels are ASIC1a/α-ENaC channels and contribute to AFC. *Am. J. Physiol. Lung Cell. Mol. Physiol.* 312, L797–L811. doi: 10.1152/ ajplung.00379.2016

Trimble, C., Lin, C.-T., Hung, C.-F., Pai, S., Juang, J., He, L., et al. (2003). Comparison of the CD8+ T cell responses and antitumor effects generated by DNA vaccine administered through gene gun, biojector, and syringe. *Vaccine* 21, 4036–4042. doi: 10.1016/s0264-410x(03)00275-5

Tseng, Y. C., Mozumdar, S., and Huang, L. (2009). Lipid-based systemic delivery of siRNA. *Adv. Drug Deliv. Rev.* 61, 721–731.

Tsuburai, T., Kaneko, T., Nagashima, Y., Ueda, A., Tagawa, A., Shinohara, T., et al. (2004). *Pseudomonas aeruginosa*-induced neutrophilic lung inflammation is attenuated by adenovirus-mediated transfer of the heme oxygenase 1 cDNA in mice. *Hum. Gene Ther.* 15, 273–285. doi: 10.1089/104303404322886129

Tsushima, K., King, L. S., Aggarwal, N. R., De Gorordo, A., D'Alessio, F. R., and Kubo, K. (2009). Acute lung injury review. *Intern. Med.* 48, 621–630. doi: 10.2169/internalmedicine.48.1741

Tzotzos, S. J., Fischer, B., Fischer, H., and Zeitlinger, M. (2020). Incidence of ARDS and outcomes in hospitalized patients with COVID-19: a global literature survey. *Crit. Care* 24:516. doi: 10.1186/s13054-020-03240-7

Unbekandt, M., and Olson, M. F. (2014). The actin-myosin regulatory MRCK kinases: regulation, biological functions and associations with human cancer. *J. Mol. Med. (Berl.)* 92, 217–225. doi: 10.1007/s00109-014-1133-6

Vadasz, I., Raviv, S., and Sznajder, J. I. (2007). Alveolar epithelium and Na,K-ATPase in acute lung injury. *Intensive Care Med.* 33, 1243–1251. doi: 10.1007/s00134-007-0661-8

Vadolas, J., Williamson, R., and Ioannou, P. A. (2002). Gene therapy for inherited lung disorders: an insight into pulmonary defence. *Pulm. Pharmacol. Ther.* 15, 61–72. doi: 10.1006/pupt.2001.0316

Vagin, O., Dada, L. A., Tokhtaeva, E., and Sachs, G. (2012). The Na-K-ATPase α1β1 heterodimer as a cell adhesion molecule in epithelia. *Am. J. physiol. Cell Physiol.* 302, C1271–C1281.

Vassiliou, A. G., Kotanidou, A., Dimopoulou, I., and Orfanos, S. E. (2020). Endothelial damage in acute respiratory distress syndrome. *Int. J. Mol. Sci.* 21:8793. doi: 10.3390/ijms21228793

Verma, I. M., and Weitzman, M. D. (2005). Gene therapy: twenty-first century medicine. *Annu. Rev. Biochem.* 74, 711–738.

Villar, J., Blanco, J., and Kacmarek, R. M. (2016). Current incidence and outcome of the acute respiratory distress syndrome. *Curr. Opin. Crit. Care* 22, 1–6. doi: 10.1097/MCC.0000000000000266

Vu, L., Ramos, J., Potta, T., and Rege, K. (2012). Generation of a focused poly(amino ether) library: polymer-mediated transgene delivery and gold-nanorod based theranostic systems. *Theranostics* 2, 1160–1173. doi: 10.7150/thno.4492

Vyas-Read, S., Vance, R. J., Wang, W., Colvocoresses-Dodds, J., Brown, L. A., and Koval, M. (2018). Hyperoxia induces paracellular leak and alters claudin expression by neonatal alveolar epithelial cells. *Pediatr. Pulmonol.* 53, 17–27. doi: 10.1002/ppul.23681

Walters, R. W., Grunst, T., Bergelson, J. M., Finberg, R. W., Welsh, M. J., and Zabner, J. (1999). Basolateral localization of fiber receptors limits adenovirus infection from the apical surface of airway epithelia. *J. Biol. Chem.* 274, 10219–10226. doi: 10.1074/jbc.274.15.10219

Wang, D., Tai, P. W. L., and Gao, G. (2019). Adeno-associated virus vector as a platform for gene therapy delivery. *Nat. Rev. Drug Discov.* 18, 358–378. doi: 10.1038/s41573-019-0012-9

Wang, G., Slepushkin, V., Zabner, J., Keshavjee, S., Johnston, J. C., Sauter, S. L., et al. (1999). Feline immunodeficiency virus vectors persistently transduce nondividing airway epithelia and correct the cystic fibrosis defect. *J. Clin. Invest.* 104, R55–R62. doi: 10.1172/JCI8390

Wang, T., Wang, L., Moreno-Vinasco, L., Lang, G. D., Siegler, J. H., Mathew, B., et al. (2012). Particulate matter air pollution disrupts endothelial cell barrier via calpain-mediated tight junction protein degradation. *Part. Fibre Toxicol.* 9:35. doi: 10.1186/1743-8977-9-35

Wang, X., Chen, Y., Lv, L., and Chen, J. (2009). Silencing CD36 gene expression results in the inhibition of latent-TGF-beta1 activation and suppression of silica-induced lung fibrosis in the rat. *Respir. Res.* 10, 36–36. doi: 10.1186/1465-9921-10-36

Ware, L. B. (2006). Pathophysiology of acute lung injury and the acute respiratory distress syndrome. *Semin. Respir. Crit. Care Med.* 27, 337–349.

Ware, L. B., Eisner, M. D., Thompson, B. T., Parsons, P. E., and Matthay, M. A. (2004). Significance of von Willebrand factor in septic and nonseptic patients with acute lung injury. *Am. J. Respir. Crit. Care Med.* 170, 766–772. doi: 10.1164/rccm.200310-1434OC

Ware, L. B., Fremont, R. D., Bastarache, J. A., Calfee, C. S., and Matthay, M. A. (2010). Determining the aetiology of pulmonary oedema by the oedema fluid-to-plasma protein ratio. *Eur. Respir. J.* 35, 331–337. doi: 10.1183/09031936.00098709

Ware, L. B., and Matthay, M. A. (2000). The acute respiratory distress syndrome. *N. Engl. J. Med.* 342, 1334–1349.

Ware, L. B., and Matthay, M. A. (2001). Alveolar fluid clearance is impaired in the majority of patients with acute lung injury and the acute respiratory distress syndrome. *Am. J. Respir. Crit. Care Med.* 163, 1376–1383. doi: 10.1164/ajrccm.163.6.2004035

Weaver, J. C., and Chizmadzhev, Y. A. (1996). Theory of electroporation: a review. *Bioelectrochem. Bioenerg.* 41, 135–160.

Weibel, E. R. (1973). Morphological basis of alveolar-capillary gas exchange. *Physiol. Rev.* 53, 419–495. doi: 10.1152/physrev.1973.53.2.419

Weinbaum, S., Tarbell, J. M., and Damiano, E. R. (2007). The structure and function of the endothelial glycocalyx layer. *Annu. Rev. Biomed. Eng.* 9, 121–167.

Weiss, D. J. (2002). Delivery of gene transfer vectors to lung: obstacles and the role of adjunct techniques for airway administration. *Mol. Ther.* 6, 148–152. doi: 10.1006/mthe.2002.0662

Weiss, Y. G., Maloyan, A., Tazelaar, J., Raj, N., and Deutschman, C. S. (2002). Adenoviral transfer of HSP-70 into pulmonary epithelium ameliorates experimental acute respiratory distress syndrome. *J. Clin. Invest.* 110, 801–806. doi: 10.1172/JCI15888

Wells, D. J. (2004). Gene therapy progress and prospects: electroporation and other physical methods. *Gene Ther.* 11, 1363–1369. doi: 10.1038/sj.gt.3302337

Wiesel, P., Patel, A. P., DiFonzo, N., Marria, P. B., Sim, C. U., Pellacani, A., et al. (2000). Endotoxin-induced mortality is related to increased oxidative stress and end-organ dysfunction, not refractory hypotension, in heme oxygenase-1-deficient mice. *Circulation* 102, 3015–3022. doi: 10.1161/01.cir.102.24.3015

Williams, R. S., Johnston, S. A., Riedy, M., DeVit, M. J., McElligott, S. G., and Sanford, J. C. (1991). Introduction of foreign genes into tissues of living mice by DNA-coated microprojectiles. *Proc. Natl. Acad. Sci. U.S.A.* 88, 2726–2730. doi: 10.1073/pnas.88.7.2726

Witzenbichler, B., Westermann, D., Knueppel, S., Schultheiss, H. P., and Tschope, C. (2005). Protective role of angiopoietin-1 in endotoxic shock. *Circulation* 111, 97–105. doi: 10.1161/01.CIR.0000151287.08202.8E

Wolff, J., Malone, R., Williams, P., Chong, W., Acsadi, G., Jani, A., et al. (1990). Direct gene transfer into mouse muscle in vivo. *Science* 247, 1465–1468. doi: 10.1126/science.1690918

Wolff, J. A., Ludtke, J. J., Acsadi, G., Williams, P., and Jani, A. (1992). Long-term persistence of plasmid DNA and foreign gene expression in mouse muscle. *Hum. Mol. Genet.* 1, 363–369. doi: 10.1093/hmg/1.6.363

Wolfson, R. K., Chiang, E. T., and Garcia, J. G. (2011). HMGB1 induces human lung endothelial cell cytoskeletal rearrangement and barrier disruption. *Microvasc. Res.* 81, 189–197. doi: 10.1016/j.mvr.2010.11.010

Worgall, S., Leopold, P. L., Wolff, G., Ferris, B., Van Roijen, N., and Crystal, R. G. (1997). Role of alveolar macrophages in rapid elimination of adenovirus vectors administered to the epithelial surface of the respiratory tract. *Hum. Gene Ther.* 8, 1675–1684. doi: 10.1089/hum.1997.8.14-1675

Wray, C., Mao, Y., Pan, J., Chandrasena, A., Piasta, F., and Frank, J. A. (2009). Claudin-4 augments alveolar epithelial barrier function and is induced in acute lung injury. *Am. J. Physiol. Lung Cell. Mol. Physiol.* 297, L219–L227. doi: 10.1152/ajplung.00043.2009

Xiong, S., Hong, Z., Huang, L. S., Tsukasaki, Y., Nepal, S., Di, A., et al. (2020). IL-1β suppression of VE-cadherin transcription underlies sepsis-induced inflammatory lung injury. *J. Clin. Invest.* 130, 3684–3698. doi: 10.1172/JCI136908

Xu, J., Qu, J., Cao, L., Sai, Y., Chen, C., He, L., et al. (2008). Mesenchymal stem cell-based angiopoietin-1 gene therapy for acute lung injury induced by lipopolysaccharide in mice. *J. Pathol.* 214, 472–481. doi: 10.1002/path.2302

Yanagi, S., Tsubouchi, H., Miura, A., Matsumoto, N., and Nakazato, M. (2015). Breakdown of epithelial barrier integrity and overdrive activation of alveolar epithelial cells in the pathogenesis of acute respiratory distress syndrome and lung fibrosis. *Biomed. Res. Int.* 2015:573210. doi: 10.1155/2015/573210

Yang, N. S., Burkholder, J., Roberts, B., Martinell, B., and McCabe, D. (1990). In vivo and in vitro gene transfer to mammalian somatic cells by particle bombardment. *Proc. Natl. Acad. Sci. U.S.A.* 87, 9568–9572. doi: 10.1073/pnas.87.24.9568

Yang, Y., Chen, Q.-h, Liu, A.-r., Xu, X.-p., Han, J.-b., and Qiu, H.-b. (2015). Synergism of MSC-secreted HGF and VEGF in stabilising endothelial barrier function upon lipopolysaccharide stimulation via the Rac1 pathway. *Stem Cell Res. Ther.* 6:250. doi: 10.1186/s13287-015-0257-0

Yang, Y., Haeger, S. M., Suflita, M. A., Zhang, F., Dailey, K. L., Colbert, J. F., et al. (2017). Fibroblast growth factor signaling mediates pulmonary endothelial glycocalyx reconstitution. *Am. J. Respir. Cell Mol. Biol.* 56, 727–737. doi: 10.1165/rcmb.2016-0338OC

Yang, Y., Hu, S., Xu, X., Li, J., Liu, A., Han, J., et al. (2016). The vascular endothelial growth factors-expressing character of mesenchymal stem cells plays a positive role in treatment of acute lung injury in vivo. *Mediators Inflamm.* 2016:2347938. doi: 10.1155/2016/2347938

Yi, Y., Noh, M. J., and Lee, K. H. (2011). Current advances in retroviral gene therapy. *Curr. Gene Ther.* 11, 218–228.

Yin, H., Kanasty, R. L., Eltoukhy, A. A., Vegas, A. J., Dorkin, J. R., and Anderson, D. G. (2014). Non-viral vectors for gene-based therapy. *Nat. Rev. Genet.* 15, 541–555. doi: 10.1038/nrg3763

You, K., Xu, X., Fu, J., Xu, S., Yue, X., Yu, Z., et al. (2012). Hyperoxia disrupts pulmonary epithelial barrier in newborn rats via the deterioration of occludin and ZO-1. *Respir. Res.* 13:36. doi: 10.1186/1465-9921-13-36

Young, J. L., Barravecchia, M. S., and Dean, D. A. (2014). "Electroporation-mediated gene delivery to the lungs," in *Electroporation Protocols: Preclinical and Clinical Gene Medicine*, eds S. Li, J. Cutrera, R. Heller, and J. Teissie (New York, NY: Springer New York), 189–204. doi: 10.1007/978-1-4614-9632-8_17

Yue, G., Russell, W. J., Benos, D. J., Jackson, R. M., Olman, M. A., and Matalon, S. (1995). Increased expression and activity of sodium channels in alveolar type II cells of hyperoxic rats. *Proc. Natl. Acad. Sci. U.S.A.* 92, 8418–8422. doi: 10.1073/pnas.92.18.8418

Zarbock, A., and Ley, K. (2009). The role of platelets in acute lung injury (ALI). *Front. Biosci. (Landmark Ed.)* 14:150–158. doi: 10.2741/3236

Zarbock, A., Singbartl, K., and Ley, K. (2006). Complete reversal of acid-induced acute lung injury by blocking of platelet-neutrophil aggregation. *J. Clin. Invest.*116, 3211–3219. doi: 10.1172/JCI29499

Zelenin, A. V., Kolesnikov, V. A., Tarasenko, O. A., Shafei, R. A. I, Zelenina, A., Mikhailov, V. V., et al. (1997). Bacterial beta-galactosidase and human dystrophin genes are expressed in mouse skeletal muscle fibers after ballistic transfection. *FEBS Lett.* 414, 319–322. doi: 10.1016/s0014-5793(97)01019-3

Zelphati, O., Uyechi, L. S., Barron, L. G., and Szoka, F. C. Jr. (1998). Effect of serum components on the physico-chemical properties of cationic lipid/oligonucleotide complexes and on their interactions with cells. *Biochim. Biophys. Acta* 1390, 119–133. doi: 10.1016/s0005-2760(97)00169-0

Zemans, R. L., and Matthay, M. A. (2004). Bench-to-bedside review: the role of the alveolar epithelium in the resolution of pulmonary edema in acute lung injury. *Crit. Care* 8, 469–477. doi: 10.1186/cc2906

Zeng, M., Huang, C., Zheng, H., Chen, Q., He, W., and Deng, Y. (2018). Effects of ghrelin on iNOS-derived NO promoted LPS-induced pulmonary alveolar epithelial A549 cells apoptosis. *Cell. Physiol. Biochem.* 49, 1840–1855. doi: 10.1159/000493630

Zhang, D., Qi, B.-Y., Zhu, W.-W., Huang, X., and Wang, X.-Z. (2020). Crocin alleviates lipopolysaccharide-induced acute respiratory distress syndrome by protecting against glycocalyx damage and suppressing inflammatory signaling pathways. *Inflamm. Res.* 69, 267–278. doi: 10.1007/s00011-019-01314-z

Zhang, H. G., Zhou, T., Yang, P., Edwards, C. K. III, Curiel, D. T., and Mountz, J. D. (1998). Inhibition of tumor necrosis factor alpha decreases inflammation and prolongs adenovirus gene expression in lung and liver. *Hum. Gene Ther.* 9, 1875–1884. doi: 10.1089/hum.1998.9.13-1875

Zhang, S., Danchuk, S. D., Imhof, K. M., Semon, J. A., Scruggs, B. A., Bonvillain, R. W., et al. (2013). Comparison of the therapeutic effects of human and mouse adipose-derived stem cells in a murine model of lipopolysaccharide-induced acute lung injury. *Stem Cell Res. Ther.* 4, 13–13. doi: 10.1186/scrt161

Zhang, Y., Jiang, G., Sauler, M., and Lee, P. J. (2013). Lung endothelial HO-1 targeting in vivo using lentiviral miRNA regulates apoptosis and autophagy during oxidant injury. *FASEB J.* 27, 4041–4058. doi: 10.1096/fj.13-231225

Zhang, Y., Satterlee, A., and Huang, L. (2012). In vivo gene delivery by nonviral vectors: overcoming hurdles? *Mol. Ther.* 20, 1298–1304. doi: 10.1038/mt.2012.79

Zhao, Y. F., Luo, Y. M., Xiong, W., Ding, W., Li, Y. R., Zhao, W., et al. (2015). Mesenchymal stem cell-based FGF2 gene therapy for acute lung injury induced by lipopolysaccharide in mice. *Eur. Rev. Med. Pharmacol. Sci.* 19, 857–865.

Zhou, G., Dada, L. A., and Sznajder, J. I. (2008). Regulation of alveolar epithelial function by hypoxia. *Eur. Respir. J.* 31, 1107–1113. doi: 10.1183/09031936.00155507

Zhou, R., and Dean, D. A. (2007). Gene transfer of interleukin 10 to the murine cornea using electroporation. *Exp. Biol. Med. (Maywood)* 232, 362–369.

Zhou, R., Norton, J. E., and Dean, D. A. (2008). Electroporation-mediated gene delivery to the lungs. *Methods Mol. Biol.* 423, 233–247.

Zhu, L., and Mahato, R. I. (2010). Lipid and polymeric carrier-mediated nucleic acid delivery. *Expert Opin. Drug Deliv.* 7, 1209–1226. doi: 10.1517/17425247.2010.513969

Ziegler, E. J., Fisher, C. J. Jr., Sprung, C. L., Straube, R. C., Sadoff, J. C., Foulke, G. E., et al. (1991). Treatment of gram-negative bacteremia and septic shock with HA-1A human monoclonal antibody against endotoxin. A randomized, double-blind, placebo-controlled trial. The HA-1A Sepsis Study Group. *N. Engl. J. Med.* 324, 429–436. doi: 10.1056/NEJM199102143240701

Zsengellér, Z., Otake, K., Hossain, S. A., Berclaz, P. Y., and Trapnell, B. C. (2000). Internalization of adenovirus by alveolar macrophages initiates early proinflammatory signaling during acute respiratory tract infection. *J. Virol.* 74, 9655–9667. doi: 10.1128/jvi.74.20.9655-9667.2000

Zuidam, N. J., and Barenholz, Y. (1998). Electrostatic and structural properties of complexes involving plasmid DNA and cationic lipids commonly used for gene delivery. *Biochim. Biophys. Acta* 1368, 115–128. doi: 10.1016/s0005-2736(97)00187-9

13

Static and Dynamic Measurements of Compliance and Driving Pressure

*Pierre Tawfik[1], Muhammad K. Hayat Syed[2], Firas S. Elmufdi[3], Michael D. Evans[4], David J. Dries[5,6] and John J. Marini[1,3]**

[1] Pulmonary, Allergy, Critical Care, and Sleep Medicine, University of Minnesota, Minneapolis, MN, United States, [2] Pulmonary and Critical Care Medicine, Baylor College of Medicine, Houston, TX, United States, [3] Department of Medicine, Regions Hospital, Saint Paul, MN, United States, [4] Clinical and Translational Science Institute, University of Minnesota, Minneapolis, MN, United States, [5] Department of Surgery, Regions Hospital, Saint Paul, MN, United States, [6] Department of Critical Care and Acute Care Surgery, University of Minnesota, Minneapolis, MN, United States

***Correspondence:**
John J. Marini
marin002@umn.edu

Rationale: Monitoring tidal cycle mechanics is key to lung protection. For this purpose, compliance and driving pressure of the respiratory system are often measured clinically using the plateau pressure, obtained after imposing an extended end-inspiratory pause, which allows for relaxation of the respiratory system and redistribution of inflation volume (method A). Alternative methods for estimating compliance and driving pressure utilize the measured pressure at the earliest instance of zero flow (method B), the inspiratory slope of the pressure-time tracing during inflation with constant flow (method C), and the expiratory time constant (method D).

Methods: Ten passive mechanically ventilated subjects, at a large tertiary referral center, underwent measurements of compliance and driving pressure using the four different methods. The inspiratory tidal volume, inspiratory to expiratory ratio, and positive end expiratory pressures were then adjusted from baseline and the measurements re-obtained.

Results: Method A yielded consistently higher compliance and lower driving pressure calculations compared to methods B and C. Methods B and C most closely approximated one another. Method D did not yield a consistent reliable pattern.

Conclusion: Static measurements of compliance and driving pressure using the plateau pressure may underestimate the maximum pressure experienced by the most vulnerable lung units during dynamic inflation. Utilizing the pressure at zero flow as a static measurement, or the inspiratory slope as a dynamic measurement, may calculate a truer estimate of the maximum alveolar pressure that generates stress upon compromised lung units.

Keywords: compliance, static compliance, dynamic compliance, driving pressure, plateau pressure, respiratory mechanics, ventilator induced lung injury, mechanical ventilation

INTRODUCTION

Measuring compliance of the respiratory system provides critical insight into the mechanics of the lungs and chest wall and the dynamics of breathing. Apart from characterizing the ease or difficulty of chest inflation, tidal compliance tracks the severity and progress of acute lung injury (ARDS). Moreover, compliance determines the driving pressure necessary to inflate the lungs with a specific tidal volume, a key indicator of the risk for ventilator-induced lung injury (VILI) (Amato et al., 2015; Goligher et al., 2021). In current clinical practice, compliance and driving pressure are commonly measured under passive conditions after an extended end-inspiratory pause is performed to obtain the stable plateau pressure ($P_{plateau}$). While this average value for driving pressure measured under "stop flow" conditions has definite worth, is simple to obtain, and is universally measured, it may underestimate the maximum stress to which some lung units are exposed under the dynamic conditions of tidally inflating the mechanically heterogeneous lungs of ARDS.

When VILI prevention is the focus of attention, $P_{plateau}$ (Method A) may not precisely reflect the maximum alveolar pressure experienced by the most vulnerable alveoli (Milic-Emili et al., 1990). The end inspiratory breath hold allows for relaxation of the respiratory system and redistribution of inflation volume and distending pressures. These processes usually decrease the measured pressure. An alternative method of measuring compliance uses the pressure measured at the first point of zero flow during the end-inspiratory pause (P_{zf}), which usually occurs about 2 s earlier than the $P_{plateau}$ (Method B) (**Figure 1**) (Milic-Emili et al., 1990). This latter method excludes the airflow resistance component from the recorded pressure measurement without allowing full relaxation and gas redistribution within the respiratory system. Measuring compliance using $P_{plateau}$ and P_{zf} may still not accurately characterize the maximum pressure experienced by some alveoli, especially in a mechanically complex environment; both are measurements made under quasi-static conditions that may or may not perfectly characterize the non-static (dynamic) tidal inflation of the lungs.

Compliance can also be measured using dynamic values obtained during inflation or deflation. One such method calculates compliance during constant flow, based on the slope of the pressure-time tracing (Method C). During inflation under constant flow conditions, time is a direct linear analog of volume. Two pressure values during inflation and their corresponding volumes can therefore be used to measure compliance using the following equation: Compliance = (V2-V1)/(P2-P1) where P1 and P2 are two pressure measurements during inflation while V1 and V2 are the corresponding tidal volumes occurring at those same time points. Another dynamic method of assessing compliance (Method D) assumes uniexponential decay of the tidal volume and computes the deflation time constant, the product of resistance and compliance (R × C) (Al-Rawas et al., 2013). Under the assumptions of uniexponential decay and unchanging resistance, the time constant is a quotient of volume at any point on the deflation curve and its corresponding instantaneous flow rate. The calculated time constant is then divided by resistance measured at end-inspiration under constant flow conditions to obtain compliance, i.e., Compliance = expiratory time constant/resistance. For each of these four methods, Driving Pressure = inspiratory volume/compliance.

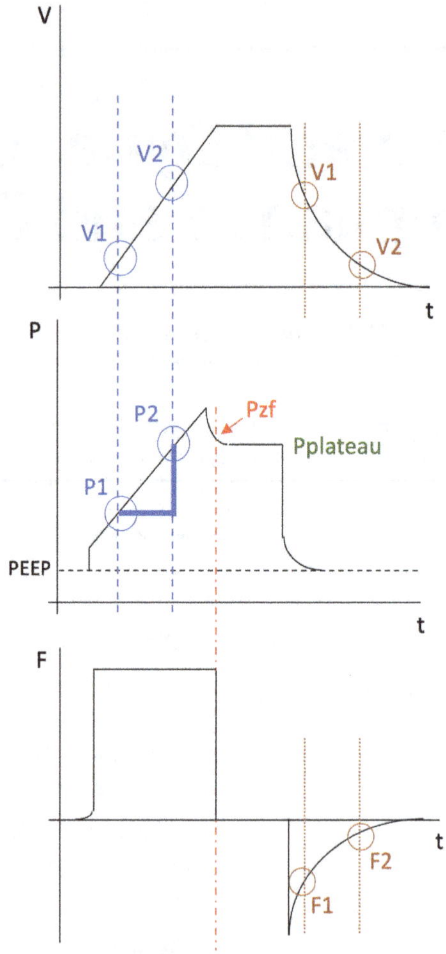

FIGURE 1 | Illustration of the inspiratory and expiratory phase of a typical breath under constant flow and the various methods for calculating compliance and driving pressure. The top waveform plots volume (V) over time (t). The middle waveform plots pressure (P) over time. The bottom waveform plots flow (F) over time. Compliance calculation in method A (green) is performed by dividing the change in volume by the change in pressure (Pplateau minus PEEP). Compliance calculation in method B (red) is performed by dividing the change in volume by the change in pressure utilizing instead the pressure at zero flow (Pzf minus PEEP). Compliance calculation in method C (blue) is performed using the following equation: [V2-V1] / [P2-P1]. Compliance calculation in method D (orange) requires measurement of multiple expiratory time constants. For example, time constant #1 equals V1/F1. Time constant #2 equals V2/F2. Compliance is then calculated by dividing the average of the different time constants by the resistance. For each of these four methods, Driving Pressure = inspiratory volume / compliance.

Although a signature property of bedside lung mechanics used in decision making, various questions arise regarding compliance and driving pressure measurements. It is unclear how these four alternative methods compare to one another in the same patient. It is also unknown how these relationships are altered by varying the ventilator settings of tidal volume and inspiratory flow. Our purpose, therefore, was to compare such methods of measuring compliance and driving pressure in the clinical setting and to explore the impact of ventilator parameters on these methods. We hypothesized that differences would arise between the inspiratory versus expiratory methods of compliance and driving pressure estimation as well as between these values obtained by the dynamic versus static methods.

MATERIALS AND METHODS

Study Design

This study was performed at Regions Hospital in St. Paul, Minnesota, and was approved by the Regions Hospital Institutional Review Board. We conducted a prospective cohort study of passive mechanically ventilated subjects. All subjects receiving mechanical ventilation in the medical intensive care unit were evaluated for inclusion. Subjects 18 years and older who were deemed to be passively ventilated, either by receiving neuromuscular blockade, or who had a Richmond Agitation-Sedation Scale (RAAS) of −3 or −4 and demonstrated no evidence of active breathing at the bedside (i.e., over-breathing, dyssynchrony), were included. Subjects who were pregnant, had undergone prior lung, chest wall or abdominal surgeries, had known deformity of the chest wall, or had known parenchymal or obstructive lung disease were excluded. Family members of subjects meeting the study criteria were approached for consent.

Study Procedures

Since deflation may not occur uniexponentially (Hamahata et al., 2020), there are potentially multiple time constants throughout expiration. For the purposes of this study, two time constants were measured, and their mean was used to obtain an average for the compliance equation.

After consent was obtained, subjects were re-evaluated at the bedside to ensure ongoing passive ventilation and stable hemodynamics. Prior to data collection, all subjects were ventilated using pressure regulated volume control. Each subject's flow profile was changed to an equivalent constant flow, maintaining the subject's same inspiratory to expiratory ratio (I:E), tidal volume (TV), respiratory rate (RR), oxygen concentration (FIO2) and positive end expiratory pressure (PEEP). At these "baseline" settings, an inspiratory breath hold was performed, followed by a breath without a hold maneuver, followed by a breath with an end expiratory hold. The ventilator screen was then frozen, and the cursor dial maneuvered to obtain the necessary measurements from the time-based tracings of pressure, volume, and flow. On the inspiratory limb of a pressure-volume display, two pressures and corresponding volumes were measured (for method C calculations). These points were chosen from the middle 80% of the inspiratory limb to avoid variability from inspiratory flow initiation and cessation. For the paused breaths, the P_{zf} was recorded, followed by the $P_{plateau}$, measured 2 s after the breath hold was initiated (for methods A and B calculations). From the second breath (without a breath hold maneuver), two expiratory flow measurements and corresponding volume measurements were obtained from the middle 50% of the generated graph (method D). For method D, the initial 25% and latter 25% of the expiratory limb of the loop were excluded to best approximate an average time constant. Compliance and driving pressure were calculated for each method.

The following ventilator setting adjustments were then performed unless they violated the prespecified protocol safety parameters. Breath holds and data gathering steps were performed as detailed above for the following variations. Tidal volume was first increased from baseline and then decreased from baseline by 2 ml/kg of ideal body weight (IBW). Next, I:E ratio was increased from the baseline ratio by 1.0 and then decreased from baseline by 1.0. Finally, PEEP was increased and then decreased from its baseline value by 2 cmH2O. After each ventilator adjustment, we allowed for a 1-min equilibration period. The ventilator was not adjusted if the following pre-specified safety parameters were surpassed: tidal volume < 4 ml/kg of IBW or > 10 ml/kg of IBW; baseline $P_{plateau}$ greater than 35 cmH2O; baseline PEEP < 5 cmH2O or PEEP > 12 cmH2O in a subject with BMI less than 30 kg/m^2; baseline PEEP < 5 cmH2O or PEEP > 16 cmH2O in a subject with BMI greater than 30 kg/m^2.

Data Collection

Study data were collected and managed using Research Electronic Data Capture (REDCap) electronic data capture tools, a secure, web-based software platform, hosted at Regions Hospital (Harris et al., 2009).

Statistical Analysis

Participants' demographic and clinical characteristics were summarized using counts and rates or medians and ranges. Radar plots were used to visualize each participant's compliance and driving pressure measurements at each ventilator setting for each of four calculation methods (**Supplementary Materials 1, 2**). To examine the average effect of ventilator setting changes on compliance and driving pressure for each calculation method, linear mixed-effects models were fit with fixed effects terms for tidal volume, I:E ratio, and total PEEP, and a random effect term for participant to account for repeated measurements within participant. To compare compliance and driving pressure between calculation methods at each ventilator setting combination, similar mixed-effects models were fit with the differences between each pair of calculation methods as the outcomes. Results are summarized using mean effects with 95% confidence intervals. Analyses were conducted using R version 4.1.1 (R Core Team, 2020).

RESULTS

The study was conducted over 8 months from October 2020 through June 2021. The study was stopped by the investigators due to low enrollment, primarily owing to a majority of considered subjects having a degree of active breathing on the ventilator (**Figure 2**). Ten subjects completed the study (**Table 1**). Five subjects underwent all ventilator settings adjustments. The remainder completed some, but not all, of the adjustments due to protocol safety limits (**Figure 2**). The subjects were primarily male (7/10, 70%) and Caucasian (8/10, 80%). The median number of days undergoing mechanical ventilation at the time of data collection was three (range 1–10 days). Reasons for intubation were COVID ARDS (5/10, 50%), encephalopathy (2/10, 20%), cardiac arrest (1/10, 10%), cardiogenic shock (1/10, 10%), and aspiration pneumonia (1/10, 10%). P/F calculations indicated a range from normal oxygenation to all degrees of ARDS severity: median P/F of 134.5 (range 75–623). Of the five subjects who completed all ventilator setting adjustments, four subjects had moderate to severe ARDS by P/F criteria. A minority of subjects received epoprostenol (2/10, 20%) and a minority were prone at the time of data collection (3/10, 30%). These two interventions did not appear to create a discernable deviation or change in the compliance or driving pressure calculations. Only two subjects were paralyzed (2/10, 20%); lack of paralysis did not appear to create a pattern of deviation or inconsistency in the calculations.

The study aimed to compare compliance and driving pressure measurement methods. Radar plots of the four methods for each subject, under baseline ventilator settings and with each ventilator adjustment, are available in **Supplementary Materials 1, 2**. A demonstrative plot for one subject is shown in **Figure 3**. Average compliance and driving pressure measurements, under baseline ventilator settings and with each adjustment, were compared. Average differences between each method were calculated along with 95% confidence intervals and Bland-Altman limits of agreements of these differences; with statistical significance indicated by confidence intervals that do not intersect the zero line (**Supplementary Material 3**). Method A consistently produced statistically significant higher values of compliance, and lower values of driving pressure, compared to method B and C. Compliance and driving pressure measurements from methods B and C most closely approximated each other; there was no statistically significant difference in method B compared to method C under baseline, volume decrease, I:E increase or decrease, PEEP increase or decrease conditions. There was a statistically significant difference between method B and C under the volume increase condition, with method C on average calculating greater compliance by 2.5 cmH2O (95% CI: −4.7 to −0.3) than Method B and lower driving pressure by 2.04 cmH2O (95% CI: 0.49 to 3.59). Method D did not show a consistent pattern, demonstrating higher measurements of compliance and lower measurements in driving pressure in eight subjects and the reverse findings in two subjects, compared to the other methods.

Linear mixed-effects regression models were used to assess the impact of each ventilator change on each measurement method (**Supplementary Material 4**). Model summaries show the average linear effect of each ventilator setting change on the compliance or driving pressure outcome; effects greater than 0 indicate that increasing that setting is associated with an increase in the outcome, and decreasing that setting with a decrease in the outcome; and, vice versa for effects less than 0. An increase in I:E resulted in a statistically significant increase in compliance and decrease in driving pressure for methods B and D, with reciprocal changes for a decrease in I:E. An increase in PEEP resulted in a statistically significant decrease in compliance and increase in driving pressure for methods A and B, with reciprocal changes for a decrease in PEEP. However, these values are averages and the patterns did not consistently hold for each individual subject. Tidal volume adjustments had

TABLE 1 | Demographics and clinical characteristics of the tested subjects.

Age (median, years)	**61.5 (range 37–81)**
Sex	
Male	7/10 (70%)
Female	3/10 (30%)
Race	
Caucasian	8/10 (80%)
Hispanic	1/10 (10%)
Southeast Asian	1/10 (10%)
Height (median, cm)	173.9 (range 154.9–188.0)
BMI (median, kg/m2)	32.3 (range 24.6–40.2)
Ventilator days at time of data collection (median, days)	3.0 (range 1–10)
Primary diagnosis requiring intubation	
Encephalopathy	2/10 (20%)
Aspiration pneumonia	1/10 (10%)
Cardiac arrest	1/10 (10%)
Cardiogenic shock	1/10 (10%)
COVID ARDS	5/10 (50%)
RAAS	
−3	2/10 (20%)
−4	4/10 (40%)
−5	4/10 (40%)
Position at time of data collection	
Supine, flat	1/10 (10%)
Supine, upright at 30–40 degrees	6/10 (60%)
Prone	3/10 (30%)
Baseline volume (median, mL)	444.5 (range 304–579)
Baseline I:E (median)	1:2.31 (range 1:1.47–1:3.29)
Baseline total PEEP (median, cmH2O)	8.57 (range 5–15)
pH (median)	7.29 (range 7.24–7.45)
PaO2/FIO2 (median, mmHg)	134.5 (range 75–623)
Hgb (median, g/dL)	9.0 (range 7.2–14.7)
WBC [median, ×10(9)/L]	11.3 (range 6.1–18.3)
Number of subjects receiving each sedative	
Hydromorphone	6/10 (60%)
Fentanyl	3/10 (30%)
Propofol	2/10 (10%)
Lorazepam	5/10 (50%)
Midazolam	4/10 (40%)
Dexmedetomidine	1/10 (10%)
Number of subjects receiving paralytics	2/10 (20%)
Number of subjects receiving inhaled epoprostenol	2/10 (20%)

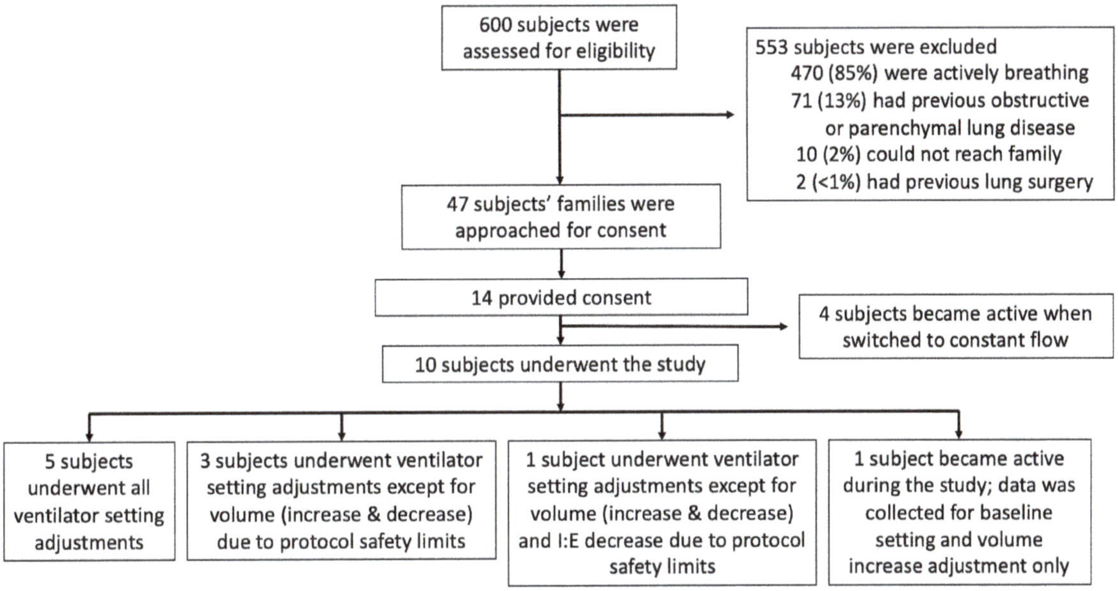

FIGURE 2 | Flow diagram outlining subjects assessed for eligibility, reasons of exclusion or inability to enroll, and breakdown of the ventilator setting adjustments that were tested.

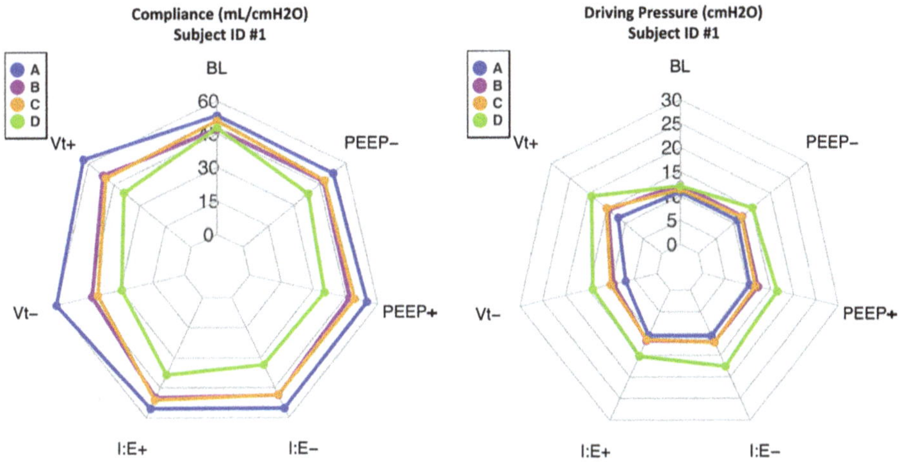

FIGURE 3 | Example radar plots for one subject (ID #1) showing compliance (mL/cmH20) and driving pressure (cmH2O) calculations. The blue line denotes calculations by method A, the pink line by method B, the orange line by method C, and the green line by method D. The baseline (BL) calculations by each of the four methods are in the top center axis. One ventilator adjustment was then performed, and the data recalculated. The changes were performed and are listed in counter-clockwise fashion: Vt+ is tidal volume increase by 2 ml/kg of ideal body weight from baseline, Vt- is tidal volume decrease by 2 ml/kg of ideal body weight from baseline, I:E+ is the ratio increase by 1.0 from baseline, I:E- is the ratio decrease by 1.0 from baseline, PEEP+ is PEEP increase by 2 cmH2O from baseline, and PEEP- is PEEP decrease by 2 cmH2O from baseline. Among the ten subjects, methods B and C best approximated one another, and Method A consistently calculated higher compliance and lower driving pressure. Method D did not demonstrate a consistent pattern.

the smallest sample size (n = 5) owing to safety limitations. An increase in tidal volume resulted in a statistically significant increase in compliance measurement for methods B, C and D and vice versa. An increase in tidal volume resulted in a statistically significant increase in driving pressure as well in all. Once again, these values were averages and the patterns of tidal volume's impact on compliance and driving pressure did not consistently hold for each individual subject. This discrepancy where tidal volume has a positive relationship with both compliance and driving pressure is due to the averaging of numerical values with different magnitudes.

Lung severity as assessed by P/F ratio, BMI, paralysis, and use of epoprostenol did not demonstrate any statistically significant impact on the measurements although the small sample size precludes any definitive statement regarding the impact of these variables.

DISCUSSION

The aim of this study was to evaluate four ways—two quasi-static methods and two dynamic methods—of measuring compliance and driving pressure of the respiratory system. In comparison to the standard method utilizing the $P_{plateau}$ minus PEEP (method A), measurements using the inspiratory slope of a constant flow pressure tracing (method C) and using the P_{zf} minus PEEP (method B) both demonstrated consistently lower compliance and higher driving pressure calculations. This would suggest that the standard method of measuring compliance and driving pressure, calculated after stress relaxation and gas re-distribution facilitated by the inspiratory hold, may overestimate the compliance and underestimate the driving pressure. Our data, therefore, suggest that utilizing the inspiratory hold may underestimate the risk to the most vulnerable lung units. Current numerical guidance for mechanical ventilation (i.e., peak pressure less than 30 cmH2O, driving pressure less than 15 cmH2O) utilizes the end-inspiratory breath hold and the resulting plateau pressure (Brower et al., 2000; Esteban et al., 2002; Amato et al., 2015). Although the numerical difference in calculations between methods A, B and C may not be dramatic, and the threshold for damage likely differs throughout regions of the heterogenous ARDS lung, these values assume significance if one aims to not surpass such numerical boundaries for safe ventilation. There was no statistically significant difference between compliance and driving pressure averages for methods B and C, except when tidal volume was increased by 2 ml/kg above baseline. Overall, method B and C most closely approximated each other compared to the other methods. P_{zf} may therefore be a better quasi-static marker for the maximum pressure experienced by the most vulnerable lung units than $P_{plateau}$. Furthermore, for purposes of lung protection, measuring compliance dynamically, utilizing the inspiratory slope during inflation by constant flow ventilation, may be a neglected but more relevant indicator than the static measure we customarily use.

Despite the small total number of subjects, the number of data points collected and the use of each subject's baseline as a self-control allow for reliable comparisons between methods. The subjects had heterogenous pathology. However, the patterns held true across this heterogenous group. Consequently, our investigation would appear to serve as a valid pilot study for larger future comparisons among these various methods. Both P_{zf} and inspiratory slopes are not commonly displayed ventilator outputs. Ventilator manufacturers may find utility incorporating P_{zf} outputs during an inspiratory hold. Likewise, although the contour-defining stress index has been incorporated into some ventilator monitoring during constant inspiratory flow, dynamic compliance and driving pressure algorithms based on the inspiratory pressure tracing are not yet available and should rather easily be programmed into any modern ventilator so as to provide relevant, intervention-free, and dynamic breath-by-breath information of additional interest.

The expiratory time constant (method D) did not provide a consistent pattern of compliance and driving pressure measurements, at times greater and at times less than the other methods. Various explanations account for this lack of precision. First, lung deflation typically is not uniexponential (Hamahata et al., 2020). There are therefore multiple time constants that apply during different phases of the expiratory cycle. Second, the speed of lung deflation is impacted by the opening of the expiratory valve and the decompression of the ventilator circuit, which further skews the data. Finally, energy can be lost between inspiration and expiration, known as lung hysteresis (Marini, 2020). As such, measures of the mechanics of lung inflation do not necessarily parallel those of deflation. Our data therefore suggest that expiratory time constant, using an average of two data points in the exhalation phase, is unlikely to be a reliable surrogate for the pressures, stress or strain experienced by the respiratory system during inflation. This method may perform better, however, if conducted using the reportedly successful Al-Rawas et al. protocol, where point-by-point values within the 0.10–0.50 s of the expiratory loop, are recorded (Al-Rawas et al., 2013). This, however, would require either a cumbersome recording process or a programmed data acquisition software that records and transfers data from the ventilator on the order of each millisecond—more frequently than currently reported or displayed.

Ventilator settings were changed (tidal volume, I:E ratio and PEEP) within a standard range of typical clinical adjustments. Some changes of settings appeared to cause statistically significant differences among methods regarding the average compliance and driving pressure measurements. It is difficult, however, to draw firm conclusions regarding predictions of machine adjustments for any given subject; the mentioned patterns of averages for machine setting adjustments did not consistently apply to each individual subject, who varied with regard to underlying lung disorder and severity.

There are various limitations to this study. First, due to judicious use of paralytic agents at our institution, most subjects were not paralyzed. However, subjects and ventilator waveforms were evaluated at the bedside by multiple clinicians to reduce the likelihood of actively initiated ventilation. Additionally, our sample size was diverse and small, owing to light sedation of many intensive care patients and difficulty consenting families of the most critically ill. The modest sample size of the study precludes more detailed conclusions from the data that might apply to disease and severity targeted populations. However, the trends discussed provide a compelling need to reevaluate $P_{plateau}$ as the standard base for compliance and driving pressure calculations that currently influence bedside decision-making. Furthermore, this study does not directly address which technique for measuring lung mechanics correlates best with VILI risk, which almost certainly varies with lung vulnerability and with the local environment of the alveoli in question. Yet, as all lung protective techniques attempt to reduce the maximum pressure applied to the alveoli, a technique that reveals higher pressure measurements does suggest that some alveoli are subjected to somewhat higher stresses and strains than previously appreciated.

In conclusion, this study serves as a pilot investigation into various methods for measuring tidal compliance and driving pressure. The standard approach utilizing $P_{plateau}$ may overestimate the compliance and underestimate the driving pressure during lung inflation. Further studies are needed to assess the impact of titrating driving pressure and compliance using these alternative methods, the influence of ventilator and patient parameters on these methods, and the potential correlation of these methods with clinical outcomes.

AUTHOR CONTRIBUTIONS

PT prepared the manuscript, participated in the study design, performed the data collection, and assisted in the data analysis. MS, DD, and JM designed the study and obtained the institutional review board approval for the project. FE participated in the study design, data collection, and data interpretation. ME performed statistical analysis of the data. JM was the principal investigator involved in all components of the project. All authors contributed to the article and approved the submitted version.

ACKNOWLEDGMENTS

We would like to acknowledge the Regions Hospital nursing staff and respiratory therapy department for their assistance in data acquisition. We would also like to acknowledge Dr. Kealy Ham for helping coordinate the study.

SUPPLEMENTARY MATERIAL

Supplementary Material 1 | Radar plots showing compliance calculations (in mL/cmH20) for each subject. The blue line denotes calculations by method A, the pink line by method B, the orange line by method C, and the green line by method D. For each subject, the baseline (BL) calculations by each of the four methods are in the top center axis. One ventilator adjustment was then performed, and the data recalculated. The changes were performed and are listed in counter-clockwise fashion: Vt+ is tidal volume increase by 2 ml/kg of ideal body weight from baseline, Vt- is tidal volume decrease by 2 ml/kg of ideal body weight from baseline, I:E+ is the ratio increase by 1.0 from baseline, I:E- is the ratio decrease by 1.0 from baseline, PEEP+ is PEEP increase by 2 cmH2O from baseline, and PEEP- is PEEP decrease by 2 cmH2O from baseline. For subject ID #14, a visual representation could not be displayed as data points were collected only for baseline and Vt+. Among the ten subjects, methods B and C best approximated one another, and Method A consistently calculated higher compliance. Method D did not demonstrate a consistent pattern.

Supplementary Material 2 | Radar plots showing driving pressure calculations (in cmH2O) for each subject. The blue line denotes calculations by method A, the pink line by method B, the orange line by method C, and the green line by method D. For each subject, the baseline (BL) calculations by each of the four methods are in the top center axis. One ventilator adjustment was then performed, and the data recalculated. The changes were performed and are listed in counter-clockwise fashion: Vt+ is tidal volume increase by 2 ml/kg of ideal body weight from baseline, Vt- is tidal volume decrease by 2 ml/kg of ideal body weight from baseline, I:E+ is the ratio increase by 1.0 from baseline, I:E- is the ratio decrease by 1.0 from baseline, PEEP+ is PEEP increase by 2 cmH2O from baseline, and PEEP- is PEEP decrease by 2 cmH2O from baseline. For subject ID #14, a visual representation could not be displayed as data points were collected only for baseline and Vt+. Among the ten subjects, methods B and C best approximated one another, and Method A consistently calculated lower driving pressure. Method D did not demonstrate a consistent pattern.

Supplementary Material 3 | Mean compliance and driving pressure measurements for methods A, B, C, and D under each ventilator setting and the differences between these means for each method under each setting. Ninety five percent confidence intervals for the differences and Bland-Altman limits of agreement (LOA) are calculated. A statistically significant difference is denoted by confidence intervals that do not intersect the "zero line."

Supplementary Material 4 | Linear mixed-effects regression models showing the average linear effect of each ventilator setting change on the compliance or driving pressure outcome; effects greater than 0 indicate that increasing that setting is associated with an increase in the outcome, and decreasing that setting with a decrease in the outcome; and, vice versa for effects less than 0. Although statistically significant patterns were sometimes noted, the values are averages and the patterns typically did not hold for each individual subject.

REFERENCES

Al-Rawas, N., Banner, M. J., Euliano, N. R., Tams, C. G., Brown, J., Martin, A. D., et al. (2013). Expiratory time constant for determinations of plateau pressure, respiratory system compliance, and total resistance. *Crit. Care* 17:R23. doi: 10.1186/cc12500

Amato, M. B., Meade, M. O., Slutsky, A. S., Brochard, L., Costa, E. L., Schoenfeld, D. A., et al. (2015). Driving pressure and survival in the acute respiratory distress syndrome. *N. Engl. J. Med.* 372, 747–755. doi: 10.1056/NEJMsa1410639

Brower, R. G., Matthay, M. A., Morris, A., Schoenfeld, D., Thompson, B. T., and Wheeler, A. (2000). Ventilation with lower tidal volumes as compared with traditional tidal volumes for acute lung injury and the acute respiratory distress syndrome. *N. Engl. J. Med.* 342, 1301–1308. doi: 10.1056/NEJM200005043421801

Esteban, A., Anzueto, A., Frutos, F., Alía, I., Brochard, L., Stewart, T. E., et al. (2002). Characteristics and outcomes in adult patients receiving mechanical ventilation - a 28-day international study. *JAMA* 287, 345–355. doi: 10.1001/jama.287.3.345

Goligher, E. C., Costa, E. L. V., Yarnell, C. J., Brochard, L. J., Stewart, T. E., Tomlinson, G., et al. (2021). Effect of lowering Vt on mortality in acute respiratory distress syndrome varies with respiratory system elastance. *Am. J. Respir. Crit. Care Med.* 203, 1378–1385. doi: 10.1164/rccm.202009-3536OC

Hamahata, N. T., Sato, R., and Daoud, E. G. (2020). Go with the flow-clinical importance of flow curves during mechanical ventilation: a narrative review. *Can. J. Respir. Ther.* 56, 11–20. doi: 10.29390/cjrt-2020-002

Harris, P. A., Taylor, R., Thielke, R., Payne, J., Gonzalez, N., and Conde, J. G. (2009). Research electronic data capture (REDCap)–a metadata-driven methodology and workflow process for providing translational research informatics support. *J. Biomed. Inform.* 42, 377–381. doi: 10.1016/j.jbi.2008.08.010

Marini, J. J. (2020). Hysteresis as an indicator of recruitment and ventilator-induced lung injury risk. *Crit. Care Med.* 48, 1542–1543. doi: 10.1097/CCM.0000000000004533

Milic-Emili, J. R., Robatto, F. M., and Bates, J. H. T. (1990). Respiratory mechanics in anesthesia. *Br. J. Anesth.* 65, 4–12.

R Core Team (2020). *R: A Language and Environment for Statistical Computing.* Vienna: R Foundation for Statistical Computing.

14

MicroRNA-7 Deficiency Ameliorates the Pathologies of Acute Lung Injury through Elevating KLF4

*Juanjuan Zhao[1†], Chao Chen[1†], Mengmeng Guo[1], Yijin Tao[1], PanPan Cui[1], Ya Zhou[2], Nalin Qin[1], Jing Zheng[1], Jidong Zhang[1] and Lin Xu[1]**

[1] *Department of Immunology, Zunyi Medical College, Guizhou, China,* [2] *Department of Medical Physics, Zunyi Medical College, Guizhou, China*

***Correspondence:**
Lin Xu
xulinzhouya@163.com

† *Juanjuan Zhao and Chao Chen contributed equally to this work.*

Recent evidence showed that microRNA-7 (miR-7) played an important role in the pathologies of lung-related diseases. However, the potential role of miR-7 in acute lung injury (ALI) still remains poorly understood. Here, we assessed the effect of miR-7 deficiency on the pathology of ALI. We, first, found that the expression of miR-7 was upregulated in lung tissue in murine LPS-induced ALI model. Notably, we generated miR-7 knock down mice by using miRNA-Sponge technique and found that miR-7 deficiency could ameliorate the pathologies of lung as evidenced by accelerated body weight recovery, reduced level of bronchoalveolar lavage (BAL) proinflammatory cytokines and decreased number of BAL cells in ALI mice. Moreover, the proportion and number of various immune cells in BAL, including innate immune cell F4/80$^+$ macrophages, γδT cells, NK1.1$^+$ T cells, and CD11c$^+$DCs, as well as adaptive immune cell CD4$^+$ T cells and CD8$^+$ T cells, also significantly changed, respectively. Mechanistic evidence showed that KLF4, a target molecule of miR-7, was upregulated in lung tissues in ALI model, accompanied by altered transduction of NF-κB, AKT, and ERK pathway. These data provided a previously unknown role of miR-7 in pathology of ALI, which could ultimately aid the understanding of development of ALI and the development of new therapeutic strategies against clinical inflammatory lung diseases.

Keywords: miR-7KD, acute lung injury, immune cells, cytokines, KLF4

INTRODUCTION

The development of acute lung injury (ALI), a clinically important complication of severe ALI in humans is a complex process, including a series of integrated steps, including the infiltration of innate and adaptive immune cells and the conversion in the balance of proinflammatory and anti-inflammatory cytokines (1–4). Recent evidence showed that microRNAs (miRNAs), small endogenous RNAs of 21–25 nucleotides capable of guiding the post-transcriptional silencing of their target mRNAs through base pairing encompassing mature mRNA 3′UTR (5, 6), played an important regulatory role in the development of ALI (7, 8). For example, Li et al. (9) reported that cardiopulmonary bypass-induced ALI could lead to dynamic changes in miRNA expression in lungs, including miR-21, miR-127, miR-145, and miR-204. Xu et al. (10) found that miR-17 expression was downregulated during development of ALI, accompanied by upregulation of its target gene FoxA1, and may play an important role in ALI. Our previously study also found that miR-155 ASO treatment could enhance the recovery of ALI through C/EBPβ, which was mediated by IL-10-secreting M2-like macrophages (Mφ) induced expansion of Tregs (11). These studies indicated that miRNAs might be a potential candidate for the therapy against ALI. Therefore, further study on the possible role of distinct miRNA molecules in the development of ALI could not only benefit the understanding of pathology of ALI but also be valuable for the development of novel clinical therapeutic strategies.

MiR-7 was a distinct miRNA family member and played an important role in the context of health, especially in organ differentiation and development (12, 13). Recent studies showed that miR-7 was involved in the development of various mammalian diseases, including lung-related diseases (14, 15). To lung cancer, accumulating evidence suggested that miR-7 was an important regulator in the development of lung cancer through controlling the growth and invasion, as well as apoptosis, of lung cancer cells and was emerged as a novel potential therapeutic target in lung cancer. Similarly, our new evidence also showed that miR-7 could regulate the proliferation and metastasis of lung cancer cells *in vitro* and *in vivo* (16). Moreover, the reduced expression of miR-7 was associated with the sites mutation of its promoter region in lung cancer tissues (17). However, the potential role of miR-7 in other lung-related diseases remains largely unknown. Interestingly, Akbas et al. (18) reported that the level of miR-7 was increased and might be a potential biomarker in chronic obstructive pulmonary disease. Moreover, Buggele et al. (19) found that influenza A virus infection could induce the expression of miR-7 in human respiratory cells, indicating miR-7 may be involved in the antivirus inflammatory reaction. Therefore, these studies raised a question regarding whether miR-7 also was involved in the development of lung-related inflammatory diseases, including ALI, which remains to be fully elucidated.

To address this aim, we generated miR-7 knock down (KD) mice by using miRNAs-Sponge technique and found that miR-7 deficiency could obviously attenuate the pathologies of lung in LPS-induced ALI mice model, which related to altered expression of related cytokines and infiltration of innate and adaptive immune cells. Of note, KLF4, a target molecule of miR-7, was upregulated in lung tissues, accompanied with reduced expression of NF-κB and phosphorylation of AKT and ERK. Thus, it is the first study showed that miR-7 played an important role in the pathology of ALI, closely correlated with upregulated expression of KLF4, which could ultimately aid the understanding of development of ALI and the development of new therapeutic strategies against clinical inflammatory lung diseases.

MATERIALS AND METHODS

Generation of miR-7 Knock Down Mice

We annealed and ligated, gel purified and cloned oligonucleotides for miR-7 binding sites with 5-nt spacers (one spacer: 5′-CGCG-3′) for 6 bulged sites (one bulged site: 5′-AACAAAATCGAGG--TCTTCCA-3′), into pEGFP-C2 vector (Invitrogen) digested with *Hind*III and *Kpn*I enzyme for the construction of pEGFP-C2-miR-7 sponge vector.

We next established miR-7 KD (miR-7KD) FVB/N mice using pEGFP-C2-miR-7 sponge vector with the help of Cyagen Biosciences Inc. To identify miR-7KD mice, we designed the primers spanning the EGFP sites and miR-7SP sequence, forward (P1): CGCACCATCTTCTTCAAGGA, reverse (P2): TGGAAGACCTCGATTTTGTTC. The predicted PCR product was 505 bp. All animals were housed under specific pathogen-free conditions at Zunyi Medical College. And all animal experiments were performed according to the guidelines for the Care and Use of Laboratory Animals (Ministry of Health, China, 1998). The experimental procedures were approved by the ethical guidelines of Zunyi Medical College laboratory Animal Care and Use committee (permit number 2013016).

LPS-Induced Murine ALI

FVB/N mice (8- to 10-week-old) and miR-7KD mice (8- to 10-week-old) were challenged with i.p. injection of 10 mg/kg LPS (*Escherichia coli* 0111:B4; Sigma) dissolved in 150 μl PBS. Then the body weight of all mice was detected for 10 consecutive days. At indicated time point, the bronchoalveolar lavage (BAL) sample, lung tissue, or spleen were obtained.

Bronchoalveolar Lavage

Immediately after euthanasia and exsanguination, 1.8 ml aliquots of PBS were slowly infused in the murine lungs through the tracheostomy and then withdrawn gently. Drainage or suction of perflubron or exudate in the airway was not performed before this lavage. This lavage was repeated four times using the same syringe. The collected lavage fluid was stored in a 2-ml tube on ice. The fluid was centrifuged at 400 × *g* and 4°C for 5 min, and the cell sediment was washed with PBS. The cell-free supernatant was centrifuged again at 16,000 × *g* and 4°C for 10 min, stored at −80°C and used for determination of cytokine content via ELISA. To the pellet, contaminating erythrocytes were lysed with 1 ml 0.15 M NH_4Cl solution for 5 min and washed with PBS. Next, the pellet was resuspended for analysis.

Histopathology

Lung tissue was fixed in 4% paraformaldehyde, embedded in paraffin, and cut into 4-μm-thick sections. Sections were stained with H&E, and images were taken with Olympus IX-71 microscope. Two investigators blinded to group assignments analyzed the samples and determined levels of lung injury. All lung fields at original magnification 200×, 100×, and 40× were examined for each sample.

Flow Cytometry

Surface markers of various immune cells were evaluated by flow cytometry (FCM) with Beckman Gallios (Beckman Coulter, Inc.). FCM was performed on Beckman Gallios (Beckman Coulter, Inc.) with CellQuest Pro software using directly anti-Mouse monoclonal conjugated mAbs against the following markers: F4/80-Percp-Cy5.5 (clone: BM8; no. 45-4801-82), γδT-APC (clone: eBioGL3; no. 17-5711-81), NK1.1-APC (clone: PK136; no. 17-5941-81), CD11c-PE (clone: N418; no. 12-0114-82), CD86-APC (clone: GL1; no. 17-0862-81) and MHC-II-PE (clone: M5/114.15.2; no. 12-5321-81), CD4-Percp-Cy5.5 (clone: GK1.5; no. 12-0041-82), CD8-Percp-Cy7 (clone: 53-6.7; no. 25-0081-81), CD62L-PE (clone: MEL-14; no. 12-0621-81), CD69-APC (clone: H1.2F3; no. 17-0691-82), with corresponding isotype-matched controls (eBioscience). To detect proportion of F4/80$^+$ cells, γδT$^+$ cells, NK1.1$^+$ cells, CD11c$^+$ DC cells, CD4$^+$ T cells, and CD8$^+$ T cells, as well as functional molecule expression of CD86 and MHC-II on F4/80$^+$ cells, and surface molecule expression of CD62L and CD69 on CD4$^+$ T cells in BAL and splenocytes, cells were stained with these corresponding Abs (1:100), respectively, at 4°C for 30 min and washed twice before analysis, according to the manufacturer's protocol.

Real-Time PCR

The conventional primers were obtained from Shanghai Sangon Biological Engineering CO., and the TaqMan probes of miR-7 (000386) and U6 (001793) were purchased from Life Technologies, the other reagents were from TAKARA Bio Inc., Reverse transcriptase reactions and real-time PCR assays were performed according to the manufacturer's protocols, all Reverse transcriptase reactions, including no-template controls and Reverse transcriptase minus controls, were run in triplicate in BIO-RAD CFX96 (Bio-Rad Laboratories). The expression of miR-7 was performed according to the TaqMan assays and samples were normalized by evaluating U6 expression. The other following primers were used: IL-6 forward: 5′-GGAAATCGTGGAAATGAG-3′, reverse: 5′-AGGACTCTGGCTTTGTCT-3′; IL-4 forward: 5′-AACG AGGTCACAGGAGAA-3′, reverse: 5′-CCTTGGAAGCCCTAC AGA-3′; IFN-γ forward: 5′-TCTGAGACAATGAACGCTAC-3′, reverse: 5′-TTCACATCTATGCCACT-3′; KLF4 forward: 5′-GCCCAACACACACGACTTC-3′, reverse: 5′-GGCAGGA AAGGAGGGTAGTT-3′; GAPDH forward: 5′-AGCAGTCCCG TACACTGGCAAAC-3′, reverse: 5′-TCTGTGGTGATGTAAA TGTCCTCT-3′. Gene expression levels were quantified using the BIO-RAD CFX96 detection system (Bio-Rad Laboratories), and the samples were normalized by evaluating GAPDH. Relative expression was calculated using the comparative threshold cycle (Ct) method.

ELISA

The BAL level of TNF-α, IL-1β, IL-6, TGF-β, IL-10, as well as IL-4, and serum level of TNF-α, IL-10 were determined using Quantikine Immunoassay kits according to the manufacturer's instructions, respectively (eBioscience).

Western Blotting

Western blotting was performed on cytosolic cellular extracts. Equal amounts of protein were resolved under reducing conditions on a 10% SDS-polyacrylamide gel. Protein migration was assessed using protein standards (Bio-Rad, CA, USA). Transfer to a nitrocellulose membrane was performed 60 min at 250 mA using a wet transfer system. Equal protein loading was confirmed with Ponceau staining. The membrane was washed in 5% skim milk in PBS plus 0.05% Tween 20 (PBST) for 2 h to block nonspecific protein-binding sites on the membrane. Immunoblotting was performed using an mAb to Rabbit-polyclonal anti-mouse KLF4 (Cell Signaling Technology; no. 4038), Rabbit-monoclonal anti-mouse NF-κB (Cell Signaling Technology; no. 4764), Rabbit-polyclonal anti-mouse p-NF-κB (Cell Signaling Technology; no. 3039), Rabbit-monoclonal anti-mouse ERK (Cell Signaling Technology; no. 4695), Rabbit-polyclonal anti-mouse p-ERK (Cell Signaling Technology; no. 4370), Rabbit-monoclonal anti-mouse AKT (Cell Signaling Technology; no. 4691) or Rabbit-monoclonal anti-mouse p-AKT (Cell Signaling Technology; no. 4060), Rabbit-monoclonal anti-mouse β-Actin (Cell Signaling Technology; no. 4970) at a dilution of 1/800 in a non-fat milk-Tris buffer. The membrane was then washed in PBST and subsequently probed with a secondary anti-rabbit Ab-conjugated to HRP (Cell Signaling Technology; no. 7074) at a dilution of 1:2000. The signal was detected and analyzed using the chemiluminescence Imaging System (ChemiScope5600, CLINX, Shanghai, China), each experiment was performed in triplicate.

Immunohistochemistry

Immunohistochemical staining was performed following standard procedures. The formalin-fixed paraffin-embedded tissues were sliced into 4-μm-thick sections, deparaffinized, and rehydrated. Then, the cells were fixed with 95% ethanol for 15 min. Antigen retrieval was performed in 10 mmol/L citric acid buffer (pH 6.0) for 10 min using a 750 W microwave. Endogenous peroxidase activity was blocked with 3% hydrogen peroxide in methanol for 15 min. After incubation with rabbit anti-mouse KLF4 antibody (1:1000 dilution; CST; no. 3087) and anti-mouse NF-κB antibody (1:100 dilution; CST; no. 4764) overnight at 4°C, the sections were washed in phosphate-buffered saline and incubated with a polymer horseradish peroxidase-conjugated secondary antibody (ZSGB-Bio, Beijing, China) for 60 min. The sections were further incubated with Liquid DAB Large-Volume Substrate-Chromogen System (ZSGB-Bio, Beijing, China) and counterstained with hematoxylin. The immunostaining was evaluated using an Olympus IX-71 light microscope (Olympus, Tokyo, Japan).

In Situ Hybridization

To evaluate the cellular distribution of miR-7 in the lungs, *in situ* hybridization was performed based as previously described (20) with some modifications. Briefly, before hybridization incubation, all solutions were prepared with diethyl pyrocarbonate-treated water. After deparaffinization and rehydration, tissue sections were treated by proteinase K digestion. After blocking with normal goat serum (1:100), sections were next incubated or microwave heating and were then incubated with hybridization cocktail containing miR-7 probe (1:1000 dilution; EXIQON; no. 38485-01) at 42°C for 16 h. Then alkaline phosphatase-labeled anti-digoxigenin antibody (1:500) (Roche Diagnostics) for 1 h, and the reaction products were colorized with nitro blue tetrazolium/5-bromo-4-choloro-3-indolyl phosphate (NBT/BCIP) (ZSGB-Bio, Beijing, China), then the tissues were counterstained with Mayer's hematoxylin and systematically viewed under a light microscope (Olympus IX-71).

Statistical Analyses

The data were analyzed with GraphPad Prism 5.0 and were presented as the mean ± SD. Student's *t*-test was used when two conditions were compared, and analysis of variance with Bonferroni or Newman–Keuls correction was used for multiple comparisons. Probability values of <0.05 were considered significant; two-sided tests were performed.

RESULTS

Generation of miR-7 Knock Down Mice

To investigate the potential role of miR-7 in the development of ALI, we detected the relative expression level of miR-7 in murine 12 organs, including heart, lung, brain, kidney, and so on. Data showed that miR-7 expression had a higher level in lung tissue (Figure S1A in Supplementary Material). Expectedly, we further found that the expression of miR-7 significantly increased in pathogenic lung tissues in LPS-induced ALI mice (Figure S1B in Supplementary Material, $p < 0.05$). Together, these data indicated that miR-7 might be involved in the development of ALI.

Accumulating evidence showed that miRNA Sponge strategy was valuable approach for the downregulation of specific miRNA expression *in vivo* (21, 22). Moreover, it is difficult to generate miR-7 deficiency mice using traditional strategies, including TALENs and CRISPR, because of mature miR-7 molecule is transcribed from three different genomic loci on chromosomes 9, 15 and 19, respectively (23). Then, we used miRNA Sponge (miR-SP) strategy to generate mice with miR-7 deficiency. The design and proof of principle of miR-SP technology is to construct a eukaryotic expression vector encoding an expression cassette for miR-7-SP sequence, the miR-7-SP elements included inserting tandemly arrayed miR-7 binding sites into the 3′UTR of a reporter gene encoding destabilized EGFP driven by the CMV promoter. Binding sites for miR-7 seed family were perfectly complementary in the seed region with a bulge at positions 9–12 to prevent RNA interference-type cleavage and degradation of the sponge RNA, the bulge contained six repetitive sequences complementary to miR-7 with mismatches for enhanced stability (**Figure 1A**). Then, transgenic mice were generated carrying one or two copies of the miR-SP cassette through putting the miR-7SP carrier to inject murine fertilized eggs, after which were transplanted into the oviduct of pseudo-pregnant mice female, and 3 weeks after birth (**Figure 1B**). To verify a special KD of miR-7 in FVB/N mice, we designed primers (P1 and P2) spanning the EGFP sites and miR-7SP sequence, and the predicted PCR product size was 505 bp. Then, we detected both wild-type (WT) mice and miR-7KD mice, while only miR-7KD mice could amplify 505 bp specific products (**Figure 1C**). Importantly, we found that the relative expression of miR-7 was obviously reduced in lung in miR-7KD mice (**Figure 1D**, $p < 0.05$). To confirm these data, we further detected the expression of miR-7 in lung tissues of miR-7KD mice using *in situ* hybridization and obtained similar results (**Figure 1E**). Consistently, the relative expression of miR-7 in other various organs and tissues in miR-7KD mice also decreased significantly (Figure S2 in Supplementary Material, $p < 0.05$). These results demonstrated that miR-7KD mice were successfully generated using miR-SP Technology.

Deficiency of miR-7 Ameliorated the Pathologies of ALI

Next, we observed the possible effects of miR-7 deficiency on the development of ALI using a murine model of LPS-induced ALI. Results showed that the loss of body weight was attenuated in LPS-treated miR-7KD group, compared with that in LPS-treated WT group (**Figures 2A,B**, $p < 0.05$). Importantly, the morphology of lung tissue of mice in LPS-treated miR-7KD group was smaller than that in LPS-treated WT group (**Figure 2C**). Furthermore, the weight and the weight index of lung tissue were also significantly reduced (**Figures 2D,E**, $p < 0.05$). Meanwhile, hematoxylin-eosin staining showed that the infiltration of inflammatory cells in lung tissue of miR-7KD ALI mice markedly decreased (**Figure 2F**). The cell apoptosis of lung tissue was involved in the pathology of lung injury (24, 25). As shown in **Figure 2G**, real-time PCR analysis further showed that the expression of anti-apoptotic proteins BCL-XL in lung tissue increased significantly in LPS-treated miR-7KD mice ($p < 0.05$), even though the expression of p53 did not change significantly ($p > 0.05$). Conversely, the expression of pro-apoptotic proteins BAX and BAD were decreased obviously ($p < 0.05$), indicating the cell apoptosis of lung tissue decreased in miR-7KD ALI mice.

To confirm this phenomenon, we further detected the level of related cytokines in ALI mice. As shown in **Figures 2H–J**, the concentration of proinflammatory factor TNF-α, IL-1β, and IFN-γ in BAL in LPS-treated miR-7KD group decreased significantly compared with those in the control group on 3 days ($p < 0.05$). By contrast, the concentration of anti-inflammatory factor IL-10 and TGF-β increased noticeably ($p < 0.05$), even though the concentration of IL-4 in BAL did not change significantly (**Figures 2K–M**, $p > 0.05$). To verify these data, we detected the relative expression of these cytokines in lung tissues, and similar results were obtained (Figure S3 in Supplementary Material). Finally, we also detected the serum level of cytokines TNF-α and IL-10, respectively. Data showed that the serum level of TNF-α decreased in LPS-treated miR-7KD mice (Figure S4A in Supplementary Material, $p < 0.05$). Conversely, the serum level of IL-10 increased significantly (Figure S4B in Supplementary Material, $p < 0.05$). Combining these data demonstrated that miR-7 deficiency could obviously ameliorate the pathologies of ALI.

miR-7 Deficiency Altered the Composition of Immune Cells in BAL of ALI Mice

The change of immune cell composition, which was closely related to inflammatory responses, plays a pivotal role in the pathology of ALI (26, 27). Hence, we examined the total number cells in BAL from LPS-treated WT and miR-7KD mice. As shown in **Figure 3A**, the total number of inflammatory cells in BAL from miR-7KD ALI mice was significantly decreased ($p < 0.05$). We further analyzed the possible changes on proportion of the innate immune cells, including F4/80$^+$ Mφ, $\gamma\delta$T cells, NK1.1$^+$ T cells, CD11c$^+$ Dendritic cells (DCs) in BAL from miR-7KD ALI mice and found that the proportion and the absolute number of F4/80$^+$ Mφ and CD11c$^+$ DCs obviously reduced in BAL (**Figures 3B,C,F,G**, $p < 0.05$). Unexpectedly, the absolute number of $\gamma\delta$T cells in BAL did not change significantly (**Figures 3B,C**, $p > 0.05$), even though the proportion of $\gamma\delta$T cells increased (**Figures 3B,C**, $p < 0.05$). Meanwhile, we also investigated the possible change on adaptive immune cells CD4$^+$ T cells and CD8$^+$ T cells, which also played important roles in the development of ALI, in BAL of LPS-treated miR-7KD mice. The results showed

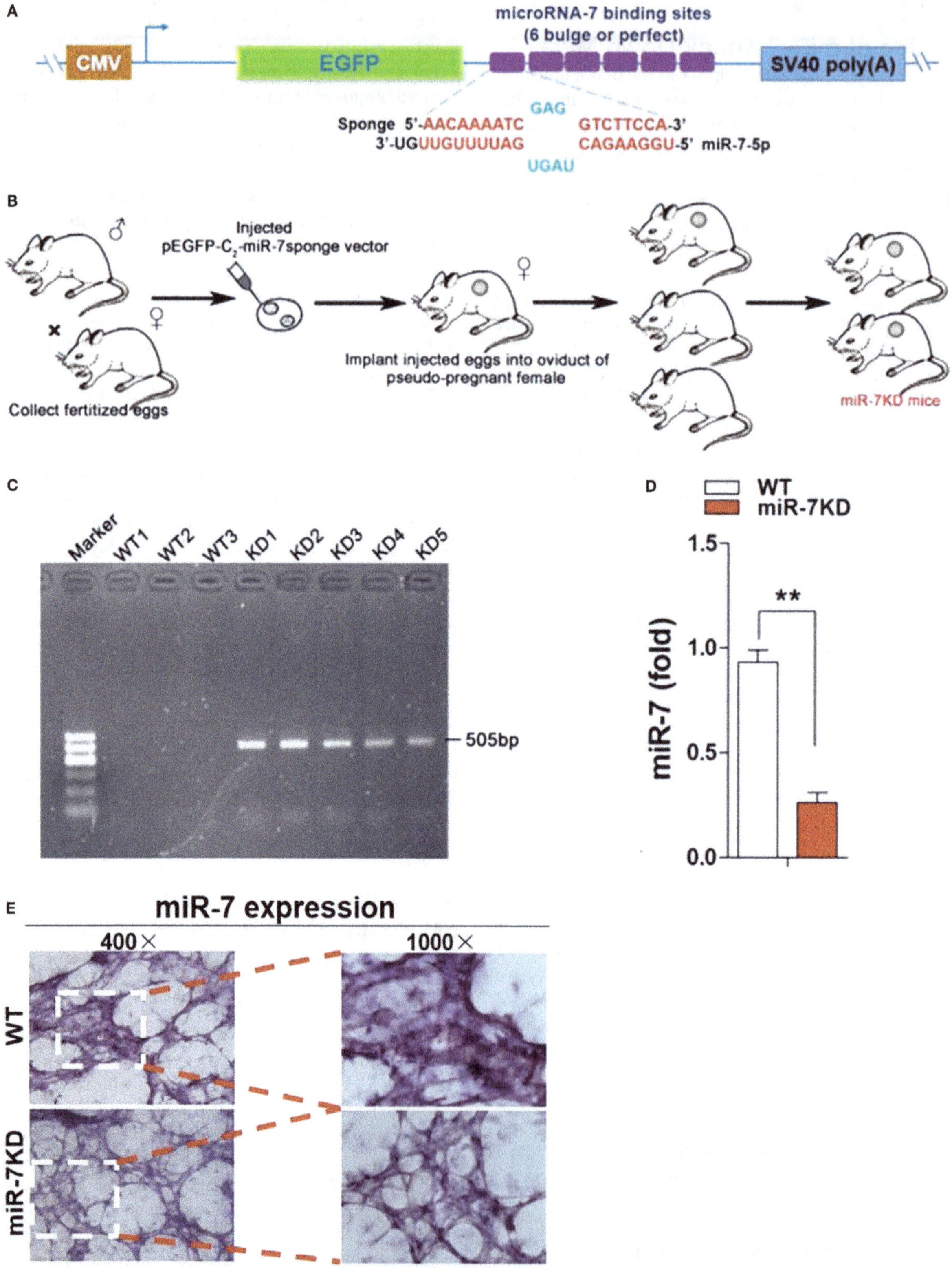

FIGURE 1 | The generation of miR-7 deficiency mice. The sketch map of construction of eukaryotic expression vector encoding miR-7-Sponge (termed as p-miR-7-Sp) **(A)** and generation of miR-7 KD mice **(B)**. **(C)** The identification of DNA. DNA was derived from wild-type (WT) or miR-7KD mice. And the expected product (505 bp size) was amplificated by PCR, respectively. **(D)** The relative expression of miR-7 in lung derived from WT mice and miR-7KD mice ($n = 6$) were detected by Real-time PCR assay. **(E)** The expression of miR-7 in lung tissue derived from WT mice and miR-7KD was analyzed by *In situ* hybridization. Representative data of three independent experiments were shown. $^{**}p < 0.01$.

that the proportion and the absolute number of $CD4^+$ T cells and $CD8^+$ T cells are also obviously reduced in BAL (**Figures 3H,I**, $p < 0.05$). To confirm this phenomenon, we also observed the total number, the proportion, and the absolute number of the innate immune cells, including F4/80^+ Mφ, γδT cells, NK1.1^+ T cells, CD11c^+ DCs, and adaptive immune cells, including $CD4^+$ T cells and $CD8^+$ T cells in the spleen. Expectedly, similar results also were obtained (Figures S5A–C,F–I in Supplementary Material).

As known, the expression of the functional membrane molecules on immune cells was closely related to the pathological status of inflammatory diseases (28); hence, the expression of CD86 and MHC-II molecule in F4/80^+ Mφ were analyzed. FCM

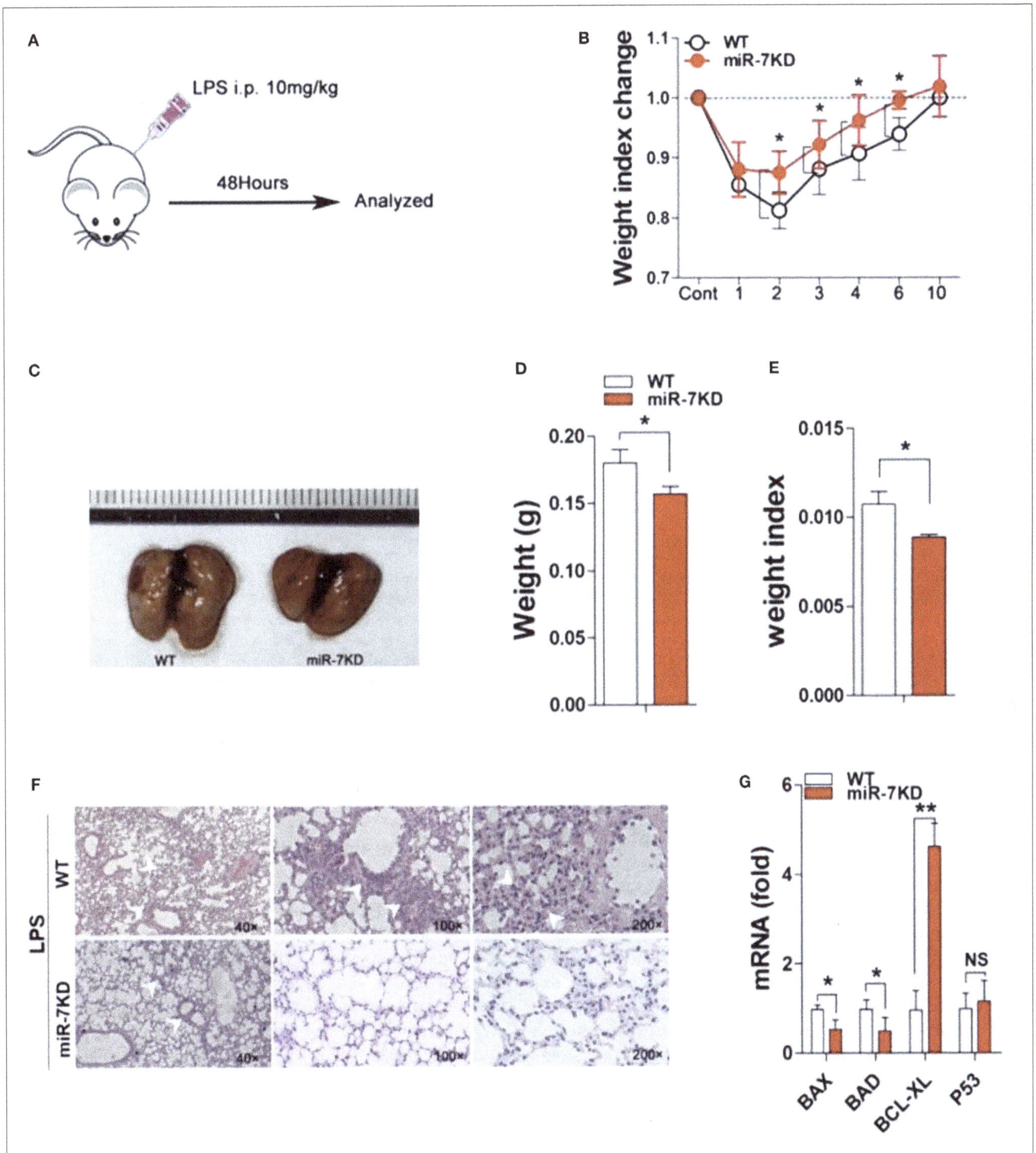

FIGURE 2 | Continued

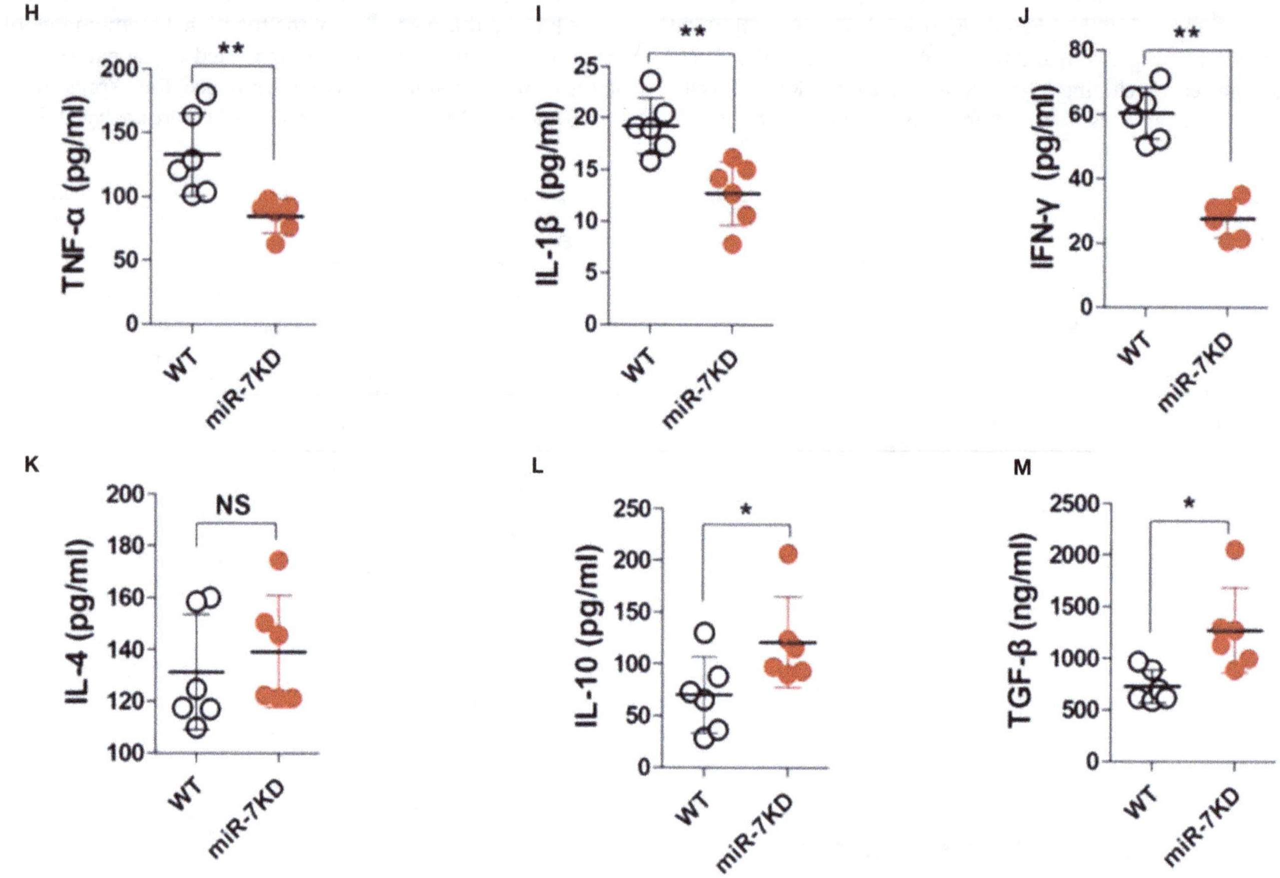

FIGURE 2 | miR-7 deficiency ameliorated the pathology of ALI. FVB/N6 mice (WT, $n = 6$) and miR-7KD mice ($n = 6$) were administered with i.p. 10 mg/kg LPS, respectively. **(A)** Schematic representation of the animal study. **(B)** The change on the body weight of WT and miR-7KD mice at indicated time point was observed. **(C)** FVB/N6 mice (WT, $n = 6$) and miR-7KD mice ($n = 6$) were administered with i.p. 10 mg/kg LPS, respectively. After 48 h, the morphology, **(D)** the body weight, and **(E)** the weight index (tissue weight/body weight), as well as **(F)** the pathology, of lung tissues were analyzed, respectively. **(G)** The relative expression of BAD, BAX, BCL-XL, and p53 in lung tissue also were analyzed by Real-time PCR assay. **(H–M)** FVB/N6 mice (WT, $n = 6$) and miR-7KD mice ($n = 6$) were administered with i.p. 10 mg/kg LPS, respectively. After 48 h, BAL was collected and the level of IFN-γ, IL-1β, TNF-α, IL-4, and IL-10, as well as TGF-β, was determined with ELISA, respectively. Representative data of three independent experiments were shown. $^{*}p < 0.05$, $^{**}p < 0.01$.

analysis showed that the proportion and absolute number of CD86 positive F4/80$^+$ Mφ obviously reduced. And the absolute number of MHC-II positive F4/80$^+$ Mφ also decreased significantly in BAL, even though the proportion of cells increased (**Figures 3D,E**). Next, we further analyzed the expression of activation molecules CD62L and CD69, respectively, in both CD4$^+$ T cells and CD8$^+$ T cells. Data showed that the expression of CD62L on CD4$^+$ T cells and CD8$^+$ T cells were significantly upregulated (**Figures 3J,K**, $p < 0.05$). Conversely, the expression of CD69 on CD4$^+$ T cells and CD8$^+$ T cells were significantly downregulated (**Figures 3J,K**, $p < 0.05$), indicating reduced activation of CD4$^+$ T cells and CD8$^+$ T cells. Consistent with above data, the absolute number of these cells were also reduced vigorously (**Figures 3J,K**, $p < 0.05$). Similarly, we also obtained the consistent results in the spleen from LPS-treated miR-7KD mice (Figures S5D,E,J,K in Supplementary Material). In summary, our results demonstrate that miR-7 deficiency could significantly affect the composition and function of various immune cells in BAL, which was closely related to ameliorated pathology of lung in ALI mice.

The Expression of KLF4 Was Upregulated in Lung Tissues in LPS-Treated miR-7KD Mice

To elucidate the potential molecular mechanism through which miR-7 deficiency affected the pathologies of lung injury, we searched for putative targets of miR-7 using computer-aided miRNA target prediction program, including TargetScan4, miRanda, and PicTar, and found 12 putative miR-7 target genes, including Snap23, TAB2, KLF4, Smad5, MAPK4, FSTL-1, Tle-4, OGT-1, RAF-1, MAPK8, MAPKAP-1, and PTK2, which also were closely associated with inflammation reaction according to previous literatures (29–34). Then, we detected the expression of these 12 predicted target genes in the lung tissues derived from LPS-treated WT mice and miR-7KD mice, respectively. Unexpectedly,

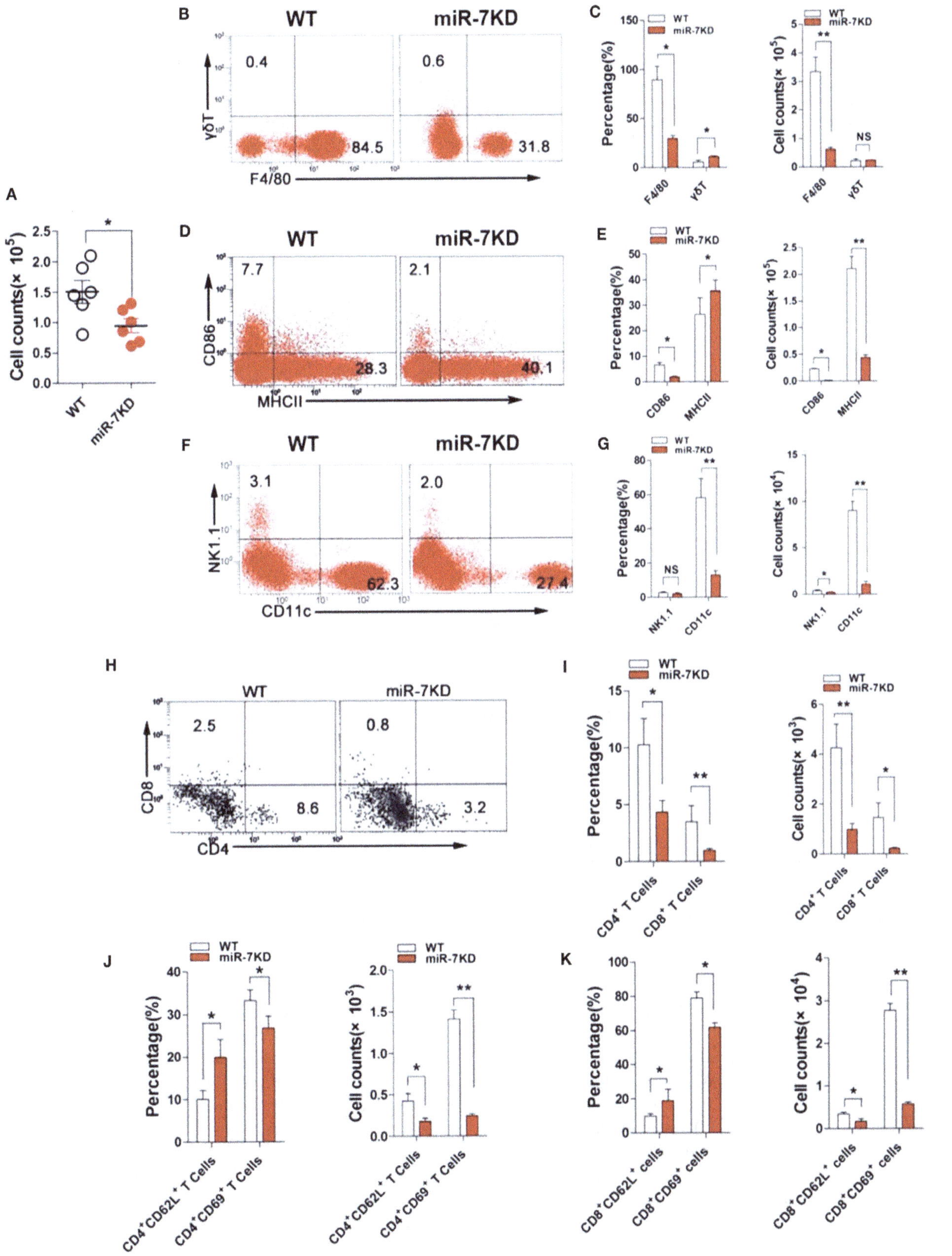

FIGURE 3 | **miR-7 deficiency altered the immune cell composition in BAL of mice from ALI.**

(Continued)

FIGURE 3 | Continued

FVB/N6 mice (WT, $n = 6$) and miR-7KD mice ($n = 6$) were administered with i.p. 10 mg/kg LPS, respectively. After 48 h, **(A)** the total numbers of BAL cells were calculated. **(B)** The proportion of F4/80+ Mφ and γδ+ T cells were analyzed by FCM. The percentage and the absolute number of cells were calculated, respectively **(C)**. **(D)** The expression of CD86 and MHC-II on F4/80+ Mφ were analyzed by FCM. The percentage and the absolute number of cells were calculated, respectively **(E)**. **(F)** The proportion of CD11c+ dendritic cells and NK1.1+ T cells were analyzed by FCM. The percentage and the absolute number of cells were calculated, respectively **(G)**. **(H)** The proportion of CD4+ T cells and CD8+ T cells were analyzed by FCM. The percentage and the absolute number of cells were calculated, respectively **(I)**. **(J)** The expression of CD62L and CD69 on CD4+ T cells were analyzed by FCM. And, the percentage and the absolute number of cells were also calculated, respectively. **(K)** The expression of CD62L and CD69 on CD8+ T cells were analyzed by FCM. And, the percentage and the absolute number of cells were also calculated, respectively. Representative data of three independent experiments were shown. $^*p < 0.05$, $^{**}p < 0.01$.

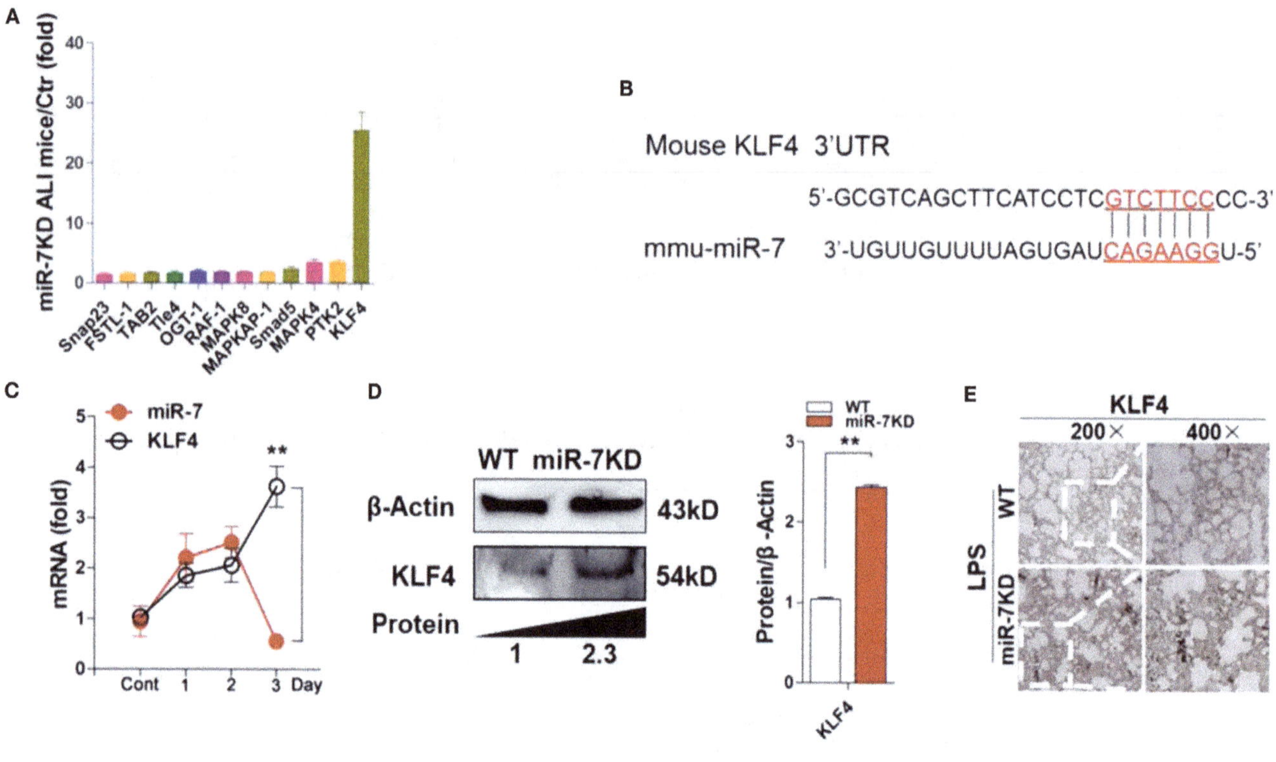

FIGURE 4 | KLF4 was upregulated in lung tissues in LPS-treated miR-7KD mice. (A) FVB/N6 mice (WT, $n = 6$) and miR-7KD mice ($n = 6$) were administered with i.p. 10 mg/kg LPS, respectively. After 48 h, the relative expression of the potential target genes of miR-7 in the lung tissue were analyzed by Real-time PCR assay. **(B)** Putative miR-7-binding sites in the 3′UTR of KLF4. **(C)** FVB/N6 mice (WT, $n = 6$) were administered with i.p. 10 mg/kg LPS. The relative expression of miR-7 and KLF4 were detected by Real-time PCR at indicated time points. **(D)** FVB/N6 mice (WT, $n = 6$) and miR-7KD mice ($n = 6$) were administered with i.p. 10 mg/kg LPS, respectively. After 48 h, KLF4 expression in lung tissue was analyzed by Western Blot and **(E)** immunohistochemical staining, respectively (original magnification 200x, 400x). Representative data of three independent experiments were shown. $^*p < 0.05$, $^{**}p < 0.01$.

Real-time PCR assay showed that only one target, KLF4, in all predicted target genes of miR-7 was significantly upregulated by more than 25-fold in the lung tissue of LPS-treated miR-7KD mice compared with LPS-treated WT mice (**Figures 4A,B**).

Recent studies showed that KLF4, a critical regulator in LPS-induced inflammatory response (35), was one of targets of miR-7 (36). Moreover, KLF4 also could promote the expression of anti-inflammatory cytokines, such as IL-10 (37). Then, to investigate the potential connection between miR-7 and KLF4 in lung injury in ALI, we further detected the relative expression of miR-7 and KLF4 in LPS-treated WT mice at different time points. As shown in **Figure 4C**, the relative expression of miR-7 increased significantly on day 1, and reached the peak on day 2, then decreased on day 3. Consistently, the relative expression of KLF4 decreased obviously in day 2 and increased significantly on day 3. Next, to verify the role of KLF4 in the effect of miR-7 deficiency on the pathology of ALI, we further detected the protein level of KLF4 in lung tissues from LPS-treated miR-7KD mice and WT mice. As shown in **Figure 4D**, the level of KLF4 protein in lung tissue was increased significantly in LPS-treated miR-7KD mice compared with that in LPS-treated WT mice ($p < 0.05$). To confirm these data, we further observed the location of KLF4 protein in the injured lung tissue. As anticipated, we found strong KLF4 protein staining on lung tissue derived from miR-7KD ALI mice compared with WT ALI mice (**Figure 4E**). Collectively, our data indicated that miR-7 deficiency could affect the pathology of ALI, which was closely due to the upregulation expression of its target KLF4.

miR-7 Deficiency Altered the Transduction of Related Signaling Pathway

The multiple signaling pathways, including AKT, ERK, and so on, were also involved in the development process of ALI (38). Moreover, KLF4 also was reported to be closely related to the transduction of these signaling pathways (39). Thus, to elucidate whether miR-7 deficiency resulted in the attenuated pathologies of ALI might be related with these signaling pathway, the expression of phosphorylation of AKT and ERK were analyzed in lung tissue derived from LPS-treated WT mice or miR-7KD mice, respectively. Data showed that there were not any change on the expression level of AKT and ERK in between miR-7KD ALI mice and WT ALI mice (**Figures 5A,B**, $p > 0.05$). However, the phosphorylation of AKT and ERK in miR-7KD ALI mice decreased significantly, compared with those in WT ALI mice (**Figures 5A,B**, $p < 0.05$).

Furthermore, we also detected the expression of NF-κB, which was critical transcription factor for inflammatory reaction, in lung tissue from miR-7KD ALI mice. Data showed that the expression of phosphorylation of NF-κB also decreased obviously

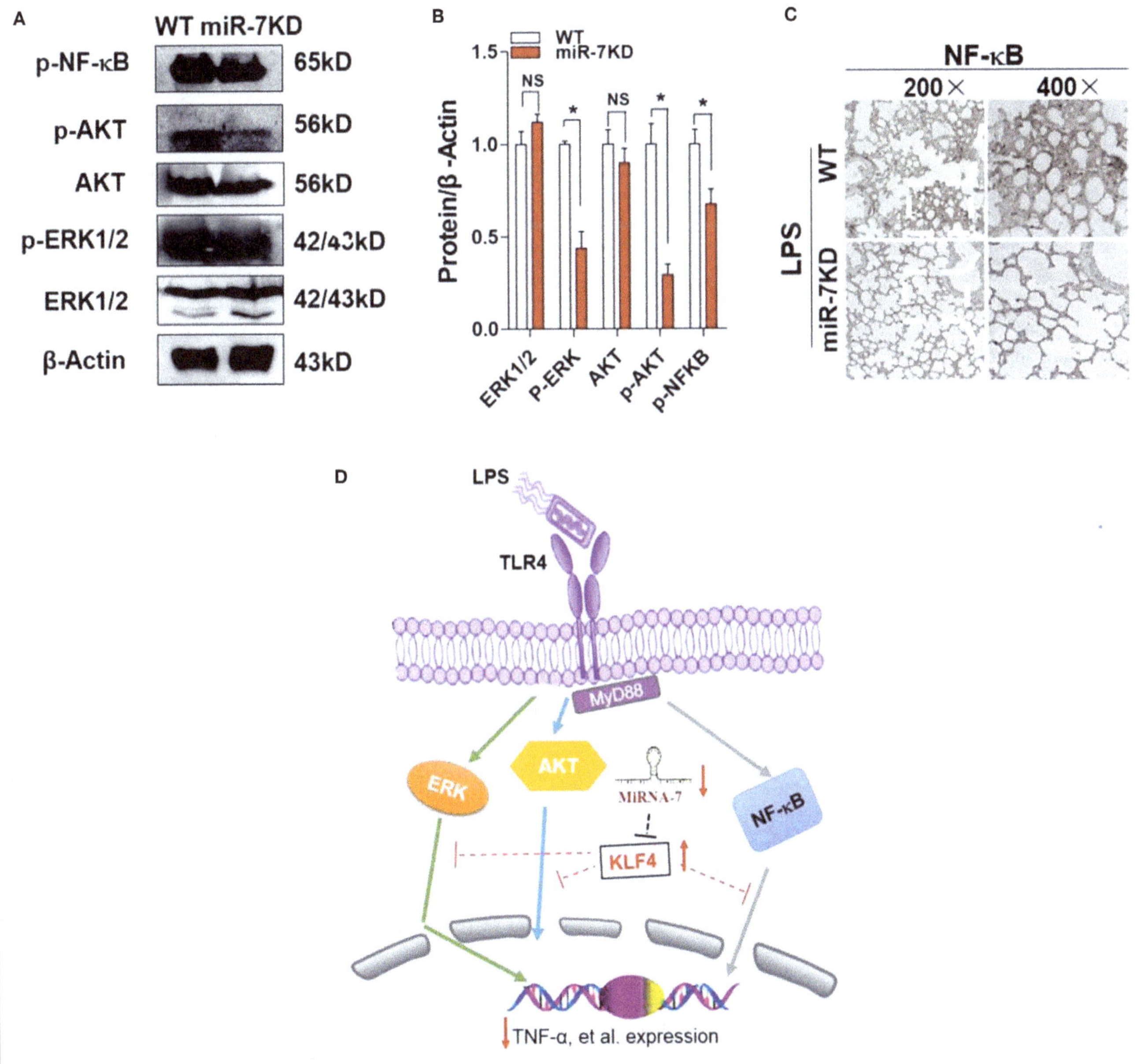

FIGURE 5 | The signaling pathway change of miR-7 deficiency in ALI. FVB/N6 mice (WT, $n = 6$) and miR-7KD mice ($n = 6$) were administered with i.p. 10 mg/kg LPS, respectively. After 48 h, the expression level of ERK, p-ERK, AKT, p-AKT, and p-NF-kB in lung tissue were determined with Western Blot **(A)** and calculated **(B)**. **(C)** The expression of NF-κB was also detected by the immunohistochemical staining. Representative data of three independent experiments were shown. $^{*}p < 0.05$, $^{**}p < 0.01$. **(D)** Schematic representation of the underlying mechanism of miR-7 deficiency on ALI. miR-7 deficiency leads to upregulation of KLF4, which could successively alter the transduction of NF-κB, ERK, and AKT signaling pathway and contribute to the ameliorated pathologies of ALI.

(**Figures 5A,B**, $p < 0.05$). To confirm this phenomenon, we further analyzed the expression of phosphorylation of NF-κB in lung tissue using immunohistochemical staining and similar result was obtained (**Figure 5C**). These results suggested that the evident effect of miR-7 deficiency on the pathology of ALI was closely correlated to the altered transduction of NF-κB and AKT, as well as ERK, signaling pathway (**Figure 5D**).

DISCUSSION

Up to now, this is the first study to explore the potential role of miR-7 in the pathologies of ALI. We, first, observed that the expression of miR-7 increased significantly in lung tissue in murine LPS-induced ALI model. Furthermore, we generated miR-7 deficiency mice by using miR-SP technology. Importantly, we found that miR-7 deficiency could significantly attenuate the pathologies of ALI, evidenced by accelerated body weight recovery, reduced infiltration of BAL cells and altered level of related cytokines, which was closely correlated to upregulation of KLF4, a target of miR-7, and altered transduction of related signaling pathway, including NF-κB, AKT, and ERK pathway.

Accumulating evidence suggested that miR-SP, which are transcripts that carry several in tandem copies of a sequence complementary to the miRNA of interest in their 3′UTRs, was a promising approach for loss-of-function strategies of distinct miRNA molecule *in vivo* (40, 41). Giusti et al developed a transgenic miRNA sponge mouse for investigation on the biological function of miR-9 in dendritic growth and synaptic transmission *in vivo* (42). Most recently, Zheng et al. constructed "Sponge" transgenic mice against miR-27a expression and found that Siglec1 and TRIM27 expression, target molecules of miR-27a, were elevated *in vivo* in antiviral innate response (43). In the current study, we generated miR-7 deficiency mice using miR-SP technology. Our data showed that the relative expression of miR-7 in various organs, including lung, spleen, brain, and so on, dramatically decreased, indicating miR-7-SP could effectively inhibit the expression of miR-7 *in vivo*. Importantly, we further found that miR-7 deficiency could obviously ameliorate the development of LPS-induced ALI, evidenced by prevention of body weight loss and reduced weight and pathological change of lung tissue. Moreover, our data further showed that, miR-7 not only was enriched in a variety of normal tissues, including brain and lung tissue, which was consistent with previous literature (44–46), but also was upregulated in lung tissue of LPS-induced ALI model. Similarly, Akbas et al. (18) reported that the level of miR-7 was increased and might be a potential biomarker in chronic obstructive pulmonary disease. These data might reflect the important role of miR-7 in the development of lung-related diseases, including ALI. Therefore, successive research work on the expression of miR-7 in clinical ALI cases, as well as the potential effect of miR-7 on other animal ALI models that were with distinct traits related to diverse pathological characters of clinical ALI, is much valuable for the validation on the role of miR-7 in pathology of ALI.

The infiltration of innate immune cells and adaptive immune cells, including Mφ, $\gamma\delta^+$ T cells, and $CD4^+$ T cells, were closely involved in the development process of ALI (47). For example, Holub and Lawrence (48) reported that the proportion of Mφ in BAL increased significantly and was contributed to the pathology of ALI. In our study, we found that the proportion and the cell absolute number of not only innate immune cells, such as $F4/80^+$ Mφ, but also adaptive immune cells, including $CD4^+$ T cells and $CD8^+$ T cells, in BAL also decreased significantly. Moreover, similar results also were obtained in splenocytes. Notably, we further reported that altered expression of activated membrane molecular, including CD86 and MHC-II, on $F4/80^+$ Mφ cells in LPS-treated miR-7 KD mice. Meanwhile, $CD4^+$ T cells and $CD8^+$ T cells also expressed lower level of CD69 and higher level of CD62L, displaying a decreased activation phenotype. Similarly, Ying et al. (49) reported that downregulation of miR-127 could impair the infiltration and function of Mφ, which was contributed to the decreased pathology of ALI. Moreover, Brusselle et al. (50) also found that the dysregulation of miRNAs could contribute to the pathogenesis of lung-associated inflammatory diseases, which were related to the impaired activation of $CD4^+$ T cells in ALI. Combining these data suggested that the change on infiltration and functional molecule of these immune cells are contributed to impaired pathologies of ALI in miR-7 KD mice. We proposed that two factors might be responsible for the change on infiltration of immune cells. First, the altered cytokine balance was important for the infiltration of immune cells because various cytokines, such as IL-10, TNF-α, and so on, could affect the migration of immune cells. Second, the potential role of miR-7 in biological function of immune cells, even was still unknown, also might be contributed to the altered migration of immune cells. It is interesting to note that recent research works showed the important role of distinct miRNA molecules in biological function of immune cells (11, 51). Therefore, our current data might provide valuable clues for the related research work on the potential function of miR-7 in immune cells, which also should be helpful for understanding the role of miR-7 in development of ALI.

It is well known that some signaling pathways, such as NF-κB, AKT, and ERK pathway, were critical for the development of inflammatory response (52–54). And KLF4, as one putative target of miR-7, played a critical role in the transduction of these signaling pathways, which were involved in the development of various diseases (55–59). To ALI, genetic analysis suggested that KLF4 was one of the leading candidate genes associated with increased susceptibility to ALI (60). And KD of KLF4 obviously augmented LPS-induced lung injury (61). In the present study, we found that the expression level of KLF4 increased in lung tissue in LPS-treated miR-7KD mice. Importantly, we further found that the transduction of NF-κB and AKT pathway, as well as ERK pathway, decreased obviously. Moreover, the level of proinflammatory cytokines, such as TNF-α, IL-1β, and IL-6, also dramatically decreased, and the level of anti-inflammatory cytokines, such as IL-10 and TGF-β1, conversely increased. Consistently, one most recent research work reported that KLF4 could potentially regulate the transduction of NF-κB pathway, which closely related to decreased levels of the pro-inflammatory cytokines TNF-α (62). Moreover, KLF4 also could bind to IL-10 and TGF-β1 promoter, as a transcriptional regulator, and upregulate the transcriptional level of IL-10 and TGF-β1, respectively (37, 63). Therefore, given the fact that regulation effect of miR-7 on KLF4 expression, these data further highlighted the critical role of miR-7/KLF4 axis in development of ALI, indicating the potential value of this axis in the development of therapeutic strategy against inflammatory lung diseases.

Taken together, as shown in **Figure 5D**, we presumed that miR-7 deficiency altered that expression of KLF4, which affected the transduction of related signaling pathway, such as NF-κB, AKT, and ERK, and successively influence on the infiltration of various immune cells and the level of inflammatory cytokines, which ultimately ameliorated the pathologies of LPS-induced ALI.

AUTHOR CONTRIBUTIONS

J Zhao and CC performed the experiments, analyzed the data, and wrote the paper; MG and YT performed the experiments and analyzed the data; PC, NQ, and J Zheng performed the experiments; YZ and J Zhang wrote the paper; LX conceived and designed the experiments, analyzed the data, and wrote the paper; and all authors reviewed the paper.

ACKNOWLEDGMENTS

We acknowledged Cyagen Biosciences Inc. for technical assistance with the generation of miR-7KD mice, and Zunyi Medical College laboratory Animal Center for providing housing and breeding places.

REFERENCES

McKenzie CG, Kim M, Singh TK, Milev Y, Freedman J, Semple JW. Peripheral blood monocyte-derived chemokine blockade prevents murine transfu- sion-related acute lung injury (TRALI). *Blood* (2014) 123(22):3496–503. doi:10.1182/blood-2013-11-536755

Zhang F, Li MY, Lan YT, Wang CB. Imbalance of Th17/Tregs in rats with smoke inhalation-induced acute lung injury. *Sci Rep* (2016) 6:21348. doi:10.1038/srep21348

Wang J, Li F, Sun R, Gao X, Wei H, Li LJ, et al. Bacterial colonization dampens influenza-mediated acute lung injury via induction of M2 alveolar macrophages. *Nat Commun* (2013) 4:2106. doi:10.1038/ncomms3106

Do-Umehara HC, Chen C, Urich D, Zhou L, Qiu J, Jang S, et al. Suppression of inflammation and acute lung injury by Miz1 via repression of C/EBP-δ. *Nat Immunol* (2013) 14(5):461–9. doi:10.1038/ni.2566

Luck ME, Muljo SA, Collins CB. Prospects for therapeutic targeting of MicroRNAs in human immunological diseases. *J Immunol* (2015) 194(11):5047–52. doi:10.4049/jimmunol.1403146

Loyer X, Mallat Z, Boulanger CM, Tedgui A. MicroRNAs as therapeutic targets in atherosclerosis. *Expert Opin Ther Targets* (2015) 19(4):489–96. doi: 10.1517/14728222.2014.989835

Zhou T, Garcia JG, Zhang W. Integrating microRNAs into a system biology approach to acute lung injury. *Transl Res* (2011) 157(4):180–90. doi:10.1016/j.trsl.2011.01.010

Rajasekaran S, Pattarayan D, Rajaguru P, Sudhakar Gandhi PS, Thimmulappa RK. MicroRNA regulation of acute lung injury and acute respiratory distress syndrome. *J Cell Physiol* (2016) 231(10):2097–106. doi:10.1002/jcp.25316

Li W, Ma K, Zhang S, Zhang H, Liu J, Wang X, et al. Pulmonary microRNA expression profiling in an immature piglet model of cardiopulmonary bypass-induced acute lung injury. *Artif Organs* (2015) 39(4):327–35. doi:10.1111/aor.12387

Xu Z, Zhang C, Cheng L, Hu M, Tao H, Song L. The microRNA miR-17 regulates lung FoxA1 expression during lipopolysaccharide-induced acute lung injury. *Biochem Biophys Res Commun* (2014) 445(1):48–53. doi:10.1016/j.bbrc.2014.01.108

Guo Z, Wen Z, Qin A, Zhou Y, Liao Z, Liu Z, et al. Antisense oligonucleotide treatment enhances the recovery of acute lung injury through IL-10-secreting M2-like macrophage-induced expansion of CD4+ regulatory T cells. *J Immunol* (2013) 190(8):4337–48. doi:10.4049/jimmunol.1203233

Zhao J, Tao Y, Zhou Y, Qin N, Chen C, Tian D, et al. MicroRNA-7: a promising new target in cancer therapy. *Cancer Cell Int* (2015) 15:103. doi:10.1186/ s12935-015-0259-0

Horsham JL, Ganda C, Kalinowski FC, Brown RA, Epis MR, Leedman PJ. MicroRNA-7: a miRNA with expanding roles in development and disease. *Int J Biochem Cell Biol* (2015) 69:215–24. doi:10.1016/j.biocel.2015.11.001

Xiong S, Zheng Y, Jiang P, Liu R, Liu X, Qian J, et al. PA28gamma emerges as a novel functional target of tumour suppressor microRNA-7 in non-small-cell lung cancer. *Br J Cancer* (2014) 110(2):353–62. doi:10.1038/bjc.2013.728

Hong CF, Lin SY, Chou YT, Wu CW. MicroRNA-7 compromises p53 protein-dependent apoptosis by controlling the expression of the chro- matin remodeling factor SMARCD1. *J Biol Chem* (2016) 291(4):1877–89. doi:10.1074/jbc.M115.667568

Xu L, Wen Z, Zhou Y, Liu Z, Li Q, Fei G, et al. MicroRNA-7-regulated TLR9 signaling-enhanced growth and metastatic potential of human lung cancer cells by altering the phosphoinositide-3-kinase, regulatory subunit 3/Akt pathway. *Mol Biol Cell* (2013) 24(1):42–55. doi:10.1091/mbc.E12-07-0519

Zhao J, Wang K, Liao Z, Li Y, Yang H, Chen C, et al. Promoter mutation of tumor suppressor microRNA-7 is associated with poor prognosis of lung cancer. *Mol Clin Oncol* (2015) 3(6):1329–36. doi:10.3892/mco.2015.648

Akbas F, Coskunpinar E, Aynaci E, Oltulu YM, Yildiz P. Analysis of serum micro-RNAs as potential biomarker in chronic obstructive pulmonary disease. *Exp Lung Res* (2012) 38(6):286–94. doi:10.3109/01902148.2012. 689088

Buggele WA, Johnson KE, Horvath CM. Influenza A virus infection of human respiratory cells induces primary microRNA expression. *J Biol Chem* (2012) 287(37):31027–40. doi:10.1074/jbc.M112.387670

Taccioli C, Garofalo M, Chen H, Jiang Y, Tagliazucchi GM, Di Leva G, et al. Repression of esophageal neoplasia and inflammatory signaling by anti- miR-31 delivery in vivo. *J Natl Cancer Inst* (2015) 107(11):djv220. doi:10.1093/ jnci/djv220

Tay FC, Lim JK, Zhu H, Hin LC, Wang S. Using artificial microRNA sponges to achieve microRNA loss-of-function in cancer cells. *Adv Drug Deliv Rev* (2015) 81:117–27. doi:10.1016/j.addr.2014.05.010

Ebert MS, Sharp PA. Emerging roles for natural microRNA sponges. *Curr Biol* (2010) 20(19):R858–61. doi:10.1016/j.cub.2010.08.052

Kalinowski FC, Brown RA, Ganda C, Giles KM, Epis MR, Horsham J, et al. microRNA-7: a tumor suppressor miRNA with therapeutic potential. *Int J Biochem Cell Biol* (2014) 54:312–7. doi:10.1016/j.biocel.2014.05.040

Lee J, Yeganeh B, Ermini L, Post M. Sphingolipids as cell fate regulators in lung development and disease. *Apoptosis* (2015) 20(5):740–57. doi:10.1007/ s10495-015-1112-6

Goldkorn T, Filosto S, Chung S. Lung injury and lung cancer caused by cigarette smoke-induced oxidative stress: molecular mechanisms and thera- peutic opportunities involving the ceramide-generating machinery and epi- dermal growth factor receptor. *Antioxid Redox Signal* (2014) 21(15):2149–74. doi:10.1089/ars.2013.5469

Connors TJ, Ravindranath TM, Bickham KL, Gordon CL, Zhang F, Levin B, et al. Airway CD8(+) T cells are associated with lung injury during infant viral respiratory tract infection. *Am J Respir Cell Mol Biol* (2016) 54(6):822–30. doi:10.1165/rcmb.2015-0297OC

Klaff LS, Gill SE, Wisse BE, Mittelsteadt K, Matute-Bello G, Chen P, et al. Lipopolysaccharide-induced lung injury is independent of serum vitamin D concentration. *PLoS One* (2012) 7(11):e49076. doi:10.1371/ journal.pone.0049076

Sun C, Beard RS Jr, McLean DL, Rigor RR, Konia T, Wu MH, et al. ADAM15 deficiency attenuates pulmonary hyperpermeability and acute lung injury in lipopolysaccharide-treated mice. *Am J Physiol Lung Cell Mol Physiol* (2013) 304(3):L135–42. doi:10.1152/ajplung.00133.2012

Zhu Q, Yamakuchi M, Lowenstein CJ. SNAP23 regulates endothelial exocy- tosis of von Willebrand factor. *PLoS One* (2015) 10(8):e0118737. doi:10.1371/ journal.pone.0118737

Moon G, Kim J, Min Y, Wi SM, Shim JH, Chun E, et al. Phosphoinositide- dependent kinase-1 inhibits TRAF6 ubiquitination by interrupting the formation of TAK1-TAB2 complex in TLR4 signaling. *Cell Signal* (2015) 27(12):2524–33. doi:10.1016/j.cellsig.2015.09.018

Hartmann P, Zhou Z, Natarelli L, Wei Y, Nazari-Jahantigh M, Zhu M, et al. Endothelial Dicer promotes atherosclerosis and vascular inflammation by miRNA-103-mediated suppression of KLF4. *Nat Commun* (2016) 7:10521. doi:10.1038/ncomms10521

George J, Lewis MG, Renne R, Mattapallil JJ. Suppression of transforming growth factor β receptor 2 and Smad5 is associated with high levels of microRNA miR-155 in the oral mucosa during chronic simian immuno- deficiency virus infection. *J Virol* (2015) 89(5):2972–8. doi:10.1128/JVI. 03248-14

Lee S, Kang J, Cho M, Seo E, Choi H, Kim E, et al. Profiling of transcripts and proteins modulated by K-ras oncogene in the lung tissues of K-ras transgenic mice by omics approaches. *Int J Oncol* (2009) 34(1):161–72. doi:10.3892/ijo_00000138

Chaly Y, Fu Y, Marinov A, Hostager B, Yan W, Campfield B, et al. Follistatin- like protein 1 enhances NLRP3 inflammasome-mediated IL-1β secretion from monocytes and macrophages. *Eur J Immunol* (2014) 44(5):1467–79. doi:10.1002/eji.201344063

Liu J, Liu Y, Zhang H, Chen G, Wang K, Xiao X. KLF4 promotes the expression, translocation, and release of HMGB1 in RAW264.7 macrophages in response to LPS. *Shock* (2008) 30(3):260–6. doi:10.1097/shk.0b013e318162bef7

Chang YL, Zhou PJ, Wei L, Li W, Ji Z, Fang YX, et al. MicroRNA-7 inhib- its the stemness of prostate cancer stem-like cells and tumorigenesis by repressing KLF4/PI3K/Akt/p21 pathway. *Oncotarget* (2015) 6(27):24017–31. doi:10.18632/oncotarget.4447

Zahlten J, Steinicke R, Bertrams W, Hocke AC, Scharf S, Schmeck B, et al. TLR9- and Src-dependent expression of Krueppel-like factor 4 controls interleukin-10 expression in pneumonia. *Eur Respir J* (2013) 41(2):384–91. doi:10.1183/09031936.00196311

Lee JP, Li YC, Chen HY, Lin RH, Huang SS, Chen HL, et al. Protective effects of luteolin against lipopolysaccharide-induced acute lung injury involves inhibition of MEK/ERK and PI3K/Akt pathways in neutrophils. *Acta Pharmacol Sin* (2010) 31(7):831–8. doi:10.1038/aps.2010.62

Gorbatenko A, Olesen CW, Mørup N, Thiel G, Kallunki T, Valen E, et al. ErbB2 upregulates the Na+,HCO3(-)-cotransporter NBCn1/SLC4A7 in human breast cancer cells via Akt, ERK, Src, and Kruppel-like factor 4. *FASEB J* (2014) 28(1):350–63. doi:10.1096/fj.13-233288

Bofill-De Ros X, Santos M, Vila-Casadesús M, Villanueva E, Andreu N, Dierssen M, et al. Genome-wide miR-155 and miR-802 target gene identi- fication in the hippocampus of Ts65Dn Down syndrome mouse model by miRNA sponges. *BMC Genomics* (2015) 16:907. doi:10.1186/s12864-015- 2160-6

Zhang ZC, Liu Y, Xiao LL, Li SF, Jiang JH, Zhao Y, et al. Upregulation of miR- 125b by estrogen protects against non-alcoholic fatty liver in female mice. *J Hepatol* (2015) 63(6):1466–75. doi:10.1016/j.jhep.2015.07.037

Giusti SA, Vogl AM, Brockmann MM, Vercelli CA, Rein ML, Trümbach D, et al. MicroRNA-9 controls dendritic development by targeting REST. *Elife* (2014) 3:e02755. doi:10.7554/eLife.02755

Zheng Q, Hou J, Zhou Y, Yang Y, Cao X. Type I IFN-inducible downregulation of MicroRNA-27a feedback inhibits antiviral innate response by upregulating Siglec1/TRIM27. *J Immunol* (2016) 196(3):1317–26. doi:10.4049/jimmunol.1502134

Choudhury NR, de Lima Alves F, de Andrés-Aguayo L, Graf T, Cáceres JF, Rappsilber J, et al. Tissue-specific control of brain-enriched miR-7 biogenesis. *Genes De* (2013) 27(1):24–38. doi:10.1101/gad.199190.112

Kredo-Russo S, Mandelbaum AD, Ness A, Alon I, Lennox KA, Behlke MA, et al. Pancreas-enriched miRNA refines endocrine cell differentiation. *Development* (2012) 139(16):3021–31. doi:10.1242/dev.080127

Baertsch MA, Leber MF, Bossow S, Singh M, Engeland CE, Albert J, et al. MicroRNA-mediated multi-tissue detargeting of oncolytic measles virus. *Cancer Gene Ther* (2014) 21(9):373–80. doi:10.1038/cgt.2014.40

Murdoch JR, Lloyd CM. Resolution of allergic airway inflammation and airway hyperreactivity is mediated by IL-17-producing {gamma}{delta} T cells. *Am J Respir Crit Care Med* (2010) 182(4):464–76. doi:10.1164/ rccm.200911-1775OC

Holub M, Lawrence DA. Influence of endotoxin-induced acute lung injury on pulmonary innate and adaptive immunity. *APMIS* (2003) 111(5):571–80. doi:10.1034/j.1600-0463.2003.1110506.x

Ying H, Kang Y, Zhang H, Zhao D, Xia J, Lu Z, et al. MiR-127 modulates macrophage polarization and promotes lung inflammation and injury by activating the JNK pathway. *J Immunol* (2015) 194(3):1239–51. doi:10.4049/ jimmunol.1402088

Brusselle GG, Joos GF, Bracke KR. New insights into the immunology of chronic obstructive pulmonary disease. *Lancet* (2011) 378(9795):1015–26. doi:10.1016/S0140-6736(11)60988-4

Shen T, Sanchez HN, Zan H, Casali P. Genome-wide analysis reveals selective modulation of microRNAs and mRNAs by histone deacetylase inhibitor in B cells induced to undergo class-switch DNA recombination and plasma cell differentiation. *Front Immunol* (2015) 6:627. doi:10.3389/fimmu.2015. 00627

Pateras I, Giaginis C, Tsigris C, Patsouris E, Theocharis S. NF-κB signaling at the crossroads of inflammation and atherogenesis: searching for new therapeutic links. *Expert Opin Ther Targets* (2014) 18(9):1089–101. doi:10.1517/14728222.2014.938051

Liu X, Cohen JI. The role of PI3K/Akt in human herpesvirus infection: from the bench to the bedside. *Virology* (2015) 47(9–480):568–77. doi:10.1016/j.virol.2015.02.040

Wang X, Tanino Y, Sato S, Nikaido T, Misa K, Fukuhara N, et al. Secretoglobin 3A2 attenuates lipopolysaccharide-induced inflammation through inhibition of ERK and JNK pathways in bronchial epithelial cells. *Inflammation* (2015) 38(2):828–34. doi:10.1007/s10753-014-9992-0

Ghaleb AM, Laroui H, Merlin D, Yang VW. Genetic deletion of Klf4 in the mouse intestinal epithelium ameliorates dextran sodium sulfate-induced colitis by modulating the NF-κB pathway inflammatory response. *Inflamm Bowel Dis* (2014) 20(5):811–20. doi:10.1097/MIB.0000000000000022

Kaushik DK, Thounaojam MC, Kumawat KL, Gupta M, Basu A. Interleukin- 1β orchestrates underlying inflammatory responses in microglia via Krüppel- like factor 4. *J Neurochem* (2013) 127(2):233–44. doi:10.1111/jnc.12382

Ohnesorge N, Viemann D, Schmidt N, Czymai T, Spiering D, Schmolke M, et al. Erk5 activation elicits a vasoprotective endothelial phenotype via induction of Kruppel-like factor 4 (KLF4). *J Biol Chem* (2010) 285(34):26199–210. doi:10.1074/jbc.M110.103127

Akalay I, Tan TZ, Kumar P, Janji B, Mami-Chouaib F, Charpy C, et al. Targeting WNT1-inducible signaling pathway protein 2 alters human breast cancer cell susceptibility to specific lysis through regulation of KLF-4 and miR-7 expression. *Oncogene* (2015) 34(17):2261–71. doi:10.1038/onc. 2014.151

Yu T, Chen X, Zhang W, Liu J, Avdiushko R, Napier DL, et al. KLF4 regulates adult lung tumor-initiating cells and represses K-Ras-mediated lung cancer. *Cell Death Differ* (2016) 23(2):207–15. doi:10.1038/cdd.2015.85

Leikauf GD, Pope-Varsalona H, Concel VJ, Liu P, Bein K, Berndt A, et al. Integrative assessment of chlorine-induced acute lung injury in mice. *Am J Respir Cell Mol Biol* (2012) 47(2):234–44. doi:10.1165/rcmb.2012-0026OC

Cowan CE, Kohler EE, Dugan TA, Mirza MK, Malik AB, Wary KK. Kruppel-like factor-4 transcriptionally regulates VE-cadherin expression and endothelial barrier function. *Circ Res* (2010) 107(8):959–66. doi:10.1161/CIRCRESAHA.110.219592

Yoshida T, Yamashita M, Iwai M, Hayashi M. Endothelial Krüppel-like factor 4 mediates the protective effect of statins against ischemic AKI. *J Am Soc Nephrol* (2016) 27(5):1379–88. doi:10.1681/ASN.2015040460

Zhang Y, Wang Y, Liu Y, Wang N, Qi Y, Du J. Krüppel-like factor 4 transcriptionally regulates TGF-β1 and contributes to cardiac myofibroblast differentiation. *PLoS One* (2013) 8(4):e63424. doi:10.1371/journal.pone.0063424

15

Aerobic Exercise Attenuates Acute Lung Injury through NET Inhibition

Yue Shi[1†], *Tingting Liu*[2†], *David C. Nieman*[3], *Yanqiu Cui*[1], *Fei Li*[4], *Luyu Yang*[5], *Hui Shi*[2*] *and Peijie Chen*[1*]

[1] *School of Kinesiology, Shanghai University of Sport, Shanghai, China,* [2] *Department of Rheumatology and Immunology, Ruijin Hospital, Shanghai Jiao Tong University School of Medicine, Shanghai, China,* [3] *North Carolina Research Campus, Appalachian State University, Kannapolis, NC, United States,* [4] *School of Physical Education and Sport Training, Shanghai University of Sport, Shanghai, China,* [5] *Department of General Surgery, Cancer Metastasis Institute, Huashan Hospital, Fudan University, Shanghai, China*

***Correspondence:**
Hui Shi
shihui_sjtu@sina.com
Peijie Chen
chenpeijie@sus.edu.cn

† *These authors have contributed equally to this work*

Introduction: Aerobic exercise improves lung inflammation in acute lung injury (ALI), but its mechanism remains unknown. Neutrophil extracellular traps (NETs) play an important role in LPS-induced ALI, and a positive correlation exists between NET formation and proinflammatory macrophage polarization. This study investigated whether aerobic exercise reduces the pro-inflammatory polarization of alveolar macrophages (AMs) by inhibiting the excessive release of NETs and then alleviating the inflammatory response of ALI.

Methods: C57BL/6 male mice were randomly divided into four groups: sedentary group (CON), sedentary and extra-pulmonary LPS injection group (LPS), 5-weeks aerobic training intervention and LPS injection group (EXE+LPS), and DNase I plus LPS injection group (DNase+LPS). Twenty-four hours after drug injection, bronchoalveolar lavage fluid (BALF), AM, and lung tissues were obtained to detect inflammatory responses, NET formation, macrophage polarization, and protein activation. In the *in vitro* study, a murine AM cell line, designated MH-S, was stimulated with LPS, purified NETs, and NETs plus DNase I.

Results: EXE+LPS and DNase+LPS mice exhibited reduced neutrophil infiltration, decreased NET release, and lower pro-inflammatory polarization of AM compared with LPS mice. Subsequently, Western blot showed inhibition of the phosphorylation of MAPK and NF-κB proteins of AMs in EXE+LPS and DNase+LPS mice compared with LPS mice. Lastly, stimulation of MH-S cells by NETs revealed a trend for pro-inflammatory cell polarization, with NF-κB protein activation at 8 h and ERK1/2 activation at 1, 2, and 8 h.

Conclusions: Aerobic exercise alleviated ALI through NET-induced AM pro-inflammatory polarization involving ERK1/2 and NF-κB signaling.

Keywords: acute lung injury, aerobic exercise, neutrophil extracellular traps, alveolar macrophages, inflammation

INTRODUCTION

Acute lung injury (ALI) is a common clinical respiratory illness characterized by acute and progressive respiratory insufficiency caused by a variety of causes. The main clinical features are respiratory distress and progressive hypoxemia (1). Due to the complex etiology and pathogenesis, the current morbidity mortality rate remains high. Excessive airway inflammatory response is regarded as the underlying cause of ALI and, when uncontrolled, leads to acute respiratory distress syndrome (ARDS) and even respiratory failure (2). Lipopolysaccharide (LPS), a main component of the gram-negative bacteria cell wall, has been identified as a key factor that activates inflammatory signaling cascades in ALI/ARDS development (3). Intratracheal instillation and intraperitoneal injection of LPS in rodents are effective methods for establishing ALI models. Aerobic exercise training for 5 weeks may inhibit extra-pulmonary LPS-induced lung inflammation by attenuating inflammatory cytokines and oxidative stress markers via IL-10 production (4). Aerobic exercise training has been widely accepted as having a positive influence on immune function and surveillance. However, the underlying molecular and signaling mechanisms of how aerobic exercise training may counter the ALI inflammation response is not well-understood.

Neutrophil extracellular traps (NETs) are released by activated neutrophils and are composed mainly of DNA, histones, myeloperoxidase (5), and neutrophil elastase (NE). The extracellular web-like structures can effectively trap invading pathogens and utilize highly localized concentrations of antimicrobial peptides to degrade virulence elements (6). Although NET formation is a potent process for host defense against foreign pathogen invasion, excessive NET release can also have adverse consequences. Proteins and dsDNA components located in NETs may be the source of key autoantigens, which lead to an inflammatory cascade in local tissues and the blood compartment. These autoantigens are involved in a variety of autoimmunity diseases such as rheumatoid arthritis (RA), systemic lupus erythematosus (SLE), psoriasis, and gout (7).

Recently, NET formation was found in LPS-induced lung inflammation and was degraded by aerosolized DNase I treatment in mice (8). The inhibition of NETs was correlated with suppression of the TLR4/NF-κB signaling pathway (9). In addition, alveolar M1 and M2 macrophages exhibit pro-inflammatory and anti-inflammatory properties, respectively. In response to LPS treatment in ALI mice, alveolar macrophages (AMs) undergo M1 activation, characterized by the expression and secretion of pro-inflammatory factors, such as TNF-α, IL-1β, and inducible nitric oxide synthase (iNOS) (10). NET levels in ARDS patients have been positively correlated with M1-like macrophage polarization (11). These studies support a linkage between NET formation and pro-inflammatory macrophage polarization, but direct evidence is lacking. Additionally, little is known regarding the beneficial role aerobic exercise training may play in attenuating AM pro-inflammatory polarization and NET formation, especially within the context of LPS-induced ALI.

In this study with ALI mice, we demonstrated that 5 weeks of aerobic treadmill exercise reduced LPS-induced lung inflammation and inhibited NET formation, similar to DNase I treatment. This beneficial response was shown to linked to alterations in the mitogen-activated protein kinase (MAPK) (ERK1/2, JNK and p38) and NF-κB signaling pathways. Additional cell culture studies with the murine AM cell line MH-S showed that NET formation was coupled to pro-inflammatory macrophage polarization and inflammation.

METHODS

Animals

Seven-week-old male C57BL/6 mice, weighing 20–25 g, were purchased from the GemPharmatec Company (Nanjing, China) and fed for 1 week to allow for acclimatization. Mice were housed in a constant temperature at 25°C with a 12-h dark/light cycle and free access to standard pellets and water. The mice were randomly divided into four groups: control (CON), intraperitoneal injection of LPS alone (LPS), 5 weeks of aerobic treadmill running plus intraperitoneal injection of LPS (EXE+LPS), and intraperitoneal injection of LPS and DNase I (DNase+LPS). All experimental protocols of this study were approved by the Ethics Committee of Shanghai University of Sport. Study procedures with the mice were in compliance with standards established by the Ethics Committee for Animal Experimentation of Shanghai University of Sport and the Guide for the Care and Use of Laboratory Animals (Institute for Laboratory Animal Research, USA). The data shown in the experiment were based on three repeated experiments.

Aerobic Exercise Protocol

The aerobic treadmill running training protocol was based on a maximal running capacity test conducted before the start of formal research, as reported previously (12). Maximum running capacity was determined as follows: 10 min warm-up (5% grade, 10 m/min) followed by an increase in the treadmill speed (3 m/min each 3 min) until exhaustion and an inability to run even after repeated mechanical stimuli. Maximal exercise capacity (100%) was set as the maximum speed reached by each mouse. EXE+LPS group mice were then trained using moderate intensity exercise (60% of average maximum speed) for 60 min/day, 5 days/week for 5 weeks (4); mice in CON, LPS, and DNase+LPS groups were all housed in the standard cages for the 5 weeks with no intervention.

Animal Exposure to LPS and DNase I Administration

Twenty-four hours after the last treadmill run of EXE+LPS group mice, mice of LPS, EXE+LPS, and DNase+ LPS groups were anesthetized and received intraperitoneal administration of 100 μl of *Escherichia coli* LPS (055: B5; Sigma-Aldrich, St. Louis, MO) diluted in saline at a dose of 1 μg/μl. Mice in the CON group were submitted to intraperitoneal injection of saline alone. To investigate the role of DNase I on reducing lung inflammation response, DNase+LPS mice received aerosolized DNase I (Sigma-Aldrich, D5025) 10 μg diluted in 100 μl of normal saline at 0 and 12 h after intraperitoneal LPS injection. Then, 24 h later, all mice were anesthetized with 2.5% chloral hydrate (0.1 ml/10 g) and the following analyses were performed (**Figure 1A**).

Collection of Bronchoalveolar Lavage Fluid (BALF)

Mice were anesthetized and the tracheae were cannulated by a 20-gauge catheter. The lungs were lavaged with 0.6 ml of ice-cold D-PBS for five consecutive washes. A total of 2.3 to 2.7 ml of BALF was recovered and centrifuged at 1,500 rpm, at 4°C, for

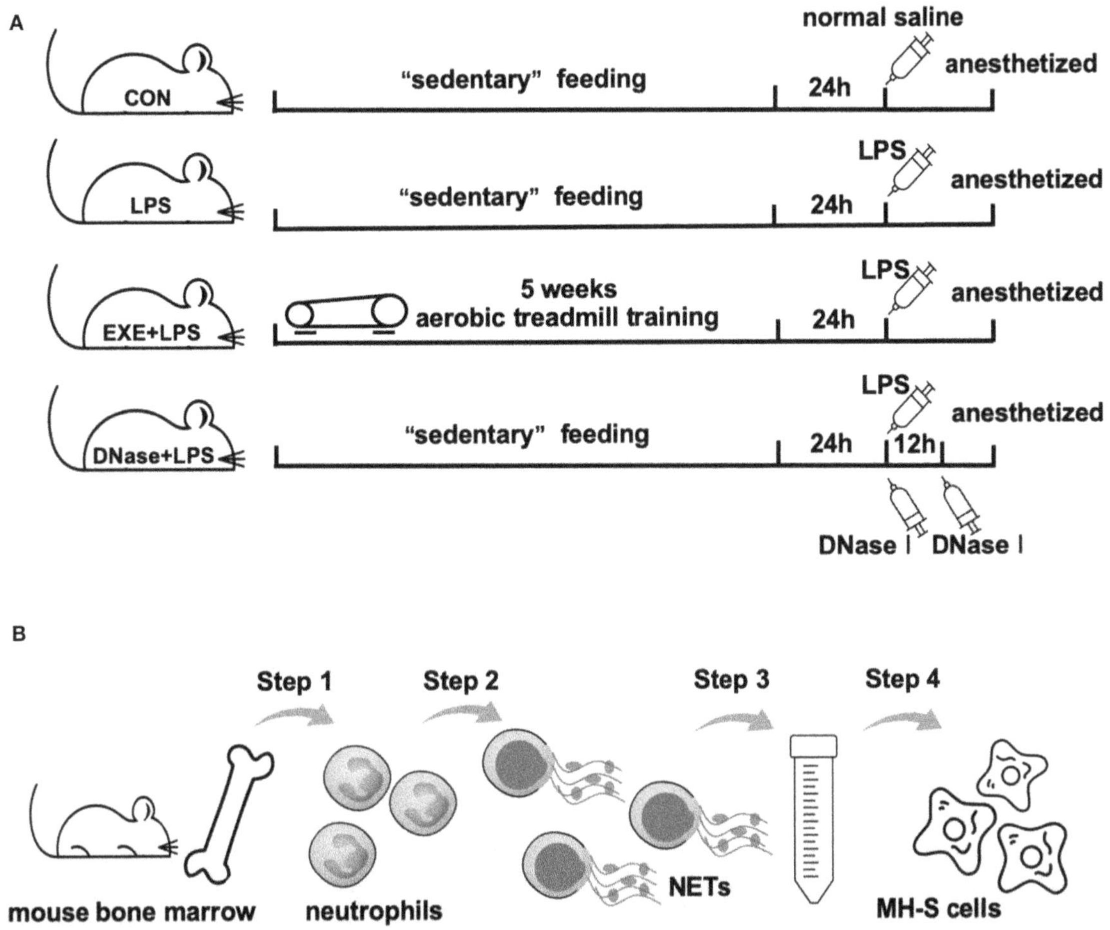

FIGURE 1 | Operational schematics of *in vivo* and *in vitro* experiments. **(A)** Schematic diagram of the time axis of intervention in each group of mice. Mice in CON, LPS, and DNase+LPS groups were housed for 5 weeks of "sedentary" feeding and mice in EXE+LPS group were engaged in 5 weeks of aerobic treadmill training. Twenty-four hours after last training, all mice except the CON group were anesthetized and received intraperitoneal administration of 100 μl of *Escherichia coli* LPS diluted in saline at a dose of 1 μg/μl. Mice in the CON group were submitted to intraperitoneal injection of saline alone, while DNase+LPS mice received aerosolized DNase I 10 μg diluted in 100 μl normal saline at 0 and 12 h after intraperitoneal LPS injection. Then, 24 h later, all mice were anesthetized with 2.5% chloral hydrate (0.1 ml/10 g), and the following analyses were performed. **(B)** General operation procedures of *in vitro* experiment: Step 1: Neutrophils were isolated from mouse bone marrow; Step 2: NET formation through PMA stimulation; Step 3: Extraction and purification of NETs by low- and high-speed centrifugation; Step 4: MH-S cells were stimulated with purified NETs to observe polarization reaction.

5 min. The supernatant was stored at −20°C for cytokine and MPO–DNA complex analysis. The cell pellet was resuspended in PBS for flow cytometry detection and acquisition of AMs.

Cell Culture and Treatment

Primary AMs were collected from C57BL/6 mice by the differential adhesion method. MH-S cells (derived from mouse AMs) were obtained from American Type Culture Collection (ATCC) (Manassas, VA, USA). Cells were cultured in RPMI 1640 medium, supplemented with 10% fetal bovine serum and 1% penicillin-streptomycin (Gibco BRL, MD, USA) at 37°C in a 5% CO_2 atmosphere. Cells were treated with media containing 100 ng/ml LPS, 1 ng/μl NETs, NETs plus DNase, and DNase alone for different time points. NETs plus DNase treatment was pre-processed as previously reported (13). NETs were digested for 15 min in 1 ml of RPMI with 10 U/ml DNase I at 37°C. Then, DNase was stopped with 2 mM EDTA. After incubation, the supernatant was collected for cytokine detection and the cells were collected for RT-PCR and Western blot analysis (**Figure 1B**).

Histology, Mucus Staining, and Immunofluorescence

The left lung lobes were fixed in 4% PFA for 48 h and then routinely processed to paraffin blocks and sectioned at ~4 μm. H&E staining of lung tissue sections was performed to evaluate the inflammatory response. The tissue sections were observed under a light microscope for the lung histopathology. To detect neutrophils and macrophages in lung tissue, paraffin-embedded mouse lung sections were permeabilized with 0.2% Triton X-100 in phosphate-buffered saline (PBS) for 15 min and blocked with 2% donkey serum. The sections were then incubated with the primary antibodies—anti-mouse myeloperoxidase (1:10000;

Servicebio) and anti-F4/80 (1:500; Servicebio) overnight at 4°C. To detect NET formation in lung tissue, the sections were incubated with anti-mouse myeloperoxidase and anti-NE (1:500; Bioss Antibodies) overnight at 4°C. Then, the slides were incubated for 2 h with secondary antibodies: Alexa Fluor 488 goat anti-rabbit (1:400; Servicebio) and HRP goat anti-rabbit (1:500; Servicebio). 4′,6-Diamidino-2-phenylindole (DAPI) was used to detect DNA. Finally, slides were visualized using a fluorescence microscope.

Flow Cytometry Detection

For the quantity and ratio of neutrophils and AMs assay, BALF cell pellets were washed with cold PBS and resuspended in 100 μl of flow buffer. Then, cells were incubated with 1 μM Ly-6G/Ly-6C Monoclonal Antibody (RB6-8C5), PE-Cyanine7 (eBioscience), 1 μM CD80 (B7-1) Monoclonal Antibody (16-10A1), FITC (eBioscience), 1 μM CD170 (Siglec F), and PE (eBioscience) at 4°C for 30 min to allow binding. Upon removal of unbound antibodies by extensive washing of the cells with PBS twice, cells were resuspended in flow buffer and placed in 4°C and blocked from light prior to measurement. All flow-cytometry-based assays were performed on a BD FACS Canto II. Data were analyzed using FlowJo software (Tree Star, Ashland, OR).

Quantitative Real-Time Reverse Transcriptase Polymerase Chain Reaction (RT-PCR)

mRNA was isolated and cDNA was prepared (Prime-Script RT Master Mix transcription kit, TaKaRa, Tokyo, Japan). RT-PCR was performed to detect NETs and LPS-stimulated MH-S macrophage genes. The RT-PCR contained 4 ng of DNA, isolated as described above, SYBR green master mix (Takara), and primers for IL-1β, IL-6, TNF-α, and β-actin. The enzyme was activated at 95°C for 30 s, followed by 40 cycles at 95°C for 15 s, and 60°C for 60 s. Primer sequences were designed as follows: 5′-TCGCAGCAGCACATCAACAAGAG-3′ (forward) and 5′-TGCTCATGTCCTCATCCTGGAAGG-3′ (reverse) for mouse IL-1β; 5′-TGGGACTGATGCTGGTGACA-3′ (forward) and 5′-ACAGGTCTGTTGGGAGTGGT-3′ (reverse) for mouse IL-6; 5′-ATGTCTCAGCCTCTTCTCATTC-3′ (forward) and 5′-GCT TGTCACTCGAATTTTGAGA-3′ (reverse) for mouse TNF-α; 5′-CTACCTCATGAAGATCCTGACC-3′ (forward) and 5′-CAC AGCTTCTCTTTGATGTCAC-3′ (reverse) for mouse β-actin.

MPO–DNA Complex ELISA

Capture ELISA was used to measure the MPO–DNA complexes as described (14). Briefly, 5 μg/ml anti-myeloperoxidase antibody (Abcam) was diluted and added into an ELISA plate (65 μl per well) overnight 4°C. After blocking with 1% bovine serum albumin, 20-μl BALF samples and the peroxidase-labeled anti-DNA monoclonal antibody (1:25; Roche) were added to each well. The plate was incubated for 2 h in a shaking table at 300 rpm and was washed three times. Finally, 100 μl of peroxidase substrate was added. The absorbance at 405 nm wavelength was measured using BioTek Synergy2 (USA).

NET Isolation and Quantification

Mouse bone-marrow-derived neutrophils were isolated and purified by density gradient centrifugation as reported (8). Briefly, the bone marrow was flushed out of the tibia and femur using a 25-gauge needle filled with RPMI supplemented with 10% FBS and 2 mM EDTA onto a 50-ml screw top Falcon tube fitted with a 100-μm filter. The red blood cells were lysed by resuspending the cell pellet in hypotonic NaCl solution. The bone marrow cells were resuspended in 1 ml of sterile PBS. Mature neutrophils were purified by centrifugation for 30 min at 2,000 rpm without braking on a Histopaque 1119 and Histopaque 1077. The neutrophils were collected at the interface of the Histopaque 1119 and Histopaque 1077, with typically >95% viable and >95% pure. Purified neutrophils were cultured in free RPMI 1640 medium (Sigma-Aldrich) and stimulated with 500 nM of PMA for 4 h on a 150 × 25 mm flat tissue culture dish. Cell culture supernatants were discarded carefully, leaving the layer of NETs and neutrophils adhered at the bottom. After washing each dish and centrifuging for 5 min at 450 *g* at 4°C, cell-free NET-rich supernatant was obtained. The supernatant was centrifuged for 10 min at 18,000 *g* at 4°C to allow NET pellets to form. The supernatant was discarded and the NET pellets were dissolved in 100 μl of PBS. The purified cell-free NETs were quantified using spectrophotometry. NETs (100–150 ng/μl) were stored at −20°C for subsequent experiments (3).

Bio-Plex Cytokine Analysis

The BALF and cell culture supernatant levels of IL-1β, IL-6, IL-10, and TNF-α were analyzed using the Bio-Plex Pro Mouse Cytokine 6-plex Assay (Bio-Rad, product No. M6000007NY) according to the manufacturer's instructions in the Bio-Plex 200 system (Bio-Rad, Hercules, CA) as previously reported (15).

Western Blot Analysis

Primary AMs and stimulated MH-S cells were lysed using RIPA buffer containing a protease inhibitor cocktail (Roche Diagnostics, Indianapolis, IN). The protein concentration was determined using BCA kits (Beyotime Technology). Protein samples (20 μg) were separated by 10% SDS-polyacrylamide gel electrophoresis and subsequently transferred onto PVDF membranes. After blocking with 5% non-fat milk in TBST (TBS with 0.1% Tween-20, pH 7.4) at room temperature for 1 h, the membranes were incubated at 4°C overnight with the following primary antibodies: anti-phospho-ERK1/2 (1:1,000; Cell Signaling Technology), anti-ERK1/2 (1:1,000; Cell Signaling Technology), anti-phospho-NF-κB (1:1,000; Cell Signaling Technology), anti-NF-κB (1:1,000; Cell Signaling Technology), anti-phospho-JNK (1:1,000; Cell Signaling Technology), anti-JNK (1:1,000; Cell Signaling Technology), anti-phospho-p38 (1:1,000; Cell Signaling Technology), and anti-p38 (1:1,000; Cell Signaling Technology). The membranes were washed three times and incubated with HRP-conjugated secondary antibody (CST) at room temperature for 1 h. Anti-GAPDH antibody was used as an internal control. Peroxidase was visualized using an enhanced chemiluminescence system (ECL) (Millipore). Bands were quantitated using ImageJ software (Bio-Rad, USA), and results are expressed as fold change relative to the internal control.

Statistical Analysis

All data were expressed as the mean ± standard deviation (SD) and statistical analyses were performed using the SPSS version 20.0 (SPSS Inc., Chicago, IL, US). Data with a Gaussian distribution were analyzed by unpaired *t*-test or ANOVA (one-way analysis of variance), while non-parametric data were assessed by Mann–Whitney *U*-test or Wilcoxon rank-sum test. $P < 0.05$ were considered statistically significant.

RESULTS

Aerobic Exercise Attenuated Airway Inflammatory Response

Twenty-four hours after the last training bout, LPS and EXE+LPS mice received the same dose of LPS intraperitoneally to establish an extra-pulmonary model of ALI, while CON mice received intraperitoneal PBS. The lung inflammation response was measured through hematoxylin and eosin (H+E) staining of lung parenchyma. The representative photomicrographs revealed a reduced presence of inflammatory cells in the alveolar spaces and in the parenchyma of EXE+LPS mice (**Figure 2A**) compared to LPS mice. To further clarify the neutrophils influx into the lung parenchyma, we utilized myeloperoxidase (MPO, neutrophil cell marker) and F4/80 (macrophage cell surface marker) to immunofluorescence staining lung tissue and also performed flow cytometry on BALF cells. An immunofluorescence photo of double-labeled lung tissue of EXE+LPS mice revealed a reduced influx of neutrophils (green light) compared to LPS mice (**Figure 2B**). Also, flow cytometry of the BALF cells showed a reduced proportion of neutrophils in the EXE+LPS mice compared to the LPS mice (**Figure 2C**).

Aerobic Exercise and DNase I Treatment Reduce NET Formation and AM Pro-Inflammatory Polarization

NETs were previously reported to participate in the LPS-induced ALI pathological process. Therefore, we explored whether aerobic exercise could reduce the formation of NETs in the injured lung. MPO and NE are the main components of the NET structure. These two immunofluorescent antibodies were stained on the lung tissue. Images from EXE+LPS mice collected by fluorescence microscope displayed less MPO and NE co-localization than with LPS mice, similar to the DNase+LPS mice (**Figure 3A**). DNase I degrades extracellular DNA structure and effectively destroys the skeleton structure of NETs. A semi-quantitative detection of the MPO–DNA complex on the supernatant of BALF was conducted. The results showed the concentration of MPO–DNA complex in BALF from LPS mice was significantly higher than in EXE+LPS mice ($p < 0.01$) and DNase+LPS mice ($p < 0.001$) (**Figure 3B**). These results demonstrated that NETs do participate in the LPS-induced ALI process and aerobic exercise can reduce the formation of NETs in the injured lung. Uncontrolled lung inflammation is the most typical feature of ALI and involves polarization of AMs. To examine this phenomenon, the pro-inflammatory macrophage phenotype cell marker (CD80) and the specific cell marker of AMs (Siglec-F) were utilized to detect the proportion of pro-inflammatory AMs (Siglec-F^+ $CD80^+$) in the BALF. The data showed that aerobic exercise and DNase injection significantly reduced pro-inflammatory AMs in the BALF during LPS-induced ALI compared to LPS alone mice ($p < 0.001$) (**Figure 3C**). At the same time, aerobic exercise and DNase administration reduced BALF levels of inflammatory cytokines including interleukin (IL) IL-1β, IL-6, and tumor necrosis factor alpha (TNF-α) in LPS-induced ALI compared to LPS alone mice ($p < 0.05$ and $p < 0.01$), with an increase in the anti-inflammatory cytokine IL-10 ($p < 0.001$ and $p < 0.01$) (**Figure 3D**).

Aerobic Exercise Reduces ALI via Suppressing MAPK and NF-κB Signaling Activation

These data confirm NET formation and AM pro-inflammatory polarization during LPS-induced ALI. However, the underlying molecular mechanism is obscure. Primary mice alveolar cells were collected from the various groups. After 1.5 h of differential adherence, the pure AMs were lysed to extract total protein. Western blotting results showed significantly increased activation levels of phospho-ERK1/2/ERK1/2 ratio, phospho-JNK/JNK ratio, phospho-p38/p38 ratio, and phosphor-NF-κB/NF-κB ratio in LPS mice compared with CON mice ($p < 0.0001$, $p < 0.0001$, $p < 0.001$, and $p < 0.0001$, respectively) (**Figure 4**). EXE+LPS mice revealed decreased activation levels both in the phospho-ERK1/2/ERK1/2 ratio, phospho-JNK/JNK ratio, phospho-p38/p38 ratio, and phosphor-NF-κB/NF-κB ratio compared to LPS alone mice ($p < 0.05$, $p < 0.001$, $p < 0.05$, and $p < 0.05$, respectively), while DNase+LPS mice showed the lowest activation levels compared to LPS mice and EXE+LPS mice (**Figure 4**).

NETs Promote AM Pro-Inflammatory Polarization via ERK1/2 and NF-κB Signaling *in vitro*

The data supported involvement of MAPK and NF-κB signaling pathways in mediating exercise-induced attenuation of the ALI inflammation response. Isolated and purified NETs were used to directly stimulate AMs *in vitro* to determine if a decrease in NETs influenced AM polarization. MH-S, a cell line of mice AMs, was stimulated with 100 ng/ml LPS, 1 ng/μl NETs, and DNase I pre-treated NETs for 8 h. The cell culture supernatant was collected for cytokine detection and cells were lysed for RT-PCR and Western blot analysis. RT-PCR results showed that LPS, NETs, and NETs+DNase stimulation all significantly increased IL-1β expression ($p < 0.001$) of MH-S cells compared to control while NETs+DNase stimulation showed the smallest increase (**Figure 5A**). IL-6 and TNF-α expression of MH-S cells were higher when stimulated with LPS and NETs ($p < 0.001$ and $p < 0.001/0.05$) compared to control. NETs+DNase stimulation showed no difference compared to control (**Figure 5A**). Cell culture supernatant levels of IL-1β, IL-6, and TNF-α revealed similar trends between the four groups. Concentrations of the four cytokines were higher under LPS compared to NET stimulation, and significantly higher compared with control ($p < 0.001$). NETs+DNase stimulation showed no difference with control (**Figure 5B**). These results support a catalytic effect of NETs on AMs pro-inflammatory phenotype polarization. To explore underlying molecular and signaling mechanisms,

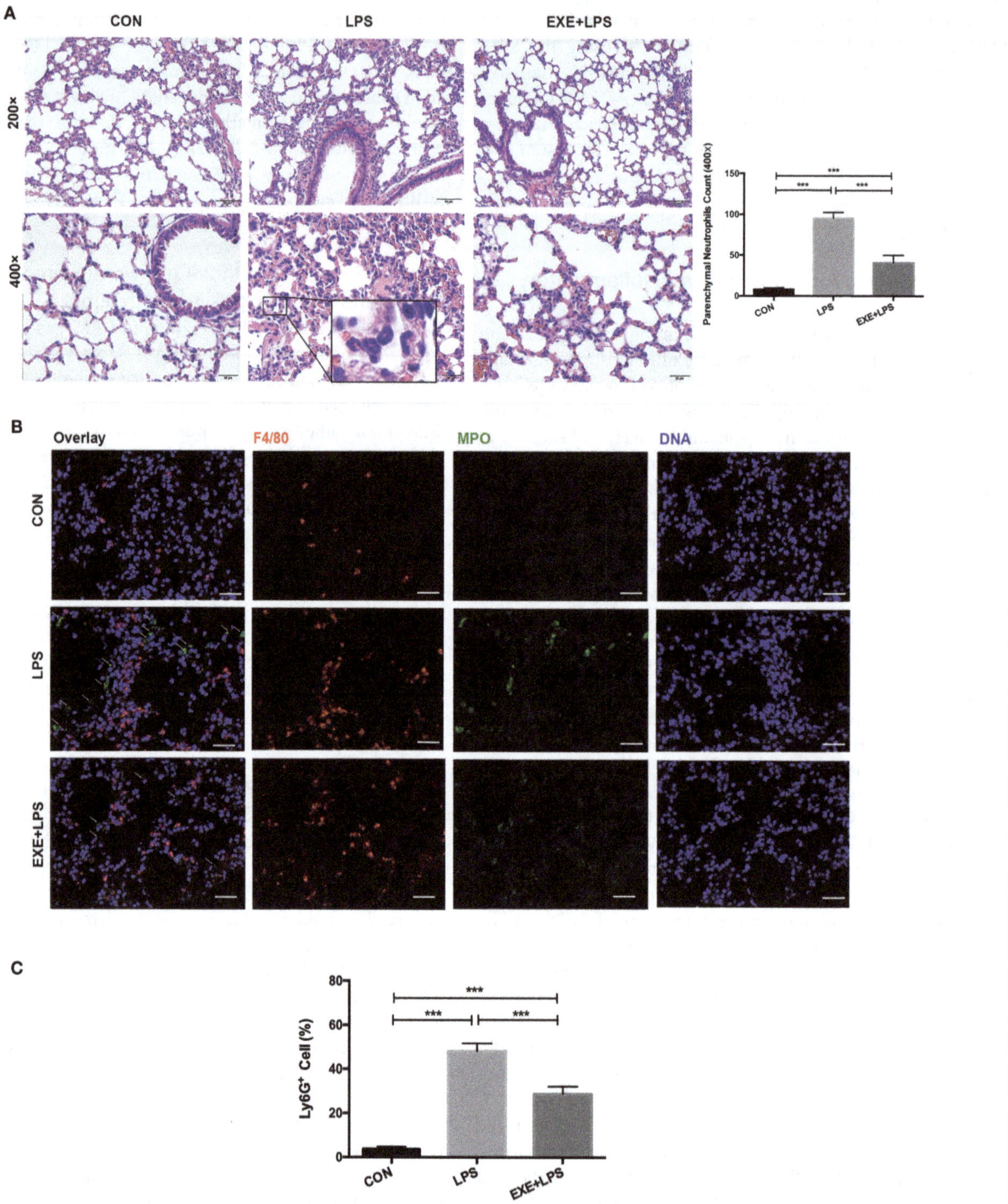

FIGURE 2 | Five weeks of aerobic exercise attenuated LPS-induced airway inflammatory response. **(A)** Images of H&E-stained lung tissue of sedentary mice (left vertical row), 24 h after intraperitoneal LPS injection of sedentary mice (middle vertical row) and 24 h after intraperitoneal LPS injection of exercised mice (right vertical row) (magnification ×200 in the first horizontal row; magnification ×400 in the second horizontal row); the neutrophils are indicated with black arrows in the enlarged black box. The right statistical chart shows parenchymal neutrophils count of three groups at 400× magnification fields. $^{***}p < 0.001$. **(B)** Representative images (magnification ×400) show merged DNA (blue), MPO (indicating neutrophils, green), and F4/80 (indicating macrophages, red) via fluorescence microscopy of lung sections from mice in the CON, LPS, and EXE+LPS groups. White arrows show the neutrophil influx. **(C)** The proportion of neutrophils in the BALF of CON, LPS, and EXE+LPS mice was determined with flow cytometry via $Ly6G^+$ antibody staining. The statistical chart shows that the percentage of neutrophils in LPS mice was significantly higher than in EXE+LPS mice and CON mice. $^{***}p < 0.001$.

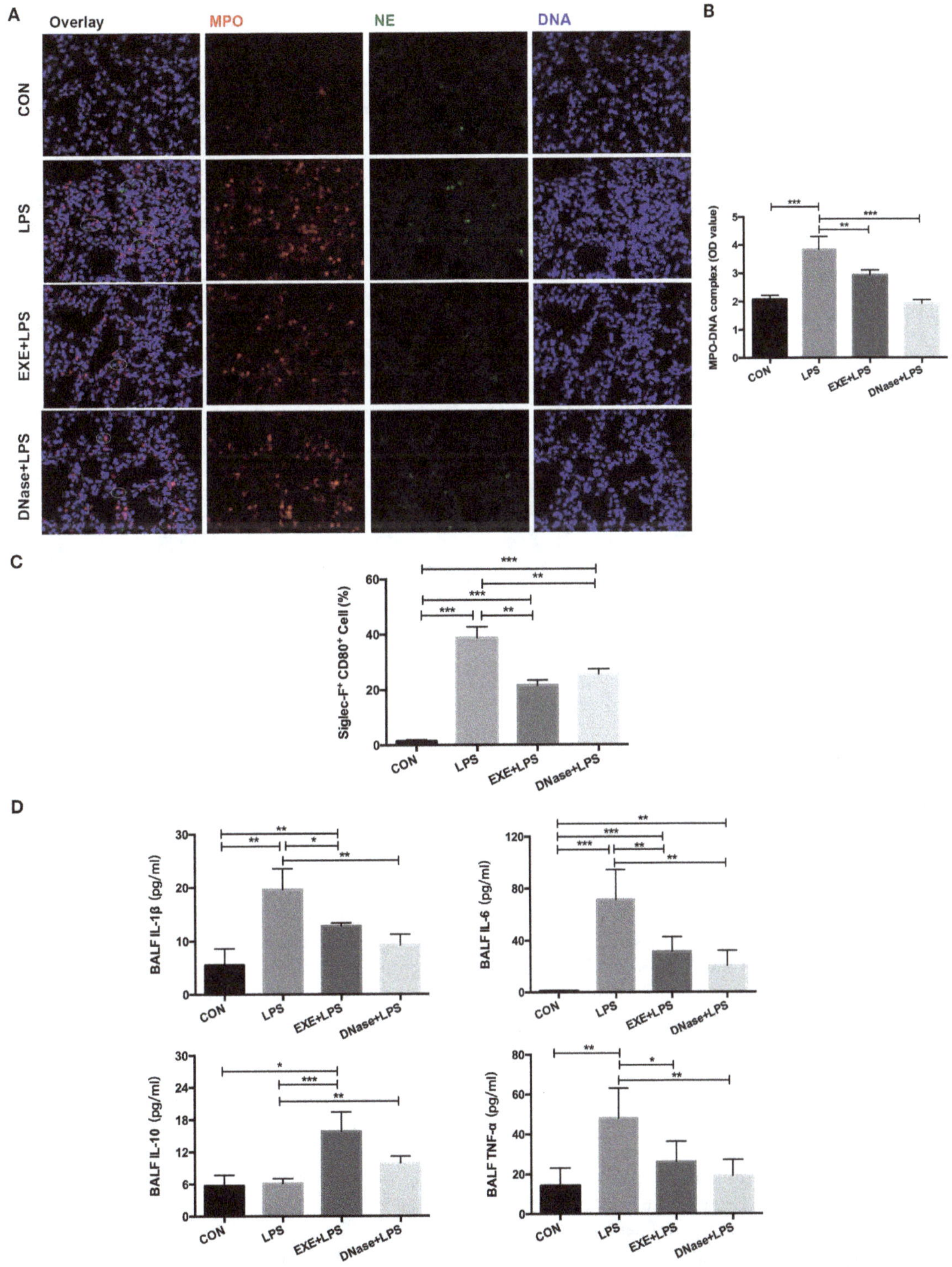

FIGURE 3 | NET formation and alveolar macrophage (AM) polarization with aerobic exercise and DNase I treatment. **(A)** Representative images (magnification ×400) show NET formation of merged DNA (blue), NE (green), and MPO (red) via fluorescence microscopy of lung sections from mice in the CON, LPS, EXE+LPS, and DNase+LPS groups. White circles indicate NETs. **(B)** MPO–DNA complex levels were detected in BALF of the CON, LPS, EXE+LPS, and DNase+LPS mice; the statistical chart shows that the MPO–DNA complex level of the EXE+LPS and DNase+LPS mice was significantly lower than LPS mice. $^{**}p < 0.01$, $^{***}p < 0.001$. **(C)** The pro-inflammatory polarization of AMs in the CON, LPS, EXE+LPS, and DNase+LPS mice were determined via flow cytometry via Siglec-F^{+} and CD80^{+} antibodies staining. The statistical chart shows that the percentage of pro-inflammatory phenotype AMs (Siglec-F^{+} CD80^{+}) in the LPS mice was higher than EXE+LPS and DNase+LPS mice. $^{**}p < 0.01$, $^{***}p < 0.001$. **(D)** Pro- and anti-inflammatory cytokines were detected in BALF. The results were expressed as picograms of cytokines per milliliter of BALF. $^{*}p < 0.05$, $^{**}p < 0.01$, $^{***}p < 0.001$.

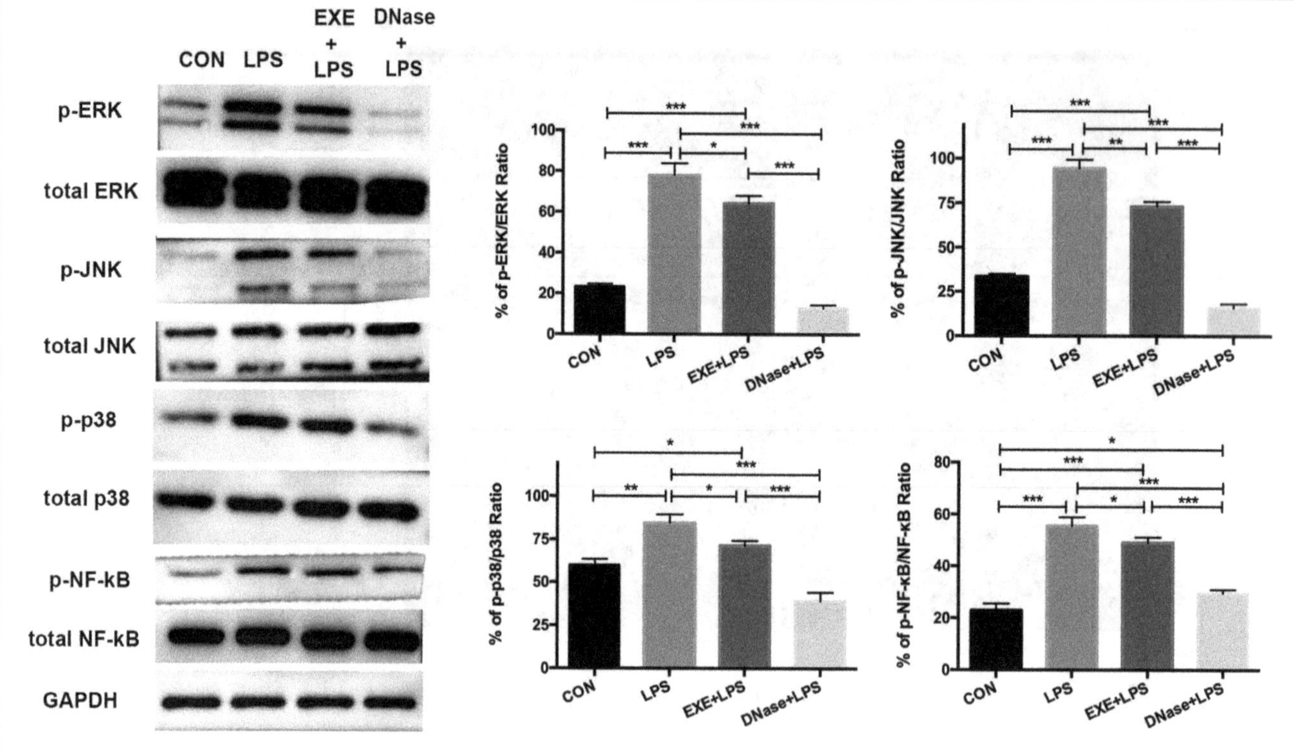

FIGURE 4 | Aerobic exercise and DNase treatment reduces lung inflammation response through MAPK and NF-κB signaling *in vivo*. The total proteins were obtained from primary AMs in the CON, LPS, EXE+LPS, and DNase+LPS mice. Representative Western blots and qualification of phospho-ERK1/2 and total-ERK1/2, phospho-JNK and total-JNK, phospho-p38 and total-p38, and phospho-NF-κB and total NF-κB expression in primary macrophages of all groups. $^{*}p < 0.05$, $^{**}p < 0.01$, $^{***}p < 0.001$.

Western blotting of the MH-S cells was conducted. The data revealed significantly increased levels of phospho-ERK/ERK ratio after 1, 2, and 8 h NET stimulation ($p < 0.001$, $p < 0.05$, and $p < 0.01$). The phosphor-JNK/JNK and phosphor-p38/p38 ratios were unaffected after NET stimulation. The phosphor-NF-κB/NF-κB ratio increased after 8 h of NET stimulation ($p < 0.001$) (**Figure 5C**). Phosphor-ERK1/2, JNK, and NF-κB, but not p38, protein activations were involved in LPS-induced MH-S cell pro-inflammatory responses (**Figure 5C**).

DISCUSSION

Our study demonstrated that 5 weeks of aerobic exercise training reduced the inflammatory response to LPS-induced ALI in mice by decreasing the excessive release of NETs and AM pro-inflammatory polarization. The beneficial influence of aerobic exercise on LPS-induced lung inflammation has been reported previously (16). These data from the current study extend these findings by improving understanding of underlying mechanisms.

The beneficial effect of aerobic exercise training on LPS-induced ALI and NET production was similar to the therapeutic effect of DNase injection. In order to cope with the invasion of pathogenic microorganisms, the body needs to find a balance between infection control and the immune response to avoid collateral damage to host tissues (17). A key feature of the LPS-induced ALI syndrome is an early, robust neutrophilic response (18). Infiltration of neutrophils and the release of NETs play a role in controlling lung infections, but at the same time, excessive formation of NETs inevitably aggravates the extent of lung injury. Our data demonstrate that 5 weeks of aerobic exercise training can help the body achieve the appropriate balance between pulmonary infection control, tissue homeostasis, and the immune response. Physical exercise improved histological and oxidative stress parameters in mice exposed to cigarette smoke (19). Exercise enhanced the activity of antioxidant enzymes (20) and up-regulated the expression of genes related to energy pathways and lipid metabolism pathways (21, 22). Additionally, exercise training reduced epithelial proliferation and mucin expression, and inhibited endothelium-dependent vasorelaxation dysfunction induced by various air pollutants in the lungs (23, 24). These findings are in good agreement with the anti-inflammatory role of exercise training in pulmonary diseases and provide evidence of exercise-mediated prevention of LPS-induced airway inflammation.

NETs have been explored extensively in the area of lung disease as contributing to the defense against bacterial respiratory infections (25). Bacterial entrapment by NETs impedes the ability of pneumococci to spread from the upper to the lower respiratory tract and to disseminate into the bloodstream (16). Mice with increased NET formation caused by a deficiency in the anti-inflammatory adenosine A2B receptor have been

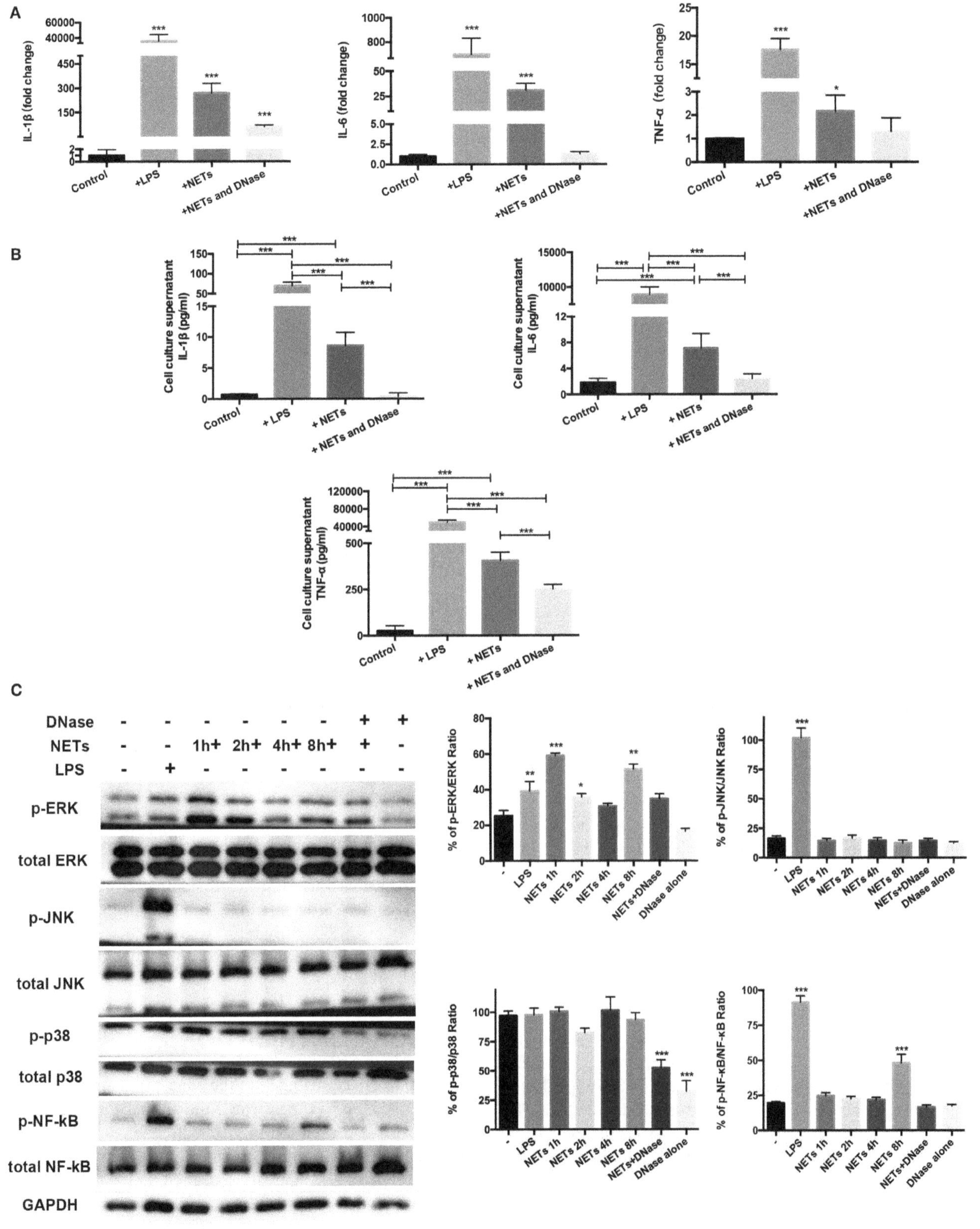

FIGURE 5 | ERK1/2 and NF-κB signaling involved in MH-S cell pro-inflammatory phenotype polarization with NET stimulation *in vitro*. Mice AM cell line MH-S cells were stimulated with 100 ng/ml LPS, 1 ng/μl isolated and purified NETs, and DNase pre-treated NETs for 8 h. **(A)** IL-1β, IL-6, and TNF-α expression in these

(Continued)

FIGURE 5 | stimulated MH-S cells was measured using PT-PCR, indicating the degree of pro-inflammatory phenotype polarization of the stimulated cells compared with the unstimulated cells. **(B)** IL-1β, IL-6, and TNF-α expression in the cell culture supernatant was determined using Bio-Plex cytokine analysis. **(C)** Representative Western blots and qualification of phospho-ERK1/2 and total-ERK1/2, phospho-JNK and total-JNK, phospho-p38 and total-p38, phospho-NF-κB, and total NF-κB expression in primary macrophages of control cells, LPS-stimulated cells, NETs+DNase-stimulated cells, DNase alone-stimulated cells for 8 h, and NET-stimulated cells for 1, 2, 4, and 8 h. All stimulated cells were statistically compared to unstimulated cells. $^{*}p < 0.05$, $^{**}p < 0.01$, $^{***}p < 0.001$.

shown to have an enhanced capacity for bacterial clearance from the lungs and increased survival when challenged with Klebsiella pneumonia (26). Although NETs have potentially beneficial anti-pathogenic functions in respiratory host defenses, protection can easily turn to injury when extensive, unbalanced NET formation occurs. NETs are embedded with potent granule proteins that are capable of killing pathogens but may also, under the right conditions, induce cell death of lung epithelial and endothelial cells (27) and contribute to certain lung diseases such as asthma (28), cystic fibrosis (29), and COPD (30). Little is known regarding the interaction between NETs and specific cells, including AMs. Recently, Song et al. (11) reported that NET levels in ARDS patients were positively correlated with M1-like macrophage polarization. Hu et al. (31) also demonstrated that NET formation may be involved in the activation of pro-inflammatory macrophages in Adult-onset Still's disease patients. These data contributed to the design of this study, with the aim of further exploring the role of NETs on macrophages. Our *in vivo* results showed a potential relationship between NETs and pro-inflammatory phenotype polarization of lung AMs. We then showed *in vitro* that extracted NETs stimulated mouse-derived AMs (MH-S) to develop in the direction of a pro-inflammatory phenotype. To a certain extent, this finding further clarifies the possible mechanism of the adverse effect of excessive NET formation in aggravating pulmonary inflammation during ALI.

LPS-induced ALI has been related to the MAPK pathways, including the extracellular signal regulated kinases ERK1/2 (32), p38, and JNK (33). These can be initiated by LPS-TLR4 receptor activation (34), leading to gene transcription and pro-inflammatory cytokine production. Others have shown that CXCR4 knockdown prevents inflammatory cytokine expression in macrophages by suppressing activation of MAPK and NF-κB signaling pathways (35). A chief aim of the current study was to explore the mechanism by which aerobic exercise training improves ALI using murine primary AMs. We found that the expression level of phosphorylated ERK1/2, JNK, p38 proteins, and phosphorylated NF-κB proteins of EXE+LPS mice was significantly suppressed when compared to the LPS mice. The expression level of these proteins was lowest in the sedentary group receiving DNase intervention (DNase+LPS group). These data provide evidence that aerobic exercise attenuates LPS-induced ALI by inhibiting NF-κB and MAPK signaling pathways, and that NETs may play a crucial role in this process. Given the pro-inflammatory effects of NETs on AMs, we sought to confirm the NET-associated molecular mechanisms by Western blot analysis. We detected a significant increase in the phosphorylated forms of both ERK1/2 and NF-κB pro-inflammatory proteins in MH-S cells when stimulated with NETs, with no effect on p38 and JNK proteins. Interestingly, the phosphorylation of ERK1/2 protein increased in the early phase of NET stimulation (at 1 and 2 h) during the 8-h period of stimulation of MH-S cells. The phosphorylated NF-κB protein ratio increased in the late stages of stimulation (at 8 h). These data suggest that NETs exert an activation of signaling pathways in a defined sequence during MH-S cell stimulation. The *in vivo* and *in vitro* data support that three key MAPK signaling pathway proteins (ERK1/2, JNK and p38) and NF-κB protein were inhibited with aerobic exercise training, and helped attenuate LPS-induced ALI. However, the *in vitro* data suggest that MH-S cells turned to M1 phenotype under NET stimulation, with an activation of ERK1/2 protein and NF-κB proteins. Thus, aerobic exercise training may reduce the production of NETs by inhibiting the ERK1/2 and NF-κB pathways, leading to a reduction in M1-type polarization of AMs and the inflammation response of ALI.

There are several limitations in our study procedure and data. We demonstrated to some extent that NETs play a key role in the attenuation of LPS-induced ALI with aerobic exercise training. However, we did not establish a direct causal relationship between these by blocking neutrophils *in vivo* or knocking out key genes that mediate NET release such as peptidylarginine deiminase 4 (PAD4) (36). Secondly, the molecular mechanism by which NETs stimulates the polarization of AMs to pro-inflammatory phenotype needs additional analysis. We verified the involvement of key proteins from the MAPK and NF-κB signaling pathways, but many others could be involved.

In conclusion, our study revealed that 5 weeks of aerobic treadmill running attenuated LPS-induced ALI in mice through inhibition of NET formation and AM pro-inflammatory phenotype polarization via suppression of ERK1/2 and NF-κB signaling pathways.

AUTHOR CONTRIBUTIONS

PC, YS, and HS contributed to the conception and design of the study. LY, YS, and FL performed the animal training program. YS and TL performed the *in vivo* experiments and cell culture studies. YS, TL, YC, and HS performed the results analysis. YS and HS prepared the figures and drafted the article. DN and PC edited and revised the article.

REFERENCES

Daniela Mokra PK. Biomarkers in acute lung injury. *Resp Physiol Neurobi.* (2015) 209:52–8. doi: 10.1016/j.resp.2014.10.006

Huang X, Xiu H, Zhang S, Zhang G. The role of macrophages in the pathogenesis of ALI/ARDS. *Mediat Inflamm.* (2018) 2018:1–8. doi: 10.1155/2018/1264913

Zhang X, Zhuang R, Wu H, Chen J, Wang F, Li G, et al. A novel role of endocan in alleviating LPS-induced acute lung injury. *Life Sci.* (2018) 202:89–97. doi:

10.1016/j.lfs.2018.04.005

Rigonato-Oliveira NC, Mackenzie B, All B, Oliveira-Junior MC, Santos-Dias A, Mar BR, et al. Aerobic exercise inhibits acute lung injury: from mouse to human evidence exercise reduced lung injury markers in mouse and in cells. *Exerc Immunol Rev.* (2018) 24:36–44. doi: 10.1183/13993003.congress-2018.pa4294

Beck KC, Hyatt RE, Mpougas P, Scanlon PD. Evaluation of pulmonary resistance and maximal expiratory flow measurements during exercise in humans. *J Appl Physiol.* (1999) 86:1388–95. doi: 10.1152/jappl.1999.86. 4.1388

Barnado A, Crofford LJ, Oates JC. At the bedside: neutrophil extracellular traps (NETs) as targets for biomarkers and therapies in autoimmune diseases. *J Leukocyte Biol.* (2016) 99:265–78. doi: 10.1189/jlb.5BT06 15-234R

Lee KH, Kronbichler A, Park DY, Park YM, Shin JI. Neutrophil extracellular traps (NETs) in autoimmune diseases: a comprehensive review. *Autoimmun Rev.* (2017) 16:1160–73. doi: 10.1016/j.autrev.2017. 09.012

Li H, Zhou X, Tan H, Hu Y, Zhang L, Liu S, et al. Neutrophil extracellular traps contribute to the pathogenesis of acid-aspiration- induced ALI/ARDS. *Oncotarget.* (2018) 9:1772–84. doi: 10.18632/oncotarget. 22744

Zou Y, Chen X, Xiao J, Zhou DB, Chen Q. Neutrophil extracellular traps promote lipopolysaccharide-induced airway inflammation and mucus hypersecretion in mice. *Oncotarget.* (2018) 9:13276–86. doi: 10.18632/oncotarget.24022

Lu HL, Huang XY, Luo YF, Tan WP, Chen PF, Guo YB. Activation of M1 macrophages play a critical role in the initiation of acute lung injury. *Biosci Rep.* (2018) 38:1–13. doi: 10.1042/BSR20171555

Song C, Li H, Li Y, Dai M, Zhang L, Liu S, et al. NETs promote ALI/ARDS inflammation by regulating alveolar macrophage polarization. *Exp Cell Res.* (2019) 382:1–11. doi: 10.1016/j.yexcr.2019.06.031

Shi Y, Shi H, Nieman DC, Hu Q, Yang L, Liu T, et al. Lactic acid accumulation during exhaustive exercise impairs release of neutrophil extracellular traps in mice. *Front Physiol.* (2019) 10:1–8. doi: 10.3389/fphys.2019. 00709

Urban CF, David E, Monika S, Ulrike AA, Christian G, Wolfgang N, et al. Neutrophil extracellular traps contain calprotectin, a cytosolic protein complex involved in host defense against *Candida albicans*. *Plos Pathog.* (2009) 5:e1000639. doi: 10.1371/journal.ppat.1000639

Kessenbrock K, Krumbholz M, Schönermarck U, Back W, Gross WL, Werb Z, et al. Netting neutrophils in autoimmune small-vessel vasculitis. *Nat Med.* (2009) 15:623–5. doi: 10.1038/nm.1959

Belzeaux R, Lefebvre MN, Lazzari A, Le CT, Consoloni JL, Zendjidjian X, et al. How to: measuring blood cytokines in biological psychiatry using commercially available multiplex immunoassays. *Psychoneuroendocrino.* (2017) 75:72–82. doi: 10.1016/j.psyneuen.2016. 10.010

Beiter K, Wartha F, Albiger B, Normark S, Zychlinsky A, Henriques- Normark B. An endonuclease allows streptococcus pneumoniae to escape from neutrophil extracellular traps. *Curr Biol Cb.* (2006) 16:401–7. doi: 10.1016/j.cub.2006.01.056

Lefrançais E, Mallavia B, Zhuo H, Calfee CS, Looney MR. Maladaptive role of neutrophil extracellular traps in pathogen-induced lung injury. *JCI Insight.* (2018) 3:1–15. doi: 10.1172/jci.insight.98178

Matthay MA, Ware LB, Zimmerman GA. The acute respiratory distress syndrome. *J Clin Invest.* (2012) 122:2731–40. doi: 10.1172/JCI60331

Menegali B, Nesi R, Souza P, Silva L, Silveira P, Valenca S, et al. The effects of physical exercise on the cigarette smoke-induced pulmonary oxidative response. *Pulm Pharmacol Ther.* (2009) 22:567–73. doi: 10.1016/j.pupt.2009.08.003

Nemmar A, Al-Salam S, Yuvaraju P, Beegam S. Exercise training mitigates water pipe smoke exposure-induced pulmonary impairment via inhibiting NF-kappaB and activating Nrf2 signalling pathways. *Oxid Med Cell Longev.* (2018) 2018:7459612. doi: 10.1155/2018/7459612

Robinson M, Dasari S, Konopka A, Johnson M, Manjunatha S, Esponda R, et al. Enhanced protein translation underlies improved metabolic and physical adaptations to different exercise training modes in young and old humans. *Cell Metab.* (2017) 25:581–92. doi: 10.1016/j.cmet.2017. 02.009

Dantas W, Murai I, Perandini L, Azevedo H, Moreira FCA, et al. Acute exercise elicits differential expression of insulin resistance genes in the skeletal muscle of patients with polycystic ovary syndrome. *Clin Endocrinol.* (2017) 86:688–97. doi: 10.1111/cen.13307

Yu Y, Liao Y, Su K, Chang T, Shyue S, Kou Y, Lee T. Prior exercise training alleviates the lung inflammation induced by subsequent exposure to environmental cigarette smoke. *Acta Physiol.* (2012) 2012:1–9. doi: 10.1111/j.1748-1716.2012.02433.x

Feng B, Qi R, Gao J, Wang T, Xu H, Zhao Q, et al. Exercise training prevented endothelium dysfunction from particulate matter instillation in Wistar rats. *Sci Total Environ.* (2019) 694:133674. doi: 10.1016/j.scitotenv.2019. 133674

Cortjens B, Woensel JBMV, Bem RA. Neutrophil extracellular traps in respiratory disease: guided anti-microbial traps or toxic webs? *Paediatr Respir Rev.* (2016) 21:54–61. doi: 10.1016/j.prrv.2016. 03.007

Barletta KE, Elaine RC, Burdick MD, Joel L, Borna M. Adenosine A(2B) receptor deficiency promotes host defenses against gram-negative bacterial pneumonia. *Am J Respir Crit Care Med.* (2012) 186:1044–50. doi: 10.1164/rccm.201204-0622OC

Mona S, Christiane J, Queisser MA, Guenter L, Guillermo B, Galuska SP, et al. Neutrophil extracellular traps directly induce epithelial and endothelial cell death: a predominant role of histones. *PLoS ONE.* (2012) 7:e32366. doi: 10.1371/journal.pone.0032366

Toussaint M, Jackson DJ, Swieboda D, Guedan A, Tsourouktsoglou TD, Ching YM, et al. Host DNA released by NETosis promotes rhinovirus- induced type-2 allergic asthma exacerbation. *Nat Med.* (2017) 23:681–91. doi: 10.1038/nm.4332

Martínez-Alemán SR, Campos-García L, Palma-Nicolas JP, Hernández-Bello R, González GM, Sánchez-González A. Understanding the entanglement: neutrophil extracellular traps (NETs) in cystic fibrosis. *Front Cell Infect Mi.* (2017) 7:1–7. doi: 10.3389/fcimb.2017.00104

Uddin M, Watz H, Malmgren A, Pedersen F. NETopathic inflammation in chronic obstructive pulmonary disease and severe asthma. *Front Immuno.* (2019) 10:1–10. doi: 10.3389/fimmu.2019.00047

Hu Q, Shi H, Zeng T, Liu H, Su Y, Cheng X, et al. Increased neutrophil extracellular traps activate NLRP3 and inflammatory macrophages in adult-onset Still's disease. *Arthritis Res Ther.* (2019) 21:1–11. doi: 10.1186/s13075-018-1800-z

de Oliveira MTP, de Sá Coutinho D, Tenório de Souza É, Stanisçuaski Guterres S, Pohlmann AR, Silva PMR, et al. Orally delivered resveratrol- loaded lipid-core nanocapsules ameliorate LPS-induced acute lung injury via the ERK and PI3K/Akt pathways. *Int J Nanomed.* (2019) 14:5215–28. doi: 10.2147/IJN.S200666

Yang L, Zhang Z, Zhuo Y, Cui L, Li C, Li D, et al. Resveratrol alleviates sepsis-induced acute lung injury by suppressing inflammation and apoptosis of alveolar macrophage cells. *Am J Transl Res.* (2018) 10:1961–75.

Qin X, Jiang X, Jiang X, Wang Y, Miao Z, He W, et al. Micheliolide inhibits LPS-induced inflammatory response and protects mice from LPS challenge. *Sci Rep.* (2016) 6:1–13. doi: 10.1038/srep 23240

Tian X, Xie G, Xiao H, Ding F, Bao W, Zhang M. CXCR4 knockdown prevents inflammatory cytokine expression in macrophages by suppressing activation of MAPK and NF-κB signaling pathways. *Cell Biosci.* (2019) 9:1–8. doi: 10.1186/s13578-019-0315-x

Perdomo JLH, Ahmadi Z, Yan F, Chong JJH, Passam FH, Chong BH. Neutrophil activation and NETosis are the major drivers of thrombosis in heparin-induced thrombocytopenia. *Nat Commun.* (2019) 10:1–14. doi: 10.1038/s41467-019-09160-7

16

Preventing Ventilator-Associated Lung Injury: A Perioperative Perspective

*Satoshi Kimura, Nicoleta Stoicea, Byron Rafael Rosero Britton, Muhammad Shabsigh, Aly Branstiter and David L. Stahl**

Department of Anesthesiology, The Ohio State University Wexner Medical Center, Columbus, OH, USA

Correspondence:
David L. Stahl
david.stahl@osumc.edu

Introduction: Research into the prevention of ventilator-associated lung injury (VALI) in patients with acute respiratory distress syndrome (ARDS) in the intensive care unit (ICU) has resulted in the development of a number of lung protective strategies, which have become commonplace in the treatment of critically ill patients. An increasing number of studies have applied lung protective ventilation in the operating room to otherwise healthy individuals. We review the history of lung protective strategies in patients with acute respiratory failure and explore their use in patients undergoing mechanical ventilation during general anesthesia. We aim to provide context for a discussion of the benefits and drawbacks of lung protective ventilation, as well as to inform future areas of research.

Methods: We completed a database search and reviewed articles investigating lung protective ventilation in both the ICU and in patients receiving general anesthesia through May 2015.

Results: Lung protective ventilation was associated with improved outcomes in patients with acute respiratory failure in the ICU. Clinical evidence is less clear regarding lung protective ventilation for patients undergoing surgery.

Conclusion: Lung protective ventilation strategies, including low tidal volume ventilation and moderate positive end-expiratory pressure, are well established therapies to minimize lung injury in critically ill patients with and without lung disease, and may provide benefit to patients undergoing general anesthesia.

Keywords: lung protective ventilation, low tidal volume ventilation, ventilator-induced lung injury, ventilator-associated lung injury, acute respiratory distress syndrome, general anesthesia

INTRODUCTION

Atelectasis is a common adverse effect of general anesthesia associated with both hypoxemia and postoperative respiratory complications (1–3). Mechanical ventilation (MV) may be used to combat atelectasis by prescribing relatively large tidal volumes (V_T) [up to 15 mL/kg predicted body weight (PBW)] (4, 5). However, we now know that using high V_T ventilation in the intensive care unit (ICU) increases mortality (6), and that MV itself can cause lung injury, through a process referred to as ventilator-induced lung injury (VILI) (7). VILI occurs through a number of different mechanisms.

Barotrauma, defined as pulmonary injury from elevated transpulmonary pressures, was the first widely recognized element of VILI (7, 8). Since it was subsequently demonstrated that humans could generate high airway pressures without causing lung injury, clinical focus shifted to volutrauma, hyperaeration caused by high V_T leading to lung injury (7, 8). Conversely, atelectrauma occurs when tidal ventilation at low airway pressures causes cyclic opening and collapse of unstable lung units (7, 9). This repeated cycling generates disruptive forces on the alveolar basement membranes and augments lung injury (7). Since the early 1990s, numerous studies have shown that MV can trigger the release of pro-inflammatory cytokines and the recruitment of neutrophils (10–13). This biological reaction in response to mechanical forces is known as biotrauma (8, 9, 14, 15).

Clinically, it can be difficult to delineate MV as the precise cause of lung injury. Therefore, when lung injury is concurrent to, but not necessarily caused by, MV, the term ventilator-associated lung injury (VALI) is used (7). The potentially detrimental effects of MV were recognized as early as 1960s (16) when canine studies demonstrated that lung overdistension resulted in an absence of surfactant and subsequent atelectasis (17). Attempts to prevent lung overdistention by therapeutically reducing V_T in humans in the ICU became feasible with acceptance of permissive hypercapnia (18).

Over the past 15 years, studies of patients with acute respiratory failure have resulted in the development of a number of lung protective strategies applied to minimize VALI. These strategies include low V_T to limit volutrauma, higher positive end-expiratory pressure (PEEP) to prevent atelectrauma, and recruitment maneuvers (i.e., application of temporary high airway pressures to reinflate collapsed lung units) (19). The successful application of these strategies in acute respiratory failure has led to increased interest in applying these principles to other patient populations. What remains controversial is whether the principles of lung protective ventilation derived from ICU patients with acute respiratory failure have applicability to otherwise healthy patients in the operating room.

MATERIALS AND METHODS

A systematic literature search was performed to identify clinical studies of lung protective ventilation strategies. We searched PubMed, EMBASE, and the Cochrane Library from inception to May 2015 with restriction to human studies published in English using a combination of standardized search terms and keywords to cover the topics of acute lung injury, acute respiratory distress syndrome (ARDS), MV, lung protective ventilation, low V_T ventilation, and general anesthesia. We reviewed articles that investigated the effects of lung protective ventilation strategies. We included randomized controlled trials (RCT), cohort, cross-sectional, and before-and-after studies. References of all studies were inspected for additional articles that were not identified by the electronic database search. We removed non-human studies, case reports, abstracts, and any other study where the full text was unavailable. Additionally, we excluded studies that specifically examined one-lung ventilation.

RESULTS

Origin of Lung Protective Strategies: Patients with ARDS and Acute Respiratory Failure in the ICU

In 1998, Amato et al. described a lung protective strategy, which included a V_T of <6 mL/kg, PEEP above the lower inflection point, and permissive hypercapnia, was associated with improved survival at 28 days, an improved rate of weaning from MV, and a lower rate of barotrauma in patients with ARDS (20). In 2000, The Acute Respiratory Distress Syndrome Network reported that lower V_T (6 mL/kg of PBW) resulted in decreased mortality and increased ventilator-free days compared with V_T of 12 mL/kg of PBW (6). An increase of 1 mL/kg PBW in initial V_T has been associated with a 23% increase in ICU mortality risk (21). In patients without ARDS, a retrospective cohort study demonstrated the use of large V_T was the main risk factor associated with the development of lung injury (odds ratio 1.3 for each milliliter/kilogram above 6 mL/kg PBW, $p < 0.001$) (22). And a prospective study conducted by the same group concluded that initial ventilator settings of high V_T (odds ratio 2.6 for $V_T > 700$ mL) and high peak airway pressure (odds ratio 1.6 for peak airway pressure >30 cmH_2O) were associated with the development of ARDS in patients without ARDS at the onset of MV (23).

Lung Protective Ventilation during General Anesthesia in Operating Room

Although lung protective ventilation strategies are widely used in the ICU, it remains unclear if these strategies can be directly translated into use in the operating room. Respiratory complications are low in patients undergoing general anesthesia, unlike the ICU (24). Therefore, it may take a much larger number of patients to improve outcomes using lung protective strategies, and there are risks associated with lung protective ventilation, including increased alveolar collapse (25), increased right ventricular afterload (26), hypercapnia and respiratory acidosis (27), and worsened metabolic acidosis (27). Studies on intraoperative MV can be divided into those that target surrogate markers of lung inflammation/injury, clinical outcomes, or systemic reviews and meta-analyses. We examine these studies to better understand the risks and benefits of lung protective ventilation in the operating room (**Table 1**).

Lung Protective Ventilation, Pulmonary Biomarkers, and Lung Mechanics

Inflammatory biomarkers can be used as surrogate outcomes for lung inflammation or injury in patients receiving MV. For example, one RCT compared 40 patients undergoing elective coronary artery bypass grafting (CABG) receiving high V_T/low PEEP or low V_T/high PEEP (28). After 6 h of MV, interleukin (IL)-6 and IL-8 levels were elevated in bronchoalveolar lavage (BAL) fluid and plasma in patients who received higher V_T/low PEEP, suggesting alveolar lung inflammation (28). The attenuation of IL-8, but not IL-6 levels by lung protective ventilation has been replicated in other surgical patients undergoing cardiopulmonary bypass (29) as well as elective surgery (30) but not in major abdominal, thoracic (31), or spinal surgery (32). IL-10 has

TABLE 1 | Randomized controlled trials comparing lung protective strategies with low tidal volumes to conservative ventilation in operating room.

Type of surgery	Source	Patients' population	Lung protective ventilation (V_T)	Conservative ventilation (V_T)	Primary outcome
Cardiac surgery	Chaney et al. (36)	Adults patients undergoing elective on-pump CABG surgery (n = 25)	6 mL/kg with 5 cmH_2O of PEEP (n = 12)	12 mL/kg with 5 cmH_2O of PEEP (n = 13)	Pulmonary mechanics
	Koner et al. (34)	Adult patients undergoing elective on-pump CABG grafting surgery (n = 44)	6 mL/kg with 5 cmH_2O of PEEP (n = 15)	10 mL/kg with 5 cmH_2O of PEEP (n = 14) or zero PEEP (n = 15)	TNF-α and IL-6 levels
	Zupancich et al. (28)	Adult patients undergoing elective on-pump CABG surgery (n = 40)	8 mL/kg with 10 cmH_2O of PEEP (n = 20)	10–12 mL/kg with 2–3 cmH_2O of PEEP (n = 20)	IL-6 and IL-8 in BAL fluid and plasma
	Reis Miranda et al. (29)	Adult patients undergoing elective on-pump CABG or valve surgery (n = 62)	4–6 mL/kg with 10 cmH_2O of PEEP during (n = 22) or after (n = 18) surgery	6–8 mL/kg (n = 22) with 5 cmH_2O of PEEP	IL-6, IL-8, IL-10, TNF-α, and interferon-γ
	Sundar et al. (43)	Adult patients undergoing elective cardiac surgery (n = 149)	6 mL/kg with PEEP according to ARDS Network investigators (6) (n = 75)	10 mL/kg with PEEP according to ARDS Network investigators (6) (n = 74)	Time to extubation
Abdominal surgery	Wrigge et al. (31)	Adult patients undergoing major abdominal surgery (n = 30)	6 mL/kg with 10 cmH_2O of PEEP (n = 15)	12 or 15 mL/kg with zero PEEP (n = 15)	TNF, IL-1, IL-6, IL-8, IL-10, and IL-12
	Weingarten et al. (37)	Adult patients aged >65 years undergoing major open abdominal surgery under general anesthesia (n = 40)	6 mL/kg with 12 cmH_2O of PEEP and recruitment maneuvers (n = 20)	10 mL/kg with no PEEP and no recruitment maneuvers (n = 20)	Oxygenation, pulmonary mechanics, hemodynamic stability
	Treschan et al. (40)	Adult patients undergoing elective upper abdominal surgery lasting ≥3 h under combined general and epidural anesthesia (n = 101)	6 mL/kg with 5 cmH_2O of PEEP (n = 50)	12 mL/kg with 5 cmH_2O of PEEP (n = 51)	Lung function
	Severgnini et al. (38)	Adult patients undergoing elective open abdominal surgery ≥2 h (n = 55)	7 mL/kg with 10 cmH_2O of PEEP and recruitment maneuvers (n = 28)	9 mL/kg with zero PEEP (n = 27)	Modified Clinical Pulmonary Infection Score, gas exchange, and pulmonary functional tests
	Futier et al. (5)	Adults patients at intermediate to high risk of pulmonary complications undergoing major abdominal surgery (n = 400)	6–8 mL/kg with 6–8 cmH_2O of PEEP and recruitment maneuvers (n = 200)	10–12 mL/kg with no PEEP and no recruitment maneuvers (n = 200)	A composite of major pulmonary and extrapulmonary complications occurring by day 7 after surgery
Others	Cai et al. (39)	Adults patients aged 20–50 years with body mass index undergoing elective excision of intracranial lesions (n = 16)	6 mL/kg without PEEP (n = 8)	10 mL/kg without PEEP (n = 8)	Atelectasis (by CT and ABG)
	Memtsoudis et al. (32)	Adult patients undergoing elective lumbar decompression and fusion in prone position under general anesthesia (n = 26)	6 mL/kg with 8 cmH_2O of PEEP (n = 13)	12 mL/kg with zero PEEP (n = 13)	Plasma levels of IL-6 and IL-8, and urinary levels of desmosine
	Choi et al. (33)	Adult patients undergoing a surgical procedure ≥5 h (n = 40)	6 mL/kg with 10 cmH_2O of PEEP (n = 21)	12 mL/kg without PEEP (n = 19)	Markers of coagulation and fibrinolysis
	Wolthuis et al. (30)	Adult patients undergoing a surgical procedure ≥5 h (n = 40)	6 mL/kg with 10 cmH_2O of PEEP (n = 21)	12 mL/kg without PEEP (n = 19)	Polymorphonuclear cell influx, changes in levels of inflammatory markers, and nucleosomes in BAL fluid and/or blood
	Determann et al. (35)	Adult patients undergoing a surgical procedure ≥5 h (n = 40)	6 mL/kg with 10 cmH_2O of PEEP (n = 21)	12 mL/kg without PEEP (n = 19)	Local and systemic levels of Clara cell protein

V_T, tidal volumes; CABG, coronary artery bypass grafting; PEEP, positive end-expiratory pressure; TNF, tumor necrosis factor; IL, interleukin; BAL, bronchoalveolar lavage; CPB, cardiopulmonary bypass; ARDS, acute respiratory distress syndrome; CT, computed tomography; ABG, arterial blood gas.

a similarly mixed profile in response to lung protective MV (29). High V_T/zero end-expiratory pressure (ZEEP) MV does appear to lead to procoagulant activation in the alveolar space (33). Many other inflammatory markers, including tumor necrosis factor-alpha (TNF-α), interferon (IFN)-γ, IL-1, IL-1α, IL-1β, IL-6, IL-12, macrophage inflammatory protein 1α, and macrophage inflammatory protein 1β, or other markers of lung epithelial injury have not been demonstrated to change in response to lung protective ventilation (29–31, 34, 35).

Other studies have demonstrated improved perioperative pulmonary mechanics as a surrogate outcome. One single-center RCT included 25 patients undergoing elective CABG showed a greater reduction in both dynamic and static lung compliance in patients receiving conventional MV, suggesting lung protective MV resulted in improved pulmonary mechanics (36). RCTs in abdominal surgery had varied results showing improved (37), unchanged (38, 39), and degraded (40) pulmonary mechanics in patients receiving lung protective MV. An improvement in the partial pressure of arterial oxygen (PaO_2)/Fraction of inspired oxygen (FiO_2) ratio in abdominal surgery patients appears to reflect the use of recruitment maneuvers more than any particular lung protective strategy (37, 40).

Lung Protective Ventilation and Clinical Outcomes

Several retrospective studies have investigated the association between MV strategies in the operating room and clinical outcomes. A retrospective evaluation of patients admitted to the ICU with postoperative hypoxemic respiratory failure, requiring MV, showed that a high V_T to ideal body weight (IBW) ratio was an independent risk factor for the development of ARDS (41). While a retrospective study of billing data for over 69,000 patients undergoing non-cardiac surgery did not show any effect of V_T on postoperative respiratory complications (24). Another retrospective study of more than 29,000 patients reported that V_T of 6–8 mL/kg IBW were associated with a significant increase in 30-day mortality compared with V_T of 8–10 mL/kg IBW (hazard ratio 1.6, $p = 0.0002$) (42). The authors hypothesized that the increased mortality may be related to the combination of lower V_T and low PEEP (≤5 cmH_2O) (42).

Prospective RCTs of MV in the operating room have specifically targeted high-risk surgical groups, primarily cardiac and abdominal surgery patients. One single-center RCT investigated duration of intubation for cardiac surgery patients by comparing ventilation with low vs. high V_T ventilation. A higher proportion of patients were extubated 6 h postoperatively in the low V_T group (37.3 vs. 20.3%; $p = 0.02$) and fewer patients in the low V_T group required re-intubation (0.3 vs. 9.5%; $p = 0.03$) (43). In two RCTs of patients undergoing open abdominal surgery, lower V_T ventilation combined with PEEP and recruitment maneuvers decreased respiratory complications as measured by two different postoperative pulmonary complication scores when compared to higher V_T ventilation with ZEEP and no recruitment maneuvers (5, 38). The IMPROVE trial also found that patients receiving lung protective ventilation and recruitment maneuvers had decreased postoperative non-invasive ventilation and intubation requirements (5.0 vs. 17.0%, $p = 0.001$), and shorter length of hospital stay (mean difference, −2.45 days, $p = 0.006$) (5). However, in 101 patients undergoing upper abdominal surgery who were randomized to low V_T ventilation (6 mL/kg PBW) with 5 cmH_2O PEEP or to higher V_T ventilation (12 mL/kg PBW) also with 5 cmH_2O PEEP, there was no significant difference in postoperative pulmonary complications (40). In the largest prospective multicenter RCT, conducted by the Protective Ventilation (PROVE) Network Investigators, 900 patients were allocated either to a high level of PEEP (12 cmH_2O) with recruitment maneuvers (higher PEEP group) or a low level of PEEP (≤2 cmH_2O) without recruitment maneuvers (lower PEEP group) while receiving 8 mL/kg V_T (PROVHILO trial). In this study, postoperative pulmonary and extrapulmonary complications were not significantly different between the two groups although hypotension happened more frequently in the higher PEEP group (relative risk 1.29; $p = 0.0016$) and those in the higher PEEP group had a greater need for vasopressors than those in the lower PEEP group (relative risk 1.20; $p = 0.0016$) (44). The results of these trials suggest an important interaction between V_T and PEEP affecting clinical outcomes.

Lung Protective Ventilation Meta-Analyses

The recently updated Cochrane meta-analysis evaluated 12 studies with 1012 participants comparing specifically low vs. high V_T ventilation in the operating room (45). They found no difference in 30-day mortality (risk ratio (RR) 0.79, 95% confidence interval (CI) 0.40-1.54), but the low V_T cohort did show a decrease in postoperative pneumonia and a decreased requirement for both invasive and non-invasive postoperative ventilation (45). Decreased rates of pulmonary infection have been confirmed by other meta-analyses of lung protective ventilation (including interventions in addition to low V_T) (46–48). These additional meta-analyses also failed to demonstrate a mortality benefit to intraoperative lung protective ventilation (46, 47).

Lung Protective Ventilation in Anesthetic Practice

While the data to support lung protective ventilation in the operating room remains unclear, it is worthwhile to examine the current state of anesthetic practice regarding MV. One cross-sectional analysis of intraoperative ventilation during elective abdominal surgery in the United States showed that ventilator settings were non-uniform and ventilation with $V_T > 10$ mL/ kg PBW is still common (17.5%). BMI ≥30, female gender, and height <165 cm may predispose certain patients to receive large V_T during general anesthesia as providers likely overestimate PBW in this patient group (49). Despite the high prevalence of high V_T ventilation in the operating room, a targeted study of the management of hypoxemic patients (defined by P/F ratio) in the operating room found V_T, and peak inspiratory pressure (PIP) have been decreasing annually while PEEP has been increasing (50). Unfortunately, worsened hypoxemia (lower P/F ratio) correlated most closely with higher FiO_2 and PIP, suggesting that patients who would most benefit from lung protective ventilation are not receiving it (50). Investigators in Australia performed an audit in 272 patients undergoing general anesthesia for three consecutive days in 2013. They showed that a median V_T was 9.5 mL/ kg PBW, suggesting that the practice of MV in the operating room does not always reflect recent studies (51). There are several ongoing studies investigating variation of MV setting within/between centers (52)[1].

DISCUSSION

The translation of research from the ICU to the operating room can be difficult for several reasons. Patients receiving MV in the

[1]IVENT. International Survery on VENTilation Practice (iVENT). In: PROVEnet [Internet]. Available from: https://sites.google.com/site/iventsurvey/.

operating room during general anesthesia commonly lack the derangements in gas exchange and pulmonary mechanics seen in the ICU. While general anesthesia does induce atelectasis, the atelectasis is well-tolerated and relatively short-lived (1–3). Rates of respiratory complications remain low in most populations and the short duration of MV likely affects lung compliance less than a prolonged course of ventilation in ICU. Furthermore, ICU patients are more likely to have comorbid illnesses, such as cardiovascular instability and shock, acid–base abnormalities, and pro-inflammatory states, such as sepsis, which affect the goals of MV.

Based on published ICU data, studies of lung protective ventilation in the operating room generally have used 6–8 mL/kg PBW as low V_T ventilation (**Table 1**), which may not be the ideal V_T for surgical patients (42). Furthermore, studies in the perioperative setting have used low V_T combined with PEEP and/or recruitment maneuvers as the lung protective strategies. Although low V_T ventilation is clearly an important factor of the lung protective ventilation (53), it is still unclear how we should combine these "lung protective strategies," including PEEP and recruitment maneuvers, into a unified best practice for MV in the operating room (44). A subsequent ongoing international multicenter RCT, aims to compare a ventilation strategy using higher levels of PEEP with recruitment maneuvers to one using lower levels of PEEP without recruitment maneuvers in obese patients at risk of postoperative pulmonary complications[2]. This study design hints at the holy grail for intraoperative ventilation: targeted interventions for specific patients. While still heterogeneous themselves, patients with acute respiratory failure and ARDS in the ICU are substantially more homogeneous than the morass of patients undergoing general anesthesia in the operating room. This heterogeneity may, in part, explain the disparate findings in previous studies. However, as we gain a better understanding of the risks and benefits of the various aspects of lung protective strategies, we can more effectively target-specific patient populations for intervention.

[2]Technische Universität Dresden. Protective Ventilation with Higher Versus Lower PEEP during General Anesthesia for Surgery in Obese Patients (PROBESE). In: ClinicalTrials.gov [Internet]. Available from: http://clinicaltrials.gov/show/NCT02148692.

CONCLUSION

As lung protective strategies, including low V_T ventilation, higher PEEP, and/or recruitment maneuvers, continue to evolve, they may also provide benefit to patients undergoing general anesthesia. Larger trials of specific ventilator strategies across different populations are required to evaluate different lung protective strategies and their interaction with different groups of surgical patients to clarify the benefit or harm of lung protective ventilation in the operating room. Furthermore, we need investigations into current practice strategies of clinical anesthesiologists, in order to help shape how new data are applied in the operating room.

AUTHOR CONTRIBUTIONS

SK made contributions to conception and design, participated in drafting the article, and revised it critically for important intellectual content. NS participated in drafting the article and revised it critically for important intellectual content. BB participated in drafting the article and revised it critically for important intellectual content. MS participated in drafting the article and revised it critically for important intellectual content. AB participated in drafting the article and revised it critically for important intellectual content. DS made contributions to conception and design, participated in drafting the article, and revised it critically for important intellectual content.

REFERENCES

Duggan M, Kavanagh BP. Pulmonary atelectasis: a pathogenic periope- rative entity. *Anesthesiology* (2005) 102(4):838–54. doi:10.1097/00000542- 200504000-00021

Gunnarsson L, Tokics L, Gustavsson H, Hedenstierna G. Influence of age on atelectasis formation and gas exchange impairment during general anaesthesia. *Br J Anaesth* (1991) 66(4):423–32. doi:10.1093/bja/66.4.423

Edmark L, Kostova-Aherdan K, Enlund M, Hedenstierna G. Optimal oxygen concentration during induction of general anesthesia. *Anesthesiology* (2003) 98(1):28–33. doi:10.1097/00000542-200301000-00008

Bendixen HH, Hedley-Whyte J, Laver MB. Impaired oxygenation in surgical patients during general anesthesia with controlled ventilation. A concept of atelectasis. *N Engl J Med* (1963) 269:991–6. doi:10.1056/ NEJM196311072691901

Futier E, Constantin JM, Paugam-Burtz C, Pascal J, Eurin M, Neuschwander A, et al. A trial of intraoperative low-tidal-volume ventilation in abdominal surgery. *N Engl J Med* (2013) 369(5):428–37. doi:10.1056/NEJMoa1301082

The Acute Respiratory Distress Syndrome Network. Ventilation with lower tidal volumes as compared with traditional tidal volumes for acute lung injury and the acute respiratory distress syndrome. *N Engl J Med* (2000) 342(18):1301–8. doi:10.1056/NEJM200005043421801

Kuchnicka K, Maciejewski D. Ventilator-associated lung injury. *Anaesthesiol Intensive Ther* (2013) 45(3):164–70. doi:10.5603/AIT.2013.0034

Oeckler RA, Hubmayr RD. Ventilator-associated lung injury: a search for better therapeutic targets. *Eur Respir J* (2007) 30(6):1216–26. doi:10.1183/09031936.00104907

Gattinoni L, Protti A, Caironi P, Carlesso E. Ventilator-induced lung injury: the anatomical and physiological framework. *Crit Care Med* (2010) 38(10 Suppl):S539–48. doi:10.1097/CCM.0b013e3181f1fcf7

Tremblay L, Valenza F, Ribeiro SP, Li J, Slutsky AS. Injurious ventilatory strategies increase cytokines and c-fos m-RNA expression in an isolated rat lung model. *J Clin Invest* (1997) 99(5):944–52. doi:10.1172/JCI119259

von Bethmann AN, Brasch F, Nusing R, Vogt K, Volk HD, Muller KM, et al. Hyperventilation induces release of cytokines from perfused mouse lung. *Am J Respir Crit Care Med* (1998) 157(1):263–72. doi:10.1164/ ajrccm.157.1.9608052

Imanaka H, Shimaoka M, Matsuura N, Nishimura M, Ohta N, Kiyono H. Ventilator-induced lung injury is associated with neutrophil infiltration, macrophage activation, and TGF-beta 1 mRNA upregulation in rat lungs. *Anesth Analg* (2001) 92(2):428–36. doi:10.1097/00000539-200102000-00029

Tsuno K, Miura K, Takeya M, Kolobow T, Morioka T. Histopathologic pulmonary changes from mechanical ventilation at high peak airway pressures. *Am Rev Respir Dis* (1991) 143(5 Pt 1):1115–20. doi:10.1164/ ajrccm/143.5_Pt_1.1115

Whitehead T, Slutsky AS. The pulmonary physician in critical care * 7: ventilator induced lung injury. *Thorax* (2002) 57(7):635–42. doi:10.1136/ thorax.57.7.635

Uhlig S. Ventilation-induced lung injury and mechanotransduction: stretch- ing it too far? *Am J Physiol Lung Cell Mol Physiol* (2002) 282(5):L892–6. doi:10.1152/ajplung.00124.2001

Greenfield LJ, Ebert PA, Benson DW. Atelectasis and surface tension proper- ties of lung extracts following positive pressure ventilation and overinflation. *Surg Forum* (1963) 14:239–40.

Greenfield LJ, Ebert PA, Benson DW. Effect of positive pressure ventilation on surface tension properties of lung extracts. *Anesthesiology* (1964) 25:312–6. doi:10.1097/00000542-196405000-00009

Hickling KG, Henderson SJ, Jackson R. Low mortality associated with low volume pressure limited ventilation with permissive hypercapnia in severe adult respiratory distress syndrome. *Intensive Care Med* (1990) 16(6):372–7. doi:10.1007/BF01735174

Zambon M, Vincent JL. Mortality rates for patients with acute lung injury/ ARDS have decreased over time. *Chest* (2008) 133(5):1120–7. doi:10.1378/ chest.07-2134

Amato MB, Barbas CS, Medeiros DM, Magaldi RB, Schettino GP, Lorenzi- Filho G, et al. Effect of a protective-ventilation strategy on mortality in the acute respiratory distress syndrome. *N Engl J Med* (1998) 338(6):347–54. doi:10.1056/ NEJM199802053380602

Needham DM, Yang T, Dinglas VD, Mendez-Tellez PA, Shanholtz C, Sevransky JE, et al. Timing of low tidal volume ventilation and intensive care unit mortality in acute respiratory distress syndrome. A prospective cohort study. *Am J Respir Crit Care Med* (2015) 191(2):177–85. doi:10.1164/ rccm.201409-1598OC

Gajic O, Dara SI, Mendez JL, Adesanya AO, Festic E, Caples SM, et al. Ventilator-associated lung injury in patients without acute lung injury at the onset of mechanical ventilation. *Crit Care Med* (2004) 32(9):1817–24. doi:10.1097/01. CCM.0000133019.52531.30

Gajic O, Frutos-Vivar F, Esteban A, Hubmayr RD, Anzueto A. Ventilator settings as a risk factor for acute respiratory distress syndrome in mechani- cally ventilated patients. *Intensive Care Med* (2005) 31(7):922–6. doi:10.1007/ s00134-005-2625-1

Ladha K, Vidal Melo MF, McLean DJ, Wanderer JP, Grabitz SD, Kurth T, et al. Intraoperative protective mechanical ventilation and risk of postop- erative respiratory complications: hospital based registry study. *BMJ* (2015) 351:h3646. doi:10.1136/bmj.h3646

Kallet RH, Siobal MS, Alonso JA, Warnecke EL, Katz JA, Marks JD. Lung collapse during low tidal volume ventilation in acute respiratory distress syndrome. *Respir Care* (2001) 46(1):49–52.

Viitanen A, Salmenpera M, Heinonen J. Right ventricular response to hypercarbia after cardiac surgery. *Anesthesiology* (1990) 73(3):393–400. doi:10.1097/00000542-199009000-00005

Wrigge H, Uhlig U, Baumgarten G, Menzenbach J, Zinserling J, Ernst M, et al. Mechanical ventilation strategies and inflammatory responses to cardiac surgery: a prospective randomized clinical trial. *Intensive Care Med* (2005) 31(10):1379–87. doi:10.1007/s00134-005-2767-1

Zupancich E, Paparella D, Turani F, Munch C, Rossi A, Massaccesi S, et al. Mechanical ventilation affects inflammatory mediators in patients undergoing cardiopulmonary bypass for cardiac surgery: a randomized clinical trial. *J Thorac Cardiovasc Surg* (2005) 130(2):378–83. doi:10.1016/j. jtcvs.2004.11.061

Reis Miranda D, Gommers D, Struijs A, Dekker R, Mekel J, Feelders R, et al. Ventilation according to the open lung concept attenuates pulmonary inflammatory response in cardiac surgery. *Eur J Cardiothorac Surg* (2005) 28(6):889–95. doi:10.1016/j.ejcts.2005.10.007

Wolthuis EK, Choi G, Dessing MC, Bresser P, Lutter R, Dzoljic M, et al. Mechanical ventilation with lower tidal volumes and positive end-expi- ratory pressure prevents pulmonary inflammation in patients without preexisting lung injury. *Anesthesiology* (2008) 108(1):46–54. doi:10.1097/01. anes.0000296068.80921.10

Wrigge H, Uhlig U, Zinserling J, Behrends-Callsen E, Ottersbach G, Fischer M, et al. The effects of different ventilatory settings on pul- monary and systemic inflammatory responses during major surgery. *Anesth Analg* (2004) 98(3):775–81, table of contents. doi:10.1213/01. ANE.0000100663.11852.BF

Memtsoudis SG, Bombardieri AM, Ma Y, Girardi FP. The effect of low versus high tidal volume ventilation on inflammatory markers in healthy individuals undergoing posterior spine fusion in the prone position: a randomized controlled trial. *J Clin Anesth* (2012) 24(4):263–9. doi:10.1016/j. jclinane.2011.08.003

Choi G, Wolthuis EK, Bresser P, Levi M, van der Poll T, Dzoljic M, et al. Mechanical ventilation with lower tidal volumes and positive end-expiratory pressure prevents alveolar coagulation in patients without lung injury. *Anesthesiology* (2006) 105(4):689–95. doi:10.1097/00000542-200610000-00013

Koner O, Celebi S, Balci H, Cetin G, Karaoglu K, Cakar N. Effects of protective and conventional mechanical ventilation on pulmonary function and systemic cytokine release after cardiopulmonary bypass. *Intensive Care Med* (2004) 30(4):620–6. doi:10.1007/s00134-003-2104-5

Determann RM, Wolthuis EK, Choi G, Bresser P, Bernard A, Lutter R, et al. Lung epithelial injury markers are not influenced by use of lower tidal volumes during elective surgery in patients without preexisting lung injury. *Am J Physiol Lung Cell Mol Physiol* (2008) 294(2):L344–50. doi:10.1152/ ajplung.00268.2007

Chaney MA, Nikolov MP, Blakeman BP, Bakhos M. Protective ventilation attenuates postoperative pulmonary dysfunction in patients undergoing cardiopulmonary bypass. *J Cardiothorac Vasc Anesth* (2000) 14(5):514–8. doi:10.1053/jcan.2000.9487

Weingarten TN, Whalen FX, Warner DO, Gajic O, Schears GJ, Snyder MR, et al. Comparison of two ventilatory strategies in elderly patients undergoing major abdominal surgery. *Br J Anaesth* (2010) 104(1):16–22. doi:10.1093/bja/ aep319

Severgnini P, Selmo G, Lanza C, Chiesa A, Frigerio A, Bacuzzi A, et al. Protective mechanical ventilation during general anesthesia for open abdom- inal surgery improves postoperative pulmonary function. *Anesthesiology* (2013) 118(6):1307–21. doi:10.1097/ALN.0b013e31829102de

Cai H, Gong H, Zhang L, Wang Y, Tian Y. Effect of low tidal volume ventilation on atelectasis in patients during general anesthesia: a computed tomographic scan. *J Clin Anesth* (2007) 19(2):125–9. doi:10.1016/j.jclinane.2006.08.008

Treschan TA, Kaisers W, Schaefer MS, Bastin B, Schmalz U, Wania V, et al. Ventilation with low tidal volumes during upper abdominal surgery does not improve postoperative lung function. *Br J Anaesth* (2012) 109(2):263–71. doi:10.1093/bja/aes140

Hughes CG, Weavind L, Banerjee A, Mercaldo ND, Schildcrout JS, Pandharipande PP. Intraoperative risk factors for acute respiratory distress syndrome in critically ill patients. *Anesth Analg* (2010) 111(2):464–7. doi:10.1213/ ANE.0b013e3181d8a16a

Levin MA, McCormick PJ, Lin HM, Hosseinian L, Fischer GW. Low intraoper- ative tidal volume ventilation with minimal PEEP is associated with increased mortality. *Br J Anaesth* (2014) 113(1):97–108. doi:10.1093/bja/aeu054

Sundar S, Novack V, Jervis K, Bender SP, Lerner A, Panzica P, et al. Influence of low tidal volume ventilation on time to extubation in cardiac surgical patients. *Anesthesiology* (2011) 114(5):1102–10. doi:10.1097/ALN.0b013e318215e254

PROVE Network Investigators for the Clinical Trial Network of the European Society of Anaesthesiology, Hemmes SN, Gama de Abreu M, Pelosi P, Schultz MJ. High versus low positive end-expiratory pressure during general anaesthesia for open abdominal surgery (PROVHILO trial): a multicentre randomised controlled trial. *Lancet* (2014) 384(9942):495–503. doi:10.1016/ S0140-6736(14)60416-5

Guay J, Ochroch EA. Intraoperative use of low volume ventilation to decrease postoperative mortality, mechanical ventilation, lengths of stay and lung injury in patients without acute lung injury. *Cochrane Database Syst Rev* (2015) 12:CD011151. doi:10.1002/14651858.CD011151.pub2

Gu WJ, Wang F, Liu JC. Effect of lung protective ventilation with lower tidal volumes on clinical outcomes among patients undergoing surgery: a meta-analysis of randomized controlled trials. *CMAJ* (2015) 187(3):E101–9. doi:10.1503/ cmaj.141005

Tao T, Bo L, Chen F, Xie Q, Zou Y, Hu B, et al. Effect of protective ventilation on postoperative pulmonary complications in patients undergoing general anaesthesia: a meta-analysis of randomised controlled trials. *BMJ Open* (2014) 4(6):e005208. doi:10.1136/bmjopen-2014-005208

Hemmes SN, Serpa Neto A, Schultz MJ. Intraoperative ventilatory strategies to prevent postoperative pulmonary complications: a meta-analysis. *Curr Opin Anaesthesiol* (2013) 26(2):126–33. doi:10.1097/ACO.0b013e32835e1242

Fernandez-Bustamante A, Wood CL, Tran ZV, Moine P. Intraoperative ventila- tion: incidence and risk factors for receiving large tidal volumes during general anesthesia. *BMC Anesthesiol* (2011) 11:22. doi:10.1186/1471-2253-11-22

Blum JM, Fetterman DM, Park PK, Morris M, Rosenberg AL. A descrip- tion of intraoperative ventilator management and ventilation strategies in hypoxic patients. *Anesth Analg* (2010) 110(6):1616–22. doi:10.1213/ ANE.0b013e3181da82e1

Karalapillai D, Weinberg L, Galtieri J, Glassford N, Eastwood G, Darvall J, et al. Current ventilation practice during general anaesthesia: a pro- spective audit in Melbourne, Australia. *BMC Anesthesiol* (2014) 14:85. doi:10.1186/1471-2253-14-85

Hemmes SN, de Abreu MG, Pelosi P, Schultz MJ. ESA clinical trials network 2012: LAS VEGAS – local assessment of ventilatory management during general anaesthesia for surgery and its effects on postoperative pulmonary complications: a prospective, observational, international, mul- ticentre cohort study. *Eur J Anaesthesiol* (2013) 30(5):205–7. doi:10.1097/ EJA.0b013e32835fcab3

Guldner A, Kiss T, Serpa Neto A, Hemmes SN, Canet J, Spieth PM, et al. Intraoperative protective mechanical ventilation for prevention of postoperative pulmonary complications: a comprehensive review of the role of tidal volume, positive end-expiratory pressure, and lung recruit- ment maneuvers. *Anesthesiology* (2015) 123(3):692–713. doi:10.1097/ ALN.0000000000000754

17

Gut-Lung Crosstalk in Sepsis-Induced Acute Lung Injury

Xin Zhou and Youxia Liao*

Department of ICU/Emergency, Wuhan University, Wuhan Third Hospital, Wuhan, China

***Correspondence:**
Xin Zhou
vgirlxin@163.com

Acute lung injury (ALI) and acute respiratory distress syndrome (ARDS) are common acute and severe cases of the respiratory system with complicated pathogenesis and high mortality. Sepsis is the leading indirect cause of ALI/ARDS in the intensive care unit (ICU). The pathogenesis of septic ALI/ARDS is complex and multifactorial. In the development of sepsis, the disruption of the intestinal barrier function, the alteration of gut microbiota, and the translocation of the intestinal microbiome can lead to systemic and local inflammatory responses, which further alter the immune homeostasis in the systemic environment. Disruption of homeostasis may promote and propagate septic ALI/ARDS. In turn, when ALI occurs, elevated levels of inflammatory cytokines and the shift of the lung microbiome may lead to the dysregulation of the intestinal microbiome and the disruption of the intestinal mucosal barrier. Thus, the interaction between the lung and the gut can initiate and potentiate sepsis-induced ALI/ARDS. The gut–lung crosstalk may be a promising potential target for intervention. This article reviews the underlying mechanism of gut-lung crosstalk in septic ALI/ARDS.

Keywords: sepsis, acute lung injury, gut-lung crosstalk, inflammation, gut microbiome

INTRODUCTION

Acute lung injury (ALI)/acute respiratory distress syndrome (ARDS) is a life-threatening condition of respiratory failure (Matthay et al., 2019). ALI/ARDS is a common clinical critical disease with rapid onset and high mortality and one of the primary causes of death in critically ill patients (Griffiths et al., 2019). According to statistics, more than three million ARDS patients are diagnosed worldwide every year, accounting for 10% of the number of people hospitalized in intensive care units (ICU) (Abe et al., 2018). The treatment of ALI/ARDS remains elusive. Despite major recent advances in the supporting care for ARDS, including the use of extracorporeal membrane oxygenation (ECMO), protective lung ventilation maneuvers, and statins (Fan et al., 2018), the mortality from ARDS is still high (34.9–46.1%) (Fernando et al., 2021). Sepsis is the leading indirect cause of ALI/ARDS in the ICU (Bellani et al., 2016), and the lung is the first affected and the most vulnerable organ during sepsis (Fan and Fan, 2018). Direct sepsis-induced ALI/ARDS arises from pulmonary infections, and indirect sepsis-induced ALI/ARDS arises from extrapulmonary infections (Bellani et al., 2016). It is worth noting that the mortality rate of ARDS caused by sepsis is higher than that of ARDS caused by other factors (Chen et al., 2019). Although the biology underlying sepsis-induced ALI/ARDS is complicated and multifactorial, our current understanding involves the release of inflammatory cytokines and the disruption of the lung microvascular barrier (Huppert et al., 2019).

Severe acute inflammation plays a crucial role in septic ALI/ARDS (Lelubre and Vincent, 2018). Pathogens activate the innate immune response of epithelial cells and alveolar macrophages, followed by migration and aggregation of neutrophils and monocytes, release of the inflammatory cytokines TNF-α, IL-1β, and IL-6, loss of alveolar-capillary barrier integrity, and increased permeability, leading to sepsis-associated ALI/ARDS (Luyt et al., 2020).

The gut microbiome coexists harmoniously with the host and plays multifarious beneficial roles in the body, such as shaping the immune system, maintaining homeostasis, and others (Morais et al., 2021). An increasing body of evidence has illustrated the role of the gut microbiome in the occurrence, development, and outcomes of sepsis (Adelman et al., 2020). Sepsis induces significantly compromised gut barrier integrity (Yoseph et al., 2016), which allows intact microbes and microbiota products to translocate, resulting in amplification of the systemic inflammatory response and contribution to multiple organ failure (Dickson, 2016). This imbalanced interaction between the gut barrier, immune system, endogenous microorganisms, and lung may lead to the deterioration of the systemic inflammatory response and the potentiation of ALI/ARDS. Hence, a better understanding of gut-lung crosstalk in sepsis-related ALI/ARDS may contribute to clarifying this complex disease and laying the foundation for new treatments.

Effect of Septic Acute Lung Injury/Acute Respiratory Distress Syndrome on the Gut

During sepsis, the onset of ALI/ARDS is related to the activation of a complex inflammatory cytokine cascade. The continuous recruitment of inflammatory cells perpetuates a vicious cycle that produces more pro-inflammatory cytokines, which interact with and influence each other to promote severe damage to the alveolar-capillary membrane as well as respiratory failure. Moreover, researchers have broadened the scope of septic ALI/ARDS to another key factor: the lung microbiome. In septic-ALI/ARDS, the inactivation of the bactericidal layer of the alveolar epithelium (Li et al., 2019), the flow of protein-rich alveolar exudate, the establishment of oxygen gradients, the surge of inflammatory mediators, and the impairment of local immune defenses (Dickson et al., 2015) may alter the lung microbiome that in turn perpetuates a positive-feedback loop of inflammation, injury, and further dysbiosis (Dickson et al., 2014). Along with an increase in inflammatory molecules and alteration of the lung flora, septic-ALI/ARDS is responsible for gut microbiota imbalance and gut barrier disruption (**Figure 1**).

Intestinal Barrier Disruption by Increased Cytokines During Sepsis

During septic ALI/ARDS, increased cytokine levels may cause impairment of the intestinal barrier. This selective barrier is composed of intestinal mucosal epithelial cells and inter-cell connections. When the selective barrier functions normally, it allows the cell-side movement of water, solutes, and immunomodulatory factors but prevents the movement of macromolecules and microorganisms (Weström et al., 2020). Tight junctions between cells play a critical role in the gut barrier function, and the cells are connected to the intracellular cytoskeleton by tight junction proteins [e.g., occludin, claudin family, junctional adhesion molecules (JAM), myosin light chain, zonula occludens (ZO); Krug and Fromm, 2020]. The increase of inflammatory cytokines during sepsis results in intestinal hyperpermeability through the up-regulation of claudin 2 and JAM and down-regulation of claudin 5 and ZO-1 (Yoseph et al., 2016). Alternatively, sepsis can also redistribute claudins 1, 3, 4, 5, and 8, resulting in intestinal barrier dysfunction (Li et al., 2009). Claudins are a protein family of up to 27 members in mammals. Expression of claudins 1–19 has been examined throughout the rat and mouse intestine and that of claudins 20–24 in the mouse upper small intestine. Members of the claudin family are major driving forces in the formation of paracellular barriers (Günzel and Yu, 2013). Claudins can be roughly divided into sealing or pore-forming claudins. Alteration of claudin expression may result in a decreased or increased paracellular transport of solutes as well as an increased permeability to macromolecules (Günzel, 2017). To date, claudin-2, -10b, and -15 qualify as cation pores and claudin-10a and -17 as anion pores, which are both acknowledged as pore-forming claudins (Odenwald and Turner, 2013). Therefore, an increase in a pore-forming protein, such as claudin-2, would directly cause hyperpermeability and deterioration of the barrier function, while a decrease in a sealing protein, such as claudin-5, would lead to the same result in a mechanistically complementary manner. Beyond that, the activation of myosin light chain kinase (MLCK) by inflammatory cytokines (TNF-α, IL-6, and IL-1β) is also associated with paracellular hyperpermeability. Cytokines further activated MLCK in a feed-forward mechanism, partly via altering ZO-1 and claudin 15 (Lorentz et al., 2017). MLCK phosphorylates the myosin regulatory light chain, which leads to contraction of the actin-myosin ring, increasing intestinal permeability (Su et al., 2020). Indeed, the significant increase of the intestinal permeability is closely interrelated to the occurrence and development of sepsis (Assimakopoulos et al., 2018), such as sepsis secondary intratracheal instillation of Pseudomonas aeruginosa due to gut mucosal and microvascular injury and gut barrier dysfunction (Yu and Martin, 2000). Recent studies have reported that gut microbes, represented by Bacteroidetes and Enterobacteriaceae, translocate across the intestinal mucosa and even enter the lung in sepsis and ARDS patients (Dickson et al., 2016; Panzer et al., 2018). However, there is no direct evidence that gut-derived bacteria or bacterial products, such as endotoxin, are present in the blood of septic patients (Haussner et al., 2019). Studies have suggested that ligation of mesenteric lymphatic vessels attenuates lung injury and neutrophil activation and improves survival in mice with endotoxemia (Badami et al., 2008). Moreover, mesenteric lymphatic vessels collected from critically ill mice induces lung injury upon intravenous injection in healthy mice (Senthil et al., 2007). Thus, translocation via intestinal lymphatic vessels is regarded (Haussner et al., 2019), which is called gut–lymph hypothesis. In detail, bacterial translocation gives rise to a local activation of the mucosal immune system (MIS). MIS stimulates the production of inflammatory substances that enter the lung and systemic circulation through the mesenteric lymphatics. These danger-associated molecular patterns (DAMPs) are recognized by innate

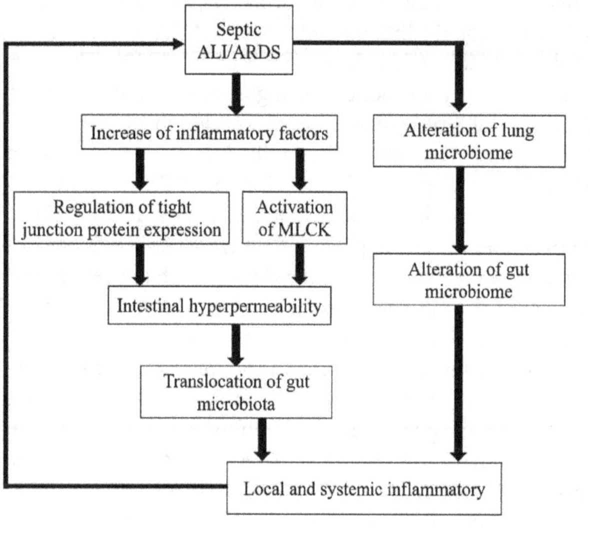

FIGURE 1 | Effect of increased inflammatory cytokines and lung microbiome alteration on the gut in septic ALI/ARDS.

immune cells to promote pro-inflammatory pathways. A massive release of DAMPs accelerates the progression of organ damage and multiple organ dysfunction syndrome (MODS), further aggravating gut injury, forming a vicious cycle (Deitch, 2012; Assimakopoulos et al., 2018; Haussner et al., 2019). Therefore, the destruction of the gut barrier contributes to the translocation of gut microbes and/or their products to the systemic circulation via the mesenteric lymphatics, exacerbating significant host inflammation and acute pulmonary edema with a positive feedback (**Figure 2**).

Notably, toll-like receptor 4 (TLR4) is widely expressed in intestinal stem cells and regulates their proliferation or apoptosis (Chen et al., 2018). During sepsis, increased cytokine levels inhibit intestinal cell regeneration and promote apoptosis in a TLR4-dependent manner (Mazmanian et al., 2008). At the cellular level, crypt cell proliferation is markedly decreased (Coopersmith et al., 2003), with increased intestinal epithelial cells (IECs; Coopersmith et al., 2002) and crypt cell apoptosis (Perrone et al., 2012) following sepsis. Although IECs migrate in a TLR-4-dependent manner (Neal et al., 2013), changes in IEC proliferation and apoptosis far exceed this slow course, leading to a shorter villi length (Dominguez et al., 2011). Moreover, cytokines cause an abnormal intestinal and barrier function of the mucous layer, characterized by reduced thickness, diminished lumen coverage, and poor adhesion (Chang et al., 2012). All of these factors further decrease the effectiveness of the gut barrier.

All in all, an increase of inflammatory cytokines induces gut barrier dysfunction, intestinal hyperpermeability, bacterial translocation, and amplification of the inflammatory responses. Subsequently, this expansion of the systemic inflammatory response contributes to lung injury.

Role of Lung Dysbiosis in the Gut–Lung Axis

Sepsis-associated ALI/ARDS results in the alteration of lung microbiota both in the mice model and in patients. The etiology of pulmonary dysbiosis in sepsis patients is complex and includes endogenous (e.g., hypoxia and ischemia-reperfusion injury) and external factors (e.g., endotracheal intubation, mechanical lung ventilation, inhaled oxygen, and antibiotics). Poroyko et al. (2015) showed in an ALI mouse model induced by the intratracheal instillation of lipopolysaccharide (LPS) that the bacterial DNA burden in bronchoalveolar lavage (BAL) was increased fivefold, whereas the community complexity measured by the Shannon diversity index was significantly decreased. The major trend in the microbial community reaction to LPS-induced ALI was the loss of Firmicutes, represented by Alicyclobacillaceae, and the bloom of Proteobacteria, represented by Brucellaceae and Xanthomonadaceae. Dickson et al. (2016) also found that the community richness was also higher in a mouse model of sepsis induced by caecal ligation and puncture (CLP). The lower respiratory tract was rapidly enriched with bacteria in the gastrointestinal tract, including members of the Bacteroidales order, Enterococcus species, and Lachnospiraceae species, and remained in this status for 5 days. Furthermore, they sequenced lung microbiota of mice exposed to intratracheal LPS to model direct lung injury and observed enrichment of Enterobacteriaceae-classified OTU in post-sepsis lungs. Based on the above experimental evidence, they further analyzed bacterial communities from the BAL fluid of 68 patients with ARDS. The gut-associated Bacteroides OTU, the most abundant genus in the human gut microbiome, were common in the lungs of ARDS patients (41%) but absent in the lungs of the healthy controls. Furthermore, the gut-associated Bacteroides OTU are most strongly correlated with the severity of systemic and alveolar inflammation. Another study conducted by Dickson reconfirmed prior findings (Dickson et al., 2020). They found the bacterial load was greater in patients with ARDS. In addition, they compared the lung bacterial community composition in BAL specimens from ARDS and non-ARDS patients. The predominant clusters in non-ARDS patients were Streptococcaceae, Veillonellaceae, Prevotellaceae, Verrucomicrobiaceae, and Flavobacteriaceae, which are common in healthy lungs and negative sequence control samples. However, in ARDS patients, the bacterial community in the lungs was characterized by Pasteurellaceae and Enterobacteriaceae. Similar to their prior results, gut-derived Enterobacteriaceae are also correlated with the ARDS status. Notably, the Enterobacteriaceae taxonomy was highly aligned with the ARDS-associated bacterial taxon, as identified by Panzer et al. (2018). They also proved that the microbiome is associated with ARDS development. A recent clinical study (Schmitt et al., 2020) compared the pulmonary microbiota in 15 patients with sepsis-induced ARDS undergoing abdominal surgery and 15 patients post esophagectomy. In the ARDS group, the α-diversity index of the pulmonary microbiome was significantly decreased, which was related to the length of the ICU stay and the need for ventilator use, suggesting that alteration of the lung microbiome may represent a mechanism of pathogenesis in septic ALI/ARDS.

Changes in the lung flora may affect the composition of the gut flora in sepsis-induced ALI/ARDS. One previous study manifested that lung microbiota imbalance in a sepsis-related ALI murine model increased the total bacterial count

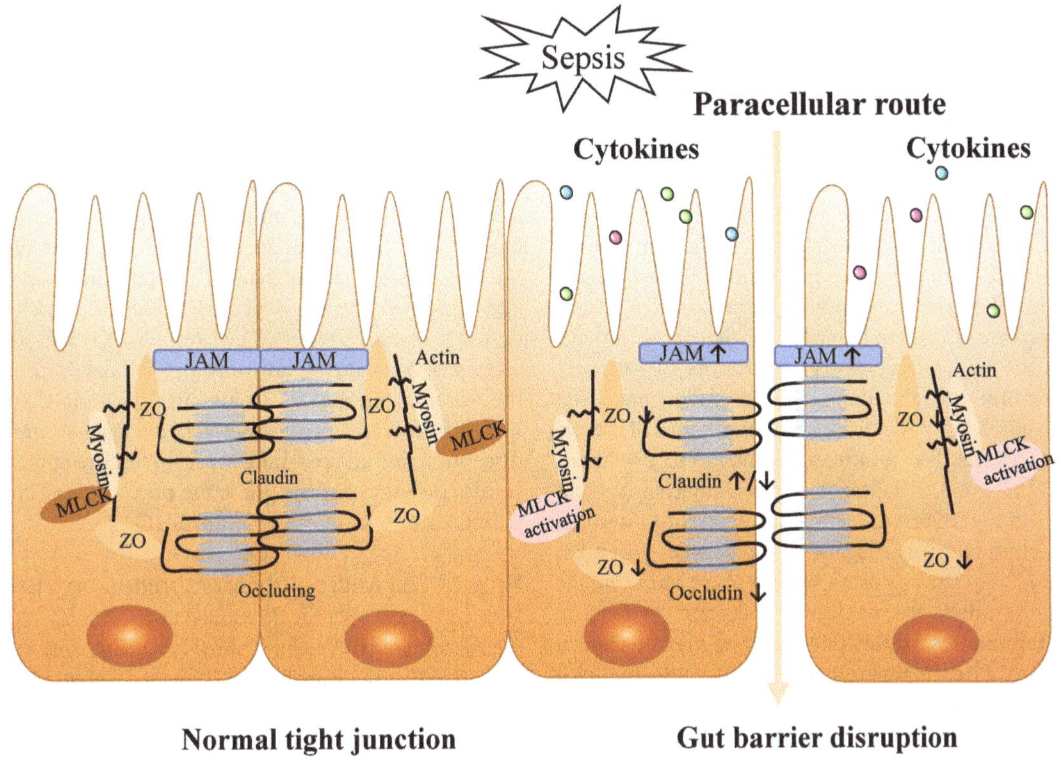

FIGURE 2 | Intestinal barrier disruption by increased cytokines during sepsis. Tight junctions between cells play a critical role in gut barrier function. In sepsis, tight junctions are destructed by inflammatory cytokines production.

in the cecum (Sze et al., 2014). In clinical cases, the most common source of sepsis is the lung (Wang et al., 2013). Rosa et al. (2020) found that Vancomycin treatment of acute Pseudomonas aeruginosa pneumonia in mice can induce intestinal dysbacteriosis, resulting in an increase in the number of Proteus, a decrease in the number of bacteroides, and inflammatory changes in the intestinal tract. After fecal microbiota transplantation, the susceptible phenotype and tissue injury phenotype were reversed in mice. Moreover, the pulmonary allergic response also influences the composition of the intestinal microbiota (Vital et al., 2015). In the context of experimental influenza infection, it has been reported that the IFN-γ produced by lung-derived CCR9 + CD4 + T cells changed the composition of the gut microbiota, and caused intestinal immune injury (Wang et al., 2014). Moreover, the pulmonary production of IFN-Is promotes the consumption of obligate anaerobic bacteria and the enrichment of proteobacteria in the gut, leading to significant intestinal dysregulation (Deriu et al., 2016). Thus, lung inflammation directly changes the intestinal bacterial community structure and further worsens lung inflammation (Vital et al., 2015). However, only very limited data have been reported on how long dysbiosis in sepsis-induced ALI/ARDS causes gut dysbiosis. The alveolo-capillary membrane becomes increasingly permeable in sepsis-induced ALI/ARDS as a result of a direct (primarily epithelial) or indirect (primarily endothelial) injury. It is reasonable to posit that alveolo-capillary permeability might be at the highest risk of gut–lung bacterial translocation. Considerable efforts are needed to increase our knowledge about the influence of post-sepsis lung injury on gut microbiota.

Effect of Gut Microbiome on Gut-Lung Crosstalk

Role of Gut Microbiota on the Sepsis

The human gastrointestinal tract is the harbor of 100 trillion bacteria, which are ten times more abundant than somatic and germ line cells of the human body (Morais et al., 2021). Regarding human health, the gut microbiota contributes to prevent infections caused by pathogens, provide nutrients, participate in metabolism, shape the immune system, and serve as a biological barrier (Haak et al., 2018). In turn, the immune system will affect the microbiota composition (Honda and Littman, 2016). In various disease states, the loss of "health-promoting" bacteria and overgrowth of "disease-promoting" pathogenic bacteria make patients more succumb to sepsis and MODS (Alverdy and Krezalek, 2017). A multi-center study has shown that patients with sepsis have an increased abundance of intestinal microbiota, which is closely related to inflammation caused by Parabacteroides, Clostridium, Bilophila, and other species. Concomitantly, researchers have detected an increased abundance of Enterococcus and other pathogenic bacteria in sepsis patients who died, suggesting that these bacteria may be potential biomarkers for ICU care (Agudelo-Ochoa et al., 2020).

It has also been shown that septic patients have a decreased abundance of Faecalibacterium associated with reduced intestinal inflammation (Lankelma et al., 2017). In a single-center case control study of children, the abundance of the following 13 bacteria in septic children were significantly higher than that in the healthy control group: Proteobacteria, Bacilli, Gammaproteobacteria, Enterobacteriales, Pseudomonadales, Lactobacillales, Enterococcaceae, Enterobacteriaceae, Moraxellaceae, Enterococcus, Clostridium innocuum group, Acinetobacter, and Enterococcus durans. Among these bacteria, Enterococcaceae, Enterococcus, and Enterococcus durans showed an increase in their abundance that is positively correlated with the inflammatory indicators CRP and WBC. Furthermore, the abundance of the following seven bacteria was significantly decreased in the guts of septic children: Bifidobacteria, Selenomonas, Aminococcus acidaceae, Daentosaceae UCG-003, Dialister, Dorea longicatena, and *Ruminococcus* sp.5_1_39bFAA. The decrease of intestinal bifidobacteria abundance is negatively correlated to WBC (Liu et al., 2021). The mechanisms behind these shifts in the microbiota composition are unclear (Haak and Wiersinga, 2017). One of the reasons for this phenomenon may be clinical intervention, such as enteral/parenteral feeding, selective oral decontamination/selective decontamination of the digestive tract, as well as the administration of antibiotics, proton pump inhibitors, opioids, catecholamines, and sedatives (Haak and Wiersinga, 2017). In addition, due to the acute phase of inflammatory response and intestinal dysfunction, critically ill patients with sepsis have a greater risk of malnutrition (Liu et al., 2014). Nutritional deficiency is associated with intestinal dysbiosis, characterized as an increase in proteus numbers and a decrease in α-diversity, and it makes epithelial barrier function weaken, which predisposes to bacterial translocation (Ralls et al., 2015; Levesque et al., 2017). And decreased gastrointestinal motility and loss of intestinal epithelial integrity in sepsis patients cause a decrease in anaerobic bacteria (e.g., Lachnospiraceae and Ruminococcaceae), which further impairs the intestinal epithelial function and allows the proliferation of opportunistic pathogenic bacteria (Haak et al., 2018). Fay et al. (2019) examined genetically identical septic C57BL/6 mice from two vendors with different microbiome compositions. Following CLP, significant differences were noted in the mortality and immunophenotype (especially splenic IFN-γ + CD4 + T cells, effector memory CD4 + T cells, central memory CD4 + T cells, and Peyer's patch effector memory CD4 + T cells). In addition, CLP was performed of naive mice from different suppliers after 3 weeks of cohousing, and the differences in the mortality and immunophenotype disappeared. These findings suggest that the microbiome plays a critical role in the survival of sepsis and the host immune response. This conclusion has also been confirmed by other studies. Depletion of intestinal microbiota with broad-spectrum antibiotics could exacerbate lung and intestinal damage and increase the mortality in sepsis (Xu et al., 2021). Notably, the differential immune responses to sepsis are determined by the microbiome (Cho and Blaser, 2012). A recent study has shown that the lung microbiome is enriched with gut-derived bacteria in murine sepsis and in human patients with ARDS. The presence of gut-specific communities (Bacteroides) is correlated with the intensity of systemic inflammation (Dickson et al., 2016). When the bacterial burden of the gut is minimized, the inflammation and injury sustained with distal organs are lessened during sepsis (Cuevas et al., 1972). Imbalance of the intestinal microbiome regulates the Toll-like receptor 4 (TLR4)/nuclear factor-κB (NF-κB) signaling pathway in the lung immune system, which activates pulmonary oxidative stress and mediates lung injury (Tang et al., 2021). Enhancing the α-diversity of the intestinal flora in mice changes the immune response to sepsis and improves the survival rate of sepsis, which is mediated by the powerful CD4 + T cell response (Fay et al., 2019). The intestinal flora affects not only the cellular immunity but also the humoral immunity. Commensal bacteria directly produce IgA, which has a protective activity against mucosal barrier disruption and the resulting sepsis (Wilmore et al., 2018). These studies indicate that the gut is the predominant motor of sepsis (Klingensmith and Coopersmith, 2016).

Role of Gut Microbiota Metabolites on the Sepsis

In recent years, with the developed in-depth understanding of gut microecology, studies have shown that not only gut microbiota itself but also the metabolites of gut microbiota are involved in various functions of the intestinal microenvironment. Bacteria can produce a variety of metabolites, including: SCFAs, vitamins, bile acids, choline metabolites, aromatic compounds, amines, etc., (Van Treuren and Dodd, 2020). In the following sections, we summarized several metabolites affecting the occurrence and development of sepsis.

Short-Chain Fatty Acids

Short-chain fatty acids (SCFAs), including butyric acid, acetic acid, and propionic acid, are the most abundant and beneficial metabolites of the intestinal flora (Zhao et al., 2018; Adelman et al., 2020). Several studies have confirmed significantly decreased SCFA concentrations in sepsis patients (Shimizu et al., 2011, 2018; Yamada et al., 2015; Valdes-Duque et al., 2020). Butyric acid reduces the nuclear NF-κB activity, IL-6 and TNF-α levels, and lung tissue neutrophil infiltration by inhibiting the expression of high mobility group protein 1, TLR4, or histone deacetylase to reduce sepsis-related ALI (Li et al., 2018; Liu et al., 2019; Parada Venegas et al., 2019). In addition, acetic acid alleviates septic ALI by regulating the mitogen-activated protein kinase (MAPK) pathway, improving the alveolar permeability, reducing inflammatory factors, and inhibiting oxygen free radical production (Xu et al., 2019). SCFA reverses the progression of sepsis by restoring host immunity and promoting pathogen clearance in an interferon regulatory factor 3-dependent manner (Kim et al., 2020). Moreover, it has been reported that SCFAs contribute to maintain intestinal barrier integrity. SCFAs enhance the immune function of intestinal mucosa by promoting the production of antimicrobial peptides (AMPs; Li et al., 2020). The underlying mechanism may be the promotion of the expression of RegIIIγ and β-defensins 1, 3, and 4 by SCFAs in a GPR43-dependent manner (Zhao et al., 2018). AMPs in the gut, including defensins, cathelicidins, and regenerating gene (Reg)IIIa/b/g, are a class of basic peptides with antibacterial activity secreted by Paneth cells and enterocytes (Zong et al., 2020). Studies have shown that gut-derived AMP deficiency is associated with intestinal barrier failure, leading to bacterial translocation (Zong et al., 2020). In CLP-induced sepsis model mice, cathelicidins gene knockout resulted in increased mortality, impaired intestinal barrier, increased permeability, increased bacterial DNA content of blood, up-regulated expression of intestinal cytokines and inflammatory pathways, and increased M1-type macrophages and neutrophils (Ho et al., 2020).

Choline Metabolites

Trimethylamine N-oxide (TMAO) derives primarily from the gut metabolite of choline, carnitine, and phosphatidylcholine (Jiang et al., 2021). Excessive increases in TMAO lead to the release of large amounts of inflammatory mediators that activate the MAPK pathway and the nuclear transcription factor (NF-κB), which mediates vascular inflammation (Kapetanaki et al., 2021). A large number of studies have shown elevated TMAO levels accelerate the progression of inflammatory diseases such as diabetes, atherosclerosis, and heart failure (Gatarek and Kaluzna-Czaplinska, 2021). However, a recent single-center prospective study reveals that TMAO may play different roles in CV and infectious diseases (Chou et al., 2021). A total of 95 patients with sepsis using mechanical ventilation were enrolled in this study and divided into three groups based on TMAO concentration. This study found that plasma TMAO concentration was an independent predictor of successful weaning in mechanically ventilated patients with sepsis after adjustment for APACHE II score and CRP concentration. Septic patients in the lowest TMAO concentrations were at greater risk of non-cardiovascular death and unsuccessful ventilator weaning than were those in higher concentrations. In addition, TMAO concentration was positively correlated with daily energy intake, albumin and prealbumin concentration. These findings suggest that TMAO may be a novel risk biomarker and nutritional indicator for patients with sepsis.

Phenolic

One of the degradation products of flavonoids and amino acids by commensal bacteria is desaminotyrosine (DAT; Steed et al., 2017). Flavonoids have anti-inflammatory properties (Peluso et al., 2015). Recently, Wei et al. conducted an experiment that LPS-induced septic mice were intraperitoneally injected with DAT and vehicle control. They found that the survival rate was significantly improved in the DAT-treated group, along with decreased hypothermia and improved clinical scores (Wei et al., 2020). It suggests that DAT modulates systemic immune homeostasis. Nonetheless, whether a flavonoid-enriched diet is a key component to sepsis remains to be studied.

Indole Derivatives

Indoles are metabolites of tryptophan metabolism by microbiota (Rattanaphan et al., 2020). It is noteworthy that indole is able to modulate expression of pro-inflammatory genes, increase expression of anti-inflammatory genes and strengthen the epithelial barrier (Nicholson et al., 2012). Researchers found that 5-Hydroxytryptamine (5-HT) significantly increase mortality in a model of sepsis in mice. Furthermore, 5-HT exacerbated the clinical symptoms, and histological damages in the lung, liver, kidney, bowel, and heart (Zhang et al., 2017). Another tryptophan metabolites, indole-3-acetate and indole-3-propionate, was significantly decreased in the both of septic mice and patients, which might result from the gut microbiome disruption in sepsis (Gao et al., 2018; Elmassry et al., 2020). These studies show that Indole derivatives may be a new therapeutic target for sepsis.

Vitamin

It is well known that gut microbiota are able to synthesize vitamin K as well as most water-soluble B vitamins such as thiamine (vitamin B1), riboflavin (vitamin B2), nicotinic acid (vitamin B3), pantothenic acid (vitamin B5), pyridoxine (vitamin B6), cobalamin (vitamin B12), biotin (vitamin H), and folates (LeBlanc et al., 2013). The potential biological functions of vitamins include enhancement of immune function, provision of complementary endogenous sources of vitamins, regulation of cell proliferation and so on. In recent years, the efficacy of B vitamins in the treatment of sepsis has received much attention. Hong et al. (2018) has found that prophylactic administration of nicotinamide riboside (NR) can protect lung and heart from injury, and improve the survival rate in sepsis mice, probably via inhibiting HMGB1 release and oxidative stress through the NAD + /SIRT1 signaling. In a rat model of polymicrobial sepsis, vitamin B6 was found to diminish neutrophil infiltration in the both of lung and liver, oxidative markers in the liver and restore catalase activity levels in the lung (Giustina et al., 2019). In addition, vitamin B1 deficiency has been found in patients with critically sepsis (Donnino et al., 2010). Several clinical trials have reported that a combination of cortisol, vitamin C, and Vitamin B1 prevent progressive organ failure, reduce mortality (Marik et al., 2017; Kim et al., 2018) and ICU length of stay (Mitchell et al., 2020) in critically ill patients with septic shock or severe pneumonia. However, an recent single center, retrospective study didn't find that vitamin B1 and C supplementation improve clinical outcomes (mortality rates, ventilator and ICU-free days) in septic ARDS patients requiring invasive mechanical ventilation (Yoo et al., 2020). Therefore, vitamin may be beneficial to the treatment of sepsis, but much more researches will be needed to verify the clinical benefit of vitamin on patients with septic lung injury.

The above discussion showed that the changes of the intestinal flora and its metabolites can affect the severity of septic ALI/ARDS by regulating the levels of local and systemic inflammation, oxidative cellular stress, and cell infiltration/activation.

Effect of Sepsis-Related Intestinal Failure on the Lung

Structural and functional disruption of intestinal barrier integrity in sepsis leads to increased intestinal permeability (Jones and Neish, 2021). Three factors contribute to intestinal barrier damage: visceral hypoperfusion or ischemia, restoration of intestinal blood flow during resuscitation leading to ischemia-reperfusion injury, and loss of the intestinal barrier function, which allows bacteria, endotoxins, or both to cross the mucosal barrier (Otani and Coopersmith, 2019). Bacterial translocation can activate local intestinal inflammatory responses, producing DAMPs, which enter the systemic circulation through mesenteric lymphatic vessels. DAMPS are recognized by cells expressing intrinsic pattern receptors in the intrinsic immune system, including macrophages, white blood cells, and dendritic cells, then secreting pro-inflammatory factors that promote lung injury and the development of MODS, which further aggravate intestinal barrier injury and lead to a vicious cycle (Pugin and Chevrolet, 1991; **Figure 3**).

Macrophages, commonly polarized into M1 (pro-inflammatory) and M2 (anti-inflammatory) types according to responses to environmental stimuli, are key orchestrators in the pathogenesis of ALI/ARDS (Shapouri-Moghaddam et al., 2018). In the acute phase of sepsis, macrophages polarize into the M1 phenotype to activate TLRs or other recognition receptors due to impaired intestinal barrier function, bacterial translocation, and increased inflammation (Osterberg et al., 1997), releasing a variety of inflammatory cytokines, such as IL-1β, IL-6, and TNF-α. Proinflammatory factors induce the recruitment of neutrophils in the blood circulation, then migrate to the lungs and alveolar cavities, resulting in lung injury. Accumulating evidence indicates that some natural or synthetic materials can ameliorate the prognosis of sepsis-induced ALI in animal models by inhibiting pulmonary M1 polarization and altering the macrophage function (Bittencourt-Mernak et al., 2017; Pinheiro et al., 2017; Wang et al., 2018, 2019; Zhuo et al., 2019). Thus, the regulation of macrophage polarization from M1 to M2 may be a novel therapeutic strategy of ALI/ARDS (Chen et al., 2020).

Prospect

As the intestinal barrier plays an important role in sepsis-induced lung injury, targeted microbiota has the potential for prevention and treatment of lung injury. Fecal microbiota transplantation (FMT) can help the recipient to establish a normal intestinal microecological environment and may be considered a useful therapy for sepsis in the future. In the last few years, FMT has made great strides in correcting microbiota disorders, repairing the intestinal barrier, and regulating immunity (Ooijevaar et al., 2019). In the intervention of FMT in lipopolysaccharide (LPS)-induced ALI, anti-inflammatory and antioxidant mechanisms may play an important role. FMT intervention could correct the changes in the intestinal flora and improve lung injury by inhibiting the activation of the PI3K/AKT/NF-κB signaling pathway and decreasing the expression of intercellular cell adhesion molecule-1 (ICAM-1; Yin et al., 2019). In addition, FMT significantly reduces the TNF-α, IL-1β, and IL-6 levels as well as inflammatory cell infiltration and interstitial exudate, thereby improving LPS-induced endotoxic ALI in rats, which is associated with the decreased expression of TGF-β1, Smad3, and P-ERK (Li et al., 2020). In the LPS-induced ALI mouse model

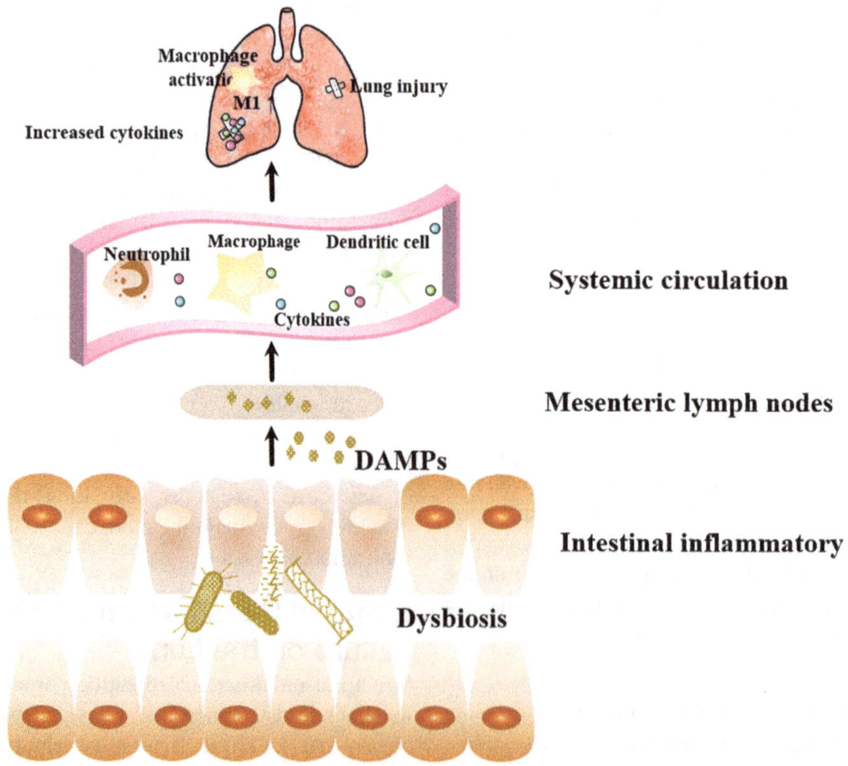

FIGURE 3 | Effect of sepsis-related intestinal failure on the lung. Bacterial dysbiosis can activate local intestinal inflammatory responses, producing DAMPs, which enter the systemic circulation through mesenteric lymphatic vessels. Immune cells recognize DAMPs and secreting pro-inflammatory factors that promote lung injury. DAMPs: danger-associated molecular patterns.

of intestinal microbiota imbalance pretreated with antibiotics, an increased diversity of the intestinal flora and abundance of beneficial bacteria producing SCFAs that antagonize acute lung injury was observed by reconstructing the intestinal flora through FMT. This inhibits the activation of the TLR4/NF-κB signaling pathway in the lung, inflammation, and the release of oxidative stress factors in ALI animals (Tang et al., 2021). Therefore, FMT therapy can be used in the treatment of lung disorder during sepsis. However, existing research in this field remains limited to animal experiments. More basic trials are needed to clarify the mechanisms of FMT in lung injury, as well as large clinical trials to evaluate the efficacy and safety of FMT therapy.

CONCLUSION

Many aspects of lung injury in sepsis have not been thoroughly studied, and the interaction between intestine and lung in sepsis is still a promising research direction. During septic lung injury, the expression of intestinal tight junction protein, the activity of MLCK, and the regulation of IECs proliferation and apoptosis are altered by cytokine storm, leading to gut hyperpermeability. Increase of the intestinal permeability leads to the translocation of gut microbiota, resulting in intestinal inflammation and a cascade of inflammatory reactions driving acute lung injury. Moreover, lung dysbiosis in sepsis-induced ALI/ARDS may cause gut dysbiosis. And the changes of the intestinal flora and reduction of beneficial metabolites in sepsis promote lung injury exacerbation by regulating local and systemic inflammation. Persistent inflammation leads to devastating consequences. Theoretically, therapies that restore the intestinal integrity, microbiome, and homeostasis balance between the two systems through FMT are efficient, but so far basic research and clinical trials are not sufficient. An in-depth understanding of gut–lung crosstalk may provide clues for the regulation of homeostasis in sepsis and contribute to the development of effective therapies to prevent sepsis-induced ALI/ARDS.

AUTHOR CONTRIBUTIONS

XZ developed the manuscript and figures. YL contributed to proofreading and revising. Both authors contributed to the article and approved the submitted version.

REFERENCES

Abe, T., Madotto, F., Pham, T., Nagata, I., Uchida, M., Tamiya, N., et al. (2018). Epidemiology and patterns of tracheostomy practice in patients with acute respiratory distress syndrome in ICUs across 50 countries. *Crit. Care* 22:195. doi: 10.1186/s13054-018-2126-6

Adelman, M. W., Woodworth, M. H., Langelier, C., Busch, L. M., Kempker, J. A., Kraft, C. S., et al. (2020). The gut microbiome's role in the development, maintenance, and outcomes of sepsis. *Crit. Care* 24:278. doi: 10.1186/s13054-020-02989-1

Agudelo-Ochoa, G. M., Valdés-Duque, B. E., Giraldo-Giraldo, N. A., Jaillier-Ramírez, A. M., Giraldo-Villa, A., Acevedo-Castaño, I., et al. (2020). Gut microbiota profiles in critically ill patients, potential biomarkers and risk variables for sepsis. *Gut Microbes* 12:1707610. doi: 10.1080/19490976.2019.1707610

Alverdy, J. C., and Krezalek, M. A. (2017). Collapse of the microbiome, emergence of the pathobiome, and the immunopathology of sepsis. *Crit. Care Med.* 45, 337–347. doi: 10.1097/CCM.0000000000002172

Assimakopoulos, S. F., Triantos, C., Thomopoulos, K., Fligou, F., Maroulis, I., Marangos, M., et al. (2018). Gut-origin sepsis in the critically ill patient: pathophysiology and treatment. *Infection* 46, 751–760. doi: 10.1007/s15010-018-1178-5

Badami, C. D., Senthil, M., Caputo, F. J., Rupani, B. J., Doucet, D., Pisarenko, V., et al. (2008). Mesenteric lymph duct ligation improves survival in a lethal shock model. *Shock* 30, 680–685. doi: 10.1097/SHK.0b013e318173edd1

Bellani, G., Laffey, J., Pham, T., Fan, E., Brochard, L., Esteban, A., et al. (2016). Epidemiology, patterns of care, and mortality for patients with acute respiratory distress syndrome in intensive care units in 50 countries. *JAMA* 315, 788–800. doi: 10.1001/jama.2016.0291

Bittencourt-Mernak, M. I., Pinheiro, N. M., Santana, F. P., Guerreiro, M. P., Saraiva-Romanholo, B. M., Grecco, S. S., et al. (2017). Prophylactic and therapeutic treatment with the flavonone sakuranetin ameliorates LPS-induced acute lung injury. *Am. J. Physiol. Lung Cell. Mol. Physiol.* 312, L217–L230. doi: 10.1152/ajplung.00444.2015

Chang, M., Alsaigh, T., Kistler, E. B., and Schmid-Schönbein, G. W. (2012). Breakdown of mucin as barrier to digestive enzymes in the ischemic rat small intestine. *PLoS One* 7:e40087. doi: 10.1371/journal.pone.0040087

Chen, H., Zhang, Y., Zhang, W., Liu, H., Sun, C., Zhang, B., et al. (2019). Inhibition of myeloid differentiation factor 2 by baicalein protects against acute lung injury. *Phytomedicine* 63:152997. doi: 10.1016/j.phymed.2019.152997

Chen, X., Tang, J., Shuai, W., Meng, J., Feng, J., and Han, Z. (2020). Macrophage polarization and its role in the pathogenesis of acute lung injury/acute respiratory distress syndrome. *Inflamm. Res.* 69, 883–895. doi: 10.1007/s00011-020-01378-2

Chen, Y., Yang, X. Q., Tseng, B. Y., Tsai, Y. H., Tseng, S. H., Lee, C. H., et al. (2018). Deferoxamine preconditioning activated hypoxia-inducible factor-1α and MyD88-dependent Toll-like receptor 4 signaling in intestinal stem cells. *J. Pediatr. Surg.* 53, 2349–2356. doi: 10.1016/j.jpedsurg.2018.01.023

Cho, I., and Blaser, M. J. (2012). The human microbiome: at the interface of health and disease. *Nat. Rev. Genet.* 13, 260–270. doi: 10.1038/nrg3182

Chou, R.-H., Wu, P.-S., Wang, S.-C., Wu, C.-H., Lu, S.-F., Lien, R.-Y., et al. (2021). Paradox of trimethylamine-N-oxide, the impact of malnutrition on microbiota-derived metabolites and septic patients. *J. Intensive Care* 9:65. doi: 10.1186/s40560-021-00581-5

Coopersmith, C. M., Chang, K. C., Swanson, P. E., Tinsley, K. W., Stromberg, P. E., Buchman, T. G., et al. (2002). Overexpression of Bcl-2 in the intestinal epithelium improves survival in septic mice. *Crit. Care Med.* 30, 195–201.

Coopersmith, C. M., Stromberg, P. E., Davis, C. G., Dunne, W. M., Amiot, D. M., Karl, I. E., et al. (2003). Sepsis from *Pseudomonas aeruginosa* pneumonia decreases intestinal proliferation and induces gut epithelial cell cycle arrest. *Crit. Care Med.* 31, 1630–1637.

Cuevas, P., De la Maza, L. M., Gilbert, J., and Fine, J. (1972). The lung lesion in four different types of shock in rabbits. *Arch. Surg.* 104, 319–322.

Deitch, E. A. (2012). Gut-origin sepsis: evolution of a concept. *Surgeon* 10, 350–356. doi: 10.1016/j.surge.2012.03.003

Deriu, E., Boxx, G. M., He, X., Pan, C., Benavidez, S. D., Cen, L., et al. (2016). Influenza virus affects intestinal microbiota and secondary *Salmonella* infection in the gut through type I interferons. *PLoS Pathog.* 12:e1005572. doi: 10.1371/journal.ppat.1005572

Dickson, R. P. (2016). The microbiome and critical illness. *Lancet Respir. Med.* 4, 59–72. doi: 10.1016/s2213-2600(15)00427-0

Dickson, R. P., Erb-Downward, J. R., and Huffnagle, G. B. (2014). Towards an ecology of the lung: new conceptual models of pulmonary microbiology and pneumonia pathogenesis. *Lancet Respir. Med.* 2, 238–246. doi: 10.1016/S2213-2600(14)70028-1

Dickson, R. P., Erb-Downward, J. R., and Huffnagle, G. B. (2015). Homeostasis and its disruption in the lung microbiome. *Am. J. Physiol. Lung Cell. Mol. Physiol.* 309, L1047–L1055. doi: 10.1152/ajplung.00279.2015

Dickson, R. P., Schultz, M. J., van der Poll, T., Schouten, L. R., Falkowski, N. R., Luth, J. E., et al. (2020). Lung microbiota predict clinical outcomes in critically ill patients. *Am. J. Respir. Crit. Care Med.* 201, 555–563. doi: 10.1164/rccm.201907-1487OC

Dickson, R. P., Singer, B. H., Newstead, M. W., Falkowski, N. R., Erb-Downward, J. R., Standiford, T. J., et al. (2016). Enrichment of the lung microbiome with gut bacteria in sepsis and the acute respiratory distress syndrome. *Nat. Microbiol.* 1:16113. doi: 10.1038/nmicrobiol.2016.113

Dominguez, J. A., Vithayathil, P. J., Khailova, L., Lawrance, C. P., Samocha, A. J., Jung, E., et al. (2011). Epidermal growth factor improves survival and prevents intestinal injury in a murine model of *pseudomonas aeruginosa* pneumonia. *Shock* 36, 381–389. doi: 10.1097/SHK.0b013e31822793c4

Donnino, M. W., Carney, E., Cocchi, M. N., Barbash, I., Chase, M., Joyce, N., et al. (2010). Thiamine deficiency in critically ill patients with sepsis. *J. Crit. Care* 25, 576–581. doi: 10.1016/j.jcrc.2010.03.003

Elmassry, M. M., Mudaliar, N. S., Colmer-Hamood, J. A., San Francisco, M. J., Griswold, J. A., Dissanaike, S., et al. (2020). New markers for sepsis caused by *Pseudomonas aeruginosa* during burn infection. *Metabolomics* 16:40. doi: 10.1007/s11306-020-01658-2

Fan, E. K. Y., and Fan, J. (2018). Regulation of alveolar macrophage death in acute lung inflammation. *Respir. Res.* 19:50. doi: 10.1186/s12931-018-0756-5

Fan, E., Brodie, D., and Slutsky, A. S. (2018). Acute respiratory distress syndrome: advances in diagnosis and treatment. *JAMA* 319, 698–710. doi: 10.1001/jama.2017.21907

Fay, K. T., Klingensmith, N. J., Chen, C.-W., Zhang, W., Sun, Y., Morrow, K. N., et al. (2019). The gut microbiome alters immunophenotype and survival from sepsis. *FASEB J.* 33, 11258–11269. doi: 10.1096/fj.201802188R

Fernando, S. M., Ferreyro, B. L., Urner, M., Munshi, L., and Fan, E. (2021). Diagnosis and management of acute respiratory distress syndrome. *CMAJ* 193, E761–E768. doi: 10.1503/cmaj.202661

Gao, J., Xu, K., Liu, H., Liu, G., Bai, M., Peng, C., et al. (2018). Impact of the gut microbiota on intestinal immunity mediated by tryptophan metabolism. *Front. Cell. Infect. Microbiol.* 8:13. doi: 10.3389/fcimb.2018.00013

Gatarek, P., and Kaluzna-Czaplinska, J. (2021). Trimethylamine N-oxide (TMAO) in human health. *EXCLI J.* 20, 301–319. doi: 10.17179/excli2020-3239

Giustina, A. D., Danielski, L. G., Novochadlo, M. M., Goldim, M. P. S., Joaquim, L., Metzker, K. L. L., et al. (2019). Vitamin B6 reduces oxidative stress in lungs and liver in experimental sepsis. *An. Acad. Bras. Cienc.* 91:e20190434. doi: 10.1590/0001-3765201920190434

Griffiths, M. J. D., McAuley, D. F., Perkins, G. D., Barrett, N., Blackwood, B., Boyle, A., et al. (2019). Guidelines on the management of acute respiratory distress syndrome. *BMJ Open Respir. Res.* 6:e000420. doi: 10.1136/bmjresp-2019-000420

Günzel, D. (2017). Claudins: vital partners in transcellular and paracellular transport coupling. *Pflugers Arch.* 469, 35–44. doi: 10.1007/s00424-016-1909-3

Günzel, D., and Yu, A. S. L. (2013). Claudins and the modulation of tight junction permeability. *Physiol. Rev.* 93, 525–569. doi: 10.1152/physrev.00019.2012

Haak, B. W., and Wiersinga, W. J. (2017). The role of the gut microbiota in sepsis. *Lancet Gastroenterol. Hepatol.* 2, 135–143. doi: 10.1016/S2468-1253(16)30119-4

Haak, B. W., Prescott, H. C., and Wiersinga, W. J. (2018). Therapeutic potential of the gut microbiota in the prevention and treatment of sepsis. *Front. Immunol.* 9:2042. doi: 10.3389/fimmu.2018.02042

Haussner, F., Chakraborty, S., Halbgebauer, R., and Huber-Lang, M. (2019). Challenge to the intestinal mucosa during sepsis. *Front. Immunol.* 10:891. doi: 10.3389/fimmu.2019.00891

Ho, J., Chan, H., Liang, Y., Liu, X., Zhang, L., Li, Q., et al. (2020). Cathelicidin preserves intestinal barrier function in polymicrobial sepsis. *Crit. Care* 24:47. doi: 10.1186/s13054-020-2754-5

Honda, K., and Littman, D. R. (2016). The microbiota in adaptive immune homeostasis and disease. *Nature* 535, 75–84. doi: 10.1038/nature18848

Hong, G., Zheng, D., Zhang, L., Ni, R., Wang, G., Fan, G. C., et al. (2018). Administration of nicotinamide riboside prevents oxidative stress and organ injury in sepsis. *Free Radic. Biol. Med.* 123, 125–137. doi: 10.1016/j.freeradbiomed.2018.05.073

Huppert, L. A., Matthay, M. A., and Ware, L. B. (2019). Pathogenesis of acute respiratory distress syndrome. *Semin. Respir. Crit. Care Med.* 40, 31–39. doi: 10.1055/s-0039-1683996

Jiang, S., Shui, Y., Cui, Y., Tang, C., Wang, X., Qiu, X., et al. (2021). Gut microbiota dependent trimethylamine N-oxide aggravates angiotensin II-induced hypertension. *Redox Biol.* 46:102115. doi: 10.1016/j.redox.2021.102115

Jones, R. M., and Neish, A. S. (2021). Gut microbiota in intestinal and liver disease. *Annu. Rev. Pathol.* 16, 251–275. doi: 10.1146/annurev-pathol-030320-095722

Kapetanaki, S., Kumawat, A. K., Persson, K., and Demirel, I. (2021). The fibrotic effects of TMAO on human renal fibroblasts is mediated by NLRP3, caspase-1 and the PERK/Akt/mTOR pathway. *Int. J. Mol. Sci.* 22:11864. doi: 10.3390/ijms222111864

Kim, S. M., DeFazio, J. R., Hyoju, S. K., Sangani, K., Keskey, R., Krezalek, M. A., et al. (2020). Fecal microbiota transplant rescues mice from human pathogen mediated sepsis by restoring systemic immunity. *Nat. Commun.* 11:2354. doi: 10.1038/s41467-020-15545-w

Kim, W. Y., Jo, E. J., Eom, J. S., Mok, J., Kim, M. H., Kim, K. U., et al. (2018). Combined vitamin C, hydrocortisone, and thiamine therapy for patients with severe pneumonia who were admitted to the intensive care unit: propensity score-based analysis of a before-after cohort study. *J. Crit. Care* 47, 211–218. doi: 10.1016/j.jcrc.2018.07.004

Klingensmith, N. J., and Coopersmith, C. M. (2016). The gut as the motor of multiple organ dysfunction in critical illness. *Crit. Care Clin.* 32, 203–212. doi: 10.1016/j.ccc.2015.11.004

Krug, S. M., and Fromm, M. (2020). Special issue on "the tight junction and its proteins: more than just a barrier". *Int. J. Mol. Sci.* 21:4612. doi: 10.3390/ijms21134612

Lankelma, J. M., van Vught, L. A., Belzer, C., Schultz, M. J., van der Poll, T., de Vos, W. M., et al. (2017). Critically ill patients demonstrate large interpersonal variation in intestinal microbiota dysregulation: a pilot study. *Intensive Care Med.* 43, 59–68. doi: 10.1007/s00134-016-4613-z

LeBlanc, J. G., Milani, C., de Giori, G. S., Sesma, F., van Sinderen, D., and Ventura, M. (2013). Bacteria as vitamin suppliers to their host: a gut microbiota perspective. *Curr. Opin. Biotechnol.* 24, 160–168. doi: 10.1016/j.copbio.2012.08.005

Lelubre, C., and Vincent, J. L. (2018). Mechanisms and treatment of organ failure in sepsis. *Nat. Rev. Nephrol.* 14, 417–427. doi: 10.1038/s41581-018-0005-7

Levesque, C. L., Turner, J., Li, J., Wizzard, P., St Pierre, B., Lim, D., et al. (2017). In a neonatal piglet model of intestinal failure, administration of antibiotics and lack of enteral nutrition have a greater impact on intestinal microflora than surgical resection alone. *JPEN J. Parenter. Enteral Nutr.* 41, 938–945. doi: 10.1177/0148607115626903

Li, N., Liu, X.-X., Hong, M., Huang, X.-Z., Chen, H., Xu, J.-H., et al. (2018). Sodium butyrate alleviates LPS-induced acute lung injury in mice via inhibiting HMGB1 release. *Int. Immunopharmacol.* 56, 242–248. doi: 10.1016/j.intimp.2018.01.017

Li, Q., Zhang, Q., Wang, C., Liu, X., Li, N., and Li, J. (2009). Disruption of tight junctions during polymicrobial sepsis in vivo. *J. Pathol.* 218, 210–221. doi: 10.1002/path.2525

Li, X. Y., He, C., Zhu, Y., and Lu, N. H. (2020). Role of gut microbiota on intestinal barrier function in acute pancreatitis. *World J. Gastroenterol.* 26, 2187–2193. doi: 10.3748/wjg.v26.i18.2187

Li, X., Jamal, M., Guo, P., Jin, Z., Zheng, F., Song, X., et al. (2019). Irisin alleviates pulmonary epithelial barrier dysfunction in sepsis-induced acute lung injury via activation of AMPK/SIRT1 pathways. *Biomed. Pharmacother.* 118:109363. doi: 10.1016/j.biopha.2019.109363

Liu, J., Chang, G., Huang, J., Wang, Y., Ma, N., Roy, A.-C., et al. (2019). Sodium butyrate inhibits the inflammation of lipopolysaccharide-induced acute lung injury in mice by regulating the toll-like receptor 4/nuclear factor κB signaling pathway. *J. Agric. Food Chem.* 67, 1674–1682. doi: 10.1021/acs.jafc.8b06359

Liu, J., Wang, M., Chen, W., Ma, J., Peng, Y., Zhang, M., et al. (2021). Altered gut microbiota taxonomic compositions of patients with sepsis in a pediatric intensive care unit. *Front. Pediatr.* 9:645060. doi: 10.3389/fped.2021.645060

Liu, M. J., Bao, S., Napolitano, J. R., Burris, D. L., Yu, L., Tridandapani, S., et al. (2014). Zinc regulates the acute phase response and serum amyloid A production in response to sepsis through JAK-STAT3 signaling. *PLoS One* 9:e94934. doi: 10.1371/journal.pone.0094934

Lorentz, C. A., Liang, Z., Meng, M., Chen, C. W., Yoseph, B. P., Breed, E. R., et al. (2017). Myosin light chain kinase knockout improves gut barrier function and confers a survival advantage in polymicrobial sepsis. *Mol. Med.* 23, 155–165. doi: 10.2119/molmed.2016.00256

Luyt, C. E., Bouadma, L., Morris, A. C., Dhanani, J. A., Kollef, M., Lipman, J., et al. (2020). Pulmonary infections complicating ARDS. *Intensive Care Med.* 46, 2168–2183. doi: 10.1007/s00134-020-06292-z

Marik, P. E., Khangoora, V., Rivera, R., Hooper, M. H., and Catravas, J. (2017). Hydrocortisone, vitamin C, and thiamine for the treatment of severe sepsis and septic shock: a retrospective before-after study. *Chest* 151, 1229–1238. doi: 10.1016/j.chest.2016.11.036

Matthay, M. A., Zemans, R. L., Zimmerman, G. A., Arabi, Y. M., Beitler, J. R., Mercat, A., et al. (2019). Acute respiratory distress syndrome. *Nat. Rev. Dis. Primers* 5:18. doi: 10.1038/s41572-019-0069-0

Mazmanian, S. K., Round, J. L., and Kasper, D. L. (2008). A microbial symbiosis factor prevents intestinal inflammatory disease. *Nature* 453, 620–625. doi: 10.1038/nature07008

Mitchell, A. B., Ryan, T. E., Gillion, A. R., Wells, L. D., and Muthiah, M. P. (2020). Vitamin C and thiamine for sepsis and septic shock. *Am. J. Med.* 133, 635–638. doi: 10.1016/j.amjmed.2019.07.054

Morais, L. H., Schreiber, H. L. T., and Mazmanian, S. K. (2021). The gut microbiota-brain axis in behaviour and brain disorders. *Nat. Rev. Microbiol.* 19, 241–255. doi: 10.1038/s41579-020-00460-0

Neal, M. D., Sodhi, C. P., Dyer, M., Craig, B. T., Good, M., Jia, H., et al. (2013). A critical role for TLR4 induction of autophagy in the regulation of enterocyte migration and the pathogenesis of necrotizing enterocolitis. *J. Immunol.* 190, 3541–3551. doi: 10.4049/jimmunol.1202264

Nicholson, J. K., Holmes, E., Kinross, J., Burcelin, R., Gibson, G., Jia, W., et al. (2012). Host-gut microbiota metabolic interactions. *Science* 336, 1262–1267. doi: 10.1126/science.1223813

Odenwald, M. A., and Turner, J. R. (2013). Intestinal permeability defects: is it time to treat? *Clin. Gastroenterol. Hepatol.* 11, 1075–1083. doi: 10.1016/j.cgh.2013.07.001

Ooijevaar, R. E., Terveer, E. M., Verspaget, H. W., Kuijper, E. J., and Keller, J. J. (2019). Clinical application and potential of fecal microbiota transplantation. *Annu. Rev. Med.* 70, 335–351. doi: 10.1146/annurev-med-111717-122956

Osterberg, J., Johnsson, C., Gannedahl, G., Westlund, A., and Haglund, U. (1997). Alterations in mucosal immune cell distribution in septic rats. *Shock* 7, 182–185. doi: 10.1097/00024382-199703000-00005

Otani, S., and Coopersmith, C. M. (2019). Gut integrity in critical illness. *J. Intensive Care* 7:17. doi: 10.1186/s40560-019-0372-6

Panzer, A. R., Lynch, S. V., Langelier, C., Christie, J. D., McCauley, K., Nelson, M., et al. (2018). Lung microbiota is related to smoking status and to development of acute respiratory distress syndrome in critically ill trauma patients. *Am. J. Respir. Crit. Care Med.* 197, 621–631. doi: 10.1164/rccm.201702-0441OC

Parada Venegas, D., De la Fuente, M. K., Landskron, G., González, M. J., Quera, R., Dijkstra, G., et al. (2019). Short chain fatty acids (SCFAs)-mediated gut epithelial and immune regulation and its relevance for inflammatory bowel diseases. *Front. Immunol.* 10:277. doi: 10.3389/fimmu.2019.00277

Peluso, I., Miglio, C., Morabito, G., Ioannone, F., and Serafini, M. (2015). Flavonoids and immune function in human: a systematic review. *Crit. Rev. Food Sci. Nutr.* 55, 383–395. doi: 10.1080/10408398.2012.656770

Perrone, E. E., Jung, E., Breed, E., Dominguez, J. A., Liang, Z., Clark, A. T., et al. (2012). Mechanisms of methicillin-resistant *Staphylococcus aureus* pneumonia-induced intestinal epithelial apoptosis. *Shock* 38, 68–75. doi: 10.1097/SHK.0b013e318259abdb

Pinheiro, N. M., Santana, F. P., Almeida, R. R., Guerreiro, M., Martins, M. A., Caperuto, L. C., et al. (2017). Acute lung injury is reduced by the α7nAChR agonist PNU-282987 through changes in the macrophage profile. *FASEB J.* 31, 320–332. doi: 10.1096/fj.201600431R

Poroyko, V., Meng, F., Meliton, A., Afonyushkin, T., Ulanov, A., Semenyuk, E., et al. (2015). Alterations of lung microbiota in a mouse model of LPS-induced lung injury. *Am. J. Physiol. Lung Cell. Mol. Physiol.* 309, L76–L83. doi: 10.1152/ajplung.00061.2014

Pugin, J., and Chevrolet, J. C. (1991). [The intestine-liver-lung axis in septic syndrome]. *Schweiz. Med. Wochenschr.* 121, 1538–1544.

Ralls, M. W., Demehri, F. R., Feng, Y., Woods Ignatoski, K. M., and Teitelbaum, D. H. (2015). Enteral nutrient deprivation in patients leads to a loss of intestinal epithelial barrier function. *Surgery* 157, 732–742. doi: 10.1016/j.surg.2014.12.004

Rattanaphan, P., Mittraparp-Arthorn, P., Srinoun, K., Vuddhakul, V., and Tansila, N. (2020). Indole signaling decreases biofilm formation and related virulence of Listeria monocytogenes. *FEMS Microbiol. Lett.* 367:fnaa116. doi: 10.1093/femsle/fnaa116

Rosa, C. P., Pereira, J. A., Cristina de Melo Santos, N., Brancaglion, G. A., Silva, E. N., Tagliati, C. A., et al. (2020). Vancomycin-induced gut dysbiosis during *Pseudomonas aeruginosa* pulmonary infection in a mice model. *J. Leukoc. Biol.* 107, 95–104. doi: 10.1002/JLB.4AB0919-432R

Schmitt, F. C. F., Lipinski, A., Hofer, S., Uhle, F., Nusshag, C., Hackert, T., et al. (2020). Pulmonary microbiome patterns correlate with the course of the disease in patients with sepsis-induced ARDS following major abdominal surgery. *J. Hosp. Infect.* doi: 10.1016/j.jhin.2020.04.028 [Epub ahead of print].

Senthil, M., Watkins, A., Barlos, D., Xu, D.-Z., Lu, Q., Abungu, B., et al. (2007). Intravenous injection of trauma-hemorrhagic shock mesenteric lymph causes lung injury that is dependent upon activation of the inducible nitric oxide synthase pathway. *Ann. Surg.* 246, 822–830.

Shapouri-Moghaddam, A., Mohammadian, S., Vazini, H., Taghadosi, M., Esmaeili, S. A., Mardani, F., et al. (2018). Macrophage plasticity, polarization, and function in health and disease. *J. Cell. Physiol.* 233, 6425–6440. doi: 10.1002/jcp.26429

Shimizu, K., Ogura, H., Asahara, T., Nomoto, K., Morotomi, M., Nakahori, Y., et al. (2011). Gastrointestinal dysmotility is associated with altered gut flora and septic mortality in patients with severe systemic inflammatory response syndrome: a preliminary study. *Neurogastroenterol. Motil.* 23, 330–335, e157. doi: 10.1111/j.1365-2982.2010.01653.x

Shimizu, K., Yamada, T., Ogura, H., Mohri, T., Kiguchi, T., Fujimi, S., et al. (2018). Synbiotics modulate gut microbiota and reduce enteritis and ventilator-associated pneumonia in patients with sepsis: a randomized controlled trial. *Crit. Care* 22:239. doi: 10.1186/s13054-018-2167-x

Steed, A. L., Christophi, G. P., Kaiko, G. E., Sun, L., Goodwin, V. M., Jain, U., et al. (2017). The microbial metabolite desaminotyrosine protects from influenza through type I interferon. *Science* 357, 498–502. doi: 10.1126/science.aam5336

Su, H., Zhao, W., Zhang, F., Song, M., Liu, F., Zheng, J., et al. (2020). cis 9, trans 11, but not trans 10, cis 12 CLA isomer, impairs intestinal epithelial barrier function in IPEC-J2 cells and mice through activation of GPR120-[Ca(2+)](i) and the MLCK signaling pathway. *Food Funct.* 11, 3657–3667. doi: 10.1039/d0fo00376j

Sze, M. A., Tsuruta, M., Yang, S. W., Oh, Y., Man, S. F., Hogg, J. C., et al. (2014). Changes in the bacterial microbiota in gut, blood, and lungs following acute LPS instillation into mice lungs. *PLoS One* 9:e111228. doi: 10.1371/journal.pone.0111228

Tang, J., Xu, L., Zeng, Y., and Gong, F. (2021). Effect of gut microbiota on LPS-induced acute lung injury by regulating the TLR4/NF-kB signaling pathway. *Int. Immunopharmacol.* 91:107272. doi: 10.1016/j.intimp.2020.107272

Valdes-Duque, B. E., Giraldo-Giraldo, N. A., Jaillier-Ramirez, A. M., Giraldo-Villa, A., Acevedo-Castano, I., Yepes-Molina, M. A., et al. (2020). Stool short-chain fatty acids in critically ill patients with sepsis. *J. Am. Coll. Nutr.* 39, 706–712. doi: 10.1080/07315724.2020.1727379

Van Treuren, W., and Dodd, D. (2020). Microbial contribution to the human metabolome: implications for health and disease. *Annu. Rev. Pathol.* 15, 345–369. doi: 10.1146/annurev-pathol-020117-043559

Vital, M., Harkema, J. R., Rizzo, M., Tiedje, J., and Brandenberger, C. (2015). Alterations of the murine gut microbiome with age and allergic airway disease. *J. Immunol. Res.* 2015:892568. doi: 10.1155/2015/892568

Wang, J., Li, F., Sun, R., Gao, X., Wei, H., Li, L. J., et al. (2013). Bacterial colonization dampens influenza-mediated acute lung injury via induction of M2 alveolar macrophages. *Nat. Commun.* 4:2106. doi: 10.1038/ncomms3106

Wang, J., Li, F., Wei, H., Lian, Z. X., Sun, R., and Tian, Z. (2014). Respiratory influenza virus infection induces intestinal immune injury via microbiota-mediated Th17 cell-dependent inflammation. *J. Exp. Med.* 211, 2397–2410. doi: 10.1084/jem.20140625

Wang, J., Li, R., Peng, Z., Zhou, W., Hu, B., Rao, X., et al. (2019). GTS-21 reduces inflammation in acute lung injury by regulating M1 polarization and function of alveolar macrophages. *Shock* 51, 389–400. doi: 10.1097/shk.0000000000001144

Wang, Y., Xu, Y., Zhang, P., Ruan, W., Zhang, L., Yuan, S., et al. (2018). Smiglaside A ameliorates LPS-induced acute lung injury by modulating macrophage polarization via AMPK-PPARγ pathway. *Biochem. Pharmacol.* 156, 385–395. doi: 10.1016/j.bcp.2018.09.002

Wei, Y., Gao, J., Kou, Y., Liu, M., Meng, L., Zheng, X., et al. (2020). The intestinal microbial metabolite desaminotyrosine is an anti-inflammatory molecule that modulates local and systemic immune homeostasis. *FASEB J.* 34, 16117–16128. doi: 10.1096/fj.201902900RR

Weström, B., Arévalo Sureda, E., Pierzynowska, K., Pierzynowski, S. G., and Pérez-Cano, F. J. (2020). The immature gut barrier and its importance in establishing immunity in newborn mammals. *Front. Immunol.* 11:1153. doi: 10.3389/fimmu.2020.01153

Wilmore, J. R., Gaudette, B. T., Gomez Atria, D., Hashemi, T., Jones, D. D., Gardner, C. A., et al. (2018). Commensal microbes induce serum IgA responses that protect against polymicrobial sepsis. *Cell Host Microbe* 23, 302–311.e3. doi: 10.1016/j.chom.2018.01.005

Xu, M., Wang, C., Li, N., Wang, J., Zhang, Y., and Deng, X. (2019). Intraperitoneal injection of acetate protects mice against lipopolysaccharide (LPS)-induced acute lung injury through its anti-Inflammatory and anti-oxidative ability. *Med. Sci. Monit.* 25, 2278–2288. doi: 10.12659/MSM.911444

Xu, Y., Zhu, J., Feng, B., Lin, F., Zhou, J., Liu, J., et al. (2021). Immunosuppressive effect of mesenchymal stem cells on lung and gut CD8(+) T cells in lipopolysaccharide-induced acute lung injury in mice. *Cell Prolif.* 54:e13028. doi: 10.1111/cpr.13028

Yamada, T., Shimizu, K., Ogura, H., Asahara, T., Nomoto, K., Yamakawa, K., et al. (2015). Rapid and sustained long-term decrease of fecal short-chain fatty acids in critically ill patients with systemic inflammatory response syndrome. *JPEN J. Parenter. Enteral Nutr.* 39, 569–577. doi: 10.1177/0148607114529596

Yin, G. F., Li, B., and Fan, X. M. (2019). [Effects and mechanism of fecal transplantation on acute lung injury induced by lipopolysaccharide in rats]. *Zhonghua Yi Xue Za Zhi* 99, 1582–1587. doi: 10.3760/cma.j.issn.0376-2491.2019.20.013

Yoo, J. W., Kim, R. B., Ju, S., Lee, S. J., Cho, Y. J., Jeong, Y. Y., et al. (2020). Clinical impact of supplementation of vitamins B1 and C on patients with sepsis-related acute respiratory distress syndrome. *Tuberc. Respir. Dis.* 83, 248–254. doi: 10.4046/trd.2020.0008

Yoseph, B. P., Klingensmith, N. J., Liang, Z., Breed, E. R., Burd, E. M., Mittal, R., et al. (2016). Mechanisms of intestinal barrier dysfunction in sepsis. *Shock* 46, 52–59. doi: 10.1097/SHK.0000000000000565

Yu, P., and Martin, C. M. (2000). Increased gut permeability and bacterial translocation in *Pseudomonas* pneumonia-induced sepsis. *Crit. Care Med.* 28, 2573–2577.

Zhang, J., Bi, J., Liu, S., Pang, Q., Zhang, R., Wang, S., et al. (2017). 5-HT drives mortality in sepsis induced by cecal ligation and puncture in mice. *Mediators Inflamm.* 2017:6374283. doi: 10.1155/2017/6374283

Zhao, Y., Chen, F., Wu, W., Sun, M., Bilotta, A. J., Yao, S., et al. (2018). GPR43 mediates microbiota metabolite SCFA regulation of antimicrobial peptide expression in intestinal epithelial cells via activation of mTOR and STAT3. *Mucosal Immunol.* 11, 752–762. doi: 10.1038/mi.2017.118

Zhuo, Y., Li, D., Cui, L., Li, C., Zhang, S., Zhang, Q., et al. (2019). Treatment with 3,4-dihydroxyphenylethyl alcohol glycoside ameliorates sepsis-induced ALI in mice by reducing inflammation and regulating M1 polarization. *Biomed. Pharmacother.* 116:109012. doi: 10.1016/j.biopha.2019.109012

Zong, X., Fu, J., Xu, B., Wang, Y., and Jin, M. (2020). Interplay between gut microbiota and antimicrobial peptides. *Anim. Nutr.* 6, 389–396. doi: 10.1016/j.aninu.2020.09.002

18

Protective Effects of Anti-IL17 on Acute Lung Injury Induced by LPS in Mice

Renato Fraga Righetti [1,2], Tabata Maruyama dos Santos [1,2], Leandro do Nascimento Camargo [1], Luciana Ritha Cássia Rolim Barbosa Aristóteles [1], Silvia Fukuzaki [1], Flávia Castro Ribas de Souza [1], Fernanda Paula Roncon Santana [1], Marcus Vinicius Rodrigues de Agrela [1], Maysa Mariana Cruz [3], Maria Isabel Cardoso Alonso-Vale [3], Isabella Santos Genaro [1,4], Beatriz Mangueira Saraiva-Romanholo [1,5], Edna Aparecida Leick [1], Milton de Arruda Martins [1], Carla Máximo Prado [6] and Iolanda de Fátima Lopes Calvo Tibério [1]*

[1] Faculdade de Medicina FMUSP, Universidade de São Paulo, São Paulo, Brazil, [2] Hospital Sírio-Libanês, São Paulo, Brazil, [3] Universidade Federal de São Paulo, Instituto de Ciências Ambientais, Químicas e Farmacêuticas, Departamento de Ciências Biológicas, Diadema, São Paulo, Brazil, [4] Public Employee of São Paulo Hospital (IAMSPE), São Paulo, Brazil, [5] University of City of São Paulo (UNICID), São Paulo, Brazil, [6] Department of Bioscience, Federal University of São Paulo, Santos, São Paulo, Brazil

***Correspondence:**
Renato Fraga Righetti
refragar@gmail.com

Introduction: T helper 17 (Th17) has been implicated in a variety of inflammatory lung and immune system diseases. However, little is known about the expression and biological role of IL-17 in acute lung injury (ALI). We investigated the mechanisms involved in the effect of anti-IL17 in a model of lipopolysaccharide (LPS)-induced acute lung injury (ALI) in mice.

Methods: Mice were pre-treated with anti-IL17, 1h before saline/LPS intratracheal administration alongside non-treated controls and levels of exhaled nitric oxide (eNO), cytokine expression, extracellular matrix remodeling and oxidative stress, as well as immune cell counts in bronchoalveolar lavage fluid (BALF), and respiratory mechanics were assessed in lung tissue.

Results: LPS instillation led to an increase in multiple cytokines, proteases, nuclear factor-κB, and Forkhead box P3 (FOXP3), eNO and regulators of the actomyosin cytoskeleton, the number of CD4+ and iNOS-positive cells as well as the number of neutrophils and macrophages in BALF, resistance and elastance of the respiratory system, ARG-1 gene expression, collagen fibers, and actin and 8-iso-PGF2α volume fractions. Pre-treatment with anti-IL17 led to a significant reduction in the level of all assessed factors.

Conclusions: Anti-IL17 can protect the lungs from the inflammatory effects of LPS-induced ALI, primarily mediated by the reduced expression of cytokines and oxidative stress. This suggests that further studies using anti-IL17 in a treatment regime would be highly worthwhile.

Keywords: acute lung injury, inflammation mediators, interleukin 17, remodeling, oxidative stress

INTRODUCTION

Acute lung injury (ALI) and acute respiratory distress syndrome (ARDS) can result from various pathologies including sepsis, microbial infection, trauma or ischemia/reperfusion, and can lead to acute respiratory failure with a mortality rate of approximately 40% (Modrykamien and Gupta, 2015). The pathogenesis of ALI/ARDS is characterized by epithelial integrity disruption and the infiltration of polymorphonuclear cells (PMNs) into the lungs, which may cause interstitial edema and alveolar collapse (Castillo et al., 2015). In addition, macrophages and neutrophils have been shown to release pro-inflammatory cytokines such as interleukin (IL)-1β, IL-6, IL-8, and tumor necrosis factor (TNF)-α and as well as profibrotic growth factors such as platelet-derived growth factor, transforming growth factor beta (TGF-β; Pinheiro et al., 2015; Blondonnet et al., 2016). Thus, macrophages and neutrophils may be important mediators in initiating the inflammatory response, regulating fibroblast function and oxidative stress in the later stage of ALI/ARDS (Pinheiro et al., 2015; Blondonnet et al., 2016).

Nitric oxide (NO) produced in large amounts by inducible nitric oxide synthase (iNOS) occurs mainly in macrophages inflammatory situations and causes lipid peroxidation and the generation of isoprostane (Villegas et al., 2014). The 8-isoprostane prostaglandin 2α (8-iso-PGF2α) is considered the predominant marker of tissue oxidative damage form generated during free radical attack of cell membranes (Elfsmark et al., 2018). Exhaled NO (eNO) has been used as a marker of both inflammation and oxidative stress (Boshier et al., 2013).

The nuclear transcription factor kB (NFkB) is a transcription factor found in the cytoplasm. The increase activation of NFkB in alveolar macrophages of patients with established ALI/ARDS, resulting in pro-inflammatory cytokines increase, such as TNF-a, IL-1β, IL-6, IL-8, and oxidative stress activation (Bittencourt-Mernak et al., 2017). The continuous inflammation and activation of matrix metalloproteinase (MMP) 9 and 12 and tissue inhibitor of metalloproteinase 1 (TIMP-1) can be followed by alterations in the lung extracellular matrix, which can occur earlier in ARDS and contribute to decreased lung function (González-López and Albaiceta, 2012; Bittencourt-Mernak et al., 2017).

Rho-kinase (ROCK) is a small GTPase and a major downstream effector of RhoA, ROCK promotes the modulating stress fiber formation, actin cytoskeleton organization, and smooth muscle cell contraction (Pigati et al., 2015). Two mammalian ROCK homologs have been identified, ROCK 1 and ROCK 2 (Defert and Boland, 2017).

T-helper (Th)-17 are a unique subset of cluster of differentiation 4 (CD4+) T-helper cells characterized by the production of pro-inflammatory IL-17A, IL-17F, and IL-22 and the their differentiation is mediated by the activation of T helper cells in the presence of a combination of TGF-β, IL-6, IL-1β, and IL-23 (Ghoreschi et al., 2010). IL-6 combined with TGF-β induces the development of Th17 effector cells. IL-17 acts by activating iNOS and inducing the expression of macrophage, IL-1β, IL-6, IL-8, TNF-α, and several chemokines, which collaborate to potentiate the inflammatory process (Gonçalves-de-Albuquerque et al., 2017).

Th17 has been implicated in the development or pathogenesis of several autoimmune and inflammatory diseases (Sakaguchi et al., 2016), including those of the lung, such as cystic fibrosis, asthma, chronic obstructive pulmonary disease and granulomatous disease (Hsu et al., 2016; Yanagisawa et al., 2017, O'Dwyer et al., 2016; Hasegawa et al., 2017). However, IL-17 also plays an important role in protective immunity against some bacterial infections, mainly through the recruitment and activation of neutrophils. Thus, the regulation of Th-17 is important in that either an excess or deficiency could result in a modulation of these diseases (Ding et al., 2017).

Mikacenic et al. (2016) shows elevated circulating and alveolar levels of IL-17 in human with ARDS, but the role of the Th-17 immune response in ALI/ARDS has not been defined. Therefore, in this study we evaluated the effect and mechanisms involved in after pretreatment with anti-IL-17 in the early phase of a mice model of ALI induced by lipopolysaccharide (LPS). Specifically we measured changes in the resistance and elastance of the respiratory system, multiple markers of inflammation, as well as oxidative stress and extracellular matrix remodeling in lung tissue. Understanding the role of IL-17 signaling in ALI/ARDS may contribute to the development of a future therapeutic target for this disease.

MATERIALS AND METHODS

Animals and Experimental Model

Thirty-two male BALB/c mice (25g to 30 g) were divided into four groups ($n = 8$ in each group):

E) SAL (saline solution-instilled),

F) LPS (LPS-instilled),

G) SAL-antiIL17 (saline solution-instilled and anti-IL17 treatment),

H) LPS-antiIL17 (LPS-instilled and anti-IL17 treatment).

All animals received humane care in accordance with the Guide for the Care and Use of Laboratory Animals (National Institutes of Health, 2011). This study was approved by the research committee of the School of Medicine at the University of São Paulo (São Paulo, Brazil) for animal studies (number 054/15).

Anti-IL17 Treatment

Anti-IL17 neutralizing antibody (R and D Systems, Abingdon, UK) was administered intraperitoneally at a dose of 7.5 μg/application, based on the protocol of Barlow et al. (2011) and Camargo et al. (2018), 1 h prior to intratracheal instillation of LPS/saline solution.

Abbreviations: ALI: acute lung injury; ARDS: acute respiratory distress syndrome; BALF: bronchoalveolar lavage fluid; BSA: bovine serum albumin; eNO: exhaled nitric oxide; Ers: respiratory elastance; Rrs: respiratory resistance; MMP-9: Metalloproteinase 9; MMP-12: Metalloproteinase 12; TIMP1: Tissue inhibitor of metalloproteinase-1; ROCK: Rho-kinase; iNOS: inducible nitric oxide synthase; TNF-α: Tumor necrosis factor - α; 8-iso-PGF2α: 8-isoprostane-PGF2α; IL: interleukin; NF: nuclear factor

Experimental Model of ALI

For intratracheal instillation (I.T.) animals were anesthetized with isoflurane (2%), then a 1 cm-long midline cervical incision was made to expose the trachea, and LPS or saline was instilled using a bent 27-gauge tuberculin needle. LPS and LPS-antiIL17 groups received a single I.T. dose of Escherichia coli LPS (026: B6L3755, Sigma Aldrich, St. Louis, MO, USA) 5 mg.kg^{-1} suspended in saline solution (total volume = 0.05 mL per animal). SAL and SAL-antiIL17 groups received a single I.T. dose of 0.05 mL saline solution. After the procedure, the cervical incision was closed with a 5.0 silk suture, and the mice were returned to their cages (Bittencourt-Mernak et al., 2017).

Exhaled Nitric Oxide (eNO)

Twenty-four hours after LPS or saline instillation, the animals were anesthetized using pentobarbital sodium (50 mg/kg i.p.), tracheostomized, connected to a Harvard 683 ventilator (Harvard Apparatus, South Natick, MA, USA) and mechanically ventilated at 60 breaths/min with a tidal volume of 10 mL/kg. A Mylar bag was connected at the expiratory port of the ventilator for 10 min by measured eNO levels and to avoid environmental contamination. This was then attached to the inspiratory breathing circuit input and NO filter. After sample collection, eNO concentrations were measured by chemiluminescence using a NOA 280 (Sievers Instruments Inc., Boulder, CO, USA). The analyzer was calibrated with an NO (nitric oxide) source certified at 47- parts per billion (ppb; White Martins, São Paulo, Brazil) and a zero NO filter (Sievers Instruments Inc.; Pigati et al., 2015).

Respiratory System Mechanics

An evaluation of respiratory system mechanics was conducted after the eNO measurement. A differential pressure transducer (Honeywell, Freeport, IL), pneumotachograph (Fleisch-4.0, OEM Medical, Richmond, VA, USA) and Honeywell 163PC01D36 differential pressure transducer were connected to the tracheal cannula to measure the tracheal pressure (Ptr) and airflow (V').

Lung volume (V) changes were determined by the digital integration of the airflow signal. Nine to ten respiratory cycles were averaged to provide one data point. The Ptr, V', and V signals were collected and stored on a microcomputer. Lung volume (V) changes were obtained by the electronic integration of V'. The respiratory system resistance (Rrs) and elastance (Ers) were computed by least squares fitting of the measured values of Ptr, V, and V. over 9 to 10 respiratory cycles using the following equation of motion of the respiratory system: $Ptr(t) = Ers \times V(t) + Rrs \times V'.(t)$, where t is time. All data were collected and processed using LABDAT software (RHT-InfoData, Montreal, Quebec, Canada; Possa et al., 2012; Pigati et al., 2015).

Bronchoalveolar Lavage Fluid (BALF) Cell Counts

After the mechanical respiratory systems evaluation, the animal's anterior chest wall was opened and it was euthanized by exsanguination *via* the abdominal aorta. The BALF was collected by flushing the lungs three times with 0.5 mL of 37°C sterile physiological saline (0.9% NaCl) via the tracheal cannula and the fluid samples were centrifuged at 420 × g at 4°C for 15 min. The cell pellets were resuspended in 1 mL of sterile physiological saline and 100 μL of each sample was cytocentrifuged in a Cytospin for 6 min at 450 rpm. The total cell counts were performed using a *Neubauer* chamber and for differential cells counts, cytospin slides were prepared and stained with *Diff-Quick* Reagent (Biochemical Sciences Inc., Swedesboro, NJ). 300 cells were counted per slide using an optical microscope, using the morphologic criteria (Vieira et al., 2007; Martins-Olivera et al., 2016).

Lung Histology

After BALF collection, the lungs were fixed dor 24 h in a sufficient volume of formalin (4%) to completely immerse the tissue, and then the lung was dehydrated in a solution of 70% ethanol, xylol, and afterwards, it was immersed in paraffin, and different regions of the lung were cut into slices to obtain 4-μm thick sections that were then mounted on to slides. The slides were stained with hematoxylin-Eosin and Picro-Sirius Red for analysis of collagen fibers, according to the following protocol:

Sections were deparaffinized, rinsed with water and hydrated in 95% alcohol before being stained with Picro-Sirius Red (Direct Red 80, C.I. 35780, Sigma Aldrich) at room temperature. Then, the slices were washed in running water for 5 min, and the sections were stained with Harris hematoxylin for 6 min and washed again in running water for 10 min. They were then dehydrated and mounted on slides (Possa et al., 2012). The histologic slides were not labeled with group information and the researcher had no knowledge of the procedures for each group.

Immunohistochemistry

The expression of positive cells was evaluated with immunohistochemistry technique. The lung sections were deparaffinized and 0.3% hydrogen peroxide was applied for 35 min to inhibit endogenous peroxidase activity. Antigen retrieval was performed using citrate solution for 45 min to inhibit endogenous peroxidase activity (Possa et al., 2012).

The sections were incubated overnight at 4°C with anti-TNF-α (1:400; R&D Systems, Minneapolis, MN, USA), anti-IL1β (1:400), anti-IL6 (1:200), anti-IL8 (1:200), anti-IL10 (1:300), anti-IL17 (1:250), anti-CD4+ (1:600), anti-iNOS (1:400), anti-forkhead box P3 (FOXP3) (1:1200), anti-p65-NF-κB (1:250), anti-8-iso-PGF2α (1:1500), anti-TGF-β (1:600), anti-MMP-9 (1:500), anti-MMP-12 (1:450), anti-TIMP-1 (1:100), anti-actin (1:1600), anti- ROCK 1 (1:50), and anti-ROCK 2 (1:100; Santa Cruz Biotechnology Inc., Santa Cruz, CA, USA). The following day, the slides were washed in PBS and incubated with a secondary antibody using the ABCKit by Vectastain (Vector Elite-PK-6105 anti-goat), PK-6101 (anti-rabbit), and PK-6102 (anti-mouse). For visualization of positive cells, the slides were washed in PBS and proteins were visualized using 3,3'-diaminobenzidine chromosome (DAB; Sigma Chemical Co., St. Louis, MO, USA). Slide sections were contrasted with Harris hematoxylin (Merck, Darmstadt, Germany) and assembled using Entellan microscopy resin (Merck; Possa et al., 2012; Righetti et al., 2014).

Quantification of Collagen Fibers, Actin and 8-Iso-PGF2α Volume Fractions

We measured the total area of lung tissue and the area of collagen fibers, actin and 8-iso-PGF2α in 15 to 20 microscopic fields per lung using a 400x magnification and the Image-ProPlus 4.5 *Image Analysis System* (Media Cybernetics, Silver Spring, USA). The amount of collagen fibers, actin or 8-iso-PGF2α was expressed as a percentage based on the relationship between the quantity of collagen fibers, actin or 8-iso-PGF2α in a specific frame and the total area of that frame (volume fraction; Prado et al., 2006).

Morphometric Analysis

We assessed the density of inflammatory cells (mononuclear and polymorphonuclear cells) that were positive for CD4+, FOXP3, TNF-α, IL-1β, IL-6, IL-8, IL-10, IL-17, iNOS, p65-NFκB, TGF-β, MMP-9, MMP-12, TIMP-1, ROCK 1, and ROCK 2 in the lung tissue using conventional morphometry. Using a 100-point grid of a known area (62,500 μm2 at × 400 magnification) attached to the ocular of the microscope; we counted the number of points covering the lung tissue and the number of inflammatory positive cells in each field. The cell density was determined as the number of positive cells in each field divided by the tissue area and expressed as positive cells/$10^4 \mu m^2$ (Weibel, 1979; Lanças et al., 2006; Righetti et al., 2014; Barreto do Carmo et al., 2016; Camargo et al., 2018). The morphometric measurements were performed on 15 fields per slices at ×1000 magnification.

Evaluation of Cytokines in Lung Tissue

Levels of TNF-α and IL-1β in the lung tissue were evaluated using ELISA in accordance with the manufacturer's instructions (Duo Set, R&D Systems, Minneapolis, MN, US) and previously used by (Bittencourt-Mernak et al., 2017).

RNA Extraction, Reverse Transcription and Quantitative Real-Time PCR (RT-PCR)

The expression level of IL-6, IL-17, and arginase 1 (ARG-1) in the lungs was evaluated using real-time PCR (polymerase chain reaction) as previously reported by our group (Pinheiro et al., 2015). Expression of GAPDH was used as an internal control. The primer sequences were: GAPDH (5′-3′ sense: CCACCAC CCTGTTGCTGTAG; 5′-3′antisense: CTTGGGCTACACTGAG GACC; 60°C; NM_008084) and IL-6 (5′-3′ sense: TTCTCTGG GAAATCGTGGAAA; 5′-3′ antisense: TCAGAATTGCCATTG CACAAC; NM_001314054); IL-17 (5′-3′ sense: TGAAGGTCA ACCTCAAAGTCT, 5′-3′ antisense: GAGGGATATCTATCAGG GTCTTCAT) and ARG-1(5′-3′ sense GCACTCATGGAAGTA CACGAGGAC, 5′-3′ antisense: CCAACCCAGTGATCTTGAC TGA). The results were obtained as the cycle number at which logarithmic PCR plots cross a calculated threshold line and used to determine ΔCt values [ΔCt = (Ct of the target gene)–(Ct of the house-keeping gene)]. The results are expressed as arbitrary units using the transformation: Expression = $1000 \times (2^{-\Delta ct})$ arbitrary units (Camargo et al., 2018).

Alveolar Collapse

The volume fraction of the lung occupied by collapsed alveoli (alveoli with rough or plicate walls) or normal pulmonary areas (those not exhibiting over distended or plicate walls) were determined by the point-counting technique (Weibel, 1963) at a magnification of ×200 across 10 random, non-coincident microscopic fields (Riva et al., 2008; Saddy et al., 2010).

Data Analysis

All analyzes were conducted using SigmaPlot 11.0 software (Systat Software, SPSS Inc., USA). Results are represented as the means ± SE and One-Way Analysis of Variance (ANOVA) followed by the Holm-Sidak method for multiple comparisons. A p-value < 0.05 was considered statistically significant.

RESULTS

Respiratory Mechanics

Figure 1 shows the functional consequences of pretreatment with anti-IL17 in this animal model of acute ling injury on Rrs (A) and Ers (B) in the four experimental groups. LPS instillation increased both pulmonary Rrs and Ers compared with the SAL and SAL-antiIL17 groups ($P < 0.05$), which was decreased by anti-IL17 in both cases ($P < 0.05$).

Exhaled Nitric Oxide

Figure 2 shows the effect of the pretreatment with anti-IL17 on the pro-inflammatory concentration of eNO in the four experimental groups. LPS instillation increased eNOS concentration compared to the SAL group and SAL-antiIL17 groups ($P < 0.05$), which was decreased by anti-IL17 ($P < 0.05$).

BALF Cell Counts

Figure 3 shows the effects of the pretreatment with anti-IL17 on the total inflammatory cells count in the BALF and the differential count for macrophages, neutrophils, lymphocytes and eosinophils.

LPS instillation increased total cell number, and the number of macrophages and neutrophils in BALF compared to the SAL and SAL-antiIL17 groups ($P < 0.05$), which were all decreased by anti-IL17 ($P < 0.05$). There was no effect of LPS or anti-IL17 on the number of lymphocytes and eosinophils in BALF. Anti-IL17 decreased 42.5% of macrophages, 80% of neutrophils, 0% of lymphocytes, and 16.6% of eosinophils compared to the LPS group.

Alveolar Collapse

Figure 4 shows the effects of the pretreatment with anti-IL17 on the evaluation of alveolar collapse in the four experimental groups. LPS instillation increased in volume fraction of alveolar collapse compared to the SAL and SAL–antiIL17group ($P < 0.05$), which was decreased by anti-IL17 ($P < 0.05$).

Determination of IL-8 and IL-10 by Immunohistochemistry

Figure 5 shows the effects of the pretreatment with anti-IL17 on the expression of inflammatory markers for IL-8 (A)

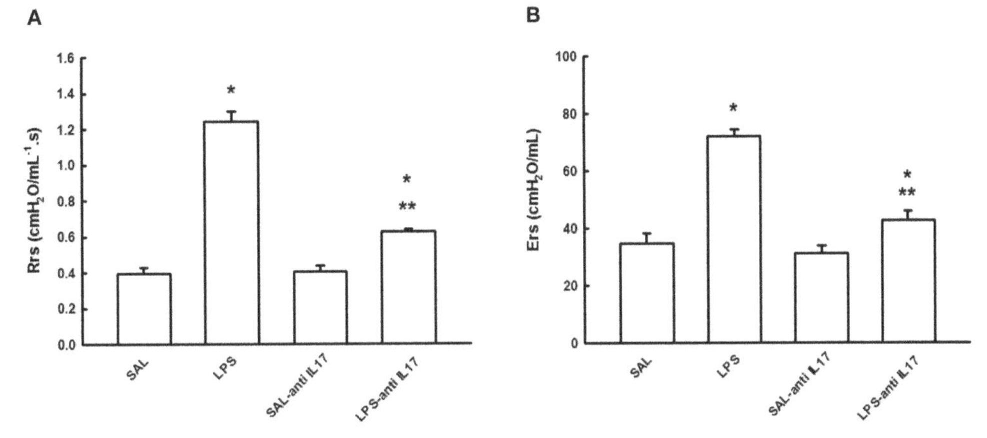

FIGURE 1 | Effects of the pretreatment with anti-IL17 on mechanical evaluation: **(A)** Respiratory system resistance and **(B)** Respiratory system elastance. **P* < 0.05 compared with SAL and SAL-antiIL17 groups; ***P* < 0.05 compared to the LPS group.

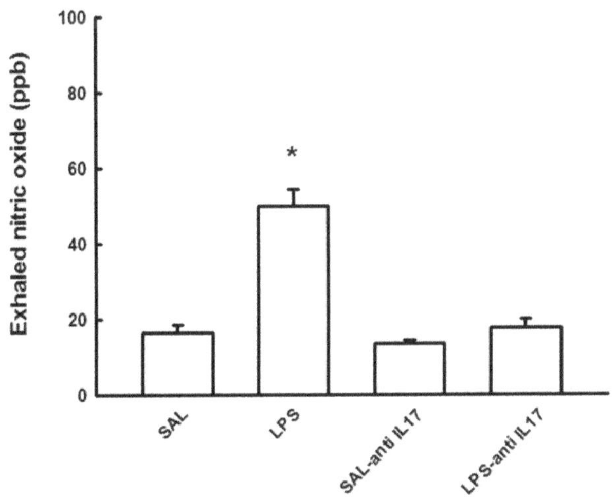

FIGURE 2 | Effects of the pretreatment with anti-IL17 on exhaled nitric oxide (ppb). **P* < 0.05 compared to the SAL, SAL-antiIL17 and LPS-antiIL17 groups.

and IL-10 (B)-positive cells in lung tissue. LPS instillation increased in the number of IL-8 and IL-10-positive cells in lung tissue compared to the SAL and SAL-antiIL17 groups ($P < 0.05$). Anti-IL17 decreased the number of IL-8 and IL-10-positive cells in lung tissue compared to the LPS group ($P < 0.05$).

Determination of IL-6 and IL-17 by Immunohistochemistry and RT-PCR

Figure 6 shows the effects of the pretreatment with anti-IL17 on the IL-6 and IL-17-positive cells and gene expression on lung tissue. LPS instillation increased IL-6 and IL-17-positive cells and gene expression compared to the SAL and SAL-antiIL17 groups ($P < 0.05$). Anti-IL17 decreased the IL-6 and IL-17-positive cells and gene expression compared to the LPS group ($P < 0.05$).

Determination of TNF-α and IL-1β by ELISA and Immunohistochemistry

Figure 7 shows the effects of the pretreatment with anti-IL17 on the TNF-α and IL-1β-positive cells (**Figures 7A,C**) and cytokines levels (**Figures 7B,D**) on lung tissue. LPS instillation increased the levels of cytokine and positive cells of TNF-α and IL-1β compared to the SAL and SAL-antiIL17 groups ($P < 0.05$). Anti-IL17 decreased the levels of cytokine and positive cells of TNF-α and IL-1β compared to the LPS group ($P < 0.05$).

CD4+ and FOXP3+ Regulatory T Cells

Figure 8 shows the effects of the pretreatment with anti-IL17 on the expression of immune cells regulation CD4+ (**Figure 6A**) and FOXP3-positive cells (**Figure 4B**) in lung tissue. We noted that the LPS group presented an increased CD4+ and FOXP3-positive cells compared to the SAL and SAL-antiIL17 groups ($P < 0.05$). Anti-IL17 (LPS-antiIL17group) decreased the CD4+ and FOXP3-positive cells compared to the LPS group ($P < 0.05$). However, LPS-antiIL17 group presented an increased FOXP3-positive cells compared to the SAL and SAL-antiIL17 groups ($P < 0.05$).

Extracellular Matrix Remodeling

Table 1 shows the effects of the pretreatment with anti-IL17 on the extracellular matrix remodeling. We observed that the LPS group presented an increased the volume fraction of collagen fibers and actin, and number of TGF-β, MMP-9, MMP-12, and TIMP-1-positive cells compared to the SAL and SAL-antiIL17 groups ($P < 0.05$). Anti-IL17 (LPS-antiIL17group) decreased the volume fraction of collagen fibers and actin, and number of TGF-β, MMP-9, MMP-12, and TIMP-1-positive cells compared to the LPS group ($P < 0.05$). However, LPS-antiIL17 group presented an increased MMP-9 and TIMP-1-positive cells compared to the SAL and SAL-antiIL17 groups ($P < 0.05$) and decreased the volume fraction of collagen fibers and actin compared to the SAL and SAL-antiIL17 groups ($P < 0.05$).

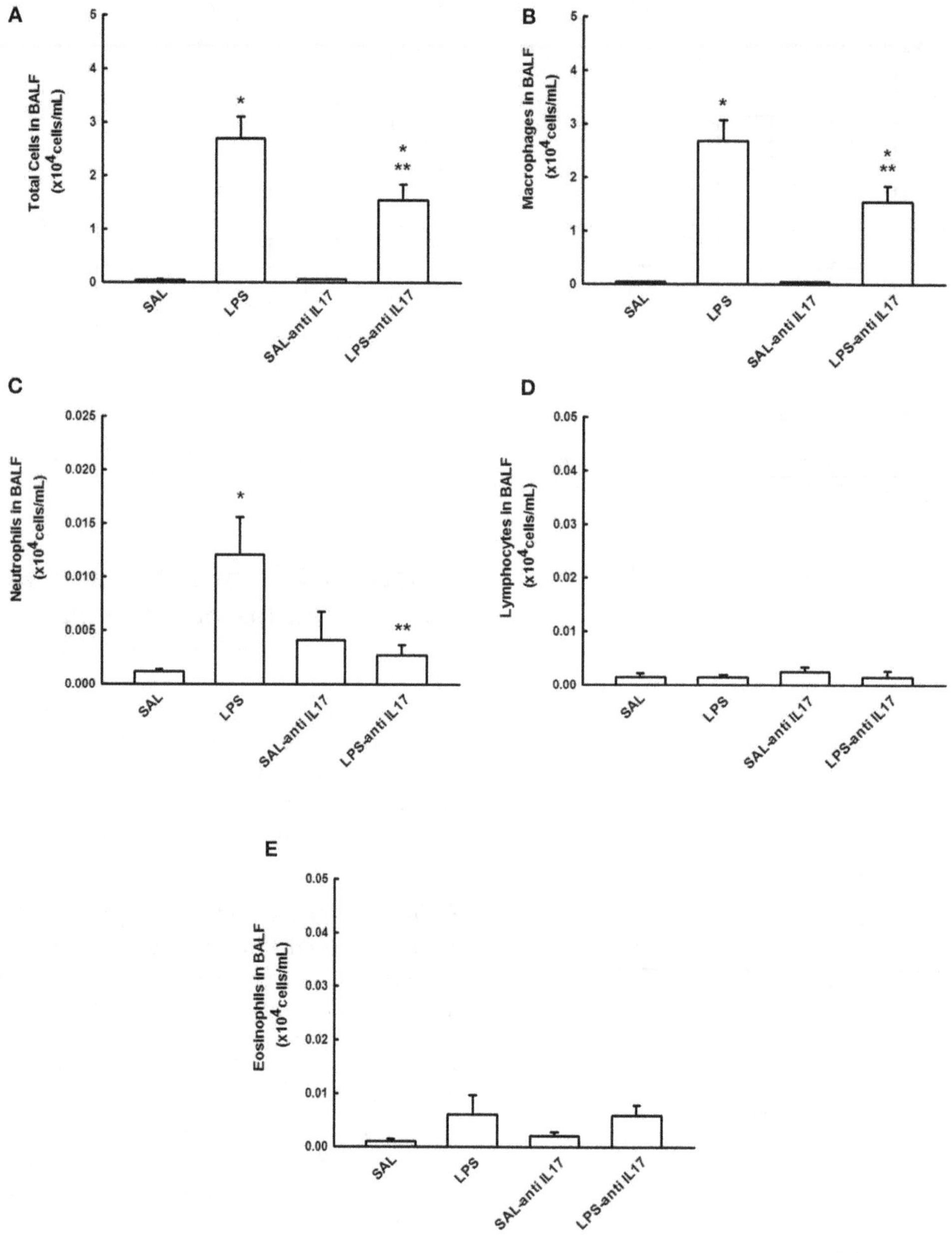

FIGURE 3 | Effects of the pretreatment with anti-IL17 on BALF. **(A)** Total cells, **(B)** cell differential for macrophages, **(C)** cell differential for neutrophils, **(D)** cell differential for Lymphocytes, and **(E)** cell differential for eosinophils. The results are expressed as x10^4 cells/mL.*$P < 0.05$ compared to the SAL and SAL-antiIL17 groups; **$P < 0.05$ compared to the LPS group.

Oxidative Stress Response

Table 2 shows the effects of the pretreatment with anti-IL17 on the oxidative stress markers. We noted that the LPS group presented an increased number of iNOS-positive cells, volume fraction of 8-iso-PGF2α and gene expression of ARG-1 compared to the SAL and SAL-antiIL17 groups ($P < 0.05$). Anti-IL17 decreased the number of iNOS-positive cells, volume fraction of 8-iso-PGF2α and gene expression of ARG-1 compared to the LPS group ($P < 0.05$).

Expression of p65-NFκB

Figure 9 shows the effect of the pretreatment with anti-IL17 on the pro-inflammatory transcription gene factor p65-NFκB in lung tissue. LPS instillation increased in the number of p65-NFκB-positive cells, compared with the SAL and SAL-antiIL17 groups ($P < 0.05$), which was decreased by anti-IL17 ($P < 0.05$).

Expression of Rock 1 and ROCK 2

Figure 10 shows the effects of the pretreatment with anti-IL17 on the expression of ROCK 1(A) and ROCK 2 (B)-positive

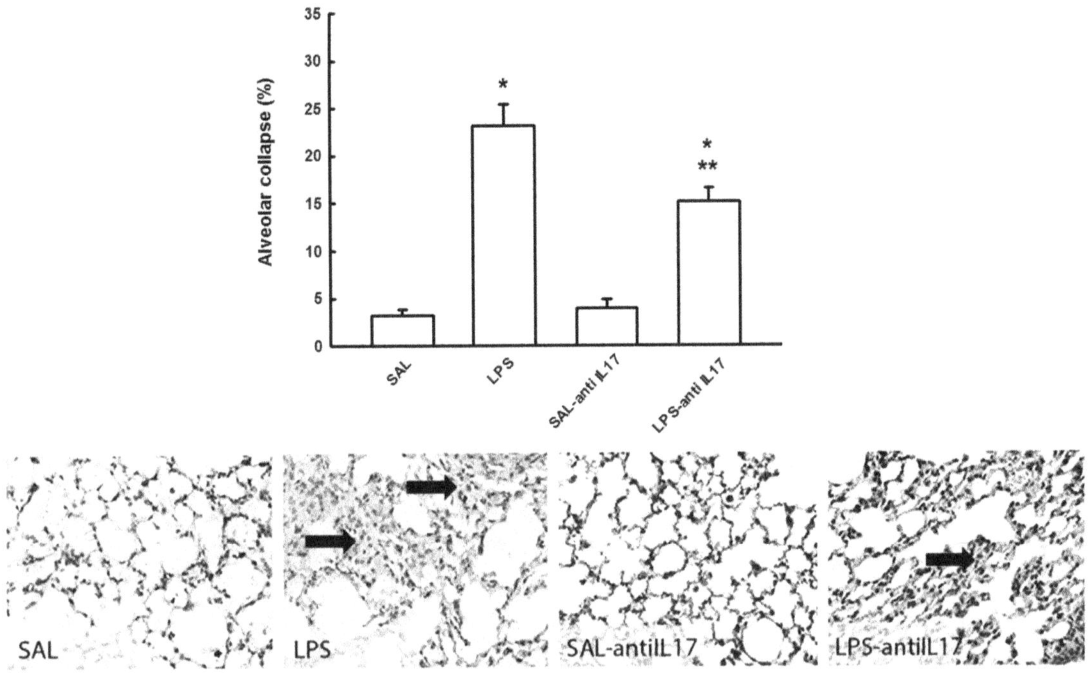

FIGURE 4 | Effects of the pretreatment with anti-IL17 on alveolar collapse (%) and photomicrographs of alveolar collapse. Magnification x1000. Arrow: alveolar collapse. All experimental groups are represented: SAL, LPS, SAL-antiIL17 and LPS-antiIL17 groups. *$P < 0.05$ compared to the SAL and SAL-antiIL17 groups; **$P < 0.05$ compared to the LPS group.

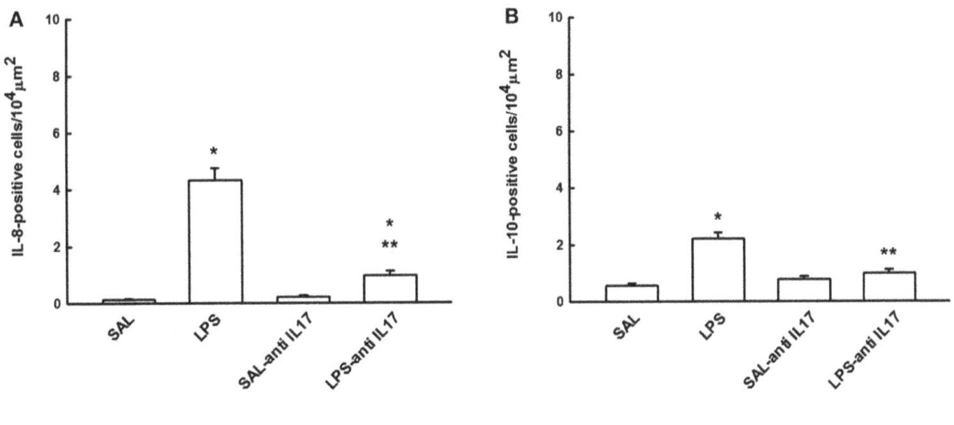

FIGURE 5 | Effects of the pretreatment with anti-IL17 on **(A)** IL-8 and **(B)** IL-10-positive cells in lung tissue. *$P < 0.05$ compared to the SAL and SAL-antiIL17 groups; **$P < 0.05$ compared to the LPS group.

cells in lung tissue to better understanding the functional lung response observed in the experimental groups. LPS instillation increased the number of ROCK 1 and ROCK 2-positive cells compared to the SAL and SAL-antiIL17 groups ($P < 0.05$), which was decreased by anti-IL17 in both cases ($P < 0.05$).

Qualitative Analysis

Representative photomicrographs are presented in **Figure 11**, and illustrate the inflammatory processes in the lung tissue. The slides were stained TNF-α, IL-1β, and IL-17-positive cells. **Figure 12** illustrates the extracellular matrix remodeling and oxidative stress processes in the lung tissue. The slides were stained for cells expressing collagen fibers, MMP-9, iNOS, and 8-iso-PGF2α. The LPS group showed an increase in the number of TNF-α, IL-1β, IL-17, MMP-9, and iNOS-positive cells and an increase in the volume fraction of 8-iso-PGF2α and collagen fibers, suggesting the presence of lung inflammation, extracellular matrix remodeling, and activation of the oxidative stress processes. Pretreatment with anti-IL17 reduced the above changes in

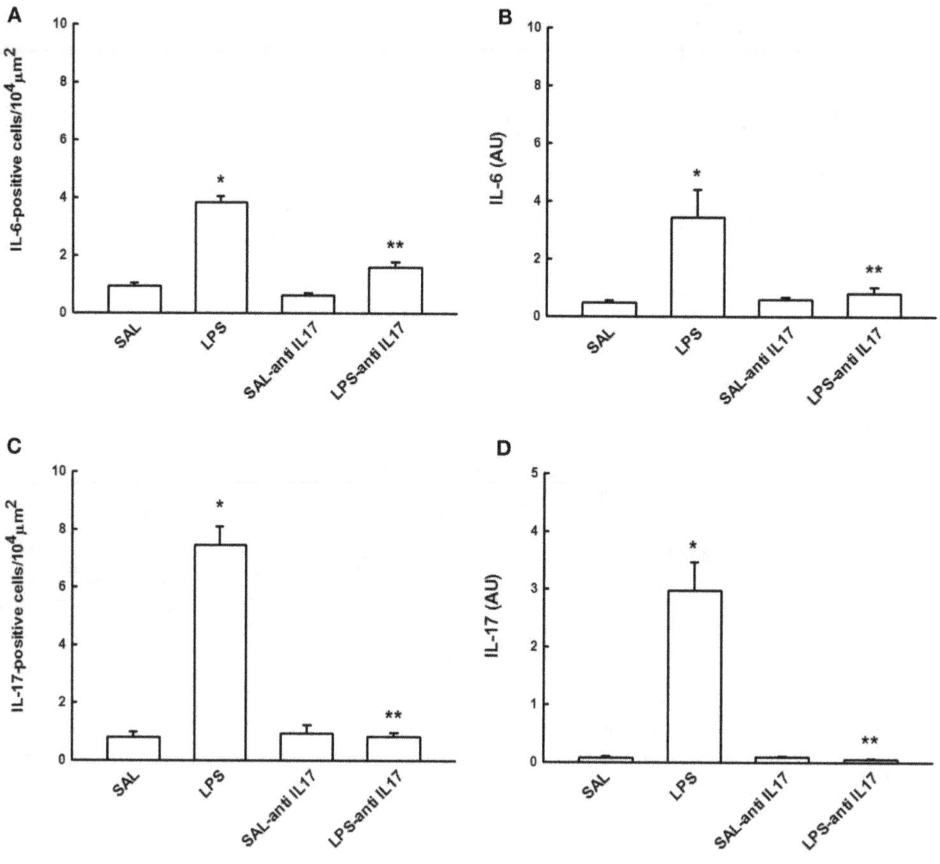

FIGURE 6 | Effects of the pretreatment with anti-IL17 on **(A)** IL-6-positive cells, **(B)** IL-6 gene expression (AU), **(C)** IL-17-positive cells and **(D)** IL-17 gene expression (AU) in lung tissue. **P* < 0.05 compared to the SAL and SAL-antiIL17 groups; ***P* < 0.05 compared to the LPS group.

lung tissue, which can be observed in the representative photomicrographs.

DISCUSSION

This study investigated the effect of and the mechanisms involved in the pretreatment with anti-IL17 in the early phase in a model of ALI induced by LPS. We demonstrated that anti-IL17 pretreatment prior to the intratracheal instillation of LPS decreased pulmonary resistance and elastance, the number of ROCK 1 and ROCK 2-positive cells, eNO concentration, neutrophilic and macrophage lung tissue infiltration, cytokine expression, extracellular matrix remodeling, and oxidative stress responses. In addition, the gene expression of ARG-1, IL-6, and IL-17 was also decreased. These results suggest that blocking the effects of IL-17 can protecting the lung from the inflammatory effects of LPS-induced ALI by altering the inflammatory, extracellular matrix remodeling, and oxidative stress profile in lung tissue.

We also showed that there was a decrease in the resistance and elastance of the respiratory system after anti-IL17. There is evidence that actin/myosin contractility is regulated by Rho-kinase (Sharanek et al., 2016). The influence of Rho-kinase on resistance and elastance of the respiratory system it is related to agonist-mediated Ca^{2+} sensitization, but the mechanisms have not been fully elucidated (Kaneko-Kawano et al., 2012; Pigati et al., 2015). Nguyen et al. (2013) evaluated IL-17 and Rho-kinase in endothelial dysfunction and hypertension and in agreement with our study, showed that IL-17 caused a threefold increase in the Rho-kinase activator RhoA, which was prevented by an IL-17 neutralizing antibody.

In this study, we also demonstrated a reduction in the number of neutrophils and macrophages in BALF. Even though neutrophils are the hallmark effector cells of acute inflammation, they also contribute to chronic inflammation and adaptive immune responses via IL-17. IL-17 secreted from neutrophils induces the release of pro-inflammatory factors (such as cytokines, chemokines and metalloproteinases) from mesenchymal and myeloid cells, leading to the further neutrophil recruitment and activation (Abraham, 2003; Ley et al., 2007; Caucheteux et al., 2017).

Cells of monocyte-macrophage lineage are another important source of and responders to IL-17 (Ge et al., 2014). In genetically modified mice IL-17 receptor A (IL-17Ra) affects monocyte homeostasis and the kidney fibrotic response to injury (Ge et al., 2014) while preventing macrophages apoptosis and

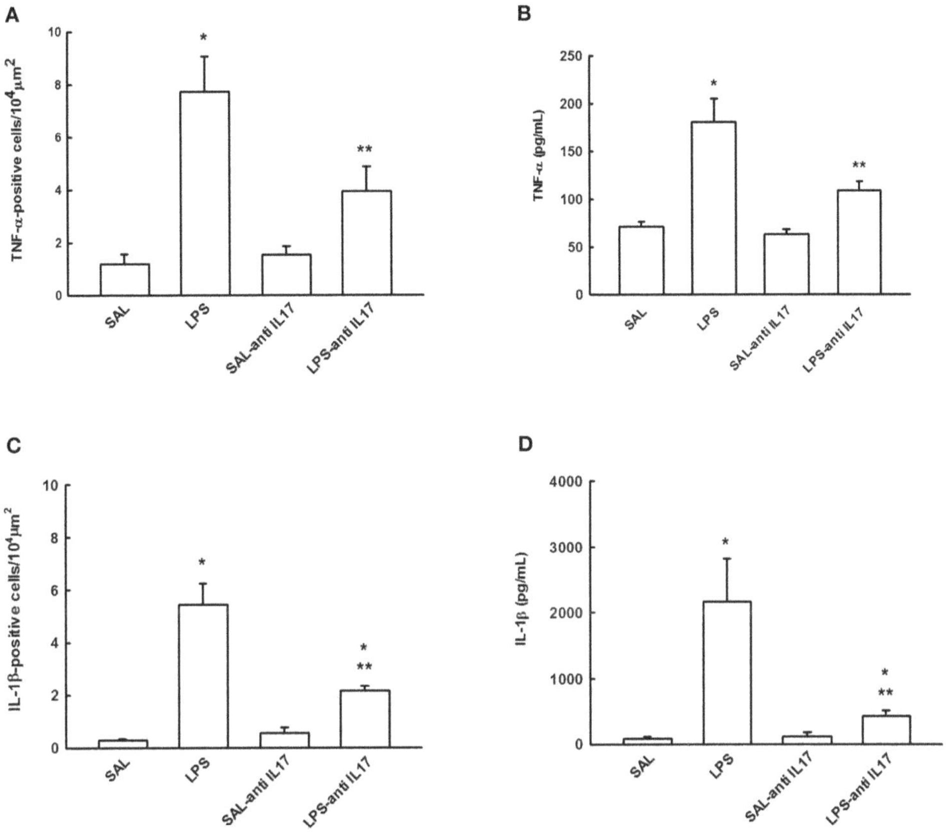

FIGURE 7 | Effects of the pretreatment with anti-IL17 on **(A)** TNF-α-positive cells, **(B)** TNF-α cytokines levels, **(C)** IL-1β-positive cells and **(D)** IL-1β cytokines levels in lung tissue.*$P < 0.05$ compared to the SAL and SAL-antiIL17 groups; **$P < 0.05$ compared to the LPS group.

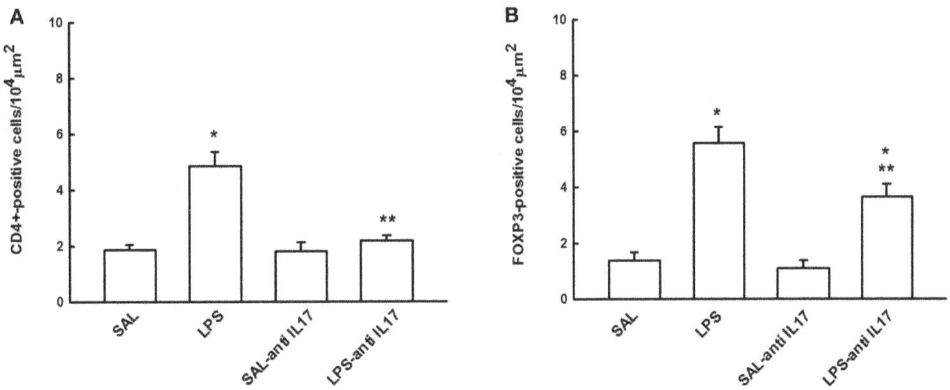

FIGURE 8 | Effects of the pretreatment with anti-IL17 on **(A)** CD4+ and **(B)** FOXP3-positive cells in lung tissue. *$P < 0.05$ compared to the SAL and SAL-antiIL17 groups; **$P < 0.05$ compared to the LPS group.

increasing their response to IL-10 and glucocorticoids (Zizzo and Cohen, 2013). In another study, IL-17 elicited a distinct transcriptional profile in mouse macrophages and contributed to monocyte attraction and adherence, while anti- IL-17 antibodies prevented atherosclerotic lesion progression (Erbel et al., 2014). In agreement with these studies, we showed that a reduction of IL-17 caused a decrease in neutrophil and macrophage cellular influx in BALF, reinforcing the importance of IL-17 signaling in neutrophilic and macrophage inflammatory processes. This inhibition with anti-IL17 was able to protect lung tissue from the inflammatory process and reduce areas of collapse.

TABLE 1 | Absolute values of the morphometric analysis of extracellular matrix remodeling markers in lung tissue.

Remodelling markers	SAL	LPS	SAL-antiIL17	LPS-antiIL17
Collagen fibers (%)	12.35 ± 1.01	23.90 ± 2.67*	11.55 ± 0.92	9.65 ± 0.37*/**
Actin (%)	17.92 ± 1.09	27.77 ± 2.38*	18.75 ± 2.46	9.14 ± 1.91*/**
MMP-9 (cells/$10^4\mu m^2$)	2.70 ± 0.46	13.10 ± 0.80*	1.89 ± 0.38	5.88 ± 0.46*/**
MMP-12 (cells/$10^4\mu m^2$)	0.32 ± 0.06	4.00 ± 0.22*	0.32 ± 0.09	0.26 ± 0.11**
TIMP-1 (cells/$10^4\mu m^2$)	1.11 ± 0.18	8.42 ± 0.95*	1.01 ± 0.25	4.59 ± 0.52*/**
TGF-β (cells/$10^4\mu m^2$)	1.65 ± 0.23	6.24 ± 0.80*	1.66 ± 0.25	1.71 ± 0.25**

*Collagen fiber and actin are expressed as percentage and MMP-9, MMP-12, TIMP-1 and TGF-β are expressed as the number of positive cells/$10^4\mu m^2$. *$P < 0.05$, compared to the SAL and SAL-antiIL17 groups; **$P < 0.05$, compared to the LPS group.*

TABLE 2 | Absolute values of the morphometric analysis of oxidative stress markers in lung tissue.

Oxidative Stress Markers	SAL	LPS	SAL- antiIL17	LPS-antiIL17
iNOS (cells/$10^4\mu m^2$)	4.52 ± 0.47	19.60 ± 2.75*	6.23 ± 1.24	9.82 ± 1.13*/**
8-iso-PGF2α (%)	0.36 ± 0.07	2.10 ± 0.21*	0.48 ± 0.06	0.19 ± 0.02**
ARG-1 (AU)	0.87 ± 0.39	6.54 ± 1.40*	1.24 ± 0.47	0.94 ± 0.18**

*iNOS is expressed as number of positive cells/$10^4\mu m^2$. 8-iso-PGF2α is expressed as percentage and gene expression arginase-1 (ARG-1) expressed in arbitrary units (AU). *$P < 0.05$, compared to the SAL and SAL-antiIL17 groups; **$P < 0.05$, compared to the LPS group.*

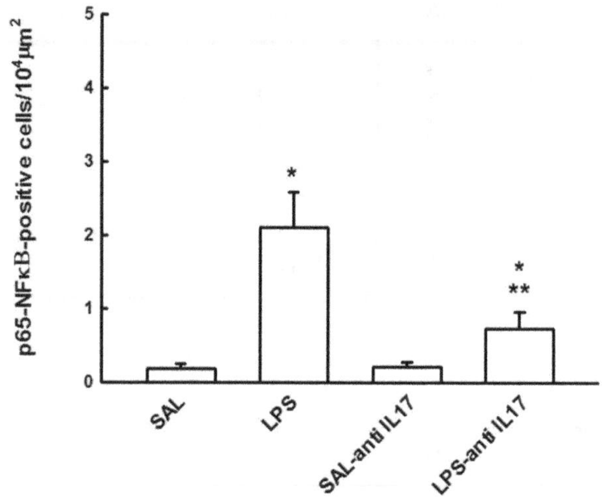

FIGURE 9 | Effects of the pretreatment with anti-IL17 on p65-NFκB-positive cells in lung tissue. *$P < 0.05$ compared to the SAL and SAL-antiIL17 groups; **$P < 0.05$ compared with LPS group.

Macrophages and neutrophils are the first line of defense and are essential for the control of common bacterial infections and provide the costimulatory and cytokine signals to promote T-cell differentiation (Witter et al., 2016). This process is essential for the differentiation process of Th17 cells and is stimulated by the activated cytokines STAT3 IL-6, IL-21 and IL-23, along with IL-1β and TGF-β (Xu and Littman, 2018). IL-6 is mainly produced by the innate immune system and is one of the first cytokines released in the acute phase of ARDS/ALI and is followed by increases in the expression of IL-1β, IL-8, TNF-α, and IL-10 (Blondonnet et al., 2016). During the initiation of Th17 cell development, IL-6 stimulates IL-21 in the early activated CD4 + T cells, thereby serving as a positive amplification loop to induce Th17 cell differentiation (Huang et al., 2012). Both IL-6 and IL-1β enhance the generation of Th17 but in contrast to this, elevated levels of TGF-β induce the differentiation of regulatory T (Treg) cells (Xu and Littman, 2018). Zhao et al. (2017) shows that Th17 inhibition with curcumin treatment was associated with a decrease in CD4 + T cell proliferation and IL-6, IL-23, IL-17A, and RORγt production. In this current study, we observed that anti-IL17 treatment inhibited Th17 cell differentiation by reducing the expression of IL-6 and TGF-β. It was demonstrated that anti-IL17 influenced both the initiation and the stabilization stages of Th17 cell differentiation.

Regarding oxidative stress, we observed a decrease in eNO, iNOS, and 8-iso-PGF2α in the lung tissue in the LPS-antiIL17 group compared to LPS group. A few studies have assessed the effects of nitric oxide synthase inhibition in modulating the inflammatory and functional responses that occur in the lung tissue (Righetti et al., 2014; Pigati et al., 2015; Camargo et al., 2018). Aristoteles et al. (2013) also found a reduction in iNOS positive cells and arginase after treatment with a specific iNOS inhibitor (1400W) and L-NAME in guinea pigs with chronic lung inflammation. Camargo et al. (2018) showed that anti-IL17 reduced iNOS-positive cells in lung tissue in a mice model of chronic allergic inflammation exacerbated induced by LPS.

It has been clearly demonstrated that iNOS activation contributes to the promotion of nitric oxide and peroxynitrite production, which leads to lipid peroxidation and 8-iso-PGF2α generation (Prado et al., 2011; Theodoro-Júnior et al., 2017). 8-iso-PGF2α generation contributes to smooth muscle contraction via tyrosine kinases and Rho/Rho-kinase, leading to the decreased activity of myosin light-chain phosphatase and increasing the level of phosphorylated myosin light chain and contraction (Righetti et al., 2014; Pigati et al., 2015). Moreover, concentrations of 8-iso-PGF2α induced a dose-dependent increase monocyte–endothelial, neutrophils recruitment and calcium release from intracellular stores (Leitinger et al., 2001). In addition, treatment of human macrophages with 8-iso-PGF2α resulted in increase in the expression of IL-8, important interleukin involved in differentiation of Th-17 and polymorphonuclear cells infiltration (Scholz et al., 2003; Gasch et al., 2014; French et al., 2018).

There have been no previous studies analyzing the effects of anti-IL17 on oxidative stress in acute lung injury, but we speculate that the reduction in macrophages, TNF-α, IL-1β,

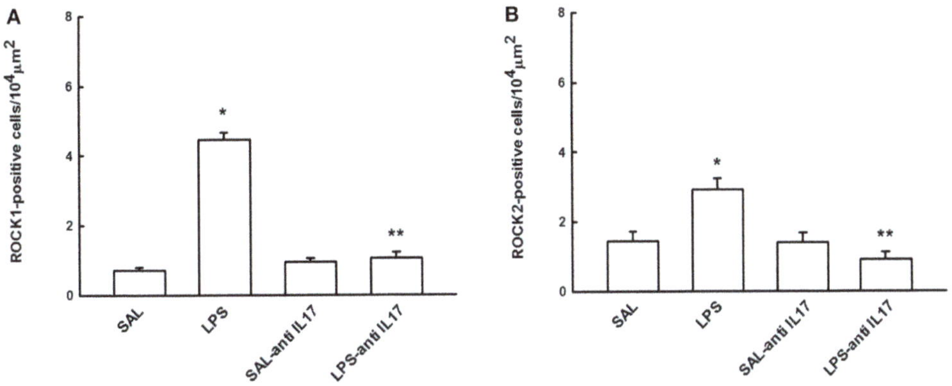

FIGURE 10 | Effects of the pretreatment with anti-IL17 on **(A)** ROCK1 and **(B)** ROCK2-positive cells in lung tissue. $^*P < 0.05$ compared to the SAL and SAL-antiIL17 groups; $^{**}P < 0.05$ compared to the LPS group.

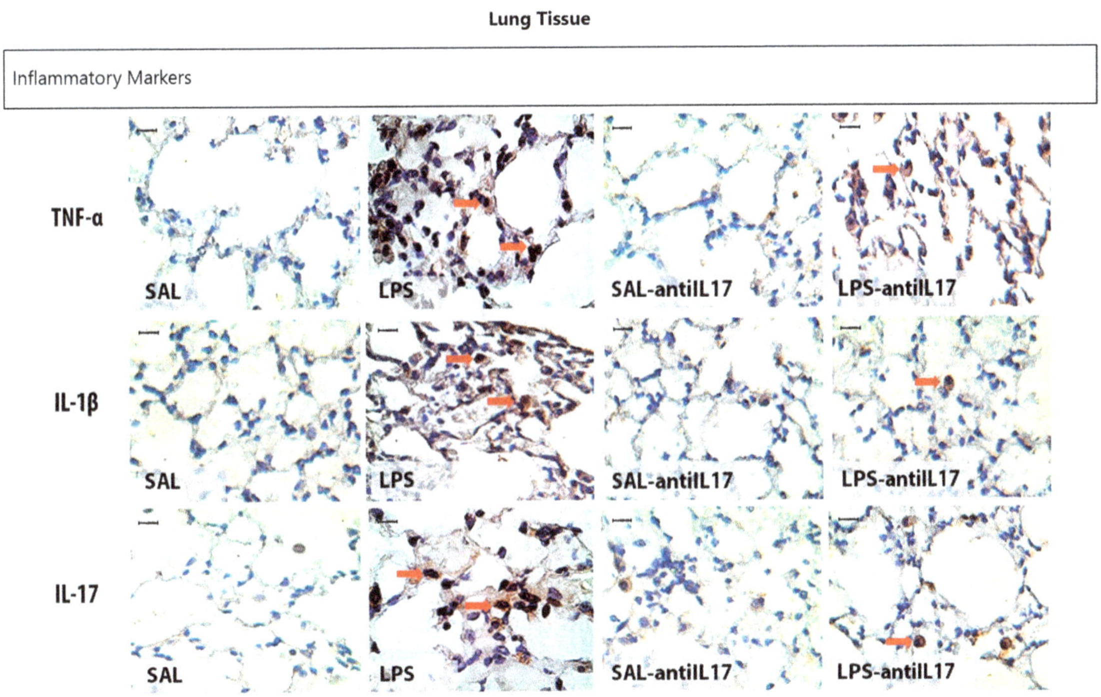

FIGURE 11 | Inflammatory markers in lung tissue: Photomicrographs of TNF-α, IL-1β and IL-17 immunohistochemical stain showing extracellular matrix inflammation in lung tissue. Magnification x1000. All experimental groups are represented: SAL, LPS, SAL-antiIL17, and LPS-antiIL17 groups. Arrow: positive cells. Scale bar = 10 µm.

and IL-17-positive cells seen in our study following IL-17 treatment could be responsible the reduction in oxidative stress, as demonstrated in other studies (Bittencourt-Mernak et al., 2017; Theodoro-Júnior et al., 2017; Camargo et al., 2018).

We assessed extracellular matrix remodeling primarily by looking at changes in volume fractions of collagen fibers, where we observed a significant reduction following anti-IL17 treatment. Acute lung inflammation is also associated with the up-regulation of MMP-9 and MMP-12, which are secretory products of activated neutrophils and macrophages (Hergrueter et al., 2011; Hsu et al., 2016). High levels of these two MMPs in BALF fluid of individuals with ALI could reflect effects of pro-inflammatory stimuli on resident alveolar macrophages and newly recruited neutrophil (Grommes and Soehnlein, 2011). In some cases, it can be directly produced by parenchymal cells in response to proinflammatory products such as bacterial LPS or immune complexes (Rosadini and Kagan, 2017). Prause et al. (2004) showed *in vivo*, that the intranasal stimulation of mice with IL-17 induced increases the concentration of biologically active MMP-9 as well as its precursor molecule in airways. In

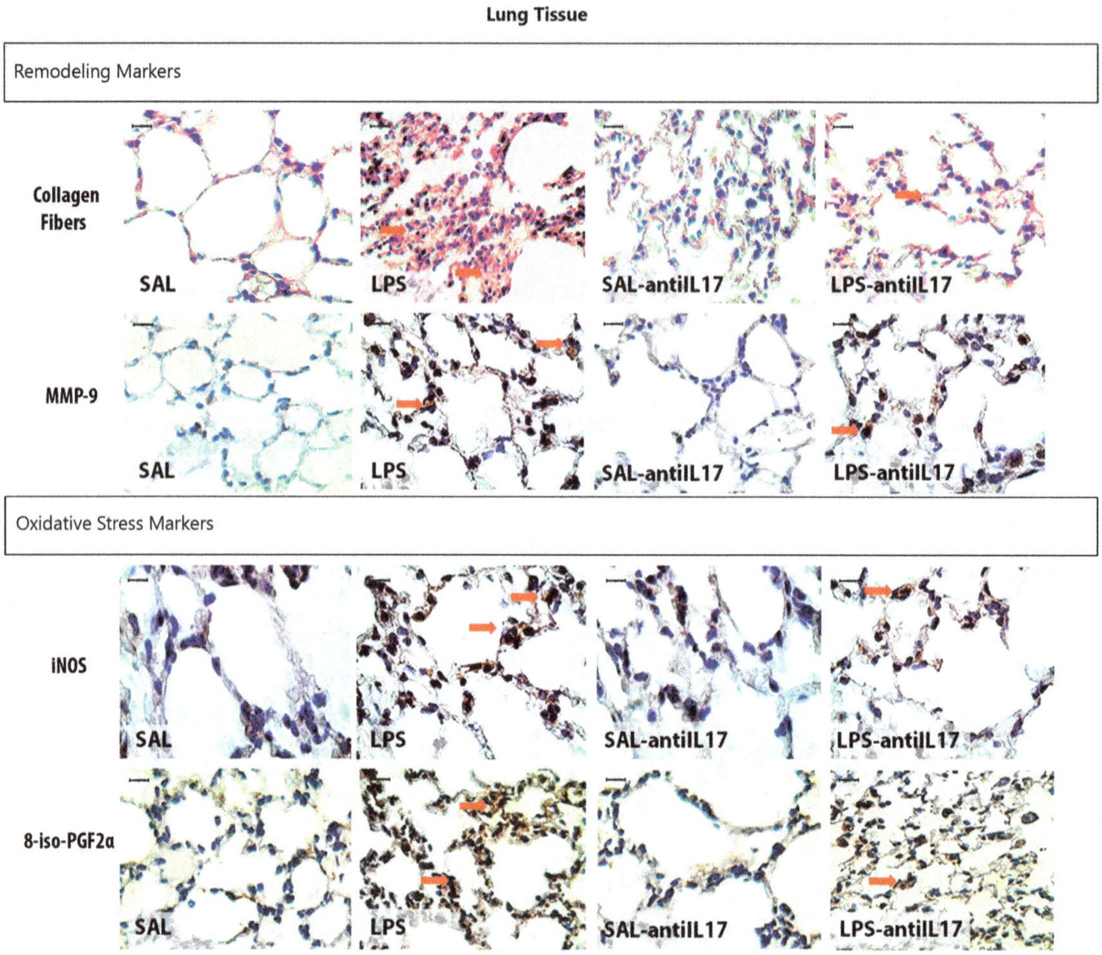

FIGURE 12 | Remodeling and oxidative stress markers in lung tissue: Photomicrographs of immunohistochemical stains showing extracellular matrix remodeling and oxidative stress in lung tissue by detecting collagen fibers, iNOS and 8-iso-PGF2α. Magnification of ×1000. All experimental groups are represented: SAL, LPS, SAL-antiIL17 and LPS-antiIL17 groups. Arrow: positive cells. Scale bar = 10 μm.

the current study, we also observed that there was augmentation of TIMP-1 in the lung parenchyma after LPS instillation. It is important to note that the specific tissue inhibitor of MMP-9, TIMP-1, has been recognized as having biologic effects independent of MMPs, such as inducing accelerate lung function decline and cellular apoptosis (Barnes, 2016; Lo et al., 2018). These results are in accordance with the idea that a process of degradation/turnover of collagen fibers in the lung parenchyma is continuously occurring, which is induced by inflammatory stimuli, as previously suggested in other studies (Righetti et al., 2014; Bittencourt-Mernak et al., 2017; Hendrix and Kheradmand, 2017). In the current study, the reduction of MMP-9, MMP-12, and TIMP-1-positive cells with anti-IL17 is associated with the reduction of the IL-17-mediated inflammatory process including the recruitment of neutrophils and macrophages.

NFκB is well characterized regulator of the expression of pro-inflammatory cytokines, including TNF-α, IL-6, and IL-1β (Li et al., 2017; Rosadini and Kagan, 2017). Li et al. (2017) showed that anti-IL17 was effectively inhibited LPS-induced expression and activation of pERK1/2 and p65-NFκB in lung tissues and suppressed nuclear translocation of p65-NFκB. Overall, our results indicated that anti-IL17 potently inhibited LPS-activated NFκB signaling in the lung tissue of ALI mice model, leading to significant suppression of inflammation and tissue injury.

Li et al. (2017) and Ding et al. (2017) evaluated the role of anti-IL-17 treatment in the activation of NFκB and inflammation in acute lung injury induced by LPS, respectively. It is important to emphasize that the our study complements the understanding of the pathophysiological process, showing the activation of signaling pathways of changes in lung functions and inflammation with the cell expression of ROCK 1, ROCK 2, CD4+, FOXP3, aspects of the extracellular matrix remodeling such as the evaluation of MMP-9, MMP-12 and TIMP-1 and cell expression as well as several markers of oxidative stress pathway activation (arginase 1, exhaled nitric oxide, iNOS and 8-iso-PGF2α).

The present study has some limitations. IL-17 was inhibited with a monoclonal antibody to IL17 in an experimental model of acute lung injury and we cannot extrapolate our findings directly to human beings. Another important point, we used a single dose of anti-IL17 prior to LPS instillation in order to clarify the role of IL-17 in the pathophysiology of acute lung injury. However, in order to determine whether anti-IL17 could be used as a potential therapeutic strategy, the treatment would need to be given following the exposure to LPS, with dosing regimens that need to be determined and including long term outcomes, such as survival. The strongly of our studies supported the importance of anti-IL-17 in the modulation of the respiratory mechanics, lung inflammatory responses, extracellular matrix remodeling, and oxidative stress pathways activation in an experimental model of acute lung injury. In addition, our results also added the importance of the control of ROCK 1, ROCK 2, and NFκB expression in these responses. Additional studies are needed to elucidate other mechanisms responsible for these changes.

CONCLUSION

In conclusion, our results show that pretreatment with anti-IL17 plays an important role in protecting the lung from the inflammatory, remodeling and oxidative stress effects of LPS-induced ALI. The effects of anti-IL17 are mainly mediated by the reduction in expression of inflammatory cytokines, neutrophils and macrophages, suggesting that anti-IL17 can modulate the inflammatory, extracellular matrix remodeling and the oxidative stress balance in ALI. This suggests that further studies using anti-IL17 in a treatment regime would be highly worthwhile.

AUTHOR CONTRIBUTIONS

IT, MM, CP, and RR conceived and designed the experiments. EL, MC, BS-R, MA-V, RR, SF, FdS, FS, MA, IG, CP, TS, LC, and LA performed the experiments. RR, MC, CP, IG, EL, and IT analyzed the data. RR, IT, MM, EL, and MA-V contributed reagents, materials, analysis tools. IT and RR wrote the paper. IG assisted in the execution of the experiments involved in the responses to the reviewers. FS, SF, and MC performed the experiments.

ACKNOWLEDGMENTS

We thank Fundação de Amparo à Pesquisa do Estado de São Paulo (FAPESP) (number: 2013/17944-1) for the financial support.

REFERENCES

Abraham, E. (2003). Neutrophils and acute lung injury. *Crit. Care Med.* 31, S195–S199. doi: 10.1097/01.CCM.0000057843.47705.E8

Aristoteles, L. R. Righetti, R. F., Pinheiro, N. M., Franco, R. B., Starling, C. M., Silva, J. C. P., et al. (2013). Modulation of the oscillatory mechanics of lung tissue and the oxidative stress response induced by arginase inhibition in a chronic allergic inflammation model. *BMC Pulm. Med.* 13:52. doi: 10.1186/1471-2466-13-52

Barlow, J. L., Flynn, R. J., Ballantyne, S. J., and McKenzie, A. N. (2011). Reciprocal expression of IL-25 and IL-17A is important for allergic airways hyperreactivity. *Clin. Exp. Allergy* 41, 1447–1455. doi: 10.1111/j.1365-2222.2011.03806.x

Barnes, P. J. (2016). Inflammatory mechanisms in patients with chronic obstructive pulmonary disease. *J. Allergy Clin. Immunol.* 138, 16–27. doi: 10.1016/j.jaci.2016.05.011

Barreto do Carmo, M. B., Righetti, R. F., Tibério, I. F., and Hunziker, M. H. (2016). The effects of prenatal "psychological" stressor exposure on lung inflammation and hyperresponsiveness in adult rat offspring. *Dev. Psychobiol.* 58, 1076–1086. doi: 10.1002/dev.21441

Bittencourt-Mernak, M. I., Pinheiro, N. M., Santana, F. P., Guerreiro, M. P., Saraiva-Romanholo, B. M., Grecco, S. S., et al. (2017). Prophylactic and therapeutic treatment with flavonone sakuranetin ameliorates LPS-induced acute lung injury. *Am. J. Physiol. Lung Cell Mol. Physiol.* 312, L217–L230. doi: 10.1152/ajplung.00444.2015

Blondonnet, R., Constantin, J. M., Sapin, V., and Jabaudon, M. (2016). A pathophysiologic approach to biomarkers in acute respiratory distress syndrome. *Dis. Markers* 2016:3501373. doi: 10.1155/2016/3501373

Boshier, P. R., Hanna, G. B., and Marczin, N. (2013). Exhaled nitric oxide as biomarker of acute lung injury: an unfulfilled promise? *J. Breath Res.* 7:017118. doi: 10.1088/1752-7155/7/1/017118

Camargo, L. D. N., Righetti, R. F., Aristóteles, L. R. C. R.B., Dos Santos, T. M., de Souza, F. C. R., Fukuzaki, S. A., et al. (2018). Effects of Anti-IL-17 on inflammation, remodeling, and oxidative stress in an experimental model of asthma exacerbated by LPS. *Front. Immunol.* 8:1835. doi: 10.3389/fimmu.2017.01835

Castillo, R. L., Carrasco Loza, R., and Romero-Dapueto, C. (2015). Pathophysiological approaches of acute respiratory distress syndrome: novel bases for study of lung injury. *Open Respir. Med. J.* 9, 83–91. doi: 10.2174/1874306401509010083

Caucheteux, S. M., Hu-Li, J., Mohammed, R. N., Ager, A., and Paul, W. E. (2017). Cytokine regulation of lung Th17 response to airway immunization using LPS adjuvant. *Mucosal. Immunol.* 10, 361–372. doi: 10.1038/mi.2016.54

Defert, O., and Boland, S. (2017). Rho kinase inhibitors: a patent review (2014 - 2016). *Expert Opin. Ther. Pat.* 27, 507–515. doi: 10.1080/13543776.2017.1272579

Ding, Q., Liu, G. Q., Zeng, Y. Y., Zhu, J. J., Liu, Z. Y., Zhang, X., et al. (2017). Role of IL-17 in LPS-induced acute lung injury: an *in vivo* study. *Oncotarget* 8, 93704–93711. doi: 10.18632/oncotarget.21474

Elfsmark, L., Ågren, L., Akfur, C., Bucht, A.,and Jonasson, S. (2018). 8-Isoprostane is an early biomarker for oxidative stress in chlorine-induced acute lung injury. *Toxicol. Lett.* 282, 1–7. doi: 10.1016/j.toxlet.2017.10.007

Erbel, C., Akhavanpoor, M., Okuyucu, D., Wangler, S., Dietz, A., Zhao, L., et al. (2014). IL-17A influences essential functions ofthe monocyte/macrophage lineage andis involved in advanced murine and human atherosclerosis. *J. Immunol.* 193, 4344–455. doi: 10.4049/jimmunol.1400181

French, B. M., Sendil, S., Sepuru, K. M., Ranek, J., Burdorf, L., Harris, D., et al. (2018). Interleukin-8 mediates neutrophil-endothelial interactions in pig-to-human xenogeneic models. *Xenotransplantation* 25:e12385. doi: 10.1111/xen.12385

Gasch, M., Goroll, T., Bauer, M., Hinz, D., Schütze, N., Polte, T., et al. (2014). Generation of IL-8 and IL9 producing CD4? T cells is affected by Th17 polarizing conditions and AHR ligands. *Mediators Inflamm.* 2014:182549. doi: 10.1155/2014/182549

Ge, S., Hertel, B., Susnik, N., Rong, S., Dittrich, A. M., Schmitt, R., et al. (2014). Interleukin 17 receptor A modulates monocyte subsets and macrophage generation *in vivo*. *PLoS ONE* 15:e85461. doi: 10.1371/journal.pone.0085461

Ghoreschi, K., Laurence, A., Yang, X. P., Tato, C. M., McGeachy, M. J., Konkel, J. E., et al. (2010). J. Generation of pathogenic T(H)17 cells in the absence of TGF-β signalling. *Nature* 467, 967–971. doi: 10.1038/nature09447

Gonçalves-de-Albuquerque, S. D. C., Pessoa-E-Silva, R., Trajano-Silva, L. A. M., de Goes, T. C., de Morais, R. C. S., Oliveira, C. N., et al. (2017). The Equivocal Role of Th17 Cells and Neutrophils on Immunopathogenesis of Leishmaniasis. *Front. Immunol.* 8:1437. doi: 10.3389/fimmu.2017.01437

González-López, A., and Albaiceta, G. (2012). M. Repair after acute lung injury: molecular mechanisms and therapeutic opportunities. *Crit. Care.* 16:209. doi: 10.1186/cc11224

Grommes, J., and Soehnlein, O. (2011). Contribution of neutrophils to acute lung injury. *Mol Med.* 17, 293–307. doi: 10.2119/molmed.2010.00138

Hasegawa, T., Uga, H., Mori, A., and Kurata, H. (2017). Increased serum IL-17A and Th2 cytokine levels in patients with severe uncontrolled asthma. *Eur. Cytokine Netw.* 28, 8–18. doi: 10.1684/ecn.2017.0390

Hendrix, A. Y., and Kheradmand, F. (2017). The Role of Matrix metalloproteinases in development, repair, and destruction of the lungs. *Prog. Mol. Biol. Transl. Sci.* 148, 1–29. doi: 10.1016/bs.pmbts.2017.04.004

Hergrueter, A. H., Nguyen, K., and Owen, C. (2011). A.Matrix metalloproteinases: all the RAGE in the acute respiratory distress syndrome. *Am. J. Physiol. Lung Cell Mol. Physiol.* 300, L512–515. doi: 10.1152/ajplung.00023.2011

Hsu, D., Taylor, P., Fletcher, D., van Heeckeren, R., Eastman, J., van Heeckeren, A., et al. (2016). Interleukin-17 Pathophysiology and Therapeutic intervention in cystic fibrosis lung infectionand inflammation. *Infect. Immun.* 84, 2410–2421. doi: 10.1128/IAI.00284-16

Huang, G., Wang, Y., and Chi, H. (2012). Regulation of TH17 cell differentiation by innate immune signals. *Cell Mol. Immunol.* 9, 287–295. doi: 10.1038/cmi.2012.10

Kaneko-Kawano, T., Takasu, F., Naoki, H., Sakumura, Y., Ishii, S., Ueba, T., et al. (2012). Dynamic regulation of myosin light chain phosphorylation by Rho-kinase. *PLoS ONE* 7:e39269. doi: 10.1371/journal.pone.0039269

Lanças, T., Kasahara, D. I., Prado, C. M., Tibério, I. F., Martins, M. A., and Dolhnikoff, M. (2006). Comparison of early and late responses to antigen of sensitized guinea pig parenchymal lung strips. *J. Appl. Physiol.* 100, 1610–1616. doi: 10.1152/japplphysiol.00828.2005

Leitinger, N., Huber, J., Rizza, C., Mechtcheriakova, D., Bochkov, V., Koshelnick, Y., et al. (2001). The isoprostane 8-iso PGF(2alpha) stimulates endothelial cells to bind monocytes: differencesfrom thromboxane-mediated endothelial activation. *FASEB J.* 15, 1254–126. doi: 10.1096/fj.00-0498fje

Ley, K., Laudanna, C., Cybulsky, M. I., and Nourshargh, S. (2007). Getting to the site of inflammation: the leukocyte adhesion cascade updated. *Nat. Rev. Immunol.* 7, 678–689. doi: 10.1038/nri2156

Li, T. J., Zhao, L. L., Qiu, J., Zhang, H. Y., Bai, G. X., and Chen, L. (2017). Interleukin-17 antagonist attenuates lung inflammation through inhibition of the ERK1/2 and NF-κB pathway in LPS-induced acute lung injury. *Mol. Med. Rep.* 16, 2225–2232. doi: 10.3892/mmr.2017.6837

Lo, C. Y., Huang, H. Y., He, J. R., Huang, T. T., Heh, C. C., Sheng, T. F., et al. (2018). Increased matrix metalloproteinase-9 to tissue inhibitor of metalloproteinase-1 ratio in smokers with airway hyperresponsiveness and accelerated lung function decline. *Int. J. Chron. Obstruct. Pulmon. Dis.* 13, 1135–1144. doi: 10.2147/COPD.S161257

Martins-Olivera, B. T., Almeida-Reis, R., Theodoro-Júnior, O. A., Oliva, L. V., Neto Dos Santos Nunes, N., Olivo, C. R., et al. (2016). The Plant-Derived Bauhinia bauhinioides Kallikrein Proteinase Inhibitor (rBbKI) attenuates elastase-induced emphysema in mice. *Mediators Inflamm.* 2016:5346574. doi: 10.1155/2016/5346574

Mikacenic, C., Hansen, E. E., Radella, F., Gharib, S. A., Stapleton, R. D., and Wurfel, M. (2016). M. Interleukin-17A is associated with alveolar inflammation and poor outcomes in acute respiratory distress syndrome. *Crit. Care Med.* 44, 496–502. doi: 10.1097/CCM.0000000000001409

Modrykamien, A. M., and Gupta, P. (2015). The acute respiratory distress syndrome. *Proc. Bayl. Univ. Med. Cent.* 28, 163–171. doi: 10.1080/08998280.2015.11929219

National Institutes of Health. (2011). *Guide for the Care and Use of Laboratory Animals, 8th Edn.* Whasington, DC: The National Academy of Science Press.

Nguyen, H., Chiasson, V. L., Chatterjee, P., Kopriva, S. E., Young, K. J., and Mitchell, B. M. (2013). Interleukin-17 causes Rho-kinase-mediated endothelial dysfunction and hypertension. *Cardiovasc. Res.* 97, 696–704. doi: 10.1093/cvr/cvs422

O'Dwyer, D. N., Ashley, S. L., and Moore, B. B. (2016). Influences of innate immunity, autophagy, and fibroblast activation in the pathogenesis of lungfibrosis. *Am. J. Physiol. Lung Cell Mol. Physiol.* 311, L590–L601. doi: 10.1152/ajplung.00221.2016

Pigati, P. A., Righetti, R. F., Possa, S. S., Romanholo, B. S., Rodrigues, A. P., dos Santos, A. S., et al. (2015). 2763 Y-2 is associated with corticosteroid-potentiated control of pulmonary remodeling and inflammation in guinea pigs with chronic allergic inflammation. *BMC Pulm. Med.* 15:85. doi: 10.1186/s12890-015-0073-4

Pinheiro, N. M., Miranda, C. J., Perini, A., Câmara, N. O., Costa, S. K., Alonso-Vale, M. I., et al. (2015). Pulmonary inflammation is regulated by the levels of the vesicular acetylcholine transporter. *PLoS ONE* 27:e0120441. doi: 10.1371/journal.pone.0120441

Possa, S. S., Charafeddine, H. T., Righetti, R. F., da Silva, P. A., Almeida-Reis, R., Saraiva-Romanholo, B. M., et al. (2012). Rho-kinase inhibition attenuates airway responsiveness, inflammation, matrix remodeling, and oxidative stress activation induced by chronic inflammation. *Am. J. Physiol. Lung Cell Mol. Physiol.* 303, L939–L952. doi: 10.1152/ajplung.00034.2012

Prado, C. M., Leick-Maldonado, E. A., Yano, L., Leme, A. S., Capelozzi, V. L., Martins, M. A., et al. (2006). Effects of nitric oxide synthases in chronic allergic airway inflammation and remodeling. *Am. J. Respir. Cell Mol. Biol.* 35, 457–465. doi: 10.1165/rcmb.2005-0391OC

Prado, C. M., Martins, M. A., and Tibério, I. F. L. C. (2011). Nitric Oxide in Asthma Physiopathology. *ISRN Allerg.* 2011:832560. doi: 10.5402/2011/832560

Prause, O., Bozinovski, S., Anderson, G. P., and Lindên, A. (2004). Increased matrix metalloproteinase-9 concentration and activity after stimulation with interleukin-17 in mouse airways. *Thorax* 59, 313–317.

Righetti, R. F., Pigati, P. A., Possa, S. S., Habrum, F. C., Xisto, D. G., Antunes, M. A., et al. (2014). Effects of Rho-kinase inhibition in lung tissue with chronic inflammation. *Respir. Physiol. Neurobiol.* 192, 134–146. doi: 10.1016/j.resp.2013.12.012

Riva, D. R., Oliveira, M. B., Rzezinski, A. F., Rangel, G., Capelozzi, V. L., Zin, W. A., et al. (2008). Recruitment maneuver in pulmonary andextrapulmonary experimental acute lung injury. *Crit. Care Med.* 36, 1900–1908. doi: 10.1097/CCM.0b013e3181760e5d

Rosadini, C. V., and Kagan, J. C. (2017). Early innate immune responses to bacterial LPS. *Curr. Opin. Immunol.* 44, 14–19. doi: 10.1016/j.coi.2016.10.005

Saddy, F., Oliveira, G. P., Garcia, C. S., Nardelli, L. M., Rzezinski, A. F., Ornellas, D. S., et al. (2010). Assisted ventilation modes reduce the expression of lung inflammatory and fibrogenic mediators in a model of mild acute lung injury. *Intensive Care Med.* 36, 1417–1426. doi: 10.1007/s00134-010-1808-6

Sakaguchi, R., Chikuma, S., Shichita, T., Morita, R., Sekiya, T., Ouyang, W., et al. (2016). Innate-like function of memory Th17 cells for enhancing endotoxin-induced acute lung inflammation through IL-22. *Int. Immunol.* 28, 233–243. doi: 10.1093/intimm/dxv070

Scholz, H., Yndestad, A., Damås, J. K., Waehre, T., Tonstad, S., Aukrust, P., et al. (2003). 8-isoprostane increases expression of interleukin-8 in human macrophages through activation of mitogenactivated protein kinases. *Cardiovasc. Res.* 59, 945–954. doi: 10.1016/S0008-6363(03)00538-8

Sharanek, A., Burban, A., Burbank, M., Le Guevel, R., Li, R., Guillouzo, A., et al. (2016). Rho-kinase/myosin light chain kinase pathway plays a key role in the impairment of bilecanaliculi dynamics induced by cholestatic drugs. *Sci. Rep.* 6:24709. doi: 10.1038/srep24709

Theodoro-Júnior, O. A., Righetti, R. F., Almeida-Reis, R., Martins-Oliveira, B. T., Oliva, L. V., Prado, C. M., et al. (2017). A plant proteinase inhibitor from enterolobium contortisiliquum attenuates pulmonary mechanics, inflammation and remodeling induced by elastase in mice. *Int. J. Mol. Sci.* 18:403. doi: 10.3390/ijms18020403

Vieira, R. P., Claudino, R. C., Duarte, A. C., Santos, A. B., Perini, A., Faria Neto, H. C., et al. (2007). Aerobic exercise decreases chronic allergic lung inflammation and airway remodeling in mice. *Am. J. Respir. Crit. Care Med.* 176, 1–7. doi: 10.1164/rccm.200610-1567OC

Villegas, L., Stidham, T., and Nozik-Grayck, E. (2014). Oxidative stress and therapeutic development in lung diseases. *J. Pulm. Respir. Med.* 4:194. doi: 10.4172/2161-105X.1000194

Weibel, E. R. (1963). Principles and methods for the morphometric study of the lungand other organs. *Lab. Investig.* 12, 131–155.

Weibel, E. R. (1979). Fleischner lecture. looking into the lung: what can it tell us? *AJR Am. J. Roentgenol.* 133, 1021–1031. doi: 10.2214/ajr.133.6.1021

Witter, A. R., Okunnu, B. M., and Berg, R. E. (2016). The essential role of neutrophils during infection with the intracellular bacterial pathogenlisteria monocytogenes. *J. Immunol.* 197, 1557–165. doi: 10.4049/jimmunol.1600599

Xu, H., and Littman, D. R. (2018). New traffic light on Th17 Avenue. *Cell Res.* 28, 139–140. doi: 10.1038/cr.2017.156

Yanagisawa, H., Hashimoto, M., Minagawa, S., Takasaka, N., Ma, R., Moermans, C., et al. (2017). Role of IL-17A in murine models of COPD airway disease. *Am. J. Physiol. Lung Cell Mol. Physiol.* 312, L122–L130. doi: 10.1152/ajplung.00301.2016

Zhao, G., Liu, Y., Yi, X., Wang, Y., Qiao, S., Li, Z., et al. (2017). Curcumin inhibiting Th17 cell differentiation by regulating the metabotropic glutamate receptor-4 expression on dendritic cells. *Int. Immunopharmacol.* 46, 80–86. doi: 10.1016/j.intimp.2017.02.017

Zizzo, G., and Cohen, P. L. (2013). IL-17 stimulates differentiation of human anti-inflammatory macrophages and phagocytosis of apoptotic neutrophils in response to IL-10 and glucocorticoids. *J. Immunol.* 190, 5237–5246. doi: 10.4049/jimmunol.1203017

19

Inflammatory Caspases Drive Pyroptosis in Acute Lung Injury

*Bohao Liu, Ruyuan He, Lin Zhang, Bo Hao, Wenyang Jiang, Wei Wang and Qing Geng**

Department of Thoracic Surgery, Renmin Hospital of Wuhan University, Wuhan, China

***Correspondence:**
Qing Geng
gengqingwhu@whu.edu.cn

Acute lung injury (ALI), a critical respiratory disorder that causes diffuse alveolar injury leads to high mortality rates with no effective treatment. ALI is characterized by varying degrees of ventilation/perfusion mismatch, severe hypoxemia, and poor pulmonary compliance. The diffuse injury to cells is one of most important pathological characteristics of ALI. Pyroptosis is a form of programmed cell death distinguished from apoptosis induced by inflammatory caspases, which can release inflammatory cytokines to clear cells infected by pathogens and promote monocytes to reassemble at the site of injury. And pyroptosis not only promotes inflammation in certain cell types, but also regulates many downstream pathways to perform different functions. There is increasing evidence that pyroptosis and its related inflammatory caspases play an important role in the development of acute lung injury. The main modes of activation of pyroptosis is not consistent among different types of cells in lung tissue. Meanwhile, inhibition of inflammasome, the key to initiating pyroptosis is currently the main way to treat acute lung injury. The review summarizes the relationship among inflammatory caspases, pyroptosis and acute lung injury and provides general directions and strategies to conduct further research.

Keywords: pyroptosis, acute lung injury, caspase, inflammasome, NLRP 3

INTRODUCTION

Acute lung injury (ALI) is a life-threatening illness syndrome in intensive care units, which often is the main cause of acute respiratory distress syndrome (ARDS) (Butt et al., 2016). ALI/ARDS is characterized by severe inflammatory processes leading to diffuse alveolar injury, varying degrees of ventilation/perfusion divergence, poor pulmonary compliance and severe hypoxemia (Matthay et al., 2012). Pulmonary edema, increased alveolar permeability, leukocyte aggregation, epithelial injury and diffuse alveolar damage are typical pathological changes of ALI (Ware, 2006). There are many precipitating factors of ALI, such as severe shock, infection, mechanical injury, etc. (Kox et al., 2011; Kao et al., 2014) Over the years, a great number of articles have revealed that gram-negative bacterial infection is one of the most important factors leading to lung injury (Aujla et al., 2008). LPS, the major component of outer membranes of gram-negative bacteria, plays a key role in the process of inducing inflammatory response and leads to lung injury. That is why LPS has gradually become a major implement for inducing acute lung injury (Burgos et al., 2019) Lately, there has been improved interest in the relationship between the inflammatory response induced by LPS and pyroptosis (Zhao et al., 2018; Qiu et al., 2019; Muendlein et al., 2020). In consequence, elucidating the correlation between acute lung injury and pyroptosis may be helpful to find a more efficient way to treat acute lung injury from the etiology.

Caspases are a family of proteolytic enzymes that induce and transmit signals leading to cell death. They can be divided into apoptotic caspases (caspase-8, 9, 10, 3, 6, and 7) for inducing apoptosis and inflammatory caspases (caspase-1, 4, 5, and 11) for mediating pyroptosis (Ramirez and Salvesen, 2018). Caspase-1, formerly named interleukin-1b converting enzyme (ICE), initiates inflammation by affecting the maturation of pre-interleukins. The closest sequence identity is exhibited between caspase-1 and other members of inflammatory caspases including caspase-4, 5 and 11 (Black et al., 1989). Both caspase-1 mediating canonical pathway and caspase-4/11 or caspase-5 mediating non-canonical pathway can induce the occurrence of pyroptosis by using Gasdermin D (GSDMD) as the direct substrate (Man et al., 2017b). This review aims to elucidate the relationship among inflammatory caspases, pyroptosis and acute lung injury and to provide the latest research progress on the underlying mechanisms.

THE FUNCTION OF CASPASES IN PYROPTOSIS

Pyroptosis is a form of programmed necrosis distinguished from apoptosis. Pyroptosis, which occurs in many types of cells in the body, is triggered for releasing inflammatory cytokines that clear cells infected by pathogen, prompting monocytes to reassemble at the site of injury (Ramirez and Salvesen, 2018). Pyroptotic cells are characterized by swollen cells with many vesicular protrusions, followed by the rupture of the cytoplasmic membrane and the flow of cytoplasmic content out of the cells. It is different from apoptosis in which cytoplasm membrane remains intact and apoptotic bodies are formed (Sangiuliano et al., 2014). Dependence on caspase-1 has long been an essential feature of pyroptosis (Bergsbaken et al., 2009). In recent years, the function of other inflammatory caspases and GSDMD, the key substrate and the direct executioner of pyroptosis, have been discovered to shed light on the mechanism of pyroptosis (Kayagaki et al., 2011; Baker et al., 2015; Pandeya et al., 2019; Xia, 2020).

Caspase-1-dependent Pathway

Inflammatory caspases are referred to as the caspase-1 subfamily before. As mentioned above, caspase-1 was originally cloned for hunting an enzyme that acts on the proteolytic and mature of the pro-inflammatory cytokine IL-1β in human monocytes (Lamkanfi and Dixit, 2014). Different from some apoptotic caspases, caspase-1 contains a caspase recruitment domain (CARD) at the N-terminal end as well as a catalytic domain whose structure is very similar to that of the apoptotic promoter caspase-9 (McIlwain et al., 2013; Van Opdenbosch and Lamkanfi, 2019). The specific domain makes procaspase-1 form a dimer and be activated by pattern-recognition receptors (PRRs), when bacteria or viruses invade the body. Caspase-1 which is locked in the active form, directly cuts its substrate GSDMD (Shi et al., 2017). And the released N domain of GSDMD combines with phosphatidylinositol in plasma membrane to form membrane pore (Shi et al., 2017). The formation of membrane pores destroys the integrity of the cell membrane and the osmotic potential of the cell, so that water molecules enter the cell, causing swelling of the cell membrane, rupture of the cell membrane, and formation of balloon-like vesicles around the nucleus, accompanied by chromatin condensation and DNA fragmentation (Man et al., 2017a). Eventually the cells undergo osmotic lysis and the release of their contents leads to inflammatory cascades that are toxic to adjacent healthy cells and the entire organism (Wang et al., 2020; Xia, 2020). Meanwhile, caspase-1 cleaves the pro-inflammatory cytokines pro-IL-1β and pro-IL-18 that promotes the formation of mature IL-1β and IL-18, which can be released from pores with the cytoplasmic content (McIlwain et al., 2013; Winkler and Rösen-Wolff, 2015).

PRRs triggered by pathogen-associated molecular patterns (PAMPs) or danger-associated molecular patterns (DAMPs) is the starting point for activating caspase -1. PRRs can be divided into two categories according to the location of the subcell (Lamkanfi and Dixit, 2014). C-type lectin receptors (CLR) and Toll-like receptors (TLRs) present on cell membranes to detect extracellular stimuli, while the nucleotide-binding domain and leucine-rich repeat-containing (NLR) proteins, the AIM2-like receptor (ALR), and RIG-I-like receptor (RLR) are present inside the cell and stimulated by PAMPs or DAMPs (Lamkanfi and Dixit, 2014).

The canonical inflammasomes that participate in caspase-1-dependent pathway are principally composed of apoptosis-associated speck-like protein (ASCs), PAMPs and DAMPs receptors such as ALRs and NLRs, and procaspase-1 (Malik and Kanneganti, 2017). Inducing activation of caspase-1 is the most important function of the canonical inflammasome during pyroptosis. ASC containing a caspase-activation and recruitment domain (CARD) is recruited to form a polymer complex called "SPECK" by NLRs or ALRs which is considered as an indication of inflammasome assembly when a particular stimulus is detected (Kesavardhana and Kanneganti, 2017; Malik and Kanneganti, 2017). The common feature of NLR family members is that they contain a central nucleotide binding domain (NBD), whereas this family is further separated into NLR family pyrin domain-containing protein (NLRP) or NLR family CARD-containing protein (NLRC) receptors due to the differences in the N-terminal PYD domain (PYD) or CARD (Malik and Kanneganti, 2017). NLRP1, NLRP3 and NLRC4 have been widely studied to induce the formation of inflammasome and participate in the activation of caspase-1. Based on the lack of CARD structure, NLRP3 must rely on ASC with both pyrin and CARD as a bridge to recruit procaspase-1, while NLRP1 and NLRC4 are not (He et al., 2016b). The inflammasome directly involved in caspase-1 activation and pyroptosis has another name: pyroptosome. Unfortunately, the activation mechanisms and exact ligands of many inflammasomes are still not fully understood and are worth exploring.

Caspase-1-independent Pathway

Caspase-1-independent pathway, named as non-canonical pyroptosis pathway, is induced by other members of inflammatory caspases including caspase-4, 5, and 11. Caspase-4/5/11, like caspase-1, structurally contains a CARD domain at the N-terminal end. Differently, human caspase-4 and 5 or their murine orthologs caspase-11 is directly stimulated by the cytoplasmic endotoxin of gram-negative bacteria, which directly lyses the substrate and leads to the occurrence of pyroptosis. Activation of non-canonical inflammasomes is required in caspase-1-independent pathway. The non-canonical inflammasome is assembled by direct interaction between procaspase-4/5/11 and the lipid A tail of LPS (Yi, 2017).

Caspase-11, which is specific to mice, is often used as a primary target for non-canonical pyroptosis pathway. Activated caspase-11 can not only induce the formation of cell membrane pores through the cleavage of GSDMD, but also promote K^+ efflux via pannexin-1/ATP/P2X7 pathway, promote the maturation and release of IL-1β, and induce the reaction of intracellular inflammatory response (Oh et al., 2020). The N-terminal produced by cleavage from GSDMD has another function for promoting the proteolytic activation of caspase-1 (Wang et al., 1998; Kayagaki et al., 2011). Thus, caspase-11 is also regarded as an upstream regulator of caspase-1 activation (Shalini et al., 2015).

Caspase-4 and caspase-5 play an important role in the caspase-1-independent pyroptosis pathway in humans. Studies have shown that caspase-4 is directly involved in the detection of LPS, while caspase-5 has no detectable role in identifying these pathogens which can be specifically regulated by IFN–γ and LPS (Lin et al., 2000; Matikainen et al., 2020). Caspase-4 promotes its own activation through direct interaction with LPS and exhibits a higher affinity with tetra-acylated LPS, showing a wider range of specificity than caspase-11 (Matikainen et al., 2020; Oh et al., 2020). However, many mechanisms of caspase-4/5/11 *in vitro* and *in vivo* remain unclear.

Other Pathway

It has been reported that caspase-3, as a key regulator of apoptosis, can also be involved in the mediation of pyroptosis. As we all know, caspase-3 is at the end of caspase cascades during the regulation of apoptosis and can be cleaved and activated by caspase-9, while caspase-3 appears as an upstream regulator in pyroptosis (Rogers et al., 2017; Frank and Vince, 2019). After induction with TNF-α or chemotherapeutic agents, GSDME, initially named as DFNA5 (Deafness Autosomal Dominant 5), is directly cleaved by caspase-3 specifically to produce the GSDME-N fragment (Wang et al., 2017a; Rogers et al., 2017). The fragment performs the same function as the activated GSDMD, penetrates the cell membrane and mediates pyroptosis (Wang et al., 2017a). Recent studies have shown that ATP induces caspase-3-induced pyroptosis after NLRP3 is blocked (Wang et al., 2017a). This pathway therefore seems to be understood as an alternative mechanism for pyroptosis. The exact mechanism of this pathway remains largely unknown.

THE ROLE OF INFLAMMATORY CASPASES AND PYROPTOSIS IN ALI

Inflammatory caspases have been proved to produce a marked effect in inducing inflammatory response in cardiovascular disease, brain injury, liver injury and kidney injury (Irrera et al., 2020; Shojaie et al., 2020). And inflammasomes are non-substitutable in the process of pyroptosis caused by inflammatory caspases in acute lung injury. Moreover, a lot of research revealed that the inducing factors and manifestations of pyroptosis are slightly dissimilar in different types of cells, including macrophages, neutrophils, and endothelial cells.

Pyroptosis in Macrophages

Macrophages are essential for natural immunity and host defense and play an important role in the lungs and the alveolar cavity. The differentiation, phenotype, function and cell-cell interaction of macrophages are indispensable in the initiation and resolution of pulmonary inflammation (Aggarwal et al., 2014). A growing body of research suggests that alveolar macrophages (AMs) have a profound impact on the development and prognosis of acute lung injury by releasing inflammatory cytokines and regulating other immune cells (Tang et al., 2017; Hung et al., 2018; Kojima et al., 2018) (**Figure 1**).

After activation of the inflammatory corpuscular pathway in pyroptosis, two lyzed subunits called p10 and p20 originate from processed procaspase-1, which is the main inducement factor of the release of IL-1β and IL-18 into the extracellular environment (Miao et al., 2011). A study has shown that p10 in the AMs activated by caspase-1 of the mice successfully induced ALI/ARDS was markedly increased after being processed by LPS, while the caspase-1 inhibitor Ac-YVAD-CMK could restrain this phenomenon (Wu et al., 2015). The authors found that NLRP3 and ASC were highly expressed following LPS through Western Blotting and immunofluorescence. In conclusion, alveolar macrophage pyroptosis may be involved in the development of acute lung injury and NLRP3/ASC inflammasomes participate in the process (Wu et al., 2015).

Moreover, the study of Lei Hou et al. indicated that NLRP3/ASC-mediated AM pyroptosis induced High-mobility group box 1 (HMGB1) secretion from AM in ALI (Hou et al., 2018). HMGB1 as one of DAMPs can promote the activation of NLRP3 and the activation of caspase-1, thus feedback positive to augment AM pyroptosis, aggravate the inflammatory response and cause the worsening of ALI (Qu et al., 2019). The study showed that knockdown of ASC or inhibiting the function of NLRP3 inflammasome can mitigate the AM pyroptosis and reduce HMGB1 release, leading to decrease the inflammation in the ALI (Hou et al., 2018). However, the secretion of HMGB1 from macrophage is seemingly independent of ASC, but dependent on NLRP4 or NLRP1b and caspase-1 (Lamkanfi et al., 2010; Van Opdenbosch et al., 2014). In addition, a study from Dandan Li et al. showed that p38-MAPK inhibitor SB203580 reverses the LPS-induced expression of caspase-1 and NLRP3 in AM. The blockage of p38-MAPK signaling pathway can reduce the expression level of pro-inflammatory cytokines and the assembling of NLRP3 inflammasomes from the lung tissues of inflammatory mice (Li et al., 2018). The authors concluded that p38-MAPK may participate in the promotion of ALI and lung inflammation through regulation of the NLRP3 inflammasome and AM pyroptosis. Double-stranded RNA-dependent kinase (PKR) has been shown in another study to

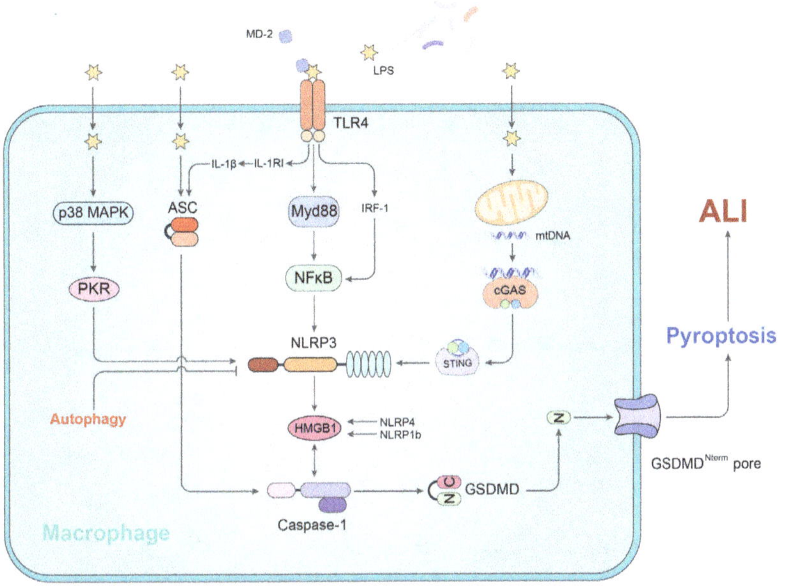

FIGURE 1 | The mechanism of pyroptosis affecting alveolar macrophages in ALI. In AMs, LPS promotes the activation of caspase-1 by regulating MD2, ASC, and NLRP3, leading to pyroptosis. P38/MAPK and TLR4-Myd88 signaling pathway participate in stimulating the development of pyroptosis via NLRP3. NLRP3, an important regulatory target, can be activated by mtDNA or cleared via autophagy pathway. HMGB1 plays a key role in this process. Stimulation of HMGB1 secretion is dependent on NLRP4/NLRP1b rather than ASC. IL-1RI regulated by TLR4 sensitizes AMs to IL-1β and facilitates to the formation of ASC pyroptosome causing the exaggeration of AMs pyroptosis. GSDMD-N fragment, derived from caspase -1's cleavage of GSDMD, is transported to the cell membrane and initiates pyroptosis in AMs.

be an effective target for blocking this pathway in alveolar macrophages (Zeng et al., 2019).

Interleukin-1β (IL-1β) is a pro-inflammatory mediator of inflammation which is released extracellular after pyroptosis occurs (Bergsbaken et al., 2009). The activation of IL-1β is closely related to the proteolysis of caspase-1 and the assembly of the inflammasomes which arises from the cutting of caspase-1 at amino acid position 116 (Delaleu and Bickel, 2004; Guo et al., 2015). It plays a main role in stimulating white blood cells to express various cytokines and chemokines and promoting the immigration of white blood cells to organs, thus exaggerating the development of inflammation (Delaleu and Bickel, 2004). A study investigated the influence of LPS-induced IL-1β release on the development of AM pyroptosis and lung inflammation (He et al., 2016a). The study showed that Toll-like receptor 4 (TLR4) up-regulates the release or expression of IL-1β and IL-1RI on the AM surface. IL-1RI upregulation sensitizes AMs to IL-1β and facilitates to the formation of ASC pyroptosome causing the exaggeration of AMs pyroptosis, which subsequently exacerbates ALI (He et al., 2016a). Xingying He et al. demonstrated a new mechanism of endotoxin induced innate immunity that a correlation between the secondary upregulation of IL-1β/IL-1RI signals and AM pyroptosis in lung injury through TLR4-MyD88-NF-κB dependent signaling (He et al., 2016a). According to their results, MyD88 is related to mediate the process of TLR4-IL-1RI cross-talk and NF-κB involves in facilitating the upregulation of IL-1RI induced by TLR4. Additionally, another article has concluded that myeloid differentiation protein 2 (MD-2), one of the core factors required for TLR4 to recognize LPS, heightens caspase-1, NF-κB p65 protein, NLRP3 and MyD88 expression and helps regulate the activation of LPS-induced NLRP3 inflammasome and the inflammatory response in AMs via MyD88/NF-κB signaling pathway (Luo et al., 2017). And this outcome eventually led to the secretion of IL-1β and pyroptosis of AMs. Coincidentally, another study also indicated that interferon regulatory factor-1 (IRF-1) plays an important role in mediating alveolar macrophage pyroptosis during acute lung injury (Wu et al., 2016). As a gene known to participate in the interferon (IFN) pathway, IRF-1 straightly adjusts alveolar macrophage pyroptosis and caspase-1 activity structurally by IRF-1-binding element (IRE) from casapse-1 gene. And the study identified that TLR4 is essential in the activation of IRF-1. MyD88 has long been proven to recruit the IRF-1 transcription factors to activate the TLR4 pathway (Harroch et al., 1995; Szekely et al., 2018). Therefore, IRF-1 may be a hub gene between LPS-TLR4 signaling and caspase-1-dependent pyroptosis pathway in alveolar macrophages.

As a highly conserved metabolic degradation system, autophagy has been shown in recent years to maintain homeostasis and protect cells under abnormal stimulation by a large amount of evidence (Duan et al., 2020). Wei Peng et al. found autophagy of alveolar macrophages played a protective role as the upstream regulator of pyroptosis in acute lung injury induced by mitochondrial damage-associated molecular patterns (MTDs) (Peng et al., 2020a). Enhanced autophagy in AMs inhibits the function of the NLRP3 inflammasome by degrading and clearing the activated NLRP3. And from that,

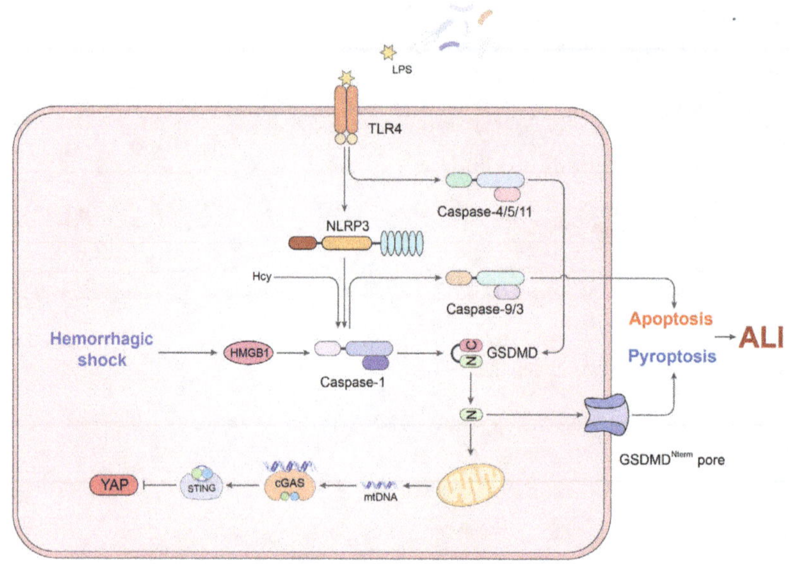

FIGURE 2 | The mechanism of pyroptosis affecting endothelial cells in ALI. In ECs, caspase-1 not only induces pyroptosis, but also participates in the regulation of apoptosis. LPS and hemorrhagic shock (HS) are two major triggers for activation of caspase-1. TLR4 on the cell membrane recognizes LPS and up-regulates NLRP3 expression, thus inducing caspase-1-mediated pyroptosis. Besides, HS promotes the formation of inflammasomes via HMGB1/RAGE signaling pathway. Cleaved caspase-1 is responsible for the downstream caspase-9 and 3 activation leading to apoptosis in EC when Hcy and LPS stimulate simultaneously. Meanwhile, non-canonical pyroptosis pathway mediated by caspase-4/5/11 also occupies a certain role in endothelial pyroptosis. GSDMD cleaved by caspase-11 has another function that promotes mtDNA releases. Through cGAS/STING axis, mtDNA inhibits the expression of YAP, resulting in endothelial cell proliferation disorders. In addition to the above, the effect of pyroptosis on the pulmonary endothelial barrier still needs to be studied.

caspase-1 and IL-1β precursors cannot be cleaved into the active form, thus inhibiting the caspase-1-mediated pyroptosis pathway (Peng et al., 2020a). It is expected that inhibition of pyroptosis by activating one of the upstream pathways of autophagy may become a new strategy for the treatment of ALI.

Our team previously illustrated that a new mechanism in macrophages to explain how mitochondrial DNA (mtDNA) activates the pyroptosis pathway to aggravate the inflammatory response of ALI (Ning et al., 2020). In our study, LPS stimulation causes mtDNA in mitochondria to leak into the cytoplasm and be identified by the sensory receptor of cytosolic DNA (cyclic GMP-AMP synthase, cGAS) (Ning et al., 2020). Stimulator of interferon gene (STING) is triggered by cGAS and its phosphorylation levels rise (Jena et al., 2020; Ning et al., 2020). LPS also upregulated the expression of transcription factor c-Myc, thus directly promoting the expression level of STING. The upregulation and activation of STING activates NLRP3 inflammasome and caspase-1, eventually leading to cell pyroptosis and ALI (Jena et al., 2020; Ning et al., 2020). Based on the CGAS-STING axis, our team will further explore the upstream mechanism of macrophage pyroptosis in acute lung injury.

In summary, the main function of macrophages in lung tissue is to preserve homeostasis and activate autoimmunity under pathogen stimulation. The suppression of inflammatory response in macrophages is crucial for the treatment of acute lung injury. There is still high research value in the field of ALI on the mechanism of inflammatory response pathway and AM.

Pyroptosis in Endothelial Cells

A single layer of fused endothelial cells (EC) covered the inner wall of pulmonary microvessels, called pulmonary endothelial barrier. ECs are responsible for the mediation of vascular tone, permeability, ventilation–perfusion matching and interactions with blood-borne cells (Maniatis and Orfanos, 2008; Muller-Redetzky et al., 2014). Pulmonary ECs account for about 50% of all lung cells, which have the function of accept total cardiac output. As a result, lung endothelial cells are most likely to be disturbed by bacterial endotoxins and circulating pathogens. Pulmonary endothelial barrier dysfunction caused by extensive ECs death is a hallmark of acute lung injury (Liu et al., 2015). Considering the induction of pyroptosis by LPS, a number of publications put attention on the impact of inflammatory caspases on ECs in ALI (**Figure 2**).

A study from Jie Yang et al. sheds light on the important role of hemorrhagic shock (HS) and EC pyroptosis in ALI (Yang et al., 2016). HS tends to make the patient more vulnerable to lung damage because an exaggerated response is initiated to respond a second infectious stimulus (Rubenfeld et al., 2005). In the study, the authors documented that the activation of caspase-1 in ECs is due to two sources. On the one hand, hemorrhagic shock promoted the secretion of HMGB1 which forms pyroptosome and activates caspase-1 through RAGE signaling and originated the endocytosis of HMGB1 by endothelial cells (Yang et al., 2016). On the other hand, caspase-1 activation was induced by LPS via TLR4-NLRP3 signaling pathway in ECs (Yang et al., 2016). More importantly, this article highlights the activation of caspase-1 in endothelial pyroptosis. Through the measurement of BALF protein concentration, lung tissue myeloperoxidase (MPO) activity and lung wet/dry ratio, they concluded that EC pyroptosis induced by HS could lead to acute lung injury (Yang et al., 2016).

Caspase-1 simultaneously plays different roles in the destruction of lung endothelial cells, not only causing pyroptosis. In a previous study, caspase-1 was related to induce ECs apoptosis and the release of IL-1β/IL-18 in lung ECs (King et al., 2003). This process seems to be connected with homocysteine (Hcy) (Xi et al., 2016). It has been reported that Hcy promotes the apoptosis of ECs and inhibits ECs growth leading to endothelial dysfunction (Tan et al., 2006; Cheng et al., 2015). In addition, Hcy can also induce inflammasome assembly and caspase-1 activation, which is synergistic with LPS. Cause it is the earliest event with higher hierarchy in caspase cascade in EC, caspase-1 activation may be responsible for mediating Hcy/LPS-induced pyroptosis/apoptosis and the downstream caspase-9 and -3 activation in EC (Xi et al., 2016). What was novel about this study was that the authors named the kind of programmed cell death which was mediated by caspase-1 through increased ROS as pyrop-apoptosis. The result also provided evidence for crosstalk between inflammatory and apoptotic caspases. It is worth mentioning that IL-33 can subdue the function of caspase-1 in ECs, which mediates Group 2 innate lymphoid cells (ILC2) expansion in the lungs acting through its receptor ST2 (Lai et al., 2018). The increase of ILC2 in the lung contribute to secrete IL-9, which inhibits the activation of caspase-1 to prevent pulmonary ECs from the occurrence of pyroptosis or apoptosis (Lai et al., 2018).

After pyroptosis occurs, the downstream pathway of caspase-1 also plays a pro-inflammatory role. Activated caspase-1 in ECs leads IL-1β to be secreted and performs its physiological functions. After binding with its specific receptor, IL-1β up-regulates the expression of adhesion factors in pulmonary capillary endothelial cells, thus promoting chemotaxis and activation of inflammatory cells into lung tissues, releasing a large number of inflammatory factors and triggering the inflammatory cascade amplification effect (Zhu et al., 2012). At the same time, IL-1β can also destroy the cell surface localization of vascular endothelial (VE)- cadherin by promoting endocytosis, and increase capillary permeability (Zhu et al., 2012).

Microparticles/microvesicles (MPs/MVs) are minor membrane-covered structures secreted from activated or dead cells (Distler et al., 2006). Microparticulate caspase-1 is a novel effective form for mononuclear macrophages to transmit death signals and caspase-1 to mediate cell death (Sarkar et al., 2009). Caspase-1 packaged into circulating microparticle is almost released from mononuclear phagocyte. The mechanism of microparticulate caspase-1 acting on lung ECs has been reported in recent years (Mitra et al., 2015; Mitra et al., 2018). Stimulated monocytic cells release activated caspase-1, GSDMD, ASC and other inflammasome proteins in target specific microparticles. This kind of exogenous caspase-1 induces endothelial cells apoptosis and pyroptosis. ASC, the inflammasome adaptor protein, and the capsulation of caspase-1 are vital for apoptotic and uptake function (Mitra et al., 2015). Once the microvesicle structure is destroyed, the novel caspase-1-dependent apoptosis is completely inhibited. In the process of microparticulate caspase-1 mediating pyroptosis of endothelial cells, cleaved GSDMD is categorically necessary (Mitra et al., 2018). As we all know, GSDMD is related to the formation of plasma membrane pores. Therefore, the authors speculated that the pore forming capacity of GSDMD is significant to the aptitude of MPs to locate the target (Mitra et al., 2018). In summary, the activation of caspase-1 regulates GSDMD cleavage, while cleaved GSDMD regulates the release of MPs encapsulating caspase-1 (Mitra et al., 2018). However, it would be further studied to confirm how does GSDMD act on MPs and whether it produces pores.

As more and more studies have been published on caspase-1-independent pathway of pyroptosis, the effect of caspase-4/5/11 in ECs draws attention recently. It was found that LPS could up-regulate the expression of caspase-11 in mouse endothelial cells via TLR4 and then induce pyroptosis of endothelial cells. In this process, caspase-11 is indispensable, nevertheless TLR4 can be substituted by TLR3 ligand poly and TLR2 ligand Pam3CSK4 (Cheng et al., 2017). Caspase-11 plays the central part in the mechanism of EC pyroptosis induced by endotoxin which is the causation of lung vascular hyperpermeability and mortality. Meanwhile, the release of MPs from pyroptotic ECs is significantly increased under the action of caspase-11.

As mentioned in the previous section, mtDNA still promotes inflammation and damage in the caspase-11-mediated pyroptosis pathway of endothelial cells. After LPS stimulation, caspase-11 is activated and participates in the assembly of atypical the non-canonical inflammasome (Huang et al., 2020). The resulting GSDMD-NT fragment not only induces the formation of plasma membrane pores, but also locates to mitochondria and induces mtDNA release into the cytoplasm (Huang et al., 2020). MtDNA, on the one hand, further promotes the process of cell pyroptosis, and on the other hand inhibits the expression of YAP through the cGAS-STING signaling pathway (Huang et al., 2020). The suppression of YAP signaling, a known pathway that regulates cell proliferation (LaCanna et al., 2019), reduces vascular repair and endothelial cell proliferation. To sum up, caspase-11 plays an important role in the anti-regeneration and pyroptosis of endothelial cells.

Pyroptosis in Neutrophil

Increasing evidence has shown that neutrophils are increasingly thought to be complex, multifaceted cells that play an important role in initiating and sustaining inflammation and promoting regression, though paradoxically (Vassallo et al., 2019). In lung injury, neutrophils not only cause lung tissue damage by mediating the inflammatory response (Summers et al., 2014), but also eliminate inflammation by recruiting monocytes and releasing a cluster of "specialized pro-resolving mediators" (SPMs) (Dalli and Serhan, 2012). As early as in 2002, the study of Sarah J. Rowe et al. found that up-regulation of the mRNA for IL-1β is significant after LPS stimulation in caspase-1-deficient mice, but their neutrophils released IL-1β minimally (Rowe et al., 2002). The authors thought the result may be related to the mice's resistance to intraperitoneal injection of endotoxin shock. However, caused by the discovery of the concept of pyroptosis, the minimum release of IL-1β from their neutrophils probably resulted on that the defect of caspase-1 inhibited the canonical pathway of pyroptosis. This is the first time that inflammatory caspases and pulmonary neutrophils have been associated with lung injury.

Recently, neutrophils was reported to achieve host protection facilitated by NLRC4/caspase-1-dependent IL-β secretion (Chen et al., 2014). In the acute lung infection induced by *P. aeruginosa* PAO1, neutrophils, rather than AMs, are indispensable for host protection. And neutrophil pyroptosis in the caspase-1-dependent manner is attributed to PAO1 flagellin for activating caspase-1 inflammasome and TLR5 which regulates PAO1 uptake under NOX2-deficient conditions (Ryu et al., 2017). The secretion of IL-1β/IL-18 increased significantly through NLRC4-caspase-1 pathway and NLRP3-caspase-11 pathway while neutrophil pyroptosis happens. It was concluded that PAO1-induced neutrophil pyroptosis may be activated by the collaborative recognition of PAO1 flagellin through TLR5 and NLRC4 (Ryu et al., 2017).

On the other hand, neutrophils, as important effector cells in immune response, recruit and exert immune function at the injured site in the process of acute lung injury (Williams and Chambers, 2014). The chemokine CXCL12 is involved in the regulation of neutrophil migration, as is its receptor CXCR4 (Tulotta et al., 2019). NLRP3-mediated pyroptosis has been shown in studies to promote the expression of CXCL12 in neutrophils, thereby inducing neutrophil migration and aggravating the severity of acute lung injury(Peng et al., 2020b). However, in the model of lung ischemia–reperfusion (IR), the recruitment of neutrophils induced by pyroptosis is a very effective defense mechanism against bacterial infections after injury (Tian et al., 2017). Minimal lung damage may follow if the post-IR pulmonary environment is sterilized (Tian et al., 2017). Otherwise dormant neutrophils would be transformed into activated neutrophils in the presence of a pathogenic toxin, which may help protect against infection (Tian et al., 2017).

THE TREATMENT OF ALI BY INHIBITING INFLAMMASOMES

As mentioned above, inflammasomes are indispensable in the process of inflammatory caspases-induced pyroptosis leading to lung injury. More recently, there has been a growing number of studies focusing on inhibition of the inflammasomes or blockage of signaling pathways to find out new treatment strategies for ALI (Samanta et al., 2018; Zhang et al., 2018; Gao et al., 2019; Wang et al., 2019; Yao and Sun, 2019; Niu et al., 2020; Shao et al., 2020).

NLRP3 Inflammasome

NLRP3 inflammasome is the most studied inflammasome, which activates caspase-1 in the caspase-1-dependent pyroptosis pathway. The activation of NLRP3 inflammasomes requires many molecular or cellular events as triggers, such as K^+ outflow, Ca^{2+} signals, reactive oxygen species stimulation or lysosome rupture, etc. (He et al., 2016b) In addition, there is the non-canonical NLRP3 inflammasome that can be triggered by caspase-11 without the regulation by TLR4 (Kayagaki et al., 2013). The inhibition of NLRP3 inflammasome is currently attracting considerable interest as an effective treatment for acute lung injury.

NLRP3 in LPS-Induced ALI

LPS-induced ALI is the most common and has the most pronounced inflammatory response in all kinds of ALI. Yu-chang Wang et al. found that dihydromyricetin (DHM) could reduce the protein expression of caspase-1, IL-18, IL-1β, NLRP3, ASC and pro-GSDMD to inhibit the inflammation in ALI and the inhibiting action was grounded on the defeat of NLRP3 inflammasome-dependent pyroptosis signaling pathway (Wang et al., 2019). Glycoprotein extracted from Chinese Yam, a kind of Chinese medicine homologous food, can also attenuate the secretion of NLRP3 in ALI and the activation of LPS-induced NF-κB/TLR4 signaling pathway can be restrained (Niu et al., 2020). Both DHM and glycoproteins are concerned because of their immunomodulatory effects, and have a negative effect on MPO activity in tissues. With the increasing research on inflammasome and lung injury, numbers of anti-inflammatory molecules including melatonin, oridonin or apocynin have been reported to suppress the NLRP3 inflammasome activation to achieve the purpose of attenuating acute lung injury (Zhang et al., 2016; Jin et al., 2019; Yang et al., 2019).

NLRP3 in Ventilator-Induced Lung Injury

Although mechanical ventilation (MV) is an effective treatment for acute lung injury at present, it will lead to the recruitment of inflammatory cells and induce the release of inflammatory mediators and cytokines, thus leading to the occurrence of acute lung injury when tidal volume is high (Liu et al., 2019). NLRP3, as an upstream regulator of caspase-1-meidated pyroptosis pathway, is an important target for reducing ventilator-induced lung injury (VILI) (Kuipers et al., 2012). Mechanical stretching induced by the ventilator induces the release of reactive oxygen species in the mitochondria of the cell (Wu et al., 2013). Mitochondrial activation and extracellular aggregation of IL-1β are highly dependent on the released mtROS (Wu et al., 2013). With one accord, a recent study suggests that oxidative stress exacerbates VILI via NLRP3 pyroptosis pathway (An et al., 2019). Therefore, inhibiting the accumulation of ROS or the occurrence of oxidative stress would be an effective way to inhibit the function of NLRP3. Moreover, salidroside and dopamine have also been reported to play a protective role in VILI by inhibiting the expression of NLRP3 and reducing the release of inflammatory factors (Wang et al., 2017b; Yang et al., 2017).

NLRP3 in Hyperoxia-Induced Lung Injury

In the hyperoxia-induced lung injury (HALI) model, NLRP3 has been shown to induce HALI by regulating chemotaxis and recruitment of immune cells and IL-1β expression levels (Fukumoto et al., 2013). P2X7, a kind of membrane receptor, is responsible for the activation of NLRP3 after exposure to hyperoxia (Galam et al., 2016). Caffeine and lycium barbarum polysaccharides (LBP) can protect hyperoxia-induced lung tissue from oxidative injury by inhibiting NLRP3 inflammasome (Hong et al., 2019; Chen et al., 2020). Interestingly, another study has shown that activated NLRP3, in addition to activating caspase-1, also plays a protective role in HALI by activating the Stats pathway in lung epithelial cells (Mizushina et al., 2015). The lack of NLRP3 greatly decreases the expression of chemokines in macrophages and neutrophils, thereby inhibiting Stat3 activation, leading to a weakening of HALI's protective mechanism (Mizushina et al., 2015). As a result, NLRP3$^{-/-}$ mice show less lung inflammation and inflammatory cell infiltration, but a higher fatality rate (Mizushina et al., 2015).

Other Inflammasome

Compared with the NLRP3 inflammasome, much less research has been done on inhibiting other inflammasomes that cause pyroptosis. A publication from Jian Gao et al. identified that AIM2 inflammasome could be inhibited by andrographolide to achieve the amelioration of acute lung injury (Gao et al., 2019). Cause for the function of preventing AIM2 from migrating to the nucleus, andrographolide significantly inhibited AIM2 inflammasome activation and lung macrophage pyroptosis (Gao et al., 2019). This is a representative study on AIM2 inflammasome for the treatment of acute lung injury in recent years. NALP3 inflammasome has the function of activating pathological processes where excessive IL-1β is produced (Campbell et al., 2016). Recently, a study from Leifang Zhang et al. revealed that suppressor of cytokine signaling-1 (SOCS-1) limits the assembly of NALP3 inflammasomes and significantly inhibits the activation of caspase-1 in smoke inhalation-induced acute lung injury as a negative regulator of pro-inflammatory cytokine signal transduction (Zhang et al., 2018). Beyond that, further research is needed on the treatment and improvement of acute lung injury by inhibiting inflammasome-induced cell death.

DISCUSSION

ALI is characterized by extensive inflammatory cell infiltration in lung tissue and damage to alveoli and endothelium resulting from an exaggerated inflammatory reaction. In the absence of a corresponding inflammatory response, apoptosis alone is undoubtedly inappropriate to describe the underlying mechanism of ALI. Pyroptosis induced by inflammatory caspases is responsible for swelling of cells and release of pro-inflammatory contents compared with apoptosis. With the increase of research on GSDMD, the process and function of pyroptosis is becoming much clearer.

Recently, a study showed that caspase-8 also mediates LPS-induced pyroptosis of macrophages, and this process does not require the involvement of other apoptotic caspases (Muendlein et al., 2020). Although the exact process and whether it occurs only in macrophages, remain unclear, the result undeniably shattered the previous understanding of pyroptosis and apoptosis. The crosstalk between inflammatory caspases and apoptotic caspases has attracted the interest of many scholars.

This review focuses on recent advances in the study of pyroptosis in ALI and the treatment via inflammasome. Although these recent advances provide evidence for the role of inflammatory caspases and pyroptosis in acute lung injury, many details remain indefinite. Most of the current studies have focused on caspase-1-dependent signaling pathways, while the non-canonical pathway induced by caspase-11/4/5 is rarely reported. Furthermore, the selection mechanism of canonical or non-canonical pyroptosis pathways in lung tissue and the role of pulmonary epithelial pyroptosis in ALI is still awaiting further study.

At present, COVID-19 is causing serious outbreaks around the globe, affecting people's health and development in many countries. Whether the resulting ALI/ARDS can be improved by blocking the pyroptosis signaling pathway deserves immediate experimental verification (López-Reyes et al., 2020). Therefore, further elucidation of the role of pyroptosis in lung injury is necessary in order to better understand its mechanism and how to use it for therapeutic purposes.

AUTHOR CONTRIBUTIONS

BL wrote the first draft. RH illustrated the draft. LZ modified the draft. The rest joined in the discussion.

REFERENCES

Aggarwal, N. R., King, L. S., and D'Alessio, F. R. (2014). Diverse macrophage populations mediate acute lung inflammation and resolution. *Am. J. Physiol. Lung Cell Mol. Physiol.* 306 (8), L709–L725. doi:10.1152/ajplung.00341.2013

An, X., Sun, X., Yang, X., Liu, D., Hou, Y., Chen, H., et al. (2019). Oxidative stress promotes ventilator-induced lung injury through activating NLRP3 inflammasome and TRPM2 channel. *Artif. Cells Nanomed. Biotechnol.* 47 (1), 3448–3455. doi:10.1080/21691401.2019.1652631

Aujla, S. J., Chan, Y. R., Zheng, M., Fei, M., Askew, D. J., Pociask, D. A., et al. (2008). IL-22 mediates mucosal host defense against Gram-negative bacterial pneumonia. *Nat. Med.* 14 (3), 275–281. doi:10.1038/nm1710

Baker, P. J., Boucher, D., Bierschenk, D., Tebartz, C., Whitney, P. G., D'Silva, D. B., et al. (2015). NLRP3 inflammasome activation downstream of cytoplasmic LPS recognition by both caspase-4 and caspase-5. *Eur. J. Immunol.* 45 (10), 2918–2926. doi:10.1002/eji.201545655

Bergsbaken, T., Fink, S. L., and Cookson, B. T. (2009). Pyroptosis: host cell death and inflammation. *Nat. Rev. Microbiol.* 7 (2), 99–109. doi:10.1038/nrmicro2070

Black, R. A., Kronheim, S. R., Merriam, J. E., March, C. J., and Hopp, T. P. (1989). A pre-aspartate-specific protease from human leukocytes that cleaves pro-interleukin-1 beta. *J. Biol. Chem.* 264 (10), 5323–5326. doi:10.1016/s0021-9258(18)83546-3

Burgos, J. R., Iresjö, B.-M., Olsson, L., and Smedh, U. (2019). LPS immune challenge reduces arcuate nucleus TSHR and CART mRNA and elevates plasma CART peptides. *BMC Neurosci.* 20 (1), 59. doi:10.1186/s12868-019-0539-z

Butt, Y., Kurdowska, A., and Allen, T. C. (2016). Acute lung injury: a clinical and molecular review. *Arch. Pathol. Lab Med.* 140 (4), 345–350. doi:10.5858/arpa.2015-0519-RA

Campbell, L., Raheem, I., Malemud, C. J., and Askari, A. D. (2016). The relationship between NALP3 and autoinflammatory syndromes. *Int. J. Mol. Sci.* 17 (5), 725. doi:10.3390/ijms17050725

Chen, K. W., Groß, C. J., Sotomayor, F. V., Stacey, K. J., Tschopp, J., Sweet, M. J., et al. (2014). The neutrophil NLRC4 inflammasome selectively promotes IL-1β maturation without pyroptosis during acute Salmonella challenge. *Cell Rep.* 8 (2), 570–582. doi:10.1016/j.celrep.2014.06.028

Chen, S., Wu, Q., Zhong, D., Li, C., and Du, L. (2020). Caffeine prevents hyperoxia-induced lung injury in neonatal mice through NLRP3 inflammasome and NF-kappaB pathway. *Respir. Res.* 21 (1), 140. doi:10.1186/s12931-020-01403-2

Cheng, K. T., Xiong, S., Ye, Z., Hong, Z., Di, A., Tsang, K. M., et al. (2017). Caspase-11-mediated endothelial pyroptosis underlies endotoxemia-induced lung injury. *J. Clin. Invest.* 127 (11), 4124–4135. doi:10.1172/JCI94495

Cheng, Z., Jiang, X., Pansuria, M., Fang, P., Mai, J., Mallilankaraman, K., et al. (2015). Hyperhomocysteinemia and hyperglycemia induce and potentiate endothelial dysfunction via μ-calpain activation. *Diabetes* 64 (3), 947–959. doi:10.2337/db14-0784

Dalli, J., and Serhan, C. N. (2012). Specific lipid mediator signatures of human phagocytes: microparticles stimulate macrophage efferocytosis and pro-resolving mediators. *Blood* 120 (15), e60–e72. doi:10.1182/blood-2012-04-423525

Delaleu, N., and Bickel, M. (2004). Interleukin-1 beta and interleukin-18: regulation and activity in local inflammation. *Periodontology* 35, 42–52. doi:10.1111/j.0906-6713.2004.003569.x

Distler, J. H. W., Huber, L. C., Gay, S., Distler, O., and Pisetsky, D. S. (2006). Microparticles as mediators of cellular cross-talk in inflammatory disease. *Autoimmunity* 39 (8), 683–690. doi:10.1080/08916930601061538

Duan, R., Xie, H., and Liu, Z. Z. (2020). The role of autophagy in osteoarthritis. *Front Cell Dev. Biol.* 8, 608388. doi:10.3389/fcell.2020.608388

Frank, D., and Vince, J. E. (2019). Pyroptosis versus necroptosis: similarities, differences, and crosstalk. *Cell Death Differ.* 26 (1), 99–114. doi:10.1038/s41418-018-0212-6

Fukumoto, J., Fukumoto, I., Parthasarathy, P. T., Cox, R., Huynh, B., Ramanathan, G. K., et al. (2013). NLRP3 deletion protects from hyperoxia-induced acute lung injury. *Am. J. Physiol. Cell Physiol.* 305 (2), C182–C189. doi:10.1152/ajpcell.00086.2013

Galam, L., Rajan, A., Failla, A., Soundararajan, R., Lockey, R. F., and Kolliputi, N. (2016). Deletion of P2X7 attenuates hyperoxia-induced acute lung injury via inflammasome suppression. *Am. J. Physiol. Lung Cell Mol. Physiol.* 310 (6), L572–L581. doi:10.1152/ajplung.00417.2015

Gao, J., Peng, S., Shan, X., Deng, G., Shen, L., Sun, J., et al. (2019). Inhibition of AIM2 inflammasome-mediated pyroptosis by Andrographolide contributes to amelioration of radiation-induced lung inflammation and fibrosis. *Cell Death Dis.* 10 (12), 957. doi:10.1038/s41419-019-2195-8

Guo, H., Callaway, J. B., and Ting, J. P. Y. (2015). Inflammasomes: mechanism of action, role in disease, and therapeutics. *Nat. Med.* 21 (7), 677–687. doi:10.1038/nm.3893

Harroch, S., Gothelf, Y., Revel, M., and Chebath, J. (1995). 5' upstream sequences of MyD88, an IL-6 primary response gene in M1 cells: detection of functional IRF-1 and Stat factors binding sites. *Nucleic Acids Res.* 23 (17), 3539–3546. doi:10.1093/nar/23.17.3539

He, X., Qian, Y., Li, Z., Fan, E. K., Li, Y., Wu, L., et al. (2016a). TLR4-Upregulated IL-1beta and IL-1RI promote alveolar macrophage pyroptosis and lung inflammation through an autocrine mechanism. *Sci. Rep.* 6, 31663. doi:10.1038/srep31663

He, Y., Hara, H., and Nunez, G. (2016b). Mechanism and regulation of NLRP3 inflammasome activation. *Trends Biochem. Sci.* 41 (12), 1012–1021. doi:10.1016/j.tibs.2016.09.002

Hong, C. Y., Zhang, H. D., Liu, X. Y., and Xu, Y. (2019). Attenuation of hyperoxic acute lung injury by Lycium barbarum polysaccharide via inhibiting NLRP3 inflammasome. *Arch Pharm. Res.* 42 (10), 902–908. doi:10.1007/s12272-019-01175-4

Hou, L., Yang, Z., Wang, Z., Zhang, X., Zhao, Y., Yang, H., et al. (2018). NLRP3/ASC-mediated alveolar macrophage pyroptosis enhances HMGB1 secretion in acute lung injury induced by cardiopulmonary bypass. *Lab. Invest.* 98 (8), 1052–1064. doi:10.1038/s41374-018-0073-0

Huang, L. S., Hong, Z., Wu, W., Xiong, S., Zhong, M., Gao, X., et al. (2020). mtDNA activates cGAS signaling and suppresses the YAP-mediated endothelial cell proliferation program to promote inflammatory injury. *Immunity* 52 (3), 475–486. doi:10.1016/j.immuni.2020.02.002

Hung, C.-M., Peng, C.-K., Wu, C.-P., and Huang, K.-L. (2018). Bumetanide attenuates acute lung injury by suppressing macrophage activation. *Biochem. Pharmacol.* 156, 60–67. doi:10.1016/j.bcp.2018.08.013

Irrera, N., Russo, M., Pallio, G., Bitto, A., Mannino, F., Minutoli, L., et al. (2020). The role of NLRP3 inflammasome in the pathogenesis of traumatic brain injury. *Int. J. Mol. Sci.* 21 (17), 6204. doi:10.3390/ijms21176204

Jena, K. K., Mehto, S., Nath, P., Chauhan, N. R., Sahu, R., Dhar, K., et al. (2020). Autoimmunity gene IRGM suppresses cGAS-STING and RIG-I-MAVS signaling to control interferon response. *EMBO Rep.* 21 (9), e50051. doi:10.15252/embr.202050051

Jin, H.-Z., Yang, X.-J., Zhao, K.-L., Mei, F.-C., Zhou, Y., You, Y.-D., et al. (2019). Apocynin alleviates lung injury by suppressing NLRP3 inflammasome activation and NF-κB signaling in acute pancreatitis. *Int. Immunopharm.* 75, 105821. doi:10.1016/j.intimp.2019.105821

Kao, R. L., Xu, X., Xenocostas, A., Parry, N., Mele, T., Martin, C. M., et al. (2014). Induction of acute lung inflammation in mice with hemorrhagic shock and resuscitation: role of HMGB1. *J. Inflamm.* 11 (1), 30. doi:10.1186/s12950-014-0030-7

Kayagaki, N., Warming, S., Lamkanfi, M., Vande Walle, L., Louie, S., Dong, J., et al. (2011). Non-canonical inflammasome activation targets caspase-11. *Nature* 479 (7371), 117–121. doi:10.1038/nature10558

Kayagaki, N., Wong, M. T., Stowe, I. B., Ramani, S. R., Gonzalez, L. C., Akashi-Takamura, S., et al. (2013). Noncanonical inflammasome activation by intracellular LPS independent of TLR4. *Science* 341 (6151), 1246–1249. doi:10.1126/science.1240248

Kesavardhana, S., and Kanneganti, T.-D. (2017). Mechanisms governing inflammasome activation, assembly and pyroptosis induction. *Int. Immunol.* 29 (5), 201–210. doi:10.1093/intimm/dxx018

King, A. R., Francis, S. E., Bridgeman, C. J., Bird, H., Whyte, M. K., and Crossman, D. C. (2003). A role for caspase-1 in serum withdrawal-induced apoptosis of endothelial cells. *Lab. Invest.* 83 (10), 1497–1508. doi:10.1097/01.lab.0000093096.62765.85

Kojima, M., Gimenes-Junior, J. A., Chan, T. W., Eliceiri, B. P., Baird, A., Costantini, T. W., et al. (2018). Exosomes in postshock mesenteric lymph are key mediators of acute lung injury triggering the macrophage activation Toll-like receptor 4. *Faseb. J.* 32 (1). doi:10.1096/fj.201700488R

Kox, M., Pompe, J. C., Peters, E., Vaneker, M., van der Laak, J. W., van der Hoeven, J. G., et al. (2011). α7 nicotinic acetylcholine receptor agonist GTS-21 attenuates ventilator-induced tumour necrosis factor-α production and lung injury. *Br. J. Anaesth.* 107 (4), 559–566. doi:10.1093/bja/aer202

Kuipers, M. T., Aslami, H., Janczy, J. R., van der Sluijs, K. F., Vlaar, A. P. J., Wolthuis, E. K., et al. (2012). Ventilator-induced lung injury is mediated by the NLRP3 inflammasome. *Anesthesiology* 116 (5), 1104–1115. doi:10.1097/ALN.0b013e3182518bc0

LaCanna, R., Liccardo, D., Zhang, P., Tragesser, L., Wang, Y., Cao, T., et al. (2019). Yap/Taz regulate alveolar regeneration and resolution of lung inflammation. *J. Clin. Invest.* 129 (5), 2107–2122. doi:10.1172/JCI125014

Lai, D., Tang, J., Chen, L., Fan, E. K., Scott, M. J., Li, Y., et al. (2018). Group 2 innate lymphoid cells protect lung endothelial cells from pyroptosis in sepsis. *Cell Death Dis.* 9 (3), 369. doi:10.1038/s41419-018-0412-5

Lamkanfi, M., and Dixit, V. M. (2014). Mechanisms and functions of inflammasomes. *Cell* 157 (5), 1013–1022. doi:10.1016/j.cell.2014.04.007

Lamkanfi, M., Sarkar, A., Vande Walle, L., Vitari, A. C., Amer, A. O., Wewers, M. D., et al. (2010). Inflammasome-dependent release of the alarmin HMGB1 in endotoxemia. *J. immunol.* 185 (7), 4385–4392. doi:10.4049/jimmunol.1000803

Li, D., Ren, W., Jiang, Z., and Zhu, L. (2018). Regulation of the NLRP3 inflammasome and macrophage pyroptosis by the p38 MAPK signaling pathway in a mouse model of acute lung injury. *Mol. Med. Rep.* 18 (5), 4399–4409. doi:10.3892/mmr.2018.9427

Lin, X. Y., Choi, M. S., and Porter, A. G. (2000). Expression analysis of the human caspase-1 subfamily reveals specific regulation of the CASP5 gene by lipopolysaccharide and interferon-gamma. *J. Biol. Chem.* 275 (51), 39920–39926. doi:10.1074/jbc.M007255200

Liu, H., Gu, C., Liu, M., Liu, G., Wang, D., Liu, X., et al. (2019). Ventilator-induced lung injury is alleviated by inhibiting NLRP3 inflammasome activation. *Mol. Immunol.* 111, 1–10. doi:10.1016/j.molimm.2019.03.011

Liu, H., Yu, X., Yu, S., and Kou, J. (2015). Molecular mechanisms in lipopolysaccharide-induced pulmonary endothelial barrier dysfunction. *Int. Immunopharm.* 29 (2), 937–946. doi:10.1016/j.intimp.2015.10.010

López-Reyes, A., Martinez-Armenta, C., Espinosa-Velázquez, R., Vázquez-Cárdenas, P., Cruz-Ramos, M., Palacios-Gonzalez, B., et al. (2020). NLRP3 inflammasome: the stormy link between obesity and COVID-19. *Front. Immunol.* 11, 570251. doi:10.3389/fimmu.2020.570251

Luo, M., Hu, L., Li, D., Wang, Y., He, Y., Zhu, L., et al. (2017). MD-2 regulates LPS-induced NLRP3 inflammasome activation and IL-1beta secretion by a MyD88/NF-kappaB-dependent pathway in alveolar macrophages cell line. *Mol. Immunol.* 90, 1–10. doi:10.1016/j.molimm.2017.06.035

Malik, A., and Kanneganti, T. D. (2017). Inflammasome activation and assembly at a glance. *J. Cell Sci.* 130 (23), 3955–3963. doi:10.1242/jcs.207365

Man, S. M., Karki, R., and Kanneganti, T.-D. (2017a). Molecular mechanisms and functions of pyroptosis, inflammatory caspases and inflammasomes in infectious diseases. *Immunol. Rev.* 277 (1), 61–75. doi:10.1111/imr.12534

Man, S. M., Karki, R., and Kanneganti, T. D. (2017b). Molecular mechanisms and functions of pyroptosis, inflammatory caspases and inflammasomes in infectious diseases. *Immunol. Rev.* 277 (1), 61–75. doi:10.1111/imr.12534

Maniatis, N. A., and Orfanos, S. E. (2008). The endothelium in acute lung injury/acute respiratory distress syndrome. *Curr. Opin. Crit. Care* 14 (1), 22–30. doi:10.1097/MCC.0b013e3282f269b9

Matikainen, S., Nyman, T. A., and Cypryk, W. (2020). Function and regulation of noncanonical caspase-4/5/11 inflammasome. *J. Immunol.* 204 (12), 3063–3069. doi:10.4049/jimmunol.2000373

Matthay, M. A., Ware, L. B., and Zimmerman, G. A. (2012). The acute respiratory distress syndrome. *J. Clin. Invest.* 122 (8), 2731–2740. doi:10.1172/JCI60331

McIlwain, D. R., Berger, T., and Mak, T. W. (2013). Caspase functions in cell death and disease. *Cold Spring Harb. Perspect. Biol.* 5 (4), a008656. doi:10.1101/cshperspect.a008656

Miao, E. A., Rajan, J. V., and Aderem, A. (2011). Caspase-1-induced pyroptotic cell death. *Immunol. Rev.* 243 (1), 206–214. doi:10.1111/j.1600-065X.2011.01044.x

Mitra, S., Exline, M., Habyarimana, F., Gavrilin, M. A., Baker, P. J., Masters, S. L., et al. (2018). Microparticulate caspase 1 regulates gasdermin D and pulmonary vascular endothelial cell injury. *Am. J. Respir. Cell Mol. Biol.* 59 (1), 56–64. doi:10.1165/rcmb.2017-0393OC

Mitra, S., Wewers, M. D., and Sarkar, A. (2015). Mononuclear phagocyte-derived microparticulate caspase-1 induces pulmonary vascular endothelial cell injury. *PloS One* 10 (12), e0145607. doi:10.1371/journal.pone.0145607

Mizushina, Y., Shirasuna, K., Usui, F., Karasawa, T., Kawashima, A., Kimura, H., et al. (2015). NLRP3 protein deficiency exacerbates hyperoxia-induced lethality through Stat3 protein signaling independent of interleukin-1beta. *J. Biol. Chem.* 290 (8), 5065–5077. doi:10.1074/jbc.M114.603217

Muendlein, H. I., Jetton, D., Connolly, W. M., Eidell, K. P., Magri, Z., Smirnova, I., et al. (2020). cFLIP protects macrophages from LPS-induced pyroptosis via inhibition of complex II formation. *Science* 367 (6484), 1379–1384. doi:10.1126/science.aay3878

Muller-Redetzky, H. C., Suttorp, N., and Witzenrath, M. (2014). Dynamics of pulmonary endothelial barrier function in acute inflammation: mechanisms and therapeutic perspectives. *Cell Tissue Res.* 355 (3), 657–673. doi:10.1007/s00441-014-1821-0

Ning, L., Wei, W., Wenyang, J., Rui, X., and Qing, G. (2020). Cytosolic DNA-STING-NLRP3 axis is involved in murine acute lung injury induced by lipopolysaccharide. *Clin. Transl. Med.* 10 (7), e228. doi:10.1002/ctm2.228

Niu, X., Zang, L., Li, W., Xiao, X., Yu, J., Yao, Q., et al. (2020). Anti-inflammatory effect of Yam Glycoprotein on lipopolysaccharide-induced acute lung injury via the NLRP3 and NF-κB/TLR4 signaling pathway. *Int. Immunopharm.* 81, 106024. doi:10.1016/j.intimp.2019.106024

Oh, C., Verma, A., and Aachoui, Y. (2020). Caspase-11 non-canonical inflammasomes in the lung. *Front. Immunol.* 11, 1895. doi:10.3389/fimmu.2020.01895

Pandeya, A., Li, L., Li, Z., and Wei, Y. (2019). Gasdermin D (GSDMD) as a new target for the treatment of infection. *Med. Chem. Comm* 10 (5), 660–667. doi:10.1039/c9md00059c

Peng, W., Peng, F., Lou, Y., Li, Y., Zhao, N., Shao, Q., et al. (2020a). Autophagy alleviates mitochondrial DAMP-induced acute lung injury by inhibiting NLRP3 inflammasome. *Life Sci.* 265, 118833. doi:10.1016/j.lfs.2020.118833

Peng, Y., Wu, Q., Tang, H., Chen, J., Wu, Q., Yuan, X., et al. (2020b). NLRP3 regulated CXCL12 expression in acute neutrophilic lung injury. *J. Inflamm. Res.* 13, 377–386. doi:10.2147/JIR.S259633

Qiu, Z., He, Y., Ming, H., Lei, S., Leng, Y., and Xia, Z.-Y. (2019). Lipopolysaccharide (LPS) aggravates high glucose- and hypoxia/reoxygenation-induced injury through activating ROS-dependent NLRP3 inflammasome-mediated pyroptosis in H9C2 cardiomyocytes. *J. Diab. Res.* 2019, 8151836. doi:10.1155/2019/8151836

Qu, L., Chen, C., Chen, Y., Li, Y., Tang, F., Huang, H., et al. (2019). High-mobility group box 1 (HMGB1) and autophagy in acute lung injury (ALI): a review. *Med. Sci. Mon. Int. Med. J. Exp. Clin. Res.* 25, 1828–1837. doi:10.12659/MSM.912867

Ramirez, M. L. G., and Salvesen, G. S. (2018). A primer on caspase mechanisms. *Semin. Cell Dev. Biol.* 82, 79–85. doi:10.1016/j.semcdb.2018.01.002

Rogers, C., Fernandes-Alnemri, T., Mayes, L., Alnemri, D., Cingolani, G., and Alnemri, E. S. (2017). Cleavage of DFNA5 by caspase-3 during apoptosis mediates progression to secondary necrotic/pyroptotic cell death. *Nat. Commun.* 8, 14128. doi:10.1038/ncomms14128

Rowe, S. J., Allen, L., Ridger, V. C., Hellewell, P. G., and Whyte, M. K. B. (2002). Caspase-1-deficient mice have delayed neutrophil apoptosis and a prolonged inflammatory response to lipopolysaccharide-induced acute lung injury. *J. Immunol.* 169 (11), 6401–6407. doi:10.4049/jimmunol.169.11.6401

Rubenfeld, G. D., Caldwell, E., Peabody, E., Weaver, J., Martin, D. P., Neff, M., et al. (2005). Incidence and outcomes of acute lung injury. *N. Engl. J. Med.* 353 (16), 1685–1693. doi:10.1056/NEJMoa050333

Ryu, J. C., Kim, M. J., Kwon, Y., Oh, J. H., Yoon, S. S., Shin, S. J., et al. (2017). Neutrophil pyroptosis mediates pathology of *P. aeruginosa* lung infection in the absence of the NADPH oxidase NOX2. *Mucosal Immunol.* 10 (3), 757–774. doi:10.1038/mi.2016.73

Samanta, S., Zhou, Z., Rajasingh, S., Panda, A., Sampath, V., and Rajasingh, J. (2018). DNMT and HDAC inhibitors together abrogate endotoxemia mediated macrophage death by STAT3-JMJD3 signaling. *Int. J. Biochem. Cell Biol.* 102, 117–127. doi:10.1016/j.biocel.2018.07.002

Sangiuliano, B., Perez, N. M., Moreira, D. F., and Belizario, J. E. (2014). Cell death-associated molecular-pattern molecules: inflammatory signaling and control. *Mediat. Inflamm.* 2014, 821043. doi:10.1155/2014/821043

Sarkar, A., Mitra, S., Mehta, S., Raices, R., and Wewers, M. D. (2009). Monocyte derived microvesicles deliver a cell death message via encapsulated caspase-1. *PloS One* 4 (9), e7140. doi:10.1371/journal.pone.0007140

Shalini, S., Dorstyn, L., Dawar, S., and Kumar, S. (2015). Old, new and emerging functions of caspases. *Cell Death Differ.* 22 (4), 526–539. doi:10.1038/cdd.2014.216

Shao, X.-F., Li, B., Shen, J., Wang, Q.-F., Chen, S.-S., Jiang, X.-C., et al. (2020). Ghrelin alleviates traumatic brain injury-induced acute lung injury through pyroptosis/NF-κB pathway. *Int. Immunopharm.* 79, 106175. doi:10.1016/j.intimp.2019.106175

Shi, J., Gao, W., and Shao, F. (2017). Pyroptosis: gasdermin-mediated programmed necrotic cell death. *Trends Biochem. Sci.* 42 (4), 245–254. doi:10.1016/j.tibs.2016.10.004

Shojaie, L., Iorga, A., and Dara, L. (2020). Cell death in liver diseases: a review. *Int. J. Mol. Sci.* 21 (24), 9682. doi:10.3390/ijms21249682

Summers, C., Singh, N. R., White, J. F., Mackenzie, I. M., Johnston, A., Solanki, C., et al. (2014). Pulmonary retention of primed neutrophils: a novel protective host response, which is impaired in the acute respiratory distress syndrome. *Thorax* 69 (7), 623–629. doi:10.1136/thoraxjnl-2013-204742

Szekely, B., Bossuyt, V., Li, X., Wali, V. B., Patwardhan, G. A., Frederick, C., et al. (2018). Immunological differences between primary and metastatic breast cancer. *Ann. Oncol.* 29 (11), 2232–2239. doi:10.1093/annonc/mdy399

Tan, H., Jiang, X., Yang, F., Li, Z., Liao, D., Trial, J., et al. (2006). Hyperhomocysteinemia inhibits post-injury reendothelialization in mice. *Cardiovasc. Res.* 69 (1), 253–262. doi:10.1016/j.cardiores.2005.08.016

Tang, L., Zhang, H., Wang, C., Li, H., Zhang, Q., and Bai, J. (2017). M2A and M2C macrophage subsets ameliorate inflammation and fibroproliferation in acute lung injury through interleukin 10 pathway. *Shock* 48 (1), 119–129. doi:10.1097/SHK.0000000000000820

Tian, X., Sun, H., Casbon, A. J., Lim, E., Francis, K. P., Hellman, J., et al. (2017). NLRP3 inflammasome mediates dormant neutrophil recruitment following sterile lung injury and protects against subsequent bacterial pneumonia in mice. *Front. Immunol.* 8, 1337. doi:10.3389/fimmu.2017.01337

Tulotta, C., Stefanescu, C., Chen, Q., Torraca, V., Meijer, A. H., and Snaar-Jagalska, B. E. (2019). CXCR4 signaling regulates metastatic onset by controlling neutrophil motility and response to malignant cells. *Sci. Rep.* 9 (1), 2399. doi:10.1038/s41598-019-38643-2

Van Opdenbosch, N., Gurung, P., Vande Walle, L., Fossoul, A., Kanneganti, T.-D., and Lamkanfi, M. (2014). Activation of the NLRP1b inflammasome independently of ASC-mediated caspase-1 autoproteolysis and speck formation. *Nat. Commun.* 5, 3209. doi:10.1038/ncomms4209

Van Opdenbosch, N., and Lamkanfi, M. (2019). Caspases in cell death, inflammation, and disease. *Immunity* 50 (6), 1352–1364. doi:10.1016/j.immuni.2019.05.020

Vassallo, A., Wood, A. J., Subburayalu, J., Summers, C., and Chilvers, E. R. (2019). The counter-intuitive role of the neutrophil in the acute respiratory distress syndrome. *Br. Med. Bull.* 131 (1), 43–55. doi:10.1093/bmb/ldz024

Wang, S., Miura, M., Jung, Y. K., Zhu, H., Li, E., and Yuan, J. (1998). Murine caspase-11, an ICE-interacting protease, is essential for the activation of ICE. *Cell* 92 (4), 501–509. doi:10.1016/s0092-8674(00)80943-5

Wang, Y. C., Liu, Q. X., Zheng, Q., Liu, T., Xu, X. E., Liu, X. H., et al. (2019). Dihydromyricetin alleviates sepsis-induced acute lung injury through inhibiting NLRP3 inflammasome-dependent pyroptosis in mice model. *Inflammation* 42 (4), 1301–1310. doi:10.1007/s10753-019-00990-7

Wang, Y., Gao, W., Shi, X., Ding, J., Liu, W., He, H., et al. (2017a). Chemotherapy drugs induce pyroptosis through caspase-3 cleavage of a gasdermin. *Nature* 547 (7661), 99–103. doi:10.1038/nature22393

Wang, Y., Liu, X., Shi, H., Yu, Y., Yu, Y., Li, M., et al. (2020). NLRP3 inflammasome, an immune-inflammatory target in pathogenesis and treatment of cardiovascular diseases. *Clin. Transl. Med.* 10 (1), e128. doi:10.1002/ctm2.13

Wang, Y., Xu, C. F., Liu, Y. J., Mao, Y. F., Lv, Z., Li, S. Y., et al. (2017b). Salidroside attenuates ventilation induced lung injury via SIRT1-dependent inhibition of NLRP3 inflammasome. *Cell. Physiol. Biochem.* 42 (1), 34–43. doi:10.1159/000477112

Ware, L. B. (2006). Pathophysiology of acute lung injury and the acute respiratory distress syndrome. *Semin. Respir. Crit. Care Med.* 27 (4), 337–349. doi:10.1055/s-2006-948288

Williams, A. E., and Chambers, R. C. (2014). The mercurial nature of neutrophils: still an enigma in ARDS? *Am. J. Physiol. Lung Cell Mol. Physiol.* 306 (3), L217–L230. doi:10.1152/ajplung.00311.2013

Winkler, S., and Rösen-Wolff, A. (2015). Caspase-1: an integral regulator of innate immunity. *Semin. Immunopathol.* 37 (4), 419–427. doi:10.1007/s00281-015-0494-4

Wu, D.-D., Pan, P.-H., Liu, B., Su, X.-L., Zhang, L.-M., Tan, H.-Y., et al. (2015). Inhibition of alveolar macrophage pyroptosis reduces lipopolysaccharide-induced acute lung injury in mice. *Chin. Med. J.* 128 (19), 2638–2645. doi:10.4103/0366-6999.166039

Wu, D., Pan, P., Su, X., Zhang, L., Qin, Q., Tan, H., et al. (2016). Interferon regulatory factor-1 mediates alveolar macrophage pyroptosis during LPS-induced acute lung injury in mice. *Shock* 46 (3), 329–338. doi:10.1097/SHK.0000000000000595

Wu, J., Yan, Z., Schwartz, D. E., Yu, J., Malik, A. B., and Hu, G. (2013). Activation of NLRP3 inflammasome in alveolar macrophages contributes to mechanical stretch-induced lung inflammation and injury. *J. Immunol.* 190 (7), 3590–3599. doi:10.4049/jimmunol.1200860

Xi, H., Zhang, Y., Xu, Y., Yang, W. Y., Jiang, X., Sha, X., et al. (2016). Caspase-1 inflammasome activation mediates homocysteine-induced pyrop-apoptosis in endothelial cells. *Circ. Res.* 118 (10), 1525–1539. doi:10.1161/circresaha.116.308501

Xia, S. (2020). Biological mechanisms and therapeutic relevance of the gasdermin family. *Mol. Aspect. Med.* 76, 100890. doi:10.1016/j.mam.2020.100890

Yang, H., Lv, H., Li, H., Ci, X., and Peng, L. (2019). Oridonin protects LPS-induced acute lung injury by modulating Nrf2-mediated oxidative stress and Nrf2-independent NLRP3 and NF-κB pathways. *Cell Commun. Signal.* 17 (1), 62. doi:10.1186/s12964-019-0366-y

Yang, J., Zhao, Y., Zhang, P., Li, Y., Yang, Y., Yang, Y., et al. (2016). Hemorrhagic shock primes for lung vascular endothelial cell pyroptosis: role in pulmonary inflammation following LPS. *Cell Death Dis.* 7 (9), e2363. doi:10.1038/cddis.2016.274

Yang, X., Sun, X., Chen, H., Xi, G., Hou, Y., Wu, J., et al. (2017). The protective effect of dopamine on ventilator-induced lung injury via the inhibition of NLRP3 inflammasome. *Int. Immunopharm.* 45, 68–73. doi:10.1016/j.intimp.2017.02.002

Yao, L., and Sun, T. (2019). Glycyrrhizin administration ameliorates Streptococcus aureus-induced acute lung injury. *Int. Immunopharm.* 70, 504–511. doi:10.1016/j.intimp.2019.02.046

Yi, Y.-S. (2017). Caspase-11 non-canonical inflammasome: a critical sensor of intracellular lipopolysaccharide in macrophage-mediated inflammatory responses. *Immunology* 152 (2), 207–217. doi:10.1111/imm.12787

Zeng, Y., Qin, Q., Li, K., Li, H., Song, C., Li, Y., et al. (2019). PKR suppress NLRP3-pyroptosis pathway in lipopolysaccharide-induced acute lung injury model of mice. *Biochem. Biophys. Res. Commun.* 519 (1), 8–14. doi:10.1016/j.bbrc.2019.08.054

Zhang, L., Xu, C., Chen, X., Shi, Q., Su, W., and Zhao, H. (2018). SOCS-1 suppresses inflammation through inhibition of NALP3 inflammasome formation in smoke inhalation-induced acute lung injury. *Inflammation* 41 (4), 1557–1567. doi:10.1007/s10753-018-0802-y

Zhang, Y., Li, X., Grailer, J. J., Wang, N., Wang, M., Yao, J., et al. (2016). Melatonin alleviates acute lung injury through inhibiting the NLRP3 inflammasome. *J. Pineal Res.* 60 (4), 405–414. doi:10.1111/jpi.12322

Zhao, L.-R., Xing, R.-L., Wang, P.-M., Zhang, N.-S., Yin, S.-J., Li, X.-C., et al. (2018). NLRP1 and NLRP3 inflammasomes mediate LPS/ATP-induced pyroptosis in knee osteoarthritis. *Mol. Med. Rep.* 17 (4), 5463–5469. doi:10.3892/mmr.2018.8520

Zhu, W., London, N. R., Gibson, C. C., Davis, C. T., Tong, Z., Sorensen, L. K., et al. (2012). Interleukin receptor activates a MYD88-ARNO-ARF6 cascade to disrupt vascular stability. *Nature* 492 (7428), 252–255. doi:10.1038/nature11603

Permissions

All chapters in this book were first published by Frontiers; hereby published with permission under the Creative Commons Attribution License or equivalent. Every chapter published in this book has been scrutinized by our experts. Their significance has been extensively debated. The topics covered herein carry significant findings which will fuel the growth of the discipline. They may even be implemented as practical applications or may be referred to as a beginning point for another development.

The contributors of this book come from diverse backgrounds, making this book a truly international effort. This book will bring forth new frontiers with its revolutionizing research information and detailed analysis of the nascent developments around the world.

We would like to thank all the contributing authors for lending their expertise to make the book truly unique. They have played a crucial role in the development of this book. Without their invaluable contributions this book wouldn't have been possible. They have made vital efforts to compile up to date information on the varied aspects of this subject to make this book a valuable addition to the collection of many professionals and students.

This book was conceptualized with the vision of imparting up-to-date information and advanced data in this field. To ensure the same, a matchless editorial board was set up. Every individual on the board went through rigorous rounds of assessment to prove their worth. After which they invested a large part of their time researching and compiling the most relevant data for our readers.

The editorial board has been involved in producing this book since its inception. They have spent rigorous hours researching and exploring the diverse topics which have resulted in the successful publishing of this book. They have passed on their knowledge of decades through this book. To expedite this challenging task, the publisher supported the team at every step. A small team of assistant editors was also appointed to further simplify the editing procedure and attain best results for the readers.

Apart from the editorial board, the designing team has also invested a significant amount of their time in understanding the subject and creating the most relevant covers. They scrutinized every image to scout for the most suitable representation of the subject and create an appropriate cover for the book.

The publishing team has been an ardent support to the editorial, designing and production team. Their endless efforts to recruit the best for this project, has resulted in the accomplishment of this book. They are a veteran in the field of academics and their pool of knowledge is as vast as their experience in printing. Their expertise and guidance has proved useful at every step. Their uncompromising quality standards have made this book an exceptional effort. Their encouragement from time to time has been an inspiration for everyone.

The publisher and the editorial board hope that this book will prove to be a valuable piece of knowledge for researchers, students, practitioners and scholars across the globe.

List of Contributors

Savino Spadaro, Gaetano Scaramuzzo, Valentina Chiavieri, Valentina Alvisi and Carlo Alberto Volta
Department of Translational Medicine, Anesthesia and Intensive Care, University of Ferrara, Ferrara, Italy

Francesca Dalla Corte
Department of Translational Medicine, Anesthesia and Intensive Care, University of Ferrara, Ferrara, Italy
Department of Anesthesia and Intensive Care Medicine, Humanitas Clinical and Research Center Istituto di Ricovero e Cura a Carattere Scientifico (IRCCS), Milan, Italy

Salvatore Grasso and Rosa Di Mussi
Department of Emergency and Organ Transplantation, University of Bari, Bari, Italy

Gilda Cinnella
Department of Medical and Surgical Sciences, University of Foggia, Foggia, Italy

Valentina Rosta, Tiziana Bellini and Alessandro Trentini
Section of Medical Biochemistry, Molecular Biology and Genetics, Department of Biomedical and Specialist Surgical Sciences, University of Ferrara, Ferrara, Italy

Egidio Beretta, Giulio Sancini and Giuseppe Miserocchi
Department of Medicine and Surgery, School of Medicine and Surgery, Università degli Studi di Milano Bicocca, Monza, Italy

Francesco Romanò
Univ. Lille, CNRS, ONERA, Arts et Métiers, Centrale Lille, FRE 2017-LMFL-Laboratoire de Mécanique des Fluides de Lille - Kampé de Fériet, Lille, France

James B. Grotberg
Department of Biomedical Engineering, University of Michigan, Ann Arbor, MI, United States

Gary F. Nieman
Department of Surgery, State University of New York Upstate Medical University, Syracuse, NY, United States

Matthieu Petit, Edouard Jullien and Antoine Vieillard-Baron
Medical Intensive Care Unit, University Hospital Ambroise Paré, APHP, Boulogne-Billancourt, France
UFR des Sciences de la Santé Simone Veil, Université Paris-Saclay, Montigny-le-Bretonneux, France

Martina Fiorito, Antonella Dall'Orto and Lorenzo Maiello
Department of Surgical Sciences and Integrated Diagnostics, University of Genoa, Genoa, Italy

Lorenzo Ball, Chiara Robba and Paolo Pelosi
Department of Surgical Sciences and Integrated Diagnostics, University of Genoa, Genoa, Italy
Anesthesia and Intensive Care, Ospedale Policlinico San Martino Istituto di Ricerca e Cura a Carattere Scientifico (IRCCS) for Oncology and Neurosciences, Genova, Italy

Iole Brunetti
Anesthesia and Intensive Care, Ospedale Policlinico San Martino Istituto di Ricerca e Cura a Carattere Scientifico (IRCCS) for Oncology and Neurosciences, Genova, Italy

Yuda Sutherasan
Division of Pulmonary and Pulmonary Critical Care Medicine, Department of Medicine, Ramathibodi Hospital, Mahidol University, Bangkok, Thailand

Maria Vargas
Department of Neurosciences, Reproductive and Odonthostomatological Sciences, University of Naples Federico II, Naples, Italy

Davide D'Antini and Pasquale Raimondo
Department of Surgical Sciences and Integrated Diagnostics, University of Genoa, Genoa, Italy
Department of Anaesthesia and Intensive Care, University of Foggia, Foggia, Italy

Robert Huhle
Mahidol Oxford Tropical Medicine Research Unit (MORU), Mahidol University, Bangkok, Thailand

Marcus J. Schultz
Mahidol Oxford Tropical Medicine Research Unit (MORU), Mahidol University, Bangkok, Thailand
Department of Intensive Care, Laboratory of Experimental Intensive Care and Anesthesiology (LEICA), Amsterdam University Medical Centers, Location Academic Medical Center (AMC), Amsterdam, Netherlands
Nuffield Department of Medicine, Oxford University, Oxford, United Kingdom

Patricia R. M. Rocco
Laboratory of Pulmonary Investigation, Carlos Chagas Filho Institute of Biophysics, Federal University of Rio de Janeiro, Rio de Janeiro, Brazil

Marcelo Gama de Abreu
Pulmonary Engineering Group, Department of Anaesthesiology and Intensive Care Medicine, University Hospital Carl Gustav Carus, Technische Universität Dresden, Dresden, Germany

Fernando Suárez-Sipmann
CIBER de Enfermedades Respiratorias, Instituto de Salud Carlos III, Madrid, Spain
Intensive Care Unit, Hospital Universitario La Princesa, Madrid, Spain
Department of Surgical Sciences, Anesthesiology & Critical Care, Hedenstierna Laboratory, Uppsala University Hospital, Uppsala, Sweden

Juan A. Sánchez-Giralt
Intensive Care Unit, Hospital Universitario La Princesa, Madrid, Spain

Jesús Villar
CIBER de Enfermedades Respiratorias, Instituto de Salud Carlos III, Madrid, Spain
Multidisciplinary Organ Dysfunction Evaluation Research Network (MODERN), Research Unit, Hospital Universitario Dr. Negrín, Las Palmas de Gran Canaria, Spain
Keenan Research Center at the Li Ka Shing Knowledge Institute, St. Michael's Hospital, Toronto, ON, Canada

Carlos Ferrando
CIBER de Enfermedades Respiratorias, Instituto de Salud Carlos III, Madrid, Spain
Department of Anesthesiology, Hospital Privado de Comunidad, Mar del Plata, Argentina
Harvard Medical School, Boston, MA, United States

Gerardo Tusman
Department of Anesthesia, Critical Care and Pain Medicine, Massachusetts General Hospital, Boston, MA, United States

Rahul Y. Mahida, Aaron Scott, Dhruv Parekh, Sebastian T. Lugg, Kylie B. R. Belchamber, Babu Naidu and David R. Thickett
Birmingham Acute Care Research Group, Institute of Inflammation and Ageing, University of Birmingham, Birmingham, United Kingdom

Rowan S. Hardy
Institute of Metabolism and Systems Research, University of Birmingham, Birmingham, United Kingdom

Michael A. Matthay
Departments of Medicine and of Anaesthesia, Cardiovascular Research Institute, University of California, San Francisco, San Francisco, CA, United States

Jing Liu and David A. Dean
Department of Pediatrics, University of Rochester, Rochester, NY, United States
Department of Pharmacology and Physiology, University of Rochester, Rochester, NY, United States

Pierre Tawfik
Pulmonary, Allergy, Critical Care, and Sleep Medicine, University of Minnesota, Minneapolis, MN, United States

Muhammad K. Hayat Syed
Pulmonary and Critical Care Medicine, Baylor College of Medicine, Houston, TX, United States

Firas S. Elmufdi
Department of Medicine, Regions Hospital, Saint Paul, MN, United States

Michael D. Evans
Clinical and Translational Science Institute, University of Minnesota, Minneapolis, MN, United States

David J. Dries
Department of Surgery, Regions Hospital, Saint Paul, MN, United States
Department of Critical Care and Acute Care Surgery, University of Minnesota, Minneapolis, MN, United States

John J. Marini
Pulmonary, Allergy, Critical Care, and Sleep Medicine, University of Minnesota, Minneapolis, MN, United States
Department of Medicine, Regions Hospital, Saint Paul, MN, United States

Juanjuan Zhao, Chao Chen, Mengmeng Guo, Yijin Tao, PanPan Cui, Nalin Qin, Jing Zheng, Jidong Zhang and Lin Xu
Department of Immunology, Zunyi Medical College, Guizhou, China

Ya Zhou
Department of Medical Physics, Zunyi Medical College, Guizhou, China

Yue Shi, Peijie Chen and Yanqiu Cui
School of Kinesiology, Shanghai University of Sport, Shanghai, China

Tingting Liu and Hui Shi
Department of Rheumatology and Immunology, Ruijin Hospital, Shanghai Jiao Tong University School of Medicine, Shanghai, China

David C. Nieman
North Carolina Research Campus, Appalachian State University, Kannapolis, NC, United States

Fei Li
School of Physical Education and Sport Training, Shanghai University of Sport, Shanghai, China

Luyu Yang
Department of General Surgery, Cancer Metastasis Institute, Huashan Hospital, Fudan University, Shanghai, China

Satoshi Kimura, Nicoleta Stoicea, Byron Rafael Rosero Britton, Muhammad Shabsigh, Aly Branstiter and David L. Stahl
Department of Anesthesiology, The Ohio State University Wexner Medical Center, Columbus, OH, USA

Xin Zhou and Youxia Liao
Department of ICU/Emergency, Wuhan University, Wuhan Third Hospital, Wuhan, China

Leandro do Nascimento Camargo, Luciana Ritha Cássia Rolim Barbosa Aristóteles , Silvia Fukuzaki, Flávia Castro Ribas de Souza, Fernanda Paula Roncon Santana, Marcus Vinicius Rodrigues de Agrela, Edna Aparecida Leick, Milton de Arruda Martins and Iolanda de Fátima Lopes Calvo Tibério
Faculdade de Medicina FMUSP, Universidade de São Paulo, São Paulo, Brazil

Fraga Righetti and Tabata Maruyama dos Santos
Faculdade de Medicina FMUSP, Universidade de São Paulo, São Paulo, Brazil, 2 Hospital Sírio-Libanês, São Paulo, Brazil
Hospital Sírio-Libanês, São Paulo, Brazil

Maysa Mariana Cruz and Maria Isabel Cardoso Alonso-Vale
Universidade Federal de São Paulo, Instituto de Ciências Ambientais, Químicas e Farmacêuticas, Departamento de Ciências Biológicas, Diadema, São Paulo, Brazil

Isabella Santos Genaro
Faculdade de Medicina FMUSP, Universidade de São Paulo, São Paulo, Brazil
Public Employee of São Paulo Hospital (IAMSPE), São Paulo, Brazil

Beatriz Mangueira Saraiva-Romanholo
Faculdade de Medicina FMUSP, Universidade de São Paulo, São Paulo, Brazil
University of City of São Paulo (UNICID), São Paulo, Brazil

Carla Máximo Prado
Department of Bioscience, Federal University of São Paulo, Santos, São Paulo, Brazil

Bohao Liu, Ruyuan He, Lin Zhang, Bo Hao, Wenyang Jiang, Wei Wang and Qing Geng
Department of Thoracic Surgery, Renmin Hospital of Wuhan University, Wuhan, China

Index

A

Acute Cor Pulmonale, 28-30, 32, 34-35

Acute Lung Injury, 23-27, 33-35, 45, 55-56, 66-69, 78, 83, 90, 93-94, 101-104, 111, 113-114, 125-127, 142, 149-150, 152-160, 162, 167-168, 179-181, 190-191, 193, 196-199, 205-210, 218, 220-222, 224-234

Acute Respiratory Distress, 9, 16-17, 24-29, 33-37, 45-47, 50, 54-57, 60, 62, 66-70, 78-80, 89-90, 92-93, 95, 101-109, 112-116, 119-121, 124-127, 129, 133, 140, 149-160, 167, 179, 182, 191-194, 196-198, 206-208, 210, 221-222, 224, 233-234

Airway Pressure, 18, 21, 23, 25-27, 38, 56, 70-71, 73, 78, 92-104, 108-109, 193

Alveolar Fluid Clearance, 19, 22-23, 27, 59, 66, 124, 127-128, 130-131, 141-142, 150-151, 153, 157, 159

Alveolar Macrophage, 115-117, 119-123, 125-126, 187, 191, 206, 227, 232, 234

Alveolar Stability, 73-74, 76-77

Assisted Mechanical Ventilation, 2-3, 8

Astrocytes, 79-82, 84, 86, 88-90

Asynchronies, 2, 36-37, 39-40, 43, 45, 106, 108

B

Biomarker, 2, 6, 59-62, 67, 130, 158, 169, 178-179, 203, 221

C

Cardiac Output, 14, 31-32, 34, 53, 56, 75, 110

Clinical Condition, 112

Clinical Trials, 57, 60-62, 65, 89, 94, 104-108, 112, 114, 133-134, 136-138, 147, 151-152, 155-156, 158, 197, 203, 205

Critical Care, 31-32, 36, 46, 57, 70-71, 75, 77, 92, 98, 100, 105, 113-114, 154, 161, 196

D

Dead Space, 31, 46-56, 105, 108, 128-129

Diaphragm, 2-3, 6-9, 18, 24, 26, 75, 96, 108

Diaphragmatic Ultrasound, 1-3, 6-7

Driving Pressure, 22, 24, 28, 30, 33-35, 51, 53-54, 60, 71-72, 74-76, 107, 110, 161-167

Dynamic Compliance, 5, 109, 114, 161, 166

E

Echocardiography, 29, 31-32, 34-35

Edema Clearance, 22, 26, 129, 134, 142, 149, 157

Efferocytosis, 115-126, 232

Electroporation, 127, 131, 136, 138, 141-145, 147-156, 159-160

Endothelial Monolayer, 158

Epithelium, 11-13, 16, 20, 22-25, 65, 68, 111, 116, 128-136, 139, 142-143, 145, 151-152, 154-155, 159-160, 180, 199, 205

Esophageal Pressure, 37-38, 40-45, 105, 110, 113-114

Expiratory Flow, 8, 71-73, 96, 98-99, 163, 191

F

Fibroblast, 23, 25, 85, 141, 146, 152, 160, 210, 222

Filtration Rate, 15-16, 19

H

Hypercapnia, 28, 31-34, 109, 129, 193, 197

Hypoxemia, 28-29, 72, 80, 89, 93, 96-97, 105-106, 108, 111-113, 128-129, 132, 181, 192, 195, 224

I

Influenza Infection, 131, 157, 201

Intensive Care Unit, 4, 8, 28, 37, 39, 46, 60, 62, 70, 93, 97, 105-107, 116, 192, 197-198, 206

Intercellular Junction, 131, 133, 146

Intubation, 6, 70, 72, 75-76, 78, 112, 164, 195, 200

L

Lentivirus, 135-136, 139, 151-152, 154-155

Lung Collapse, 8, 18, 47, 109-110, 197

Lung Injury, 8, 10-12, 16, 18-20, 22-27, 31-35, 45-47, 55-60, 63, 65-69, 71, 78-80, 82-83, 90, 92-94, 96-98, 100-106, 111-114, 124-129, 132-136, 139-162, 167-169, 171, 174, 176, 178-181, 188, 190-193, 196-200, 202-210, 218, 220-222, 224-234

Lung Lesion, 16, 18-19, 23, 205

Lung Mechanics, 46-47, 51, 54-55, 106, 109-110, 162, 166, 193

Lung Parenchyma, 47, 51, 70, 76, 90, 150, 185, 220

Lung Perfusion, 47, 54-55

Lung Tissue, 10-11, 14, 17-18, 24-25, 47, 53, 59, 63-64, 89, 115-118, 124, 131, 149, 168-169, 171-172, 174, 176-178, 183-186, 202, 209, 212-222, 224, 229, 231

Lysosomal Degradation, 131, 137

M

Mass Spectrometry, 57, 60, 65, 132

Matrix Fragmentation, 16, 21-22

Membrane Localization, 132, 145

Mortality, 3-4, 18, 27-29, 31, 33-35, 45, 47, 54-55, 57, 59-61, 63-64, 66, 68-70, 72, 78, 80, 89, 92-98, 100, 102, 104, 106-114, 116, 121, 124, 127-128, 133-134, 139, 141, 146, 149-150, 152, 155-156, 158-159, 167, 181, 192-193, 195, 197-198, 202-203, 205, 207-208, 210, 224, 229

N

Neuromuscular Blockade, 95-96, 106, 108, 114, 163

Norepinephrine, 3, 32, 34, 75-77

O

Oscillation, 14, 78, 92, 102, 104, 107-109, 113-114

Oscillatory Ventilation, 92, 95-98, 101-105, 108

Oxygenation, 28-29, 31-37, 43-45, 59, 69, 71, 73-76, 80, 93-94, 96-100, 102-111, 113, 132, 134, 140, 149, 164, 194, 196, 198

P

Pathogenesis, 23, 25, 60, 67-68, 90, 115-116, 125, 127-128, 133, 146-147, 149-150, 155, 159, 178, 181, 190-191, 198, 200, 204-207, 210, 222, 232, 234

Pathophysiology, 11, 28-29, 34-35, 68, 70, 78, 92-93, 100-101, 124, 127, 142, 149, 152-153, 159, 205, 221-222, 234

Pediatric Population, 93, 100

Peptide, 25, 57-58, 63, 67-68, 145, 156, 208

Phagocytosis, 115, 117-122, 125-126, 135, 223

Phenotype, 24, 60, 88, 101, 115-116, 118, 120-122, 124, 139, 180, 185, 187, 189-190, 201, 204, 226

Plateau Pressure, 17, 21, 34, 58, 74, 76, 96, 106, 147-148, 161-162, 166

Predicted Body Weight, 37, 39-41, 44, 58, 106, 192

Pressure Ventilation, 34, 55, 58, 196

Prone Ventilation, 106, 108-109

Pulmonary Circulation, 28-30, 32-33, 35, 46

Pulmonary Edema, 16, 23-27, 33, 58-59, 80, 105-106, 128, 135, 139, 144-145, 147, 149, 151-152, 155-156, 158, 160, 200, 224

R

Reactive Oxygen Species, 10, 16, 59, 129, 151, 230

Recruitment Maneuver, 71, 109, 222

Renin-angiotensin System, 57, 60, 62-63, 66-69

Respiratory Failure, 1-4, 7-8, 24, 34-35, 37, 39, 44-45, 47, 61, 63, 66, 70, 78, 80, 99, 101-108, 110, 113, 121, 127-128, 182, 192-193, 195-196, 198-199, 210

Respiratory Mechanics, 6, 14, 25, 36-37, 39-44, 54, 103, 161, 167, 209, 212, 221

Retrovirus, 135, 139

Rho-associated Kinase, 115-116, 120, 123

S

Sepsis, 4, 16, 35, 39, 57, 63-64, 68-69, 78, 80, 102, 112, 116, 118-119, 127, 130-131, 133-134, 140-141, 143-144, 146-147, 149, 152-153, 155-158, 160, 196, 198-208, 210, 232, 234

Skeletal Troponin, 1-9

T

Tidal Volume, 17, 30, 34, 37, 39-41, 44-46, 48-49, 53, 58-59, 70-71, 76, 92, 94, 96-99, 102, 113, 132, 140, 147, 161-167, 192, 197, 211, 230

Transfection Efficiency, 135-139, 151

V

Vasoconstriction, 19-20, 29, 31, 33

Ventilatory Strategy, 17-18, 23, 31, 71

Viral Vectors, 127, 135-137, 139, 150, 154, 156-157, 160

Volumetric Capnography, 46-48, 51, 54-56

W

Weaning, 1-2, 6-9, 45, 73, 77, 112-113, 193, 203